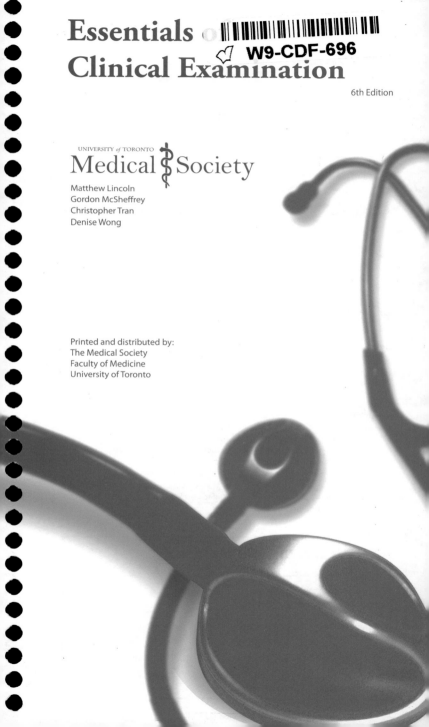

Essentials of Clinical Examination

6th Edition

UNIVERSITY *of* TORONTO
Medical Society

Matthew Lincoln
Gordon McSheffrey
Christopher Tran
Denise Wong

Printed and distributed by:
The Medical Society
Faculty of Medicine
University of Toronto

Sixth Edition Copyright © 2010
Essentials of Clinical Examination Handbook

Editors:
Matthew Lincoln   Christopher Tran
Gordon McSheffrey   Denise Wong

Cover Design: Lauren O'Malley

Fifth Edition   Editors:
Copyright © 2005   Woganee Filate   Dawn Ng
                         Rico Leung   Mark Sinyor

Fourth Edition   Editors:
Copyright © 2002   Sonial Butalia   Catherine Lam
                         Hin Hin Ko   Jensen Tan

Third Edition   Editors:
Copyright © 2000   Tyler Rouse   Cory Torgerson
                         Gilbert Tang   Hariette Van Spall

Second Edition   Editors:
Copyright © 1999   Ashis Chawla and Rizwan Somani

First Edition   Editors:
Copyright © 1997   Shane Burch and Derek Plausinis

Library and Archives Canada Cataloguing in Publication

Main entry under title:

Essentials of clinical examination handbook /Matthew Lincoln ... [et al.].
– 6th ed.

Includes bibliographical references and index.
ISBN 978-0-7727-8736-1

I. Physical diagnosis – Handbooks, manuals, etc. I. Lincoln, Matthew
II. University of Toronto. Medical Society

RC76.E87 2010   616.07'54   C2010-900331-4

Contributors

Chief Editors

Matthew Lincoln (1T1)
Gordon McSheffrey (MD/PhD)

Christopher Tran (1T1)
Denise Wong (1T0)

Chapter Editors

Ishtiaq Ahmed (1T0)
Ravi Bajaj (1T0)
Emily Baker (1T0)
Henry Becker (MD/PhD)
Pearl Behl (1T0)
Sarah Blissett (1T0)
Michal Bohdanowicz (MD/PhD)
Kimberly Bremer (1T0)
Caroline Chan (1T0)
Yingming Chen (1T1)
Alex Cheng (1T1)
Homan Cheng (1T0)
Derek Chew (1T1)
Amanda Cipolla (1T0)
Katie Connolly (1T1)
Sarah Erdman (1T1)
Antoine Eskander (1T0)
Hana Farhang Khoee (1T0)
Vinay Fernandes (1T0)
Alyse Goldberg (1T0)
Weronika Harris-Thompson (1T0)
Michael Hill (1T1)
Carlo Hojilla (1T0)
Janine Hutson (MD/PhD)
Michael Jurkiewicz (1T0)
Christopher Kandel (1T1)
James Kennedy (MD/PhD)
Kevin Koo (1T0)
Yonah Krakowsky (1T1)
Allison Kwan (1T0)
Emilie Lam (1T0)

Grace Lam (MD/PhD)
Christine Law (1T0)
Joanna Lazier (1T0)
Lik Hang Lee (1T0)
Jo Jo Leung (1T0)
Vincent Leung (1T0)
Fiona Lovegrove (MD/PhD)
Lea Luketic (1T0)
Lindsay MacKenzie (1T1)
Alfonse Marchie (1T0)
Moises Maria (1T0)
Monique Martin (1T1)
Ian Mayne (1T0)
Amy Ng (1T0)
Ali Okhowat (1T0)
Modupe Oyewumi (1T1)
Sylvia Papp (1T1)
Elena Qirjazi (1T1)
Varinder Randhawa (MD/PhD)
Roshan Razik (1T0)
Ilana Saltzman (1T0)
Caroline Scott (1T1)
Amy Shafey (1T0)
Marat Slessarev (1T0)
Gursharan Soor (1T0)
Sarah Troster (1T1)
Eric Tseng (1T0)
Jenny Wang (1T0)
Bertha Wong (1T1)
Grace Yeung (1T0)
Julia Zhu (1T0)

Illustrators

Jennifer Belanger (BMC)
Simon Ip (BMC)
Pina Kingman (BMC)
Diana Kryski (BMC)
Tabetha Lulham (BMC)
Niraj Mistry (0T7)
Caitlin O'Connell (BMC)
Tess Peters (BMC)

Varinder Randhawa (MD/PhD)
John Sauve (1T1)
Marta Scythes (BMC)
Krista Shapton (BMC)
Kaiyan Su (1T2)
Gilbert Tang (0T2)
Lorraine Trecroce (BMC)

Preface and Acknowledgements

A thorough history and physical examination is essential to the management of any patient in a clinical setting. The *Essentials of Clinical Examination Handbook* was created by University of Toronto medical students to provide their colleagues with a comprehensive yet concise and efficient resource for practicing clinical examinations.

Originally used by Canadian medical students, the *Essentials of Clinical Examination Handbook* is now sold in the United States and internationally. It has proven to be an excellent resource not only for the medical student, but for trainees in many allied health professions such as nursing and naturopathic medicine. A common approach is taken to develop skills in a variety of clinical settings, so this handbook can be used as a valuable reference for any clinically oriented course of study.

The *6th Edition* continues the University of Toronto's undergraduate medical students' illustrious tradition of producing medical education texts and their strong commitment to improving medical education. When resources in a particular area are found wanting, our students do not hesitate to produce a resource designed specifically to enhance their education and that of their colleagues in the healthcare professions.

In this edition of the *Essentials of Clinical Examination Handbook*, we have sought to maintain the concise yet comprehensive nature of this work, while enhancing areas in response to feedback from the first five editions. Each chapter has been rigourously edited to ensure that only the most essential, up-to-date and evidence-based information has been included. We have streamlined many chapters and added several new ones including sections on Oncology and Pain Management. We acknowledge the tremendous work done by our predecessors in creating an excellent foundation and establishing this work as a favourite resource of health professions trainees.

The *Essentials of Clinical Examination Handbook* would not have been possible without the outstanding support and contributions of the faculty associated with the University of Toronto's network of teaching hospitals. We are privileged to have access to these leaders in the fields of medicine.

We would like to recognize the contribution of the following to this work:
- The undergraduate medical classes of 1T0, 1T1 and the MD/PhD program
- The illustrators from the Biomedical Communications Program and the undergraduate medical classes of 1T0, 1T1, 1T2 and the MD/PhD program
- The Faculty Reviewers
- Type & Graphics
- The University of Toronto Medical Society

The Editors-in-Chief would like to express their deepest gratitude to the above groups for allowing us to produce the 6th Edition of the *Essentials of Clinical Examination Handbook*. We hope that you find this text to be a useful and invaluable addition to your medical education.

The Editors-in-Chief,

Matthew Lincoln, D.Phil   **Christopher Tran**, B.Sc.
Gordon McSheffrey, B.Sc.   **Denise Wong**, B.A.Sc., M.Sc.

Table of Contents

The General History and Physical Exam 5

The Abdominal Exam 27

The Breast Exam 49

The Cardiovascular Exam 59

The Geriatric Exam 79

The Gynecological Exam 91

The Head and Neck Exam 107

The Lymphatic System and Lymph Node Exam 131

The Musculoskeletal Exam 141

The Neurological Exam 177

The Obstetric Exam 203

The Ophthalmological Exam 227

The Pediatric Exam 247

The Peripheral Vascular Exam 299

The Psychiatric Exam 317

The Respiratory Exam 335

The Urological Exam 353

The Essentials of Clinical Pharmacology 373

The Essentials of Dermatology 385

The Essentials of Emergency Medicine 399

The Essentials of Endocrinology 415

The Essentials of Fluids, Electrolytes, and Acid/Base Disturbances 427

The Essentials of General Surgery 441

The Essentials of Infectious Diseases 447

The Essentials of Medical Imaging 477

The Essentials of Oncology 507

The Essentials of Pain Management 515

Appendix 1: Concepts in Evidence-Based Medicine 529

Appendix 2: Commonly Used Drugs 535

Appendix 3: Common Laboratory Values 543

Index 551

The General History and Physical Exam

Editors:
Gursharan Soor &
Grace Yeung

Faculty Reviewer:
Daniel M. Panisko, MD, MPH, FRCP(C)
Spousal Abuse Section:
Patricia Windrim, MD, MHSc, MRCP

TABLE OF CONTENTS

Approach to the Interview   5
Introduction   5
General History   8
General Physical Exam – Overview   12
Preparation for Physical Exam   12
General Physical Exam   13
General Inspection   14
Vital Signs   19
Spousal Abuse   23

APPROACH TO THE INTERVIEW

The Medical Interview serves to:
- Collect information about the patient and his or her illness
- Establish a therapeutic contract
- Understand the patient's environment
- Establish lists of problems that should be solved
- Develop problem-specific plans that encompass diagnostic studies, therapy, and education of the patient and their family

> **Evidence-Based Medicine: Accuracy of the History and Physical Exam**
> One study in a general medical clinic found that 56% of patients had been assigned correct diagnoses by the end of the history, and that number rose to 73% by the end of their physical examination.
>
> Sackett DL, Rennie D. 1992. *JAMA* 267(19):2650-2652.

INTRODUCTION

- The beginning of the interview sets the tone for the rest of your history and physical examination. During the introduction, it is essential to clearly define the nature of the relationship and to be respectful of the patient's wishes and concerns such that both you and the patient are comfortable (see below)

Setting
- Start by choosing a time and place for your interview that allows for *privacy* and minimal distraction
- Remember to **draw the curtain** around the bed and *close the window blinds*

Interviewer
- *Introduce yourself* and explain your role: e.g. "Hello, my name is X. I am a Y-year medical student and I'd like to talk to you today in order to get

some information about why you're in the hospital, and then to examine you. Will that be alright? If you feel uncomfortable at any point or have any questions, please feel free to stop and let me know."

- *Be honest* with your level of training – state the year of medical school or residency in which you are currently enrolled
- If a third party (evaluator) is present, explain his/her role in the interview
- *Define* the *time* allotted for, and *purpose* of the encounter
- Be aware of *posture* and *positioning*: sit at the same or lower level than the patient, in a position that permits but does not force eye contact; preferably on the patient's right side
- Be aware of your tone of voice, dressing and grooming
- Maintain good *eye contact* and show interest
- *Take notes*: they are essential for recording a detailed and precise history; explain to the patient why you are taking notes and ensure they are comfortable with this. Mention that the notes will be kept confidential and not be shared with anyone outside of those caring for the patient

Patient

- Ask the patient how he/she would like you to address them; use his/her first name only if he/she asks you to
- Ensure that the patient is positioned comfortably and draped appropriately
- If there are visitors, suggest that they wait outside while you conduct the interview and physical exam; this is particularly important while interviewing adolescents as they may be hesitant to share personal information if their parent/guardian is in the room

> **Evidence-Based Medicine: Perspective on Greetings in Medical Encounters**
> Physicians should be encouraged to shake hands with patients but remain sensitive to nonverbal cues that might indicate whether patients are open to this behaviour. Given the diversity of opinion regarding the use of names, coupled with national patient safety recommendations concerning patient identification, physicians should initially use patients' first and last names and introduce themselves using their own first and last names.
>
> Makoul G, Zick A, Green M. 2007. *Arch Intern Med* 167(11):1172-1176.

Questioning Techniques

- *Focusing*: progressing from open-ended questions to direct questions allows for broad answers and keeps the interviewer's mind open
- *Open-ended questions*: "What is the reason you have come in today?", "Can you describe the pain?"
- *Facilitation*: encourages the patient to continue – "uh-huh", "yes", "tell me more", gentle nodding of the head
- *Repetition*: highlights important or last words spoken by rephrasing and reiterating
- *Clarification and directive questions*: "You mentioned that you were having pain..."
- *Check accuracy of your understanding*: relate symptoms to events or place, e.g. previous episodes: "was it the same as when...", "what was different about this episode?"
- *Create hypothetical situations to clarify*: "suppose that..."
- *Summarizing and paraphrasing*: shows the patient you are listening, provides focus, acts as a transition, clarifies any inconsistencies, and provides organization

Hints

- *Quantify*: when did it happen? how long was each episode?
- If patient rambles, do not be afraid to *redirect the patient back to the pertinent issue*: "it seems like this is important to you and maybe we can discuss it further, but right now I would like to focus on..."
- *Precision*: define vague terms (qualitative), have the patient describe what he/she means by sudden, a little, tired, dizzy, hurts, sick, weak, gas, pain etc.
- Inquire about *what made them decide to seek help*: do not limit attention to one problem; the presenting complaint may not be their main concern, as they may initially be afraid to reveal the actual reason for their visit
- *Avoid rapid-fire, complex/multiple-part and leading questions*: e.g. avoid "you've never had X, have you?"; instead provide a list of useful descriptors
- *Avoid jargon, vague terms, and social judgments*

Empathy

Empathy: the mental capacity to understand the suffering of others
Sympathy: the emotional capacity to care about that suffering

- It strengthens the doctor-patient relationship and facilitates cooperation
- Strive for basic understanding and respect for patients' experience: e.g. explore and acknowledge patient's concerns and how the illness has affected them:
    - "That sounds like it would be very uncomfortable" may let the patient know you sympathize with what has happened to him/her
- Non-verbal skills:
    - Be aware of your *own* and the *patient's* facial expressions, intonation, body language, posture, and eye contact: leaning away? toward? fidgeting?

Evidence-Based Medicine: Verbal and Non-verbal Behaviour in Medical Encounters

Verbal behaviour associated with positive health outcomes include empathy, support, patient-centered questioning techniques, encounter length, explanations, positive reinforcement, humour, health education, information sharing, friendliness, courtesy, summarization, and clarification. Non-verbal behaviours associated with positive health outcome include forward leaning, head nodding, uncrossed arms and legs, arm symmetry, and less mutual gaze.

Beck RS, Daughtridge R, Sloane PD. 2002. *JABFP* 15(1):25-38.

Confidentiality

- All patient information is confidential
- Patients have the right to view their records
- Patient's consent is required for sharing information with outsiders
- Avoid discussing patient information in public areas where you can be easily overheard (e.g. elevator, cafeteria)
- See *Personal Health Information Protection Act, 2004* for Ontario guidelines on collection, use, retention, transfer, disclosure, access and disposal of patients' personal health information

Breaking Bad News: SPIKES Approach

The SPIKES approach has four goals:

1. *Information gathering*: To determine how much the patient knows and how much they want to know

2. *Information delivery*: To provide intelligent information in line with the patient's preferences and needs
3. *Support*: To deliver the news in a manner that lessens the emotional difficulty in accepting the news
4. *Strategy*: To develop a shared treatment plan that is in line with the patient's goals and values

Six Steps of SPIKES

S: *SETTING UP* the Interview
  - Anticipate time constraints or interruptions
  - Deliver the news while sitting
  - Ensure the setting allows for privacy and the involvement of significant others

P: *PERCEPTION* of the Patient
  - Use open-ended questions to assess the patient's understanding of the severity of his/her condition and how much is known regarding the diagnosis and prognosis

I: *INVITATION* to Disclose Information
  - Inquire as to how much information the patient would like to know
  - Ideally, pose this question when ordering tests. If less information is desired, treatment plans and follow-up may be addressed instead

K: *KNOWLEDGE* and Information Sharing with the Patient
  - Deliver information in small chunks using non-technical words
  - Refrain from excessive bluntness

E: *EMPATHIZING* with and Addressing Patients' Emotions
  - Identify the specific reason the patient is experiencing an emotion (it may not always be the bad news) and employ empathy techniques to help them feel understood and to validate their emotions

S: *STRATEGIZE* and *SUMMARIZE*
  - Once the emotion has sufficiently cleared, discuss the treatment plan and have the patient summarize their understanding of what was discussed

GENERAL HISTORY

The general history is organized into a series of sections, which when taken together, should form a comprehensive review of the patient's entire medical history. The format of the history is typically as follows:

1. Identifying data (ID)
2. Chief complaint (CC)
3. History of the present illness (HPI)
4. Past medical history (PMHx)
5. Family history (FMHx)
6. Social history (SocHx)
7. Sexual history (SexHx)
8. Review of systems or functional inquiry (ROS/FI)

Identifying Data (ID)
  - Patient's *name, age, relationship status, dependents, occupation,* and *ethnicity*
  - If family members contribute to the history, document their names and relationships and note if a *translator* is used

Chief Complaint (CC)
  - Brief statement of why he or she *sought medical attention*, usually recorded in the patient's own words, and the duration of symptoms
  - A good question to ask is "What is the reason you have come to the hospital/clinic today?"

History of Present Illness (HPI)

- Elaborates on the CC through *relevant past and family history*
- Any information relevant to the patient's current medical problem should be included in the HPI
- Ensure a clear understanding of the *chronology* and *progression* of the symptoms leading to the CC
- **OPQRSTUVW** is an acronym used to characterize symptoms:
  O = **O**nset and duration (circadian pattern)
  P = **P**rovoking and alleviating factors
  Q = **Q**uality of pain (e.g. "Is the pain sharp or dull? Is it throbbing?")
  R = **R**adiation of pain
  S = **S**everity (on a scale from 1 to 10, 10 being the worst pain ever experienced)
  T = **T**iming and progression (e.g. "Is the pain constant or intermittent?")
  U = "How does it affect '**U**' in your daily life?"
  V = déjà **V**u? (e.g. "Has it happened before?")
  W = "**W**hat do you think is causing it?"
- Explore associated symptoms and inquire about relevant risk factors
- The interviewer should be able to compose a differential diagnosis (DDx) at the end of an HPI

Past Medical History (PMHx)

- A review of all medical events during the patient's lifetime:
  - *General state of health*: "How has your health been in the past?"
  - *Past illnesses*: including childhood illnesses such as measles, mumps, whooping cough, rheumatic fever, chickenpox, polio, and scarlet fever
  - *Injuries*: type and date(s)
  - *Hospitalizations*: reasons for admission and date(s)
  - *Surgery*: type of procedure, date, hospital, and surgeon's name
  - *Psychological history*
  - *Immunization history*
  - *Substance use*
    - *Cigarette smoking*: number of *pack-years* and the type of nicotine (e.g. cigarettes, cigars, chewing tobacco)
    - Pack-year = (number of years a patient has smoked cigarettes) x (number of packs per day)
    - *Alcohol*: type of alcohol consumed and weekly consumption amounts should be inquired about in a non-judgmental manner (e.g. "How many alcoholic *drinks* do you have *in a week*?"). If alcohol abuse is suspected, the CAGE questionnaire should be asked (see **Psychiatric Exam** p. 319)
    - *Recreational drugs*: document quantity and type of drug used
  - *Diet*: ask for a description of food eaten the day before, including all meals and snacks

Medications (MEDS)

- *Prescription drugs* (name, dosage, and route of administration)
- *Compliance* (e.g. count pills)
- *Over-the-counter medications* (e.g. vitamins and herbal remedies)

Allergies (ALL)

- All *environmental, ingestible*, and *drug-related* allergies, particularly the response and its timing (i.e. immediate, delayed, etc.)

Family History (FMHx)

- Health status of *immediate family members, living* and *deceased*
- The *age* and *health* of all immediate family members and the age and *cause of death* of family members if applicable
- In general, inquire about family history of:

cancer	anemia	tuberculosis (TB)
diabetes mellitus	arthritis	mental illness
hypertension	asthma	any history of abuse
heart disease	epilepsy	(sexual, emotional, physical)
hypercholesterolemia	headaches	
stroke	kidney diseases	

- Document in the form of a *family tree* or *pedigree*:
  - e.g. Mrs. Jill Hill, a consultant, and Mr. Jack Hill are consanguineous in that their mothers are sisters. They have a healthy son and a healthy daughter who is 16 weeks pregnant. Jack has one older sister and an older brother who died of an autosomal recessive (AR) disease. Jill has a younger brother. Jill's uncle (mother's youngest brother) had a son who passed away of the same AR disease and two other healthy boys

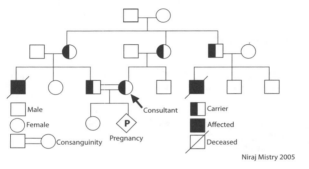

Niraj Mistry 2005

Figure 1. Family Tree

Social History (SocHx)

- Education (highest grade/degree/training attained)
- Occupation (past, present and long range goals and ambitions)
- Marital status and other personal relationships with family and friends
- Home structure (type, location, occupants, privacy)
- Finances (source and amount; public assistance)
- Religious beliefs (in relation to the perceptions of health and treatment)
- Effect of the patient's illness on his/her daily life
- Patient attitude, outlook and insight

Sexual History (SexHx)

- The *sexual, reproductive*, and *gynecological* history has traditionally been part of the social history or review of systems
- Approaches differ depending on whether the patient is an adult, adolescent or child

- In adults and adolescents, they should include the following:
  - Does the patient have sex with men, women, or both? (avoid the terms homosexual, heterosexual)
  - Is the patient currently sexually active and with how many partners?

- Are safe sex practices and contraceptive methods being used? Types?
- Does the patient have a sexually transmitted disease?
- Has the patient ever been sexually abused or raped?

A. Sexual History of the Adult:
- Is the patient having any sexual problems (e.g. ejaculating, achieving and maintaining an erection, reaching orgasm, lubrication)?
- *For males, the reproductive history also includes:*
  - Sexual interest, function, and satisfaction
  - Fertility
- *For females, the reproductive and gynecological history also includes:*
  - Age at menarche, menstrual regularity and duration
  - GTPALM status (see *Obstetric Exam* p. 210)

B. Sexual History of the Adolescent
- Interview without parents unless patient requests otherwise
- State interview is confidential but that incidents of abuse or self-inflicted harm must be reported

C. Sexual History of the Child (see *Pediatric Exam*)
- Self-exploration/masturbation is normal (peaks at 3-5 years and may continue into school age)
- Inappropriate or aggressive behaviour may suggest sexual abuse

Review of Systems/Functional Inquiry (ROS/FI)
- General inquiry into the functioning of all the body systems
- Serves to address symptoms that may have been overlooked or are unrelated to the CC
- Best organized in a head-to-toe fashion. The patient should be instructed to answer simply 'yes' or 'no' to the questions. If the response is 'yes', more detail should be sought
  - *General*: weight gain/loss, loss of appetite, fever, chills, fatigue, night sweats
  - *Dermatological (DERM)*: rashes, skin discolorations, pruritus (itchiness)
  - *Head (HEENT):* headaches, dizziness, masses, seizures
  - *Eyes*: visual changes, visual field deficits
  - *Ears*: tinnitus (sensation of sound in one or both ears), vertigo (sense of spinning or turning while in a resting position), hearing loss
  - *Nose*: epistaxis (nosebleeds), discharge, sinus diseases
  - *Mouth & Throat*: dental disease, hoarseness, throat pain
  - *Respiratory (RESP)*: cough, shortness of breath, sputum (consistency and colour), hemoptysis (blood in sputum)
  - *Cardiovascular (CV):* chest pain, orthopnea (difficulty in breathing while lying flat), paroxysmal nocturnal dyspnea (sudden onset of shortness of breath during sleep), dyspnea on exertion, claudication, edema, palpitations
  - *Gastrointestinal (GI):* dysphagia (difficulty swallowing), abdominal pain, nausea, emesis (vomiting), change in bowel habits, diarrhea, constipation, melena (black, tarry stool), hematochezia (bright red blood per rectum)
  - *Genitourinary (GU):* dysuria (pain on urination), frequency of urination, hesitancy, hematuria, discharge
  - *Gynecological (OBGYN):* number of pregnancies and children, abortions, last menstrual period (frequency, duration), age of menarche, age of menopause; dysmenorrhea (painful menstruation), contraception, vaginal bleeding, breast masses

- *Endocrine (ENDO):* polyuria (voiding large amounts of urine), polydipsia (excessive thirst), skin or hair changes, heat intolerance
- *Musculoskeletal (MSK):* joint pain, swelling, arthritis, myalgias (muscle pain or tenderness)
- *Lymphatics:* easy bruising, lymphadenopathy
- *Neuropsychiatric (PSYCH):* weakness, seizures, problems with gait, parasthesia (numbness or tingling), memory changes, depression

Geriatric and Pediatric History
- See *Geriatric Exam* and *Pediatric Exam*

GENERAL PHYSICAL EXAM – OVERVIEW

Preparation for the Physical Exam
1. Ensure that the patient is comfortable (e.g. draping, positioning, minimize movement, address pain)
2. Ensure that the examiner is comfortable (e.g. lighting, positioning, equipment, infection control)

GENERAL PHYSICAL EXAM (SYNOPSIS OF EACH SYSTEM)
- General Inspection
  - General Appearance
  - General Colour
  - Face
  - Mouth
  - Skin
  - Hands and nails
  - Hair
- Vitals (Some people include pain as 5th vital sign)
  - Temperature
  - Pulse
  - Respiration
  - Blood Pressure
- Body Mass Index
- Waist Circumference

PREPARATION FOR PHYSICAL EXAM

Draping, Positioning and Lighting
- Ensure good lighting, appropriate bed height, and incline
- Ensure that the patient is comfortable (positioning)
- Ensure that the patient is appropriately draped
- By convention, examine from the right side of the patient

Required Equipment
- Stethoscope
- Ophthalmoscope/otoscope
- Reflex hammer (Queen square hammer recommended)
- Tape measure
- Pocket flashlight
- Tuning forks (128 and 512 Hz)
- Pocket visual acuity card

Infection Control – Body Substance Protocols (BSPs):

Basic Priniciples:

1. Hand hygiene
2. Barriers
3. Minimize needlestick injury
4. Added precautions for airborne pathogens and antibiotic-resistant organisms

- Medical personnel are the #1 route of transmission of nosocomial infections, which affect 5-15% of all hospitalized patients
- Sources for nosocomial pathogens included endogenous (patient's own microflora) and exogenous (hands of staff, staff carriers, environment, such as water, food, air, and contaminated equipment/fluids)
- Assume all patients are potentially infected with pathogens and all body substances/fluids are sources of transmission
- Body substances include blood, oral secretions, sputum, emesis, urine, feces, wound drainage, and any additional moist body substances (not tears or sweat)
- Handwash with alcohol-based hand cleanser both before and after seeing patient to remove transient bacteria (if hands are not heavily soiled); use soap and warm water for 15 seconds when hands are soiled (dirt, blood, etc.)
- Use barriers (gloves, gowns, mask, eyewear) when appropriate (e.g. gloves when in contact with any body substances, mask when with patient with respiratory infection)
- Minimize risk of needlestick injury (never recap needles; immediately dispose of any sharps in designated sharps container)
- For airborne pathogens use high efficiency filter masks
- Maintain immunizations in order to prevent spread (e.g. flu vaccination to benefit elderly and immunocompromised patients)

GENERAL PHYSICAL EXAM

Four Principles of Physical Exam for Each Body System

- **I**nspection
- **P**alpation
- **P**ercussion
- **A**uscultation

The following is a guideline for screening exam

- *General Appearance*: note whether the patient looks ill, well, or malnourished, and if there are any IV lines or tubes present
- *Vitals*: temperature, pulse, respiration, blood pressure
- *Lymph Nodes*: occipital, posterior and pre-auricular, tonsillar, submandibular, submental, cervical (superficial, deep, posterior), supra- and infra-clavicular, epitrochlear, axillary, inguinal nodes; note size, shape, tenderness (see *Head & Neck Exam* and *Lymphatic System & Lymph Node Exam*)
- *Head*: bruising, masses; check fontanelles in infants/young children
- *Eyes*: pupils (equal, round, pupillary light and accommodation reflexes), extraocular movements, visual fields and acuity, ptosis, fundoscopy (red reflex, optic disc, retinal vessels), scleral icterus (see *Ophthalmological Exam*)
- *Ears*: external ear, auditory acuity, tympanic membranes (shiny, dull, intact, injected, bulging), tenderness (see *Head & Neck Exam*)

- *Nose, Mouth & Throat*: nasal discharge, sense of smell, mucous membrane colour and moisture, oral lesions, dentition, pharynx, tonsils, tongue, palate, uvula (see **Head & Neck Exam**)
- *Neck*: thyroid disease, lymphadenopathy, masses, carotid or thyroid bruits (see **Head & Neck Exam**)
- *Resp*: can divide into I, P, P, A; chest configuration, clubbing, central cyanosis, chest expansion, tactile fremitus, percussion, diaphragmatic excursion, auscultation for adventitious sounds, egophony, whispered pectoriloquy (see **Respiratory Exam**)
- *Heart*: JVP at 30° incline, hepatojugular reflux, point of maximal impulse (PMI or apex beat), regular rate and rhythm (RRR), first and second heart sounds (S1, S2), gallops (S3, S4), murmurs and thrills (graded 1-6), pulses (graded 0-4), (see **Cardiovascular Exam**)
- *Breast*: dimpling, tenderness, lumps, nipple discharge, axillary masses (see **Breast Exam**)
- *Abdomen*: IPPA or IAPP – contour (flat, obese, distended), scars, bowel sounds, bruits, tenderness, guarding, masses, liver and spleen size, ascites, costovertebral angle tenderness (see **Abdominal Exam**)
- *Urological*: inguinal masses, hernias, penis, scrotum, varicoceles, anal sphincter tone, rectal masses, prostate gland (nodules, tenderness, size) (see **Urological Exam**)
- *Gynecological*: external genitalia, vaginal mucosa, cervical discharge and colour, lesions, uterine size and shape, masses, adnexal masses, ovaries (see **Gynecological Exam**)
- *Extremeties or MSK*: can divide into I, P, ROM, special tests e.g. for joint stability: joint swelling, erythema, muscle atrophy, deformities, range of motion, edema, clubbing, peripheral cyanosis and pulses (see **Musculoskeletal Exam** and **Peripheral Vascular Exam**)
- *Neuropsychiatric*: level of consciousness, mood, cranial nerve exam, mental status, thought process, speech, mood and affect; Sensory – primary and secondary modalities – 1° sensory modalities (light touch, pain (sharp vs. dull), vibration, proprioception), 2° sensory modalities (stereognosis, graphesthesia, 2-pt discrimination); Motor – inspect, tone, power, reflexes – muscle tone and power (graded 0-5), reflexes (biceps, brachioradialis, triceps, patellar, ankle, Babinski; graded 0-4+), Romberg test for balance, gait, coordination, (see **Neurological Exam** and **Psychiatric Exam**)

GENERAL INSPECTION

General Appearance
- Acute distress, very ill, or well? Any lines or tubes present (e.g. Foley catheter, IV tubes)? Rapidly peruse the room (bedside items, number of pillows for orthopnea, etc.) for "clues"
- *Physical appearance*: skin colour (jaundice, cyanosis, pallor, plethora), diagnostic facies, level of consciousness, appears stated age
- *Body structure*: height (within normal range for age and culture), fat distribution, symmetry, posture (sitting erect as appropriate to age), position (comfortable with arms relaxed at sides), physical deformities
- *Mobility*: gait (normally, base as wide as shoulder width, with smooth, even walk), range of motion, no involuntary movement (e.g. tremor, twitching) (see **Neurological Exam** and **Geriatric Exam**)
- *Behaviour*: facial expression (eye contact, but consider cultural context), mood, affect, speech (articulation clear and understandable, fluency, hoarseness)

General Colour

Table 1. General Abnormalities of Colour

Colour Abnormality	Where to Look	Examples of Possible Causes
Blue	Tongue and mouth	Central cyanosis (pulmonary and/or cardiac disease)
	Lips, hands and feet	Peripheral cyanosis
Blue-grey	General appearance	Hemochromatosis
Pale	Conjunctiva and oral mucosa	Anemia
Red	Distinguish flushing from plethora	Polycythemia
	Plethora and erythema (inflammation)	Infections, drug reactions
Yellow	Sclera (jaundice)	Cholestasis, hepatic failure, hemolysis

Table 2. Common Signs of the Face

Signs and Symptoms	Examples of Disease States
Thick dry skin, loss of hair on head and lateral eyebrows	Hypothyroidism
Lid retraction, exophthalmos, sweating	Hyperthyroidism
Moon facies, acne, hirsutism, thinning of skin, and erythema	Cushing's syndrome
Large protruding jaw, wider spacing of teeth, protruding tongue, thick skin, prominent supraorbital ridges	Acromegaly
Periorbital edema (puffy eyes)	Nephrotic syndrome or thyroid disorder
Sunken eyes, wasting along temporal bones	Malignancy, AIDS, advanced peritonitis
Dry sunken eyes, dry mucous membranes, reduced skin turgor	Dehydration
Malar flush with facial telangiectasias	Alcoholism
Expressionless face, depressed affect, infrequent blinking	Parkinson's disease
Flat occiput and forehead, downslanting palpebral fissures, low nasal bridge, large tongue	Down syndrome

Face
- Look first for overall dysmorphic features, then for manifestations of disease such as colour changes and edema
- Special attention should be given to the eyes and the mouth

Mouth
- See *Head & Neck Exam* p. 116 for a description of a systematic oral cavity exam

Table 3. Common Signs of the Mouth

Signs and Symptoms	Examples of Disease States
Herpetic lesions	Fever, pneumonia, immunocompromised state
Aphthous ulcers (oral lesion)	Associated with celiac disease or IBD
Gum hypertrophy	Leukemia
Leukoplakia	Neoplasms, HIV
Angular stomatitis	Vit. B12 or folate deficiency
Tongue telangiectasias	GI bleeding
Peutz-Jeghers spots (brown spots on lips and oral mucosa)	Intestinal polyps and GI bleeding
Glossitis	Vitamin B12 deficiency

IBD = inflammatory bowel disease

Hands and Nails

Inspect and palpate hands for the following:

- Hand colour:
  - Paleness in the nailbeds and palmar creases: suggests anemia
  - Blue: suggests peripheral cyanosis
  - Pigmented: suggests jaundice (palmar creases may be yellow)
  - Dorsal ecchymoses: associated with steroid use, old age, bleeding disorders
  - Palmar erythema: suggests hyperestrogenism (pregnancy, liver disease)
- Hand morphology/pathology:
  - Enlarged or wasted
  - Localized joint swelling
  - Heberden's nodes (DIP)
  - Bouchard's nodes (PIP)
  - Asterixis (flapping tremor): associated with metabolic encephalopathy (e.g. uremia, hepatic failure, hypercapnia)
- Nails
  - Shape, size, colour, consistency and hemorrhages
  - Nail-bed changes are usually not pathognomonic for a specific disease, but may still provide important clues about systemic illnesses

---

Evidence-Based Medicine: Precision of the Clinical Examination for Clubbing

Studies have shown that interobserver agreement on clubbing is only fair to moderate, and that the accuracy of techniques to detect clubbing has not been well established. In cases of diagnostic uncertainty, in disease-free populations the phalangeal depth ratio rarely exceeds 1.0, and a profile nail-fold angle that approaches a straight line (180°)

Myers KA, Farquhar DRE. 2001. *JAMA* 286(3):341-347.

Table 4. Typical Nail Changes Associated with Medical Diseases

Abnormality	Characteristics	Common Associations
Clubbing	**Nail-fold Angles**: nail projects from the nailbed at an angle of ~160°, but this angle approaches 180° in clubbed fingers. This is the hyponychial angle	**Lungs**: bronchial cancer; bronchiectasis, lung abscess, CF, idiopathic pulmonary fibrosis, asbestosis
	Phalangeal Depth Ratio: in the normal finger, distal phalangeal depth is smaller than the interphalangeal depth. Ratio is reversed in clubbing	**Heart**: congenital cyanotic heart disease; infective endocarditis
	Schamroth Sign: normal fingers create a diamond-shaped window when the dorsal surfaces of terminal phalanges of similar fingers are opposed. Clubbing obliterates the diamond	**GI**: cirrhosis (esp. primary biliary cirrhosis); IBD, celiac disease
	Palpation: clubbed nails perceived as "floating" within soft tissues, and in advanced cases examiner may even be able to feel the proximal edge of the nail. Elicited by rocking the nail	**Others**: hyperthyroidism, subclavian artery stenosis, familial, idiopathic
Splinter hemorrhages	Longitudinal red-brown flecks on nailbed	<1 mm, in nail itself (i.e. will grow out): trauma (e.g. manual work) >1 mm, in nailbed: infections (e.g. endocarditis, septicemia)
Leukonychia (White nails)	White marks across nailbed	Fungal infections TB Chemotherapy Cirrhosis
Koilonychia	Spoon-shaped nails	Iron deficiency anemia
Onycholysis	Separation of nail from nailbed	Fungal infection Thyrotoxicosis Psoriasis Drugs
Pitting	Slight depression (<1 mm diameter) in nailbed	Psoriasis and psoriatic arthritis
Beau's lines	Single transverse, non-pigmented ridge	Past debilitating illness – distance from cuticle corresponds to time since recovery from illness

Table 4. Typical Nail Changes Associated with Medical Diseases (continued)

Abnormality	Characteristics	Common Associations
Mees' bands	White lines across pink nailbed	Arsenic poisoning
Lindsay's nails	"½ and ½ nails", pink-white proximally and brown distally	Chronic liver disease Azotemia
Terry's nails	White nailbeds with 1-2 mm of distal border of the nail	Cirrhosis Hypoalbuminemia

Legend: CF = cystic fibrosis; IBD = inflammatory bowel disease; TB = tuberculosis

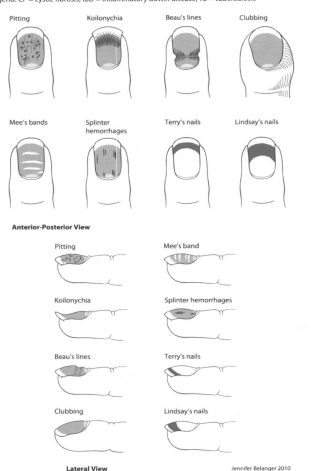

Anterior-Posterior View

Lateral View

Jennifer Belanger 2010

Figure 2. Common Nail Changes Associated with Systemic Disease

Hair

- Inspect and palpate texture, distribution (alopecia, hirsutism), scalp lesions

VITAL SIGNS

Table 5. Normal Values for Vitals

Age Group	Temperature (oral, °C)	Pulse (bpm)	Respiration (breaths per minute)	Blood Pressure (mmHg)
Adult	37.0 (range: 35.8-37.3)	80 (range: 60-100)	10-14	120/80
Child† (6yr, male)	36.5 (range: 35.5-37.3)	95 (range: 65-125)	15-25	110/70
Older adult	36.0*	70 (range: 50-90)	10-14	120/80 (diastolic may increase)

† see **Pediatric Exam** p. 256 for more detailed vitals for each pediatric age group
* for FRAIL elderly (e.g. in nursing home), upper limit of normal: 37.3°C

Temperature
- Normal oral temp in resting adult is 37°C (range: 35.8°-37.3°C)
- Rectal temp 1°C higher, axillary temp 1°C lower
- Normal temperature is influenced by:
    - Diurnal cycle (± 0.5°C, with lowest in early morning and peak in late afternoon)
    - Menstrual cycle (0.5°C rise with progesterone increase between ovulation and menses)
    - Age (in infants and young children, wider normal range because of less effective heat control mechanisms; older adults, temperature is usually lower, mean of 36.2°C)
    - Exercise

Pulse Measurement
Determine the following:
1. *Rate*: count the pulse for 30 seconds, especially if patient is bradycardic
2. *Rhythm*: regular, regularly irregular, or irregularly irregular
3. *Magnitude*: normal, diminished, or increased
4. *Shape*: how steep is the upstroke/downstroke, single/double peaked pulse
5. *Symmetry*: left vs. right
- A normal pulse will have a:
    - Steep upstroke
    - Slow decline
    - Dicrotic notch (rarely palpable)

Radial Artery
- Palpate left and right pulses simultaneously
- Use pads of first 3 fingers (not thumb since it has its own pulse), palpate just medially along radius
- 3 types of rhythm:
    - *Regular*: count number of beats in 30s and multiply by 2; (remember to start count with "zero" for first pulse felt)
    - *Regularly irregular*: count for 1 full minute
    - *Irregularly irregular*: you need to do an apical heart beat measurement, since patient has a "pulse deficit" (not all of the contractions are transmitted to peripheral pulses)

Carotid Artery
- Inspect for apparent carotid pulse, differentiate from JVP (see **Cardiovascular Exam** p. 62)
- First auscultate for bruit below angle of the jaw; if bruit is present, *do not palpate*
- *Never press on both carotids simultaneously*
- Palpate between the sternocleidomastoid and trachea, low in neck and hence away from carotid sinus
- Use 2nd and 3rd digits to palpate

Respiratory Assessment

Measure respiratory rate while pretending to still palpate the pulse; breathing will be altered if the patient is aware that they are being observed. Count for 30 seconds if breathing is normal and for 1 full minute if you suspect an abnormality
- Normal adult respiratory rate is 10-14 breaths per minute
  - *Bradypnea*: an abnormal slowing of respiration
  - *Tachypnea*: an abnormal increase
  - *Apnea*: absence of breathing, either periodic or sustained (i.e. cardiac arrest, CNS lesion)
- Breathing abnormalities (see **Respiratory Exam** p. 340)
  - Biot's breathing
  - Cheyne-Stokes breathing
  - Kussmaul's breathing

Blood Pressure Measurement

Physiology
- Systolic blood pressure (SBP): maximum pressure felt on an artery during left ventricular contract (systole)
- Diastolic blood pressure (DBP): elastic recoil (resting pressure that blood constantly exerts between each contraction)
- Pulse pressure = (SBP) – (DBP)

Brachial Artery Blood Pressure (BP) Measurement
- The patient should be relaxed, note the side and position (e.g. left arm, sitting) for which BP was measured
- The cuff bladder is centered over the brachial artery. Use the appropriate cuff size (e.g. for obese and for children). BP cuff bladder should cover 80% of biceps
- Wrap the cuff at least 2.5 cm above the antecubital fossa
- Palpate for the brachial pulse medial to the biceps tendon; use this area for auscultation
- Patient's arm should be relaxed and supported at, not above, the level of the heart
- The systolic pressure should be assessed first by palpation of the radial artery to avoid the auscultatory gap (which is sometimes present in patients with hypertension or aortic stenosis)
- In order to do this, palpate the radial (or brachial) while the cuff is inflated above the pressure needed to obliterate the pulse. Next, slowly begin to deflate the cuff; the reappearance of the radial pulse is the systolic pressure
  - Blood pressure by auscultation is assessed by inflating cuff to about 20 mmHg above systolic pressure that was determined by palpation. Deflate the cuff slowly (2 mmHg/sec). Korotkoff sounds are evaluated
  - The systolic blood pressure is the point at which the initial tapping sounds are heard. The diastolic pressure is the point at which the sounds disappear

Check Pulsus Paradoxus
- Inflate the cuff beyond systolic pressure
- Reduce pressure until systolic Korotkoff sounds are heard during expiration only
- Further deflate the cuff until sounds are also heard during inspiration
- The difference between these two pressures, called the Pulsus Paradoxus, is normally 5-10 mmHg
- An exaggerated Pulsus Paradoxus (drop in systolic blood pressure during inspiration >5-10 mmHg) is associated with: cardiac tamponade, pericardial effusions, constrictive pericarditis, asthma, emphysema, increased ventilation effort

Orthostatic Hypotension Measurement
- To assess, measure the patient's BP supine, ask them to stand, wait a couple of minutes and then remeasure the BP; consider measuring BP in both arms
- Positive for orthostatic hypotension with one or more of:
  - ≥20 mmHg fall in systolic pressure
  - ≥10 mmHg fall in diastolic pressure
  - Symptoms of cerebral hypoperfusion upon sitting/standing: dizziness, weakness, lightheadedness, visual blurring, darkening of visual fields, syncope (due to abrupt peripheral vasodilation without compensatory increase in cardiac output)
- Associated (especially in elderly) with prolonged bedrest, autonomic dysfunction, hypovolemia

Auscultatory Gap
- Transient loss of Korotkoff sounds below systolic pressure and above the diastolic pressure
- May result in missed hypertension
- When inflating the cuff, ensure that the radial artery is occluded before deflating and aucultation

Blood Pressure Classification
- Note: if the patient's systolic and diastolic categories are not the same, classify them according to the more severe category
- Varies with:
  - Age (gradually rises through childhood until adult)
  - Sex (in general, lower in females than males, until menopause, after which females have higher BP)
  - Diurnal rhythm (early morning low, late afternoon high)
  - Weight (higher in obese people)
  - Exercise
  - Stress
  - Ethnicity

Table 6. Blood Pressure Levels for Adults

Classification	Systolic Pressure (mmHg)	Diastolic Pressure (mmHg)
Normal	<120	<80
Prehypertension	120-139	80-89
Hypertension Stage 1	140-159	90-99
Hypertension Stage 2	>160	>100

Chobanian AV et al. 2003. *JAMA* 289(19):2560-2572.

Errors in BP Measurements
- Falsely *high* readings:
  - Cuff too narrow
  - Recording BP just after meal, smoking, or with distended bladder
  - Mercury column not vertical
  - Deflating cuff too slowly (produces venous congestion, falsely elevating diastolic pressure)

Evidence-Based Medicine: Benefits of Home-Blood Pressure Monitoring

Compared to office blood-pressure measurement, home measurement is a better predictor of cardiovascular events. It can also be used to confirm the diagnosis of hypertension, improve blood pressure control, reduce the need for medications, screen for masked and white coat hypertension, and improve medication adherence in non-adherent patients.

The 2008 Canadian Hypertension Education Program recommendations: the scientific summary – an annual update. 2008. *Can J Cardio* 24(6):447-452.

- Falsely *low* readings:
  - Cuff too large or loose
  - Having person's arm above heart level (hydrostatic pressure can cause error up to 10 mmHg in both systolic and diastolic pressures)
  - Failure to notice auscultatory gap (esp. in hypertension)
  - Diminished hearing acuity of health care professional
  - Stethoscope too small/large
  - Inability to hear faint Korotkoff sounds
- Falsely *low or high* readings:
  - Inaccurately calibrated sphygmomanometer
  - Defective equipment (e.g. valve)
  - Failure to have meniscus of mercury at eye level
  - Too little attention to detail

Body Mass Index Measurement
- BMI is an internationally designated measure of nutritional status used in adults and is based on height and weight
  - Advantage: Easy to calculate
  - Disadvantage: It does not take into consideration body composition (percent body fat/muscle/fluid) and may result in an inaccurate interpretation. It does not provide information about body fat distribution

$$BMI = weight\ (kg)/height\ (m^2)\ or\ BMI = weight\ (lbs)/height\ (inches^2)\ X\ 703$$

Table 7. BMI Classifications for Adults (Male and Female)

Classification	Body Mass Index (kg/m²)
Healthy Weight	18.5-25.0
Overweight	25.0-29.9
Obese	>30

Waist Circumference Measurement
- For any given BMI value, there is considerable variation in waist circumference, and an increased waist circumference predicts increased morbidity and mortality beyond those indicated by BMI alone

- Waist circumference should be measured while the patient is in the standing position. The measuring tape should be positioned in a horizontal plane at the level of the top of the iliac crest, which is used as a landmark to standardize measurement
- The person should be standing with their feet 25-30 cm apart and arms hanging naturally at the sides. The measurer should stand to the side of the patient and fit the tape snugly around the waist, horizontal to the floor
- The circumference should be measured to the nearest 0.5 cm, with the patient's abdominal muscles relaxed at the end of a normal expiration

Table 8. Ethnic-Specific Values for Waist Circumference

Ethnicity/Country*	Waist Circumference (as a measure of central obesity), cm	
	Male	Female
European	≤94	≤80
South Asian/Chinese	≤90	≤80
Japanese	≤85	≤90

*Since ethnic-specific data is not available for all groups, it is suggested that South Asian cutoffs be used for individuals from South and Central America, and European cutoffs be used for individuals from Sub-Saharan Africa, Eastern Mediterranean, and the Middle East.
Lau DC et al. 2007. *CMAJ* 176(8):S1-13.

SPOUSAL ABUSE

Definition
- Physical, sexual or psychological abuse directed against one individual by another individual in an attempt to control his/her behaviour or intimidate him/her. Perpetrators are most often men abusing female partners, but abuse can also occur in other family situations, including child and elder abuse, and abuse in same-sex relationships

Types of Abuse
- Physical: including pushing, shoving, choking or battering
- Sexual: forced sex, imposed pregnancy/abortion
- Emotional: verbal denigration, name-calling
- Psychological: social isolation, controlling the victim's behaviour through jealousy or threats to the individual, their children or other family members including pets
- Financial control

Prevalence
- 27% of all violent crimes are due to family violence
- 62% of incidents of family violence is spousal abuse
- Young females aged 25-35 experience the highest rates of spousal abuse
- 85% of the victims of spousal abuse are female
- The lifetime prevalence of sexual assault is 1 in 4 for women (and 1 in 6 for men)
- 25% to 45% of abused women are beaten during pregnancy (physical abuse may start or increase during pregnancy)
- Rates highest among those with unemployed and "heavy drinker" partners
- Spouses in step families and in families with children younger than 15 years old are more likely to be victims
- Harassment and violence may increase after the relationship ends

Physician's Role

- Identification
- Assessment/Examination
- Documentation
- Medical care
- Safety planning
- Referral
- Respect for doctor/patient confidentiality (doctor cannot notify police unless permission is given by patient)

Common Chief Complaints

- Patients rarely identify abuse as their CC, therefore be alert to the following:
  - Unexplained traumatic injuries or explanations that do not match injury patterns
  - Chest pain, GI pain, pelvic pain, back pain
  - Multiple visits for specific and often stress-related complaints
  - Headache, insomnia, anxiety, depression
  - Suicidal ideation, suicide attempts
  - Chronic pain syndromes
  - Substance abuse
  - Eating disorders

Common Disorders

- *Obstetrics*: miscarriage, stillbirth, abruptio placentae, premature labor and delivery
- *Gynecology*: dyspareunia, chronic pelvic pain, trauma and STDs from sexual assault
- *Emergency*: facial lacerations, fractures, head or neck injury, burns
- *Ophthalmology*: retinal detachment, orbital blow-out fracture, retinal hemorrhages

---

Evidence-Based Medicine: Interventions For Intimate Partner Violence Against Women

Insufficient evidence is available to recommend for or against routine screening for violence against women who are pregnant or who are not pregnant, or of men. This is distinct from the need for clinicians to include questions about exposure to domestic violence as part of their diagnostic assessment of women. This information is important in caring for the patient and may influence assessment and treatment of other health problems.

Wathen CN, MacMillan HL. 2003. *CMAJ* 169(6):582-584 .

- *Neurology*: skull fracture, subdural and epidural hematoma, "shaken adult syndrome"
- *Mental Health*: chronic anxiety and/or depression, post-traumatic stress disorder, substance abuse

Approach to History

- Interview the patient alone (if this is impossible, document)
- Be non-judgmental; avoid "why" questions
- Provide and ensure confidentiality (highest incidence of life threatening abuse occurs after seeking professional help or leaving the relationship)
- Have a list of community resources available or give 211 for community resources
- Ask direct and specific questions
- Include an empathetic response to descriptions of violence humiliation
- Believe reports of abuse

- Reassure them it is not their fault and they are not alone
- Arrange for follow-up
- Document in writing treatment given: antibiotics etc. and give a copy to the patient
- Do risk assessment and safety planning before they leave the medical setting
- Do not be frustrated if abuse is denied or help is declined

History: Sample Questions

- Questions assessing domestic violence exposure should be asked of all women, because women rarely disclose abuse spontaneously:
  - How are things in your relationship?
  - What happens when your partner loses his/her temper?
  - Do you feel safe at home?
- Direct questions should be asked:
  - Sometimes when people feel the way you do it may be because they are being yelled at or hit at home. Is this happening to you?
  - Do arguments ever reult in pushing or shoving?
  - Many patients with similar injuries have been hit by someone - is this what happened to you?
  - Has anyone ever forced you to have sex against your wishes?
  - Does your partner ever hit or abuse your children? (Inform them that suspected or confirmed child abuse must be reported to Children's Aid Society – CAS)

Approach to Physical Examination

- Reassure patient, inform them of examination procedures and involve them in decision-making
- Complete physical exam including neurological exam

Physical Signs of Abuse

- Injuries inconsistent with history
- Injury to head, face, neck, breasts, abdomen most common (especially if bilateral)
- Injuries during pregnancy
- Multiple bruises, bruises at different stages of healing, or tenderness to any part of the body
- Burns from cigarettes, electrical appliances or acids
- Perforated eardrums
- Fractured teeth and soft tissue injuries to mouth
- Old bruises or untreated fractures
- Recovery from illness/injury inappropriately delayed
- Indications of substance abuse

Other Clues

- Non-adherence with medications, treatment or follow-up appointments
- Overly "supportive" partner
- Cancelled appointments, especially if cancellation call was made by partner

Interpretation of Findings

- Multiple injuries are more likely in abused individuals compared to accident victims
- Spousal abuse is a cycle that usually escalates over time; be alert for repeated injuries
- Physicians significantly underestimate abuse, thus assess all women for abuse
- People with addictions are abused more often than those without
- Chronic abuse often leads to substance abuse

Safety Planning

- Has there been an increase in severity/frequency of assaults?
- Have there been new or increasing threats of homicide or suicide by their partner?
- Have there been new or increasing threats to any children? (Including pets that may pose a threat to children – report all threats to CAS)
- Does their partner have access to a firearm?
- Do they know where to call for help in an emergency?
- Write emergency numbers on a piece of paper
- Never tell an abusive partner that abuse has been disclosed
- Developing a safety plan includes making provision for escape including what documents they need to have with them, money, birth certificates, keys, change of clothes, children's favorite toys, etc.
- Consult Best Practice Guidelines by the Woman Abuse Council of Toronto for more information

Documentation

- Detailed history – reported cause of injury in patient's own words
- Avoid using terms such as "patient alleges" or "patient claims" in documentation
- Physical findings – body map of bruises and tender areas
- Photographs (can use a polaroid camera), with a ruler or other measurements and physical evidence (with consent)
- Your own suspicion of abuse – including physical injuries or chronic stress-related complaints

After Disclosure

- Documentation
- Support
- Make A Safety Plan

REFERENCES

Beck RS, Daughtridge R, Sloane PD. 2002. Physician-patient communication in the primary care office: a systematic review. *J Am Board Fam Pract* 15(1):25-38.

Bickley LS, Szilagyi PG, Bates B. 2007. *Bates' Guide to Physical Examination and History Taking*. Philadelphia: Lippincott Williams & Wilkins.

Canadian Hypertension Education Program. 2008. The 2008 Canadian Hypertension Education Program recommendations: the scientific summary – an annual update. *Can J Cardiol* 24(6):447-452.

Chobanian AV et al. 2003. The Seventh Report of the Joint National Committee on Prevention, Detection, Evaluation, and Treatment of High Blood Pressure: the JNC 7 report. *JAMA* 289(19): 2560-2572.

Lau DC, Douketis JD, Morrison KM, Hramiak IM, Sharma AM, Ur E. 2006. Canadian clinical practice guidelines on the management and prevention of obesity in adults and children [summary]. *CMAJ* 176(8):S1-13.

Makoul G, Zick A, Green M. 2007. An evidence-based perspective on greetings in medical encounters. *Arch Intern Med* 167(11):1172-1176.

Miller GF. 2000. *The Mating Mind: How Sexual Choice Shaped the Evolution of Human Nature*. New York: Doubleday.

Myers KA, Farquhar DR. 2001. The rational clinical examination. Does this patient have clubbing? *JAMA* 286(3):341-347.

Orient JM, Sapira JD. 2005. *Sapira's Art & Science of Bedside Diagnosis*. Philadelphia: Lippincott Williams & Wilkins.

Sackett DL, Rennie D. 1992. The science of the art of the clinical examination. *JAMA* 267(19):2650-2652.

Statistics Canada. *Family Violence in Canada: A Statistical Profile 2004*. Ottawa: Canadian Centre for Justice Statistics.

Wathen CN, MacMillan HL. 2003. Prevention of violence against women: recommendation statement from the Canadian Task Force on Preventive Health Care. *CMAJ* 169(6):582-584.

The Abdominal Exam

Editors:
Antoine Eskander &
Christopher Kandel

Faculty Reviewers:
Gabor Kandel, MD FRCP(C)
Peter Rossos, MD, MBA, FRCP(C)

ABDOMINAL

TABLE OF CONTENTS

Essential Anatomy 27
Approach to the Abdominal History and Physical Exam 28
Common Chief Complaints 30
Common Disorders 30
Focused History 30
Focused Physical Exam 33
Common Investigations 41
Common Clinical Scenarios 42

ESSENTIAL ANATOMY

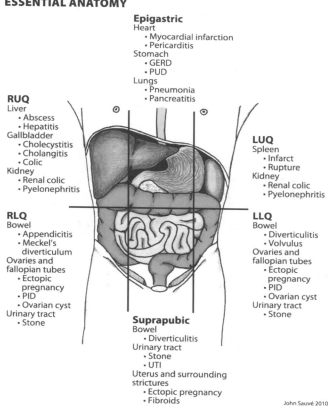

Epigastric
Heart
- Myocardial infarction
- Pericarditis
Stomach
- GERD
- PUD
Lungs
- Pneumonia
- Pancreatitis

RUQ
Liver
- Abscess
- Hepatitis
Gallbladder
- Cholecystitis
- Cholangitis
- Colic
Kidney
- Renal colic
- Pyelonephritis

LUQ
Spleen
- Infarct
- Rupture
Kidney
- Renal colic
- Pyelonephritis

RLQ
Bowel
- Appendicitis
- Meckel's diverticulum
Ovaries and fallopian tubes
- Ectopic pregnancy
- PID
- Ovarian cyst
Urinary tract
- Stone

LLQ
Bowel
- Diverticulitis
- Volvulus
Ovaries and fallopian tubes
- Ectopic pregnancy
- PID
- Ovarian cyst
Urinary tract
- Stone

Suprapubic
Bowel
- Diverticulitis
Urinary tract
- Stone
- UTI
Uterus and surrounding strictures
- Ectopic pregnancy
- Fibroids

John Sauvé 2010

Figure 1. Differential Diagnosis of Abdominal Pathology by Location

APPROACH TO ABDOMINAL HISTORY AND PHYSICAL EXAM

Approaching an abdominal complaint varies depending on its severity, character, and duration

Acute GI Symptoms

Acute abdominal pain

- *Assess vital signs* (including body temperature) while taking history
  - In addition to OPQRSTUVW, consider underlying diseases (e.g. think of ischemic bowel if history of heart disease, perforated ulcer if arthritis treated by NSAIDs, pancreatitis if alcoholism, cholangitis if gallstones)
- *Search for signs of peritonitis* (in the elderly signs may be less apparent)
  - Position favoured by patient to minimize pain is a clue to its origin (e.g. sitting forward suggests pancreatitis, immobile suggests peritonitis, sitting with hips constantly flexed suggests renal colic)
  - Look for guarding
  - Assess for exacerbation of pain when patient coughs or when shaking the bed
  - If no pain elicited from coughing or shaking bed, palpate gently for area of maximum tenderness
  - If no tenderness elicited by gentle palpation, push deeply, withdraw your hand suddenly – pain more severe when your hand is withdrawn than during palpation suggests peritonitis ("rebound tenderness")
  - If signs elicited, CT usually indicated along with surgical consultation
- *Auscultation*
  - Least useful sign: if increased think of mechanical bowel obstruction, if decreased think of non-mechanical bowel obstruction or peritonitis
- *Palpation and Percussion*
  - Identify the area of maximal tenderness to ensure it is examined last
  - Assess for signs of peritonitis, masses, dullness
  - Estimate the size of the spleen or liver
- *Acute GI Bleed*
  - Upper or lower GI source: proximal or distal to ligament of Treitz, respectively
  - Hematochezia: either lower or massive upper
  - Hematemesis: always due to upper GI tract source
  - Classify upper as variceal or non-variceal
    - Look for signs of portal hypertension (especially splenomegaly) as clues to varices
  - Prioritize large bore IV catheter, stabilization with IV fluids, endoscopy when ABCs addressed – immediate vs. urgent (<24h); remember to measure hemoglobin, platelet count, INR/PTT, take a bleeding and drug hx (ASA, NSAIDS, other anti-platelet agents, anti-coagulants)
- *Acute Vomiting*
  - Think bowel obstruction if vomiting develops after meals, food in vomitus, abdominal pain relieved by vomiting
  - Non-gut causes: pregnancy, alcoholism, chronic renal failure, medications, hepatitis
  - Think pancreatitis, cholecystitis, if associated abdominal pain not relieved by vomiting
  - Look at ocular fundus for papilledema from increased intracranial pressure
  - Remember to search for succussion splash (place stethoscope in epigastrium shake patient, consider gastric outlet obstruction if you hear "whoosh" sound)

Subacute/Chronic Alarm GI Symptoms

In addition to general history taking, important aspects of the abdominal history include:

Abdominal Pain	Jaundice
Vomiting	Timing of symptoms
Weight change	Food intolerance
Bowel habits	Medications
GI bleeding	Family history
	Social history

Overview of the physical exam:
- Vitals
- Inspection
  - Skin, hands and nails (peripheral signs of liver disease)
  - Peripheral edema
  - Abdomen
  - JVP (if ascites, liver disease)
- Auscultation
  - Bowel sounds
  - Bruits
  - Miscellaneous (succussion splash)
- Percussion
  - Quadrants
  - Liver
  - Spleen
  - Ascites
- Palpation
  - Light palpation
  - Deep palpation
- Special Tests and Signs
- Digital Rectal Exam

Well Patient Visit

History
- In addition to routine functional inquiry focus on:
  - Family history of cancer, especially colon (to determine whether screening indicated), also inflammatory bowel/autoimmune disease, malabsorption (celiac disease)
  - Use of NSAIDs (others as above)
  - Dietary history
  - Estimate alcohol intake (CAGE questionnaire if indicated) (see *Psychiatric Exam* p. 319)

Physical
- Subjective global nutritional assessment
- Pallor
- Jaundice
- Lymphadenopathy
- Hepatomegaly
- Splenomegaly
- Digital rectal exam

COMMON CHIEF COMPLAINTS

- Abdominal pain
- Fever
- Jaundice (yellowing skin)
- Dysphagia (difficulty swallowing)
- Odynophagia (painful swallowing)
- Vomiting
- Hematemesis (vomiting blood)
- Nausea
- Gas/bloating
- Abdominal distension
- Reflux (heartburn)
- Mass
- Diarrhea
- Constipation
- Irregular bowel habits (alternating constipation and diarrhea)
- Melena or hematochezia (blood in stool)
- Weight loss

COMMON DISORDERS

Disorders marked with (✓) are discussed in **Common Clinical Scenarios**

- ✓ Alcoholic Liver Disease
- ✓ Appendicitis
- ✓ Celiac Disease
- ✓ Cirrhosis – including complications (ascites, encephalopathy, variceal bleeding, spontaneous bacterial peritonitis)
- ✓ Colorectal Cancer
- ✓ Diarrhea
- ✓ Gallstones
- ✓ GI Bleeding
- ✓ Pancreatitis
- ✓ Inflammatory Bowel Disease
- ✓ Irritable Bowel Syndrome
- ✓ Peptic Ulcer Disease
- Diverticulitis
- Hemochromatosis
- Hepatitis – alcoholic, viral, drug-related/toxic
- Gastroesophageal Reflux Disease (GERD)
- Other GI Malignancies (esophageal cancer, gastric carcinoma, pancreatic cancer and hepatocellular carcinoma)
- Vascular Disease of the Bowel

FOCUSED HISTORY

1) Pain

- OPQRSTUVW (see *General History and Physical Exam* p. 9)
- Location and character are especially important

> **Clinical Pearl**
> Diseases of the heart and lungs, such as coronary artery disease and pneumonia, can present with upper abdominal pain.

Table 1. Area of Pain May Suggest Its Cause

Location of Pain	Possible Pathology
RUQ	Cholecystitis, hepatitis, pancreatitis, hepatic abscess, choledocolithiasis, cholangitis, tumour (e.g. colon, kidney, liver)
Epigastric	PUD (complicated or perforated), pancreatitis, thoracic causes (pericarditis, aortic aneurysm, MI), gallstones
LUQ	Splenic infarct, ruptured spleen, pancreatitis, abscess, gastric ulcer, gastric cancer
Flank	Pyelonephritis, nephrolithiasis, retrocecal appendicitis, retroperitoneal bleeding, sarcoma, abscess
Lower abdomen	Aortic aneurysm, appendicitis, diverticulitis, colorectal cancer, PID, bowel perforation, sigmoid volvulus
Variably located	Gastroenteritis, GI obstruction, IBD, ischemic colitis, visceral angina
Diffuse, steady or sharp	Peritonitis

Legend: R/LUQ = right/left upper quadrant, PUD = peptic ulcer disease, MI = myocardial infarction, GI = gastrointestinal, IBD = inflammatory bowel disease, PID = pelvic inflammatory disease

Table 2. Character of Pain Suggests Its Cause

Character	Possible Pathology
Abrupt, excruciating	MI, perforated ulcer, ruptured aneurysm, ureteral colic, biliary colic
Rapid onset, steady and severe	Acute pancreatitis, strangulated bowel, ectopic pregnancy, mesenteric ischemia (may present with pain disproportionate to signs),
Gradual, steady	Acute cholecystitis, acute cholangitis, acute hepatitis, appendicitis
Colicky	Small bowel obstruction, IBD

2) Bowel Habits

- Chronic or acute change in bowel patterns
- Change in number of stools per day
- Constipation, diarrhea, tenesmus (straining, passing little or no feces, sense that all stool has not been passed)
- Character of stools: solid/loose, floating, malodorous, bloody, mucous, colour and intensity of colour (pale/dark)
- Rectal bleeding
- Association with:
    - Weight loss
    - Pain (aggravating or alleviating)
    - Meals
- Risk of food poisoning
- Travel history

3) GI Bleeding
- Hematemesis – vomiting of blood from gut
- Melena – black stools
- Hematochezia – blood in stools

4) Jaundice and Scleral Icterus
- Best seen in full spectrum natural light (artificial lighting may impair detection of cyanosis, pallor and jaundice)
- Inquire especially about associated symptoms, duration, fever, medications, alcohol
- Pruritus (indicates chronic cholestasis)
- Pale stools (can be due to any cause of an increased direct bilirubin fraction, i.e. biliary obstruction, acute hepatitis)
- Dark urine (increased passage of bilirubin, more sensitive for cholestasis than visible icterus)
- Industrial chemicals

5) Medications
- Non-steroidal anti-inflammatory drugs (NSAIDs), steroids, ulcer medications, laxatives

6) Family History
- Colorectal cancer
- Gallstones
- Inflammatory Bowel Disease (IBD) – Ulcerative Colitis (UC) or Crohn's Disease (CD)
- Celiac Sprue or other autoimmune diseases
- Functional Bowel Disease
- Family history of similar symptoms

7) Social History
- Sexual practices (e.g. anal intercourse)
- Decreased libido
- Menstrual patterns
- Alcohol intake – CAGE questionnaire* (see *Psychiatric Exam* p. 319)
  *to be used for screening only and not for diagnosis

Clinical Pearl
In a patient with jaundice, long-standing history of decreased libido and abnormal menstruation points toward chronic liver disease.

FOCUSED PHYSICAL EXAM

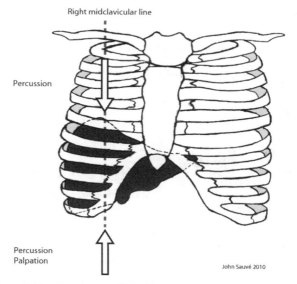

Figure 2. Liver Percussion and Palpation

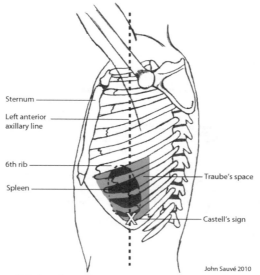

Figure 3. Spleen Percussion

Prepare the Patient

- Adequate lighting, warm room, comfortable environment
- Adjust bed to flat position

- Patient lying supine, arms at his/her side
- Appropriate draping
- Stand on the patient's right
- If abdominal wall is tense, it can be relaxed by maximally flexing knees (heels close to buttocks), by placing a pillow under patient's head and/or knees or by placing patient's hand onto your palpating hand (this may also help with "ticklish" patients, and children)

Vital Signs
- BP, HR, RR, T°

Inspection
Most commonly missed: nail and skin changes, subtle edema, elevated neck veins

- *State of the patient*
    - Completely still: suggests peritonitis
    - Curled up in fetal position: suggests visceral pain
    - One hip flexed: suggests splinting
    - Sitting up and leaning forward suggests retroperitoneal irritation
- *Skin*
    - Skin colour
        + Jaundice, pallor, cyanosis, erythema
        + Ecchymoses of the abdomen and flanks (Grey-Turner's Sign, Cullen's Sign, see **Table 3**)
    - Skin Abnormalities
        + Striae (recent = pink, blue; purple = Cushing; old = silver, obese, post-partum)
        + Keloid, hyperplastic surgical scars
        + Spider angiomas (due to elevated estrogen)
- *Hands & Nails*
    - Thenar wasting
    - Palmar erythema
    - Dupuytren's contracture
    - Clubbing
    - Leukonychia (white spots, streaks on nails)
- *Abdomen* – look at the abdomen from the foot of the bed
    - Contour
        + Normal – note symmetry
        + Scaphoid – normal, malnourished
        + Protuberant – 6 F's (Fat, Fluid, Feces, Flatus, Fetus, Fatal growth)
        + Distended lower half: suggests pregnancy, leiomyoma (fibroid), ovarian tumour
        + Distended upper half: suggests gastric dilatation, enlarged lobe of liver
        + Bulging flanks – suggests ascites but need to differentiate from obesity
    - Umbilicus
        + Everted – increased abdominal pressure: suggests fluid, mass
        + Umbilical hernia
        + Bluish (Cullen's Sign, see **Table 3**)
        + Nodular: suggests metastatic cancer
    - Hernias (see *Urological Exam*)
    - Superficial veins
        + Visible in thin patients and in vena cava obstruction
        + Caput medusae (surrounding umbilicus)

      ◆ Cephalad drainage pattern in IVC obstruction, caudad drainage in SVC obstruction, normal flow pattern (cephalad above umbilicus and caudad below umbilicus) in portal hypertension without caval obstruction
- *JVP* (see ***Cardiovascular Exam*** p. 62)

Clinical Pearl
An elevated JVP may be the only clinical clue to a cardiac cause of liver disease (tricuspid insufficiency, pericarditis), whereas in other causes of cirrhosis, JVP is low. Look for a pulsatile liver.

- *Stigmata of chronic liver disease*
  - Spider angioma
  - Gynecomastia
  - Testicular atrophy
  - Frontal balding

Auscultation
- Bowel sounds (least useful portion of the physical exam)
  - Listening to one quadrant is sufficient
  - Listen for 2 min before concluding absent
- Bruits
  - Vascular (remember to listen over the flanks as well)
    - ◆ Aortic
    - ◆ Renal artery
    - ◆ Bifurcation of the common iliac arteries
  - Liver
    - ◆ Bruit: suggests hepatic carcinoma, alcoholic hepatitis
- Miscellaneous
  - Succussion splash (assess distension of abdominal viscera)
    - ◆ Gently shake patient from side to side and auscultate for "whoosh" sound of air or fluid moving in a distended abdomen (suggests colon or stomach distension)

Percussion
- Percuss all 4 quadrants (usually tympanic; note any dullness)
- Liver
  - Lower border: start below umbilicus (tympanic) and percuss upward in right mid-clavicular line (MCL) or mid-sternal line (MSL) until liver dullness
  - Upper border: start from lung resonance in MCL or MSL and percuss downward to liver dullness
  - Measure the span
    - ◆ Normal: 9-11 cm MCL, 4-8 cm MSL
    - ◆ Falsely increased span (lung dullness, e.g. right pleural effusion)
    - ◆ Falsely decreased span (gas in the RUQ, e.g. gas in the colon)
- Spleen
  - *Traube's Space*
    - ◆ "The patient is supine with the left arm slightly abducted for access to the entire Traube's space, defined by the sixth rib superiorly, the mid-axillary line laterally, and the left costal margin inferiorly. With the patient breathing normally, this triangle is percussed across one or more levels from its medial to lateral margins. Normal percussion yields a resonant or tympanic note. Splenomegaly is diagnosed when the percussion note is dull" *(Grover SA et al, 1993)*

- *Castell's Sign*
  - ◆ Have the patient lie supine and breathe in and out deeply in a continuous manner
  - ◆ While patient is breathing continuously percuss the lowest intercostal space in the left anterior-axillary line
  - ◆ Normal or small spleen sounds tympanic
  - ◆ Enlarged spleen will be dull on inspiration

Clinical Pearl
Since food in the stomach causes dullness in the left upper quadrant interpret dullness cautiously if patient has eaten within the past four hours.

Evidence-Based Medicine: Splenomegaly
Percussion is more sensitive but less specific than palpation as a diagnostic test for splenomegaly. Percussion (Castell's Sign) should therefore be done first, followed by palpation. If both percussion and palpation are positive, the diagnosis of splenomegaly can be ruled in, provided there is a pre-test probability of at least 10%.

Grover SA et al. 1993. *JAMA* 270(18):2218-2221.

- **Ascites**
  - Shifting Dullness
    - ◆ Determine the border of tympany and dullness by percussion in supine position (mark this spot with a pen) and then repeat with the patient on his/her side
      - In the presence of ascites, the tympany-dullness margin will move 'upward' (towards the umbilicus)
      - In the absence of ascites, the margin does not move
- **Fluid Wave**
  - Ask the patient to place the ulnar side of his/her hand in the midline of the abdomen (this prevents a false positive due to the patient's fat and flatus)
  - Tap on lateral side of abdomen and assess the transmission of a wave to contralateral side using the other hand – if the fluid thrill can be palpated by this hand, the abdominal distension is due to ascites

Palpation
- Warm hands
- Ask the patient to locate the area of maximum tenderness; examine this area last

Clinical Pearl
Watch the face not their abdomen while palpating. A grimace suggests pathology in the palpated area.

Light Palpation
- Detects abdominal tenderness, areas of muscle spasm/rigidity
  - Lightly palpate entire abdomen using flat part of the right hand (fingers joined)
  - Lift hand entirely from the skin when moving from area to area
  - In the case of a ticklish patient try placing the patient's hand on top of your hand while palpating

- If an area of tenderness is found, perform a one finger palpation to delineate the specific area of tenderness
- If hernia suspected, examine inguinal hernial rings and male genitalia
- Palpate costovertebral angle tenderness:
  - Place one hand flat on the costovertebral angle to assess for tenderness
  - If pain not elicited, attempt fist palpation (use of the ulnar surface of fist to strike your hand lying flat on the costovertebral angle)
  - For assessment of retroperitoneal abscess, retrocecal appendicitis and pyelonephritis
- Elicit cough tenderness (examine this last)
  - Coughing often elicits localized pain in an inflamed area
- Shake tenderness – shake the bed

Deep Palpation
- Detects presence of masses, inflamed gallbladder, appendiceal abscess, etc.
- Rest right hand on the abdomen while left hand exerts gentle but steady pressure
- Ask patients to breathe through their mouths

Clinical Pearl
To differentiate between involuntary or malingering pain try to distract patient by pretending to auscultate but pushing in the stethoscope (Note: Do not do this routinely, only when pain is questionable!)

Palpation of Liver, Spleen, and Kidney
- Determines presence of organ enlargement and/or tenderness
  - Ask patient to breathe deeply through their mouth
  - Palpate during inspiration; move hand during expiration
  - Palpate for the liver beginning at the pelvic brim
  - Palpate for the spleen beginning at the umbilicus
  - May feel the liver or spleen slip over the fingertips

Palpation of Liver Edge
Note: the edge of an enlarged liver may be missed by starting palpation too high on the abdomen
- *Method 1:*
  - Place the right hand on the abdomen with fingertips positioned superiorly (parallel to the rectus abdominus muscle) and push inwards and upwards towards patient's head during each inspiration until the liver edge is felt
  - The hand inches forward/upward during expiration
  - To check for tenderness, the examiner's left hand is placed on the liver while the ulnar side of the right fist strikes the left hand
- *Method 2:* (useful method if a patient is obese)
  - Stand near the head of the patient with examiner facing patient's feet
  - Place both hands below the right costal margin to "hook" over the liver edge
  - The examiner pushes inward and toward the patient's head during inspiration

- When describing your examination of the liver, always include:
  - Length of liver below costal margin
  - Total liver span
  - Texture of liver edge (i.e. smooth or nodular)
  - Consistency of liver edge (i.e. firm or soft)
  - Tenderness of liver edge
  - Presence of bruits

Evidence-Based Medicine: Hepatomegaly
Combined results of 3 studies:

Palpability	Hepatomegaly		LR	95% CI
	Yes	No		
Yes	231	301	LR+ 2.5	2.2 – 2.8
No	112	818	LR- 0.45	0.38 - 0.52

A palpable liver is not necessarily enlarged, but increases the likelihood of hepatomegaly. A non-palpable liver edge does not rule out hepatomegaly, but reduces its likelihood.

Naylor CD. 1994. *JAMA* 271(23):1859-1865.

Palpation of Spleen
- Stand on the right side of the supine patient
- Place left hand behind the patient's left rib cage and right hand in the right lower quadrant (area of the appendix) angled towards the anterior axillary line
- As patient inspires deeply, palpate for the spleen with the right hand searching for a massively enlarged spleen
- Then incrementally move the right hand diagonally upward to the left costal margin all the while palpating for the spleen
- When the right hand reaches the left costal margin, gently dig deep under the left costal margin while the patient inspires deeply, searching for a minimally enlarged spleen (i.e. palpate for the tip of the spleen coming forward)

Palpation of Kidney
- The kidney is not usually palpable in an adult except in polycystic kidney disease
- Stand on the patient's right side
- Palpate deeply with the right hand below the right costal margin
- Left hand is placed on the patient's back between the right costal margin and the right iliac crest and is used to lift upwards
- For the left kidney, stand on the left side of the patient and repeat the maneuvers switching hands
- To check for tenderness, ask patient to sit up; strike the two costovertebral angles with the ulnar side of your fist (lightly)
  - Proceed in a downward vertical direction

Table 3. Specific Signs and Their Possible Interpretation

Sign/Special Test	Description	Possible Pathology
Rovsing's sign	RLQ pain on LLQ palpation	Appendicitis
McBurney's sign	Tenderness at McBurney's Point ($^1/_3$ along line extending from the ASIS to the umbilicus)	Appendicitis
Rebound tenderness	Pain on quick withdrawal of palpation *check for peritonitis before assessing rebound tenderness by asking patient to cough or by lightly jarring the bed; if this reproduces the abdominal pain, there is no need to maximize the pain by demonstrating rebound tenderness	Peritonitis
Murphy's sign	Arrest of deep inspiration on RUQ palpation (hand contact with gallbladder elicits pain)	Cholecystitis
Courvoisier's sign	Painless, palpable distended gallbladder	Pancreatic cancer
Cullen's sign	Blue discolouration of periumbilical area caused by retroperitoneal hemorrhage tracking around to anterior abdominal wall	Acute hemorrhagic pancreatitis Ectopic pregnancy
Grey-Turner's sign	Blue discolouration of the flank area caused by retroperitoneal hemorrhage	Acute hemorrhagic pancreatitis Ruptured abdominal aortic aneurysm Strangulated bowel
Kehr's sign	Severe left shoulder pain exacerbated by elevating foot of bed (referred pain; diaphragmatic involvement)	Splenic rupture
Psoas test	Pain on flexion of the hip against resistance	Appendicitis Other causes of inflammation in region of psoas muscle (e.g. retroperitoneal abscess)
Obturator test	Pain when thigh is flexed to a right angle and gently rotated, first internally then externally	Pelvic Appendicitis Diverticulitis PID Other causes of inflammation in region of obturator internus muscle

ABDOMINAL

Table 3. Specific Signs and Their Possible Interpretation (continued)

Sign/Special Test	Description	Possible Pathology
Positive Carnett's sign	Abdominal pain/ tenderness exacerbated when patient lifts feet above the bed without bending knees	Source of pain is abdominal wall (strain/sprain/ abdominal wall hernia), because stretching of abdominal wall worsens any lesion within wall (positive Carnett's sign)
Negative Carnett's sign	Abdominal pain/ tenderness alleviated when patient lifts feet above the bed without bending knees	Source of pain is inside abdominal cavity because stabilizing abdominal wall protects the organs within the abdominal cavity (negative Carnett's sign)

R/LUQ = right/left upper quadrant, PID = pelvic inflammatory disease

Evidence-Based Medicine: Appendicitis

Sign	Sensitivity (%)	Specificity (%)	LR+
RLQ pain	81	53	8.0
Rigidity	27	83	3.76
Pain Migration	64	82	3.18
Psoas Sign	16	95	2.38

Wagner JM et al. 1996. *JAMA* 276(19):1589-1594.

ABDOMINAL AORTIC ANEURYSM
- See *Peripheral Vascular Exam* p. 309

DIGITAL RECTAL EXAM (DRE)
- Male
  - See *Urological Exam* p. 359

- Female
  - See *Gynecological Exam* p. 98

Clinical Pearl
- Most common cause of an epigastric mass is an enlarged liver
- Most common cause of epigastric tenderness is tenderness of the aortic thrust, which has no clinical significance
- Always check JVP in ascites to rule out tricuspid insufficiency and pericardial disease as a cause of the ascites

COMMON INVESTIGATIONS

Table 4. Common GI Investigations

Test	Description	Indication for Test
Stool C/S and/or microscopy	Detection of microbes in stool	To rule or infection (ask specifically for *Clostridium difficile* toxin assay if patient has been on antibiotics or recent hospitalization)
FOBT	Detects small volumes of blood in the stool	Colon cancer screening
Colonoscopy*	Provides best view of colon mucosa and opportunities for biopsy	Used to rule out or establish diagnosis of multiple mucosal conditions (e.g. colorectal cancer, IBD)
Upper endoscopy*	Provides a view of the esophagus, stomach, and duodenum	Look for esophageal varices, peptic esophagitis, peptic ulcer, small bowel biopsy to rule out intestinal diseases such as celiac disease
CT Colonography	CT examination of colon after introduction of air into anorectum	To detect diverticula, fistulae, look of intrinsic compression of the colon or if a colonoscopy indicated but cannot be completed
MRCP	MRI evaluation of the bile duct, gallbladder, and pancreatic duct	To diagnose biliary obstruction as a cause of jaundice or elevated liver enzymes
ERCP*	Endoscopic procedure to examine the common bile duct, and pancreatic duct	Suspect bile duct obstruction requiring intervention such as sphincterotomy, stent, biopsy
Schilling test*	Measurement of urinary radioactive labeled vitamin B12 following oral ingestion	Evaluate vitamin B12 absorption to test for pernicious anemia, ileal disease, bacterial small bowel overgrowth, pancreatic insufficiency
C-14 Urea breath test C-13 Non-radioactive	Detection of the enzyme urease, produced by *Helicobacter pylori*. If gastric urease present, then orally administered C-14 urea will be hydrolyzed into ammonia and $^{14}CO_2$. The $^{14}CO_2$ can be detected in the expired breath. Analogous test possible with non-radioactive $^{13}CO_2$, but is more expensive	*Helicobacter pylori* infection of stomach
H_2 Breath test	Measures H_2 content of expired air	Lactose intolerance, bacterial overgrowth

* gold standard for the indicated pathology
Legend: C/S = culture and sensitivity; FOBT = fecal occult blood test; ERCP= endoscopic retrograde cholangiopancreatography; MRCP= magnetic resonance cholangiopancreatography

COMMON CLINICAL SCENARIOS

Acute Diarrhea

- *History*
  - Associated signs and symptoms include vomiting, fever, arthritis, skin rash, anorexia and weight loss
  - Onset (abrupt onset suggests infection) and duration (longer duration suggests initial phase of a chronic illness)
  - Urgency to defecate points toward rectal involvement
  - Frequency of movements (Does it wake you at night?) indicates severity of diarrhea and rectal involvement
  - Quantity of each bowel movement:
    - The small bowel tends to be the source if the bowel movements are large and relatively infrequent
    - The colorectum is the more likely source of disease if the feces are small in volume, passed frequently, and are mixed with blood, mucus or pus
  - Quality:
    - Bloody (bright red) suggests large bowel problem, black suggests upper GI problem, watery suggests small bowel problem; mucus, foul smelling, floating in toilet, difficult to flush all suggest steatorrhea
  - Abdominal pain: cramping before defecation has no diagnostic significance but abdominal pain between movements suggests involvement of bowel serosa
- *Risk Factors*
  - Antibiotic history (*Clostridium difficile*)
  - Food history, especially potential for undercooked poultry or eggs (*Campylobacter, Salmonella*), beef products (*E. coli* O157:H7), seafood (*Vibrio parahaemolyticus*, cholera, viral agents), food poisoning due to *S. aureus* or *Clostridium perfringens*, fresh fruits such as raspberries (*Cyclospora*)
  - Contact with infected person (all bacterial and viral agents), exposure to healthcare, chronic care, childcare facilities
  - Travel history
  - Immunosuppression
  - Laxative use
  - Anal intercourse
  - Malignancy
- *Physical Exam*
  - Assessment of extracellular volume by blood pressure/pulse with postural changes, JVP evaluation, capillary refill, skin turgour (recognizing that this is a crude test and useless in adults)
  - Hydration status is essential especially in infants, children and the elderly, all of whom can potentially die from diarrhea by dehydration
  - Is patient in distress? (toxic?)
  - *GI*: peritonitis (guarding), masses, tenderness, sigmoidoscopy or proctoscopy with appropriate swabs and cultures if rectal urgency not yet diagnosed and/or question of anorectal problems associated with anal intercourse
  - *MSK*: myalgias and arthritis

Acute Pancreatitis

- Upper abdominal pain, usually with fever, vomiting
- Characterized by elevated serum lipase or amylase, often with increase in liver enzymes/serum glucose, dilated loop of bowel visualized radiologically

- First step: rule out syndromes other than pancreatitis, such as bowel perforation, infarction, obstruction, since pancreatitis itself not amenable to specific therapy
- Ultrasound searching for gallstones, dilated bile duct suggesting obstructing stone as a cause of the pancreatitis, followed by ERCP if gallstone pancreatitis suspected
- CT with contrast (exercise caution if serum creatinine elevated) rules out complications such as pseudocyst, determines severity by estimating proportion of pancreatic gland involved in inflammation (inflamed gland does not take up the contrast)

Alcoholic Liver Disease
- *Spectrum*: fatty liver, alcoholic hepatitis, and cirrhosis
- *Fatty liver*: characteristically asymptomatic, but hepatomegaly may be present
- *Alcoholic hepatitis*: variable symptoms and signs but characteristically presents as dull RUQ discomfort, anorexia, jaundice, fever, etc.
- *Cirrhosis*: irreversible stage of chronic liver disease
- Signs and symptoms (by etiology)
  - Hyperestrogenism: palmar erythema, gynecomastia, spider nevi, altered hair distribution (frontal balding), pectoral alopecia and testicular atrophy
  - Portal hypertension (increasing back pressure on various organs): splenomegaly (sometimes with petechiae secondary to splenomegaly-associated thrombocytopenia), encephalopathy, ankle edema, esophageal variceal bleeding, caput medusae, hemorrhoids and ascites
  - Liver insufficiency (i.e. decreased nitrogenous waste removal, decreased albumin production, decreased bilirubin processing, decreased clotting factor production) leading to encephalopathy, edema, jaundice, ecchymoses, respectively
  - Systemic/non-specific: anorexia, clubbing, fatigue, fever

Appendicitis
- Fever, typically low grade, unless there is a perforation
- Worsening of symptoms is the most reliable feature
- Typical presentation includes vague dull constant periumbilical pain initially which then gradually localizes to McBurney's Point
- Positive Rovsing's sign
- May also have a positive psoas sign or a positive obturator sign (depending on location of appendix)
- Peritonitis if there is a perforation
- Ultrasound and CT scan now considered to have high positive and negative predictive values

Celiac Disease
- Most common presentation is mimicker of Irritable Bowel Syndrome
- Anemia and osteopenia are key presentations
- Diagnostic testing with tissue transglutaminase (tTG) antibodies reported to have positive and negative predictive values
- Prevalence varies according to geographic location (more prevalent in Europe and North America with a Caucasian predilection)
- IgA levels must be checked to exclude a false negative tTG related to selective IgA deficiency. 1-2% of people with Celiac Disease have selective IgA deficiency

Cirrhosis and its Complications (ascites, encephalopathy, variceal bleeding and spontaneous bacterial peritonitis)

1. Ascites

- Suspect free fluid in the peritoneal cavity when there has been an increase in abdominal girth
- Causes can be grouped as hepatic and non-hepatic
  - Hepatic causes (portal hypertension):
    - Cirrhosis (most common)
  - Non-hepatic causes:
    - Fluid retention due to congestive heart failure
    - Cancer – second most common cause of ascites after portal hypertension
    - Constrictive pericarditis, tricuspid regurgitation
- Ascites can be detected clinically by
  - Detection of shifting dullness on abdominal percussion (most reliable physical examination maneuver)
  - Elicitation of a fluid wave (with larger collections of fluid)
  - Examination for bulging or fullness of the flanks and elicitation of a fluid thrill
  - Abdominal ultrasound/CT (gold standard; recommended in all cases but especially for detection of smaller fluid volumes)

Evidence-Based Medicine: Ascites

		Sens (%)	Spec (%)	LR+	LR-
History	Increased abdo. girth	87	77	4.16	
	Hepatitis	27	92		
	Ankle swelling	93	66		
Physical	Bulging flanks	81	59	2.0	0.3
	Flank dullness	84	59	2.0	0.3
	Shifting dullness	77	72	2.7	0.3
	Fluid wave	62	90	6.0	0.4

- Useful in ruling out ascites:
  - history negative for ankle swelling and negative for increased abdominal girth
  - physical exam negative for bulging flanks, flank dullness, or shifting dullness
- Useful for ruling in ascites:
  - presence of a fluid wave, shifting dullness, or peripheral edema

Williams Jr. JW, Simel DL. 1992. *JAMA* 267(19):2645-2648.

2. Encephalopathy

- Increased amount of toxins (particularly ammonia) in blood due to shunting around hepatocytes
- 4 Stages
  - I: reversal of sleep rhythm (earliest sign)
  - II: asterixis, lethargy ± disorientation
  - III: stupor (rousable only by pain), hyperreflexic
  - IV: coma
- Can be precipitated by an increase in nitrogen load, medications, electrolyte disturbance, infection or a worsening of hepatic function (any change in steady state)

ABDOMINAL

3. *Variceal Bleeding*
- Due to portal hypertension
- Often worsened by hypocoagulability (as all clotting factors except for VIII are exclusively made in the liver)
- See GI bleed below

4. *Spontaneous Bacterial Peritonitis*
- Consider in a patient with increasing abdominal discomfort and ascites, even if afebrile, WBC normal
- Diagnosis made by diagnostic paracentesis (look for neutrophils in ascetic fluid)

Note: liver transplantation is only definitive therapy for end-stage liver disease. Candidates should be referred for assessment at signs of early decompensation since wait times are long and mortality rates for advanced disease with late features are high.

Colorectal Cancer
- Primarily a disease of middle aged, older adults: 99% >40 years old and 85% >60
- Primary symptoms
  - Rectal bleeding persistently without anal symptoms
  - Change in bowel habit persistently over six weeks – most commonly increased frequency or looser stools (or both)
  - Abdominal pain characteristically with weight loss
- Secondary effects
  - Iron deficiency anemia
  - Intestinal obstruction
  - Clinical examination may show an abdominal mass or rectal mass
- In work up, use flexible colonoscopy or CT colonography

Gallstones
- Ultrasound best test to visualize gallstones
- Gallstones are often an incidental finding on an ultrasound done to investigate non-biliary symptoms such as dyspepsia
- Cause biliary colic, cholecystitis, cholangitis, pancreatitis, gallstone ileus – but do not cause dyspepsia
- Biliary colic: a "set piece" – pain starts suddenly, most often late afternoon/evening, RUQ or epigastrium, radiates to back, associated with vomiting, lasts ~3 to 6 hours
- If unsure whether gallstones seen on ultrasound are the cause of the pain, perform biliary HIDA scan – presence of nucleotide in gallbladder on this scan indicates that the cystic duct is patent, virtually ruling out biliary colic/cholecystitis. Cholecystitis = upper abdominal pain, usually but not always associated with vomiting and fever, liver enzymes only slightly elevated, ultrasound shows stones in the gallbladder and also a thickened gallbladder wall, fluid around gallbladder
- Cholangitis = fever, upper abdominal pain, jaundice, requires urgent ERCP and sphincterotomy

GI Bleeding

- 3 factors determine stool colour: bleed location, bleed rate, stool/blood transit time
- In an upper GI bleed, the presentation can be a clue to the severity of the bleeding: hematochezia indicates fastest bleeding, melena the slowest bleeding; hence, upper GI source can cause hematochezia if bleeding massive, transit time rapid
- Resuscitation is key to management
- Octreotide infusion – variceal, non-variceal upper GI bleeds
- Proton pump inhibitor infusion for bleeding ulcers
- Urgent gastroscopy for significant upper GI bleeds
- If lower GI bleed: do sigmoidoscopy without preparation to rule out mucosal disease/anal source. However, colonoscopy without preparing the colon by lavage is likely to reveal nothing but blood, hence colonic lavage before colonoscopy
- If lower GI bleed does not stop spontaneously, consider angiography

Inflammatory Bowel Disease

- Chronic, relapsing inflammatory disorders of unknown etiology
- Rectal exam and visualization of the bowel (barium studies and/or sigmoid/colonoscopy) are indicated
- Stool culture and microscopy required to rule out enteric infection
- Divided into 2 primary diseases (Crohn's and Ulcerative Colitis)
  - *Crohn's (granulomatous) Disease*
    - Affects any portion of GI tract, but most often in small intestine and colon
    - Transmural inflammation
    - Symptoms: fever, malaise, abdominal pain, diarrhea, vomiting
    - Signs: fever/temperature increase, weight loss, nutritional problems, anemia, lower-right abdominal mass and/or tenderness, extraintestinal manifestations (eye, MSK, hepatobiliary, skin)
  - *Ulcerative (nongranulomatous) Colitis*
    - Limited to colon (mucosal inflammation)
    - Rectum always involved and disease progresses proximally
    - Symptoms: bloody diarrhea, lower abdominal cramps, urgency
    - Signs: anemia, low serum albumin, negative stool cultures

Irritable Bowel Syndrome (IBS)

- 15% of U.S. adults report symptoms that are consistent with IBS
  - 3:1 female to male (in countries such as India the ratio is reversed)
- IBS is the most common diagnosis made by gastroenterologists in the U.S.
- IBS is defined as the presence:
  - For at least 12 weeks (not necessarily consecutive) in the preceding 12 months of abdominal discomfort or pain that cannot be explained by structural or biochemical abnormalities
  - Of at least two of the following three features:
    - Pain is relieved with defecation
    - Onset associated with a change in the frequency of bowel movements (diarrhea or constipation)
    - Onset associated with change in form of stool (loose, watery, or pellet-like often with bloating, mucus in stool)

- Diagnosis
  - After complete history and physical exam, the following tests should be ordered: CBC, blood chemistry, liver function, thyrotropin, albumin, amylase, flexible sigmoidoscopy, stool microscopy and culture if diarrhea; ESR is of limited use

Peptic Ulcer Disease (PUD)

- Burning, epigastric pain
- Onset: 1-3 hrs after meal
- $^1/_3$ of patients awakened at night by pain
- Pain relieved by food or antacid
- Intermittent and may return in several months
- May present with complications: bleeding, perforation
- *H. pylori* and ASA/NSAID use are the major risk factors
- Cannot distinguish by history from functional dyspepsia

Primary Biliary Cirrhosis

- Predominantly middle-aged women (mean age at diagnosis 51 years). Up to 10% are male and 10% are <35. Males and females follow similar clinical course, characterized by elevated serum alkaline phosphatase, positive anti-mitochondrial antibody

Table 7. Symptoms and Frequency of Occurrence in Primary Biliary Cirrhosis

Symptom	Frequency of Occurrence
Pruritus (severe itching)	47%; usually first symptom
Non-specific symptoms – fatigue, right upper quadrant pain and dyspepsia	22%
Typical late features (though may appear earlier) – jaundice, GI bleeding or ascites	19%

REFERENCES

Bickley LS, Szilagyi PG, Bates B. 2007. *Bates' Guide to Physical Examination and History Taking*. Philadelphia: Lippincott Williams & Wilkins.

Canadian Hypertension Education Program. 2008. *The 2008 Canadian Hypertension Education Program recommendations: the scientific summary – an annual update*. *Can J Cardiol* 24(6):447-452.

Feighery C. 1999. Fortnightly review: coeliac disease. *BMJ* 319(7204):236-239.

Grover SA, Barkun AN, Sackett DL. 1993. The rational clinical examination. Does this patient have splenomegaly? *JAMA* 270(18):2218-2221.

Hobbs FD. 2000. ABC of colorectal cancer: the role of primary care. *BMJ* 321(7268):1068-1070.

Horwitz BJ, Fisher RS. 2001. The irritable bowel syndrome. *N Engl J Med* 344(24):1846-1850.

Moayyedi P, Talley NJ, Fennerty MB, Vakil N. 2006. Can the clinical history distinguish between organic and functional dyspepsia? *JAMA* 295(13):1566-1576.

Naylor CD. 1994. The rational clinical examination. Physical examination of the liver. *JAMA* 271(23):1859-1865.

O'Donohue J, Williams R. 1996. Primary biliary cirrhosis. *QJM* 89(1):5-13.

Trowbridge RL, Rutkowski NK, Shojania KG. 2003. Does this patient have acute cholecystitis? *JAMA* 289(1):80-86.

Wagner JM, McKinney WP, Carpenter JL. 1996. Does this patient have appendicitis? *JAMA* 276(19):1589-1594.

Williams JW, Jr., Simel DL. 1992. The rational clinical examination. Does this patient have ascites? How to divine fluid in the abdomen. *JAMA* 267(19):2645-2648.

The Breast Exam

Editors:
Katie Connolly &
Caroline Scott

Faculty Reviewers:
Robert A. Mustard, MD, FRCS(C)
Sandra Messner, MD, FCFP

TABLE OF CONTENTS

Essential Anatomy   49
Approach to the Breast History and Physical Exam   49
Common Chief Complaints   50
Common Disorders   50
Focused History   50
Focused Physical Exam   51
Common Investigations   54
Common Clinical Scenarios   55

BREAST

ESSENTIAL ANATOMY

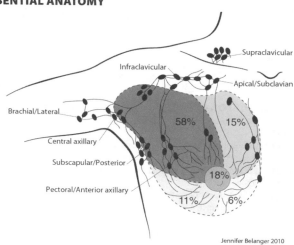

Jennifer Belanger 2010

Figure 1. Lymph Nodes of the Breast and Frequency of Disease by Quadrant

APPROACH TO THE BREAST HISTORY AND PHYSICAL EXAM

In addition to general history taking, important aspects of the breast history include:

- History of the chief complaint (breast pain/tenderness, breast mass, nipple changes/discharge, skin changes)
- Past breast history (surgeries, breast diseases, etc.)
- Assessment of risk factors (age, family history, obstetrical history, gynecological history)

Overview of the physical exam

- Exam should be done in the upright and supine positions
- Inspection of the breasts (size, symmetry, shape, skin changes, secretion)
- Palpation of the breasts (radial vector method, vertical strip method)
- Palpation of regional lymph nodes (axillary, supraclavicular, infraclavicular)

COMMON CHIEF COMPLANTS

- Breast pain/tenderness
- Breast mass
- Nipple changes (retraction, ulceration, scaling)
- Nipple discharge (spontaneous, upon compression)
- Change in skin of breast
- Change in size of breast

COMMON DISORDERS

Disorders marked with (✓) are discussed in **Common Clinical Scenarios**

✓ Fibroadenoma (benign; accounts for 75% of solitary breast lumps in women)
✓ Fibrocystic condition (benign; occurs to some extent in 50% of women)
✓ Mastitis (common during breast feeding)
- Breast carcinoma
- Fat necrosis
- Intraductal papilloma
- Gynecomastia (breast enlargement in males)
- Mastalgia

FOCUSED HISTORY

CC and HPI

- Breast pain (mastalgia): onset, bilateral or unilateral, intermittent or constant, changes with menstrual cycle, recent trauma
- Breast mass: onset, location, changes with menstrual cycle, recent trauma
- Nipple changes:
  - Changes since first noticed
  - Changes with menstrual cycle
  - Recent injury or trauma to breast
  - Nipple retraction – often exaggerated on arm elevation
  - Ulceration/scaling – may be Paget's disease
  - Bilateral or unilateral (bilateral discharge indicates physiological cause, e.g. fibrocystic condition)
  - Colour, consistency, spontaneity of discharge (cancer may be associated with spontaneous bloody or watery discharge, galactorrhea has hormonal/pharmacologic causes)
  - Skin changes (erythema, dimpling suggests tumour, ulceration/scaling may be Paget's disease)

Risk Factor Assessment (Past Medical History, Family History

- Major risk factors for breast cancer
  - Age (>50)
  - Female
  - Personal history of breast cancer, ovarian cancer

- Maternal or paternal family history of breast and/or ovarian cancer in 1st or 2nd degree relatives, especially if early onset (<50 years old)
  - Genetics – mutations in the tumour suppressor genes BRCA-1, BRCA-2
  - History of atypical hyperplasia or lobular carcinoma in situ (LCIS)
  - History of high dose radiation (e.g. mantle radiation for Hodgkin's)
- Minor risk factors for breast cancer
  - Nulliparity
  - Menarche <12 years old
  - Menopause >55 years old
  - Hormone replacement therapy
  - Obesity
  - Excessive alcohol intake
  - Previous history of breast biopsy regardless of findings
- 75% of women diagnosed with breast cancer do not have identifiable risk factors
- Negative mammogram does not rule out breast cancer

FOCUSED PHYSICAL

- Purpose: Identify features that distinguish malignant vs. benign lumps (refer to **Table 1**)
- The patient must be draped appropriately
- Male doctors should have a female witness in the room when possible
- Always examine both breasts, even if complaints are localized to one side
- Clinical breast examination (CBE) can detect up to 50% of cancers not detected by mammography alone

---

Evidence-Based Medicine: Breast Cancer

6 human studies were considered strong enough to pool results relating to the sensitivity and specificity of CBE in detecting breast cancer. The gold standard used (although acknowledged to be inadequate) was clinical follow-up. The women in these studies ranged from 35 to 74 years of age.

Sensitivity = 0.54 (0.48 – 0.60)   LR+ = 10.6 (5.8 to 19.2)
Specificity = 0.94 (0.90 – 0.97)   LR- = (0.47 (0.40 to 0.56)

Spending adequate time on the CBE (3 minutes per breast), and using proper technique improves breast lump detection.

Barton MB, Harris R, Fletcher SW. 1999. *JAMA* 282(13):1270-1280.

- Cancer cannot be ruled out on the basis of clinical exam alone; other diagnostic tests must be performed (see **Common Investigations**, p. 55)
- Increase in breast size, density, nodularity, and tenderness occur 3-5 days prior to menses – the most appropriate time for a breast exam is 7-10 days post menses
- Breasts normally involute and are less dense following menopause
- Document breast, quadrant, and distance from nipple of any mass noted on exam
- Document qualities of mass: size, shape, consistency, delineation of borders, tenderness, mobility, and menstrual changes (refer to **Table 1**)

Inspection

- Inspect both breasts with the patient in each of the following positions:
  - Patient sitting with hands resting on thighs
  - Patient sitting with arms raised above head
  - Patient sitting with hands pressing against hips
  - Patient sitting and leaning forward
- Inspection of the breast: 4 S's
  - *Size* of each breast
  - *Symmetry* of two breasts (some variability is normal)
  - *Shape* and contour: bulges, flattening, skin dimpling, retraction
  - *Skin changes*:
    - Inflammation
    - Erythema
    - Peau d'orange (edema in skin – indicative of advanced cancer)
    - Abnormal vascularity (increased visibility of blood vessels)
    - Thickening
- Inspection of nipple: 6 S's
  - *Size*
  - *Symmetry*
    - Ask patient to raise arms – one nipple may deviate due to a small cancer in breast (caused by tethering)
  - *Shape*
    - Inversion (sunken inward) or eversion
    - Direction
  - *Skin changes*: eczema or ulceration/scaling
  - *Spontaneous secretion*: serous, bloody, or coloured discharge
  - *Supernumerary nipples*:
    - Most commonly in axilla or below breasts, along milk line
    - Developmental variant – no prognostic significance

- In males:
  - Inspect the nipple and areola for swelling, ulceration or nodules
  - Inspect the axilla for rashes, infection, abnormal pigmentation (may suggest internal malignancy)

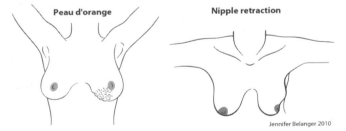

Jennifer Belanger 2010

Figure 2. Positions for Breast Inspection

Palpation

Axillae and Supraclavicular Area

- Three key groups of lymph nodes: axillary, supraclavicular, and infraclavicular (see **Figure 1**)
  - Check for size, location, consistency, and mobility
  - Palpate above and below clavicle with patient's arms resting on thighs

- Partially abduct patient's arm and support it on your arm to assess axilla
- Palpate deeply into axilla, along posterior surface of pectoralis muscles, and up along inferior surface of upper arm

Palpation of Breasts
- Performed with patient in sitting position, and again with patient in supine position
    - In supine position, breast tissue stretches more evenly across chest wall for easier deep palpation
- If breasts are large, or for more effective deep palpation, also palpate with patient in oblique position (supine, arm raised on side of breast being examined, hips turned away from examiner; cushions may assist positioning in less mobile patients)
    - Always palpate both breasts
    - If patient has complaint involving one breast, begin with opposite breast
- Use fleshy pads of three middle fingertips
    - Systematically cover entire breast area: from 2nd to 6th rib, sternum to midaxillary line
    - At each new point of contact, use light then increasingly stronger pressure
- Two possible patterns of palpation (see **Figure 3**):
    - Radial vector pattern
        - Palpation at each location in small circular motion
        - Begin at "12 o'clock" position at outer edge of breast and move inwards along all "spokes of wheel" with nipple as central point; end with palpation of areolar area and nipple
        - Continue with next vector, partially overlapping with previous one, and work inwards to nipple
    - Vertical strip pattern
        - Palpate each location with small circular motions
        - Mentally divide breast area into a series of vertical regions, and palpate each one thoroughly from top to bottom
        - Begin at axilla and palpate downward along midaxillary line to 6th rib
        - For next strip, work upward from 6th rib to top of breast and partially overlap with first strip
        - Continue in this antiparallel fashion until the entire breast is examined

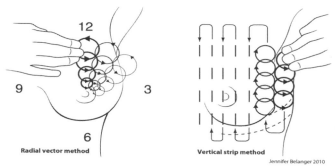

Radial vector method

Vertical strip method

Jennifer Belanger 2010

Figure 3. Common Approaches to Breast Palpation

- Distinguish between abnormal mass and normal compressed tissue ridge (inframammary fold) which may be found along lower border of breast, particularly with large breasts

- If a mass is detected:
    - Determine distance from nipple
    - Gently elevate breast near the mass and watch for dimpling (suggests an underlying cancer)
- Nipple distortion may be a sign of underlying cancer
- In males:
    - Distinguish between obesity (soft fatty tissue enlargement)

Table 1. Interpretation of Findings

	Carcinoma	Fibroadenoma	Fibrocystic Condition
Location of mass	Unilateral and solitary	Unilateral and solitary (85%)	Multiple and bilateral
Size	Variable	1-3 cm (may be larger)	Variable
Shape	Irregular	Round	Round
Consistency	Firm or hard	Firm and rubbery	Nodular (may be firm)
Delineation	Ill-defined	Discrete	Region of nodular thickening
Tenderness	Non-tender	Non-tender	Tender
Mobility	May be tethered	Mobile	Mobile
Menstrual Changes	No	May change in size with menstrual cycle	Increased tenderness pre-menstrually
Age Group	80% >40 years	Usually <30 years	30-50 years
Investigations	Mammography, ultrasound for palpable findings or to further evaluate mammography findings, core needle biopsy for definitive diagnosis	Ultrasound, mammography if > age 30, core biopsy if indicated by imaging findings	Mammogram if > age 30, ultrasound for discrete masses, aspirate dominant or symptomatic cysts

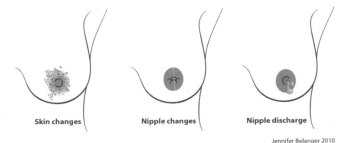

Jennifer Belanger 2010

Figure 4. Visible Signs of Breast Disease

BREAST

COMMON INVESTIGATIONS
- Refer to **Flowchart** on p. 57

Mammography
- Indications:
  - Diagnosis and screening
  - Evaluation of new or worrisome palpable mass in any woman > age 30
  - May start any time after age 30 if sufficiently increased risk (e.g., BRCA positive)
  - Optional between 40-50 years old – harms/benefits should be discussed
  - All women over 50 every 2 years
  - Best modality for picking up ductal carcinoma in situ (DCIS, earliest stage of breast cancer), often before a mass is palpable (presents with microcalcifications)
- Non-palpable malignancies <1 cm in size may be detected
  - 1/3 of all malignancies detected by mammography are non-palpable

Ultrasound
- In general, for diagnosis rather than screening
- Indications:
  - Evaluate palpable masses or mammographic abnormalities
  - Determine distance of lesion from nipple
  - Differentiate cystic masses from solid masses
  - Frequently diagnostic for fibroadenomas
    - Highly operator-dependent, requires special breast expertise
    - False positives common and can generate significant anxiety

Fine Needle Aspiration Biopsy (FNAB)
- Smears prepared from aspirate for cytologic evaluation
- If aspirated fluid is non-bloody and mass completely disappears following aspiration, diagnosis is simple cyst and cytology is not required
- If aspirated fluid is bloody or only cells present, send for cytology
- A negative FNAB does NOT rule out cancer

Core Needle Biopsy
- If available, core biopsy is the preferred method for tissue diagnosis
- Provides better sample and pathology (tissue architecture, staining, hormone receptor status) compared with cytology
- Provides information for planning procedures
- Core biopsy results MUST be concordant with imaging findings (radiologist should dictate addendum after reviewing path results)

Excisional Biopsy
- When core biopsy is not concordant or clinical suspicion high even if core biopsy is negative
- When core biopsy is not possible or available

COMMON CLINICAL SCENARIOS

Fibroadenoma (most common benign solid breast mass)

History
- Single non-tender lump, 15% are multiple, especially on U/S
- Lump more noticeable in the 2nd half of menstrual cycle
- Usually develop in young women (<30 years old)

- About 1/3 get smaller, 1/3 stay the same, 1/3 grow
- May regress with menopause

Physical
- Palpable breast lump 1-2 cm in size
- Well-defined, non-tender, round or lobulated with firm or rubbery consistency
- No tethering to underlying tissue, very mobile

Investigations
- Mammography, U/S ± core needle biopsy for tissue diagnosis

Management
- Consider excision of fibroadenomas more than 3 cm or if enlarging

Fibrocystic Condition

History
- Bilaterally tender breasts, exaggerated premenstrually
- Nodular breasts or solitary mass of recent onset
- Cysts may increase in size rapidly, may decrease or disappear
- Bilateral, non-spontaneous nipple discharge, colour can be murky or greenish-black
- Affected females often 30-50 years old
- Estrogen therapy may cause cyst development in menopausal women

Physical
- Breast mass which is firm, smooth, tender, mobile and well-defined

Investigations
- Mammography, ± ultrasound and fine needle aspiration (FNA) ± cytological studies
- Ultrasound (U/S) is the best way to differentiate cystic from solid masses
- Simple cysts do not need any treatment or special follow-up
- Complicated cysts followed with repeat U/S at 6 months
- Complex cysts require FNA and tissue diagnosis
- Aspirate dominant or bothersome cysts

Mastitis/Superficial Cellulitis of the Breast

History
- Occurs around the time of childbirth, in nursing mothers, or after injury
- Fever, malaise

Physical
- Unilateral erythema, swelling, tenderness, and warmth

Investigations
- *S. aureus* almost always the etiologic agent
- In non-lactating women, need imaging to rule out cancer

Management
- Drain and incise abscess if present
- Antibiotics
- Continue breast feeding

Clinical Presentation of Breast Disease

Symptomatic (50%)
- Palpable lump
- Skin change
- Nipple discharge

Screen Detected (Mammography) (50%)
- Mass
  - 1/3 detected not palpable
- Calcification
  - Ductal carcinoma in situ – earliest stage of breast cancer, "microcalcifications"
- Density
- Asymmetry
- Architectural distortion

Who is Screened
- All women >50, every 2 yr
- Women >30 with risks
- Harms/Benefits should be discussed

Further Investigation of Breast Disease
1. Mammography in women >30 years with palpable breast mass
2. Ultrasound
   - Evaluate borders of mass
   - Determine cystic or fibrous character of mass
   - Diagnostic of fibroadenoma (but high false positive and generates significant anxiety)

Diagnostic Modalities
1. Fine needle aspiration (FNA)*
   - Cytology for a palpable mass
2. Core needle biopsy*
   - Pathology for a non palpable mass detected by screening
   - Radiologically assisted
   - Distinguishes between non-invasive and invasive disease

*Important to know laboratory results before surgery to plan treatment

Notes on FNA
- If fluid non-bloody and mass disappears after aspiration → cyst, no cytology needed
- If fluid is bloody → cytology
- No fluid, cells → cytology
- Negative FNA does not rule out cancer

Assessment of Extent of Disease Imaged by MRI

Develop Treatment Plan for Suspected Cancer
1. Surgery
   - Treat local and region disease
   - Staging
2. Radiotherapy
   - Minimize local and regional recurrence
   - Breast, chest wall
3. Systemic Therapy
   - Minimize distant recurrence
   - Chemo, endocrine, others

Clinical Pearls
- Breast radiation always after lumpectomy
- Large extent of disease indicative for mastectomy
- Sentinel lymph node biopsy is 98% accurate and reduces post-surgical mobidity (e.g. lymphedema)

REFERENCES

Barton MB, Harris R, Fletcher SW. 1999. The rational clinical examination. Does this patient have breast cancer? The screening clinical breast examination: should it be done? How? *JAMA* 282(13): 1270-1280.

Bickley LS, Szilagyi PG, Bates B. 2007. *Bates' Guide to Physical Examination and History Taking*. Philadelphia: Lippincott Williams & Wilkins.

Bilimoria MM, Morrow M. 1995. The woman at increased risk for breast cancer: evaluation and management strategies. *CA Cancer J Clin* 45(5):263-278.

Pruthi S. 2001. Detection and evaluation of a palpable breast mass. *Mayo Clin Proc* 76(6):641-647; quiz 647-648.

BREAST

The Cardiovascular Exam

Editors:
Ravi Bajaj, Michael Jurkiewicz &
Marat Slessarev

Faculty Reviewer:
Andrew Yan, MD

TABLE OF CONTENTS

Essential Anatomy 59
Approach to the Cardiovascular History 60
Common Chief Complaints 60
Focused History 60
Focused Physical Exam 62
Common Investigations 67
Common Clinical Scenarios 67
Review of Anatomy and Physiology 70
ECG Interpretation 71
Approach to the ECG 72

ESSENTIAL ANATOMY

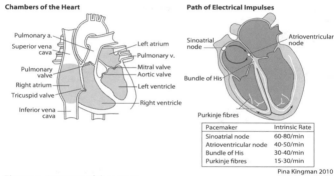

Figure 1. Anatomy of the Heart

Pacemaker	Intrinsic Rate
Sinoatrial node	60-80/min
Atrioventricular node	40-50/min
Bundle of His	30-40/min
Purkinje fibres	15-30/min

Pina Kingman 2010

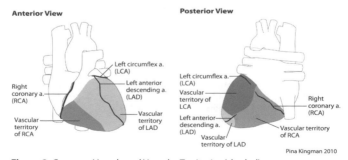

Figure 2. Coronary Vessels and Vascular Territories (shaded)

Pina Kingman 2010

APPROACH TO THE CARDIOVASCULAR HISTORY

In addition to general history-taking, important aspects of the cardiovascular history are outlined below:

- Chest pain (OPQRST)
- Dyspnea, orthopnea, paroxysmal nocturnal dyspnea (PND)
- Past cardiac history (e.g. rheumatic fever), respiratory history
- Chronic medical conditions, Hx of GERD, Hx of stroke/TIA
- Cardiac investigations (e.g. angiography, stress test)
- Previous admissions to hospital, ER
- Risk factors for cardiovascular disease
- Medications: prescribed vs. OTC, antiplatelets, antithrombin therapies, β-blockers, ACE inhibitors, ARBs, CCBs, diuretics, antiarrhythmics, lipid-modifying agents
- Social history: occupation (sedentary), stress (physical vs. emotional), access to family doctor, psychiatric history (depression, anxiety)

COMMON CHIEF COMPLAINTS

- Chest pain (angina)
- Shortness of breath (dyspnea)
    - At rest, on exertion, when supine (orthopnea), upon waking up at night (PND)
- Heart pounding (palpitations)
- Swelling (edema), especially in lower extremities
- Fainting/Light-headedness (syncope/presyncope)
- Fatigue, exercise intolerance
- Coughing up blood (hemoptysis)
- Blue lips/fingers/toes (cyanosis)

FOCUSED HISTORY

Chest Pain

- Onset/duration: sudden vs. gradual, hours vs. days, previous similar symptoms, frequency, progression, course (constant vs. intermittent), pleuritic, after meals (post-prandial)
- Precipitating and relieving factors: better or worse with exercise/rest/sleep/position
- Quality: crushing, pressing, squeezing, burning, stabbing, tightening
- Location: epigastric, peri-umbilical, flank, back
- Radiation: to neck, jaw, axilla, back, arm; usually left-sided but can be right-sided
- Associated symptoms: fatigue, palpitations, diaphoresis, peripheral edema, N/V, dyspnea
- Stable vs. unstable angina:
    - **Stable angina** is intermittent chest pain during exertion or emotional stress, relieved by rest
    - **Unstable angina** is considered one of:
        1. New onset (<2 months) that is severe (CCS III or IV) and/or frequent
        2. Progression of symptoms
        3. At rest or nocturnal
        4. Post-MI
    - Note: always assess functional class of angina (see **Table 1** and **Table 2**)
- See *Essentials of Emergency Medicine* p. 410 for differential diagnosis of chest pain

CARDIOVASCULAR

Table 1. Canadian Cardiovascular Society (CCS) Functional Classification of Angina

Class	Activity Evoking Angina	Limits to Physical Activity
I	Prolonged exertion	None
II	Walking >2 blocks or >1 flight of stairs	Slight
III	Walking <2 blocks or <1 flight of stairs	Marked
IV	Minimal activity or at rest	Severe

Table 2. New York Heart Association (NYHA) Functional Classification of Congestive Heart Failure

Class	Activity Evoking Angina	Limits to Physical Activity
I	None	None
II	Ordinary physical activity	Slight
III	Walking <2 blocks or <1 flight of stairs	Marked
IV	Minimal or at rest	Severe

Cardiac Risk Factors

- Major risk factors:
  - Family history (MI <55 in male relatives, <65 in female relatives)
  - Hypertension (BP >140/90 mmHg or taking antihypertensive medications)
  - Hypercholesterolemia
  - Diabetes mellitus
  - Smoking
- Minor risk factors:
  - Age (male ≥45, female ≥55)
  - Male
  - Post-menopausal
  - Obesity
  - Sedentary lifestyle
  - Stress
  - Alcoholism
  - Depression
  - Hyperhomocysteinemia

Dyspnea

- See *Respiratory Exam* p. 338

Peripheral Vascular Disease

- Peripheral edema
- See *Peripheral Vascular Exam*

FOCUSED PHYSICAL EXAM

General
- Patient's level comfort/distress
- Skin colour (pale vs. pink)
- Cyanosis: central (blue mucous membranes) vs. peripheral (blue fingers/toes)
- Respiratory distress (tachypnea, accessory muscle use, intercostal indrawing, position)
- Presence of edema in lower limbs
- Extra-cardiac features: xanthomata, rash, petechiae, nail splinter hemorrhages

Vitals
- HR – rate, rhythm (regular vs. regularly irregular vs. irregularly irregular), amplitude (strong vs. soft)
- BP – both arms
- RR, O_2 saturation
- Temperature
- Orthostatic vitals (HR, BP)

Jugular Venous Pressure (JVP)
- Direct assessment of the pressure in the right atrium (i.e. central venous pressure)
- Assessment includes four parameters: height, waveform, Kussmaul's sign, hepatojugular reflux
- Differentiate internal jugular pulse from carotid pulse (**Table 3**)

Table 3. Characteristics of Internal Jugular vs. Carotid Pulse

Feature	Internal Jugular Pulse	Carotid Pulse
Palpable	No	Yes
Number of waveforms	Multiple	Single
Finger pressure above clavicle	Disappears	Persists
Inspiration/Elevation of bed	↓	No change
Hepatojugular reflux/Lowering of bed	↑	No change

JVP Height (see **Figure 3**)
- Position the patient at 30° elevation and turn the patient's head slightly to the left, then adjust the angle of elevation until jugular pulsations are observed
- Look between the two heads of the sternocleidomastoid for pulsations. If difficult to observe, shine a light tangentially across the right side of the patient's neck and look for shadows of pulsations
    - The JVP is more of an inward, multiple waveform movement and will cast a shadow with tangential light
- Determine JVP by measuring the *vertical* distance from the sternal angle to a horizontal line drawn from the top of the jugular pulsation
- **Normal JVP: ≤4 cm**

- Elevated JVP suggests increased pressure in the right atrium due to:
  - Obstruction of SVC
  - Right heart failure (may be secondary to left heart failure)
  - Constrictive pericarditis

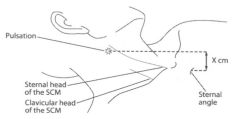

Pina Kingman 2010

Figure 3. Measuring JVP Height

Kussmaul's Sign
- Rising of JVP with inspiration (paradoxical) suggests that the blood flow into the right heart is impaired. This could result from:
  - Constrictive pericarditis
  - Right heart failure
  - SVC obstruction
  - Tricuspid stenosis
  - Restrictive cardiomyopathy

Hepatojugular/Abdominal Reflux
- To assess high JVP and RV function:
  - Position the patient so that the top of the JVP is visible with his/her mouth open and while he/she is breathing normally (prevents Valsalva maneuver)
  - Place the right hand over the liver in the right upper quadrant or anywhere in the abdomen
  - Apply moderate pressure (25-30 mmHg) and maintain compression for 10 seconds
  - The JVP may rise or remain unchanged; a sustained elevation of the JVP height (>4 cm) after 10 seconds is pathological

Waveforms
- The JVP is a multiple waveform entity. An understanding of each of the wave components is essential to conceptualizing how certain diseases are reflected by changes in the JVP:
  - a-wave: atrial contraction
  - x-descent: atrial relaxtion following contraction
  - c-wave: closing of the tricuspid valve increases atrial pressure during relaxation
  - v-wave: increasing atrial pressure with venous return
  - y-descent: opening of the tricuspid valve decreases atrial pressure

Precordial Exam

- Divide the precordium into 4 zones where sounds from the heart valves are best auscultated (**Figure 4**)

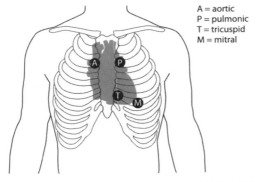

A = aortic
P = pulmonic
T = tricuspid
M = mitral

Pina Kingman 2010

Figure 4. Anatomical Positions of the Heart Sounds

Inspection
- Chest shape: normal vs. excavatum (hollow) vs. carinatum (pigeon-like)
- Apex beat (5th intercostal space, mid-clavicular line)
- Abnormal motions (heaves, lifts)
- Scars

Palpation
- Palpate over the 4 valve zones and along the sternum
- Palpate for **heaves** (sustained outward motion), **thrills** (vibration over area of turbulent blood flow) and **impulses** (systolic vs. diastolic)
- Palpate over the apex beat and describe it in terms of LADS (location, amplitude, duration, size)

Table 4. Palpable Findings in Precordial Exam

Valve Zone	Abnormal Findings	Possible Pathology
A	Systolic impulse	Systemic HTN Dilated aortic aneurysm
P	Systolic impulse	Pulmonary HTN
T	Heave, thrill	RV enlargement (2° to pulmonary HTN or left-sided heart disease)
M	Heave, thrill	LV enlargement

Auscultation
- Auscultate over the 4 valve zones for heart sounds and murmurs
- Focus on identifying S1 and S2 first, then listen between (systole) and after (diastole)

Table 5. Heart Sounds

Timing	Valve Zone	Sound	Significance	Pathology
Systolic	A, P	Ejection sound		Congenital AS/PS Bicuspid AV Aortic root or PA dilatation Physiologic
	T, M	**S1**	Normal closure of MV and TV	**Loud S1**: ↑ HR ↑ LAP (early MS), ↓ PR interval **Soft S1**: calcified MV (late MS), CHF, 1° heart block **Variable S1**: AF, conduction heart block **Split S1**: RBBB/LBBB
		Non-ejection click		MV/TV prolapse
Diastolic	A, P	**S2**	Normal closure of AV and PV	**Loud S2**: Systemic/Pulmonary HTN, Ao. Root or PA dilatation **Soft S2**: AS or PS **Split S2**: Wide: RBBB, PS, Pulmonary HTN, MR Fixed: ASD Paradoxical: LBBB, AS, HCM
		Knock		Chronic constrictive pericarditis Severe MR
	T, M	Opening snap	Abrupt opening of MV due to ↑ LAP	MS
	M	Plop		Atrial myxoma
		S3	Children: normal Adults: ventricle volume overload	MR, TR CHF
		S4	Normal in athletes, elderly ↑ resistance to ventricular filling due to ↓ ventricular compliance	**LVH**: AS, systemic HTN, CAD, cardiomyopathy **RVH**: PS, pulmoic HTN, IHD, angina, MI
		S3 + S4	Summation gallop	Chronic HTN, CHF

Murmurs

- Describe murmurs in terms of:
    - Timing: systolic, diastolic, continuous
    - Shape: crescendo, decrescendo, crescendo-decrescendo, plateau
    - Location of maximal intensity
    - Radiation: axilla, back, neck
    - Duration

CARDIOVASCULAR

- Intensity:
  - 6-point scale
  - Intensity of murmur not necessarily related to clinical severity
- Pitch: high, medium, low
- Quality: blowing, harsh, rumbling, musical, machine-like or scratchy
- Relationship to respiration
- Relationship to body position
- Effect of special maneuvers
- Murmur is likely nonpathological if:
  - Early systolic, short duration and low intensity (usually grade 1-2/6)
  - Nonradiating, not associated with other CV abnormalities/murmurs
  - Found in otherwise healthy children, especially in states of hyperdynamic blood flow (e.g. exercise, fever, anxiety)
  - Decreases or disappears on sitting

Table 6. Examples of Murmurs

Timing	Zone	Radiation	Quality	Pitch	Pathology
Mid-systolic	A	Neck	Harsh	Medium	Aortic stenosis
	P	Neck, back	Harsh	Medium	Pulmonic stenosis
	T	LLSB	Harsh	Medium	Hypertrophic cardiomyopathy
	M	Axilla			MV prolapse
Pan-systolic	M	L axilla	Blowing	High	MR
	T	RLSB	Blowing	High	TR
		Wide	Harsh	High	VSD
Diastolic	T	Apex, RSB	Blowing	High	AR
	M	None	Rumbling	Low	Mitral stenosis

LLSB = left lower sternal border, RSB = right sternal border, MV = mitral valve, MR = mitral regurgitation, TR = tricuspid regurgitation, VSD = ventriculo-septal defect, AR = aortic regurgitation

- Special maneuvers for auscultation:

Table 7. Special Positions and Maneuvers for Auscultation of Heart Sounds

Position	Effect on Heart Sounds
Sitting upright, leaning forward, holding exhalation	↑ AS, AR, pericardial rubs
Left lateral decubitus (LLD) (use bell of stethoscope)	S3, S4, MS

Maneuver	Physiological Effect	Effect on Heart Sounds
Quiet inspiration-sustained abdominal pressure, leg elevation	↑ venous return	↑ right-sided murmurs, TR, PS
Fist-clenching (isometrics)	↑ systemic arterial resistance	↑ some left-sided murmurs (MR, AR, VSD) ↓ AS
Standing (Valsalva strain)	↓ venous return, ↓ vascular tone	↑ MVP, HCM ↓ AS
Squatting (Valsalva release)	↑ venous return, ↑ vascular tone	↓ MVP, HCM ↑ AS

AS = aortic stenosis, AR = aortic regurgitation, MS = mitral stenosis, TR = tricuspid regurgitation, PS = pulmonic stenosis, MR = mitral regurgitation, VSD = ventricular septal defect, MVP = mitral valve prolapse, HCM = hypertrophic cardiomyopathy

Respiratory Exam
- See *Respiratory Exam*

Peripheral Vascular Exam
- See *Peripheral Vascular Exam*

COMMON INVESTIGATIONS

Table 8. Cardiac Investigations

Study Type	Test	Description
ECG	Resting	Normal 12 lead ECG
	Stress tests	**Treadmill exercise test (GXT)**: ECG monitoring during progressively increasing treadmill speed until chest discomfort, inordinate dyspnea, abnormal ECG changes or target HR is observed **Pharmacologic stress testing**: in patients who are unable to exercise maximally, medications such as dobutamine, dipyridamole and adenosine can be used
Anatomy/ Function	Echocardiography	Beams of ultrasonic waves that record the position and motion of heart wall and internal structures
Perfusion studies	Coronary angiography	Radiographic visualization of coronary vessels following introduction of contrast material
	Radionuclide angiography	First-pass radionuclide angiography analyzes rapidly acquired image frames to observe a bolus of 99mTc as it traverses the venous system to the right side of the heart, pulmonary artery, lungs, left atrium and left ventricle
	Nuclear perfusion	Heart function and coronary blood flow studied using injected radioactively labelled tracers
Enzymes	CK-MB, troponin	Enzymes released into circulation following damage to cardiac muscle; used to diagnose myocardial injury/infarctions

GXT = graded exercise test

CARDIOVASCULAR

COMMON CLINICAL SCENARIOS

Acute Myocardial Infarction (AMI)
- Symptoms:
  - *Pain*: classically retrosternal, heavy, squeezing or crushing pain, radiating to arm, abdomen, back, neck, jaw, prolonged (often lasting >30 min)
  - *Atypical pain*: "silent" AMI (more often in patients with DM, hypertension, increased age)
  - *Associated symptoms*: diaphoresis, nausea, vomiting, weakness, pallor, dizziness, palpitations, cerebral symptoms, sense of impending doom

- Physical examination
    - *JVP*: normal, ↑ with RV infarct
    - *Pulse*: variable, most commonly rapid and regular, may be normal, ↓ pulse volume, variable BP
    - *Palpation*: ↓ PMI, abnormal systolic pulsation 3rd-5th left intercostal space
    - *Auscultation*: S3, S4, ↓ intensity of heart sounds, paradoxical split S2, transient apical systolic murmur, mitral regurgitation, pericardial rub
    - *Extra-cardiac findings*: ↑ RR, pulmonary crackles, signs of arteriosclerosis

Congestive Heart Failure – Left and Right Heart
- Symptoms:
    - Dyspnea, orthopnea, PND, cough, Cheyne-Stokes respiration, fatigue, weakness, abdominal symptoms (anorexia, nausea, abdominal pain), cerebral symptoms, nocturia, peripheral edema, weight gain
- Physical examination:
    - *JVP*: ↑, positive hepatojugular reflux
    - *Pulse*: ↓ pulse volume, ± pulsus alternans (alternating stronger and weaker beats), sinus tachycardia
    - *Palpation*: PMI may be sustained, diffuse and displaced, S3 may be palpable, ± left parasternal lift
    - *Auscultation*: S3, S4; S2 may be paradoxically split (often associated with LBBB), murmurs often associated with mitral regurgitation and tricuspid regurgitation
    - *Extra-cardiac*: systemic hypotension, diastolic pressure may be ↑, pulmonary HTN, peripheral cyanosis, pulmonary crackles, hepatomegaly, ascites, edema, pleural effusion, cachexia

Mitral Stenosis
- Symptoms:
    - Pulmonary edema, atrial arrhythmias, fatigue, abdominal discomfort, edema, hemoptysis, recurrent pulmonary emboli, pulmonary infection, systemic embolization
- Physical examination:
    - *JVP*: elevated if RHF has occurred, no "a" wave if in AF
    - *Pulse*: normal contour, normal volume, may be irregularly irregular as in atrial fibrillation (AF)
    - *Palpation*: PMI normal, S1 may be palpable
    - *Auscultation*: loud S1, opening snap, mid-diastolic decrescendo murmur with pre-systolic accentuation (lost in AF), possible PR (Graham-Steell's murmur)
    - *Extra-cardiac*: ± evidence of pulmonary HTN

Aortic Stenosis
- Symptoms:
    - Dyspnea, angina pectoris, exertional syncope, congestive heart failure signs and symptoms in later course
- Physical examination:
    - *JVP*: normal or prominent "a" wave (septal hypertrophy)
    - *Pulse*: pulsus parvus et tardus (slow-rising and small volume pulse), apical-carotid delay
    - *Palpation*: sustained apical beat, systolic thrill may be palpable over aortic area

- *Auscultation*: soft S2, delayed A2, S2 splitting may be lost or paradoxical, systolic crescendo-decrescendo ejection murmur radiating to neck/sternal border, S4 (late peaking correlates with severe AS)

Evidence-Based Medicine: Aortic Stenosis

Effort syncope, slow rate of rise of the carotid artery pulsation, timing of peak murmur intensity in mid or late systole and decreased intensity of S2 are all associated with an increased likelihood for aortic stenosis.

Absence of a systolic murmur or murmur radiating to the right common carotid artery are associated with a decreased likelihood of aortic stenosis.

Etchells E et al. 1997. *JAMA* 277(7):564-571.

Atrial Fibrillation (AF)

- Symptoms:
  - Pulmonary congestion, angina pectoris, syncope, fatigue, anxiety, dyspnea, cardiomyopathy, signs of pulmonary emboli
- Physical examination:
  - *JVP*: absent "a" wave
  - *Pulse*: irregularly irregular pulse, often tachycardic, variable pulse pressure in the carotid arterial pulse
  - *Palpation*: S1 usually varies in intensity
- Investigations:
  - *ECG*: P waves not discernable, undulating baseline or sharply inscribed atrial deflections with varying amplitude and frequency (350-600 bpm)
  - *Echocardiogram*: left atrium is sometimes enlarged

Mitral Regurgitation (MR)

- Symptoms:
  - Fatigue, exertional dyspnea, orthopnea, symptoms of right-sided heart failure and LV failure
- Physical examination:
  - *JVP*: abnormally prominent "a" waves in patients with sinus rhythm and marked pulmonary hypertension and prominent "v" waves in those with accompanying severe TR
  - *Pulse*: usually normal, arterial pulse may show a sharp upstroke in patients with severe MR
  - *Palpation*: systolic thrill often palpable at cardiac apex, brisk systolic impulse and a palpable rapid-filling wave, apex beat often displaced laterally, RV tap and the shock of pulmonary valve closure may be palpable in patients with marked pulmonary hypertension
  - *Auscultation*: systolic murmur of at least grade 3/6 intensity, may be holosystolic or decrescendo, S1 generally absent, soft or buried in the systolic murmur, wide splitting of S2, a low-pitched S3 occurring 0.12 to 0.17 s after the aortic valve closure sound, S4 often audible
  - *Extra-cardiac*: pulmonary edema, hepatic congestion, ankle edema, distended neck veins, ascites

Infective Endocarditis (IE)

- Life-threatening infection of the endocardial surface of the heart, usually on the valves
  - Duke's criteria may be helpful in diagnosis

Table 9. Infectious Endocarditis

History	Signs/Symptoms
Rheumatic fever	Constitutional: fever, chills, malaise, night sweats, anorexia, arthralgias
Prosthetic valves	
Previous IE	Cardiac: murmur, palpitations, heart failure
IV drug users	Pulmonary: septic pulmonary embolism
Intravascular devices (e.g. arterial lines)	Neurological: focal deficit, headache, meningitis
Most congenital heart malformations	Metastatic infection: organ infarction
	Embolic manifestations
Valvular dysfunction	Peripheral signs:
HCM	Petechiae: conjunctivae, buccal mucosa, palate
MVP with MR	Splinter hemorrhages: linear dark red streaks under nails
Recent surgeries	Janeway lesions: nontender hemorrhagic macules on palm and soles
Indwelling catheters or hemodialysis	Osler's nodes: small painful nodules on fingers, toe pads, lasting hours to days
	Roth spots: retinal hemorrhage with pale center near optic disc
	Immune-mediated phenomena: vasculitis, glomerulonephritis, splenomegaly, synovitis

HCM = hypertrophic cardiomyopathy, MVP = mitral valve prolapse, MR = mitral regurgitation

REVIEW OF ANATOMY AND PHYSIOLOGY

- Circulatory pathway has two components: pulmonary (low pressure) system (RV → pulmonary arteries → lungs for oxygenation → pulmonary veins → LA) and systemic (high pressure) system (LV → aorta → body tissues for oxygen delivery → caval system → RA)
- **Blood supply** to the heart is regulated by the right and left coronary arteries (RCA and LCA) which are the first branches of the aorta; the left coronary system is comprised of a short left main artery (LMA) which bifurcates into the left anterior descending artery (LAD) and left circumflex artery (LCX). The RCA is longer than the LMA and bifurcates into the posterior descending artery (PDA) and the posterior lateral artery (PLA). The venous drainage occurs through the coronary sinus, which empties into the RA and enters the pulmonary circulation. Anatomic variants of the coronary system are common
- **Electrical conduction system** begins at the sino-atrial (SA) node located between the SVC and right atrial appendage → depolarizes both atria (LA via Bachmann's bundle) → internodal branches → atrio-ventricular (AV) node located between the coronary sinus and septal leaflet of tricuspid valve → His-Purkinje system → RBB and LBB → Purkinje fibres (see **Figure 1**)
- Neural innervation of heart from both sympathetic and parasympathetic nervous systems (SNS and PSNS)
    - SNS causes ↑ HR and ↑ AV node conduction rate
    - PSNS causes to ↓ HR and ↓ AV node conduction rate

ECG INTERPRETATION

ECG Leads

- Six limb leads record voltages from the heart directed onto the frontal plane of the body (3 bipolar leads I, II and III; 3 augmented unipolar leads aVL, aVR, aVF)
- The six chest leads (V1 to V6) record voltages from the heart directed onto the horizontal plane of the body
- A wave of depolarization moving towards an electrode will record a positive deflection on an ECG; a negative deflection represents a wave of depolarization moving away from an electrode
- Direction of atrial depolarization down and right
- Direction of septal depolarization down and left
- Direction of verticular depolarization down and right

Table 10. Anatomical Correspondence of the ECG Leads

Leads	Anatomical View
V1-V2	Right ventricle, posterior heart, septum
V3-V4	Interventricular septum, anterior LV wall
V5-V6	Anterior and lateral LV walls
V1-V2	Posterior part of the heart
V1-V4	Anterior part of the heart
R chest leads	Right side of the heart
I, aVL, V5-V6	Lateral part of the heart
II, III, aVF	Inferior part of the heart

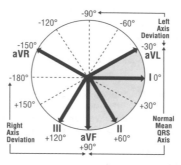

Gilbert Tang 2005

Figure 5. Axial ECG Leads and their Normal Ranges

APPROACH TO THE ECG

1. Heart Rate
2. Rhythm
3. Mean QRS Axis
4. Waves and Segments
5. Hypertrophy and Chamber Enlargement
6. Ischemia/Infarction

Heart Rate (HR)

- Each small box is 0.04 s; each large box is 0.2 s
- If HR is regular, divide 300 by the number of large squares between two consecutive R waves (e.g. HR is 60 if 5 large squares between consecutive R waves since 300/5 = 60)
- If a rough estimate of HR is required, simply count off the number of large boxes between two consecutive QRS complexes, using the sequence 300, 150, 100, 75, 60, 50 – this corresponds to the HR in beats/min
- If HR is irregular, multiply the number of complexes in 6 sec (30 large squares) by 10 to determine the average ventricular rate
- Normal sinus rhythm = 60-100 bpm (beats per minute); sinus bradycardia <60 bpm; sinus tachycardia >100 bpm

Rhythm

- Rhythm is considered regular if both RR and PP intervals are all equal:
  - Sinus rhythm (i.e. every P wave followed by QRS and every QRS preceded by P, P wave is positive in leads II or I and aVF)
  - QRS complex – wide or narrow
  - Relationship between P waves and QRS complexes, prolonged PR intervals
  - Ectopic beats
  - Pattern – regular or irregular
  - If irregular, note if regularly irregular or irregularly irregular

Means QRS Axis

- Many methods are available for a fast approximation of the mean QRS axis
- Normal mean QRS axis falls between –30° and +90° (up to +105°)

2-Lead Method (I, II)

1. Is the QRS complex of lead I positive or negative?
2. Is the QRS complex of lead II positive or negative?
3. Determine in which quadrant the mean QRS axis lies (e.g. if I is positive and II is positive, then the mean QRS lies between –30° and +90°, which is normal)

Isoelectric Lead Method (more precise)

1. Look for the most isoelectric lead (i.e. the net QRS complex is 0 in amplitude)
2. Find the perpendicular lead – is it positive or negative?
3. If positive, the mean QRS complex lies in the positive direction of that lead
   - **Left Axis Deviation**: mean axis between –30° and –90°
     - Common causes: LVH, LBBB, inferior MI
     - Associated causes: heart movement during respiration or an elevated left diaphragm associated with pregnancy, ascites or abdominal tumours
   - **Right Axis Deviation**: mean axis between +90° and 180°
     - Common causes: RVH, RBBB, dextrocardia, acute heart strain (e.g. massive pulmonary embolism), may also be seen in thin individuals

Table 11. Important ECG Characteristics

P Wave	PR Interval	QRS Complex	ST Segment	T Wave
Represents atrial depolarization	Measured from beginning of P wave to beginning of QRS complex	Represents ventricular depolarization	Normally at same level as the TP segment	Represents ventricular repolarization
Usually <2.5 mm in height and <0.12 s (3 small squares) in duration	Represents the time taken for the impulse to travel from the SA node to the ventricles	Narrow QRS complex (<0.12 s or <3 small squares) reflects normal rapid activation of ventricles via the His-Purkinje system	Shortens as heart rate increases	Usually positive in all leads except aVR
Should always be positive in leads I, II, aVF 0.12 s to 0.2 s (3-5 small squares)		Wide QRS complex (>0.12 s or >3 small squares) reflects abnormally slow ventricular activation	Ensures complete emptying of ventricles	May be inverted in leads III, aVF, V1 and V2 in normal individuals
				An inverted T wave in leads I, II, V3-V6 is usually abnormal

CARDIOVASCULAR

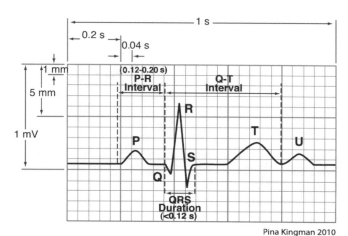

Pina Kingman 2010

Figure 6. ECG and Normal Values

Table 12. Common Arrhythmias (not inclusive)

Location	Example	
Atrium		
Premature atrial contractions (PAC)		*
Atrial flutter		**
Atrial fibrillation (AFib)		**
Supraventricular tachycardia (SVT)		**
AV node		
Conduction blocks:		
1° atrioventricular block (↑ P-R interval)		*
2° atrioventricular block (Wenckebach) shown to the right – Mobitz Type 1 (Wenckebach) – Mobitz Type 2 (Classic)		*
3° atrioventricular block (complete heart block)		*
Ventricle		
Premature ventricular contractions (PVC)		*
Ventricular tachycardia (VTach)		**
Torsades de pointes		**
Ventricular fibrillation (VFib)		**

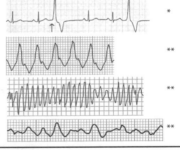

*Adapted from GE Marquette, 2000; **Adapted from patient samples

CARDIOVASCULAR

Waves and Segments (P Wave Abnormality)
- **Left atrial enlargement**
  - LA enlarges posteriorly (downward deflection in V1)
  - In V1 a deep terminal component that is at least 1 square wide (0.04 s) and 1 square deep (1 mm)
  - P wave has two peaks (p mitrale) in lead II
- **Right atrial enlargement**
  - RA enlarges vertically (tall P wave in inferior leads)
  - In V1 a large positive wave >1.5 mm
  - Large P wave >2.5 mm (height) in leads II, III or aVF may be seen

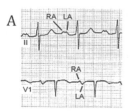 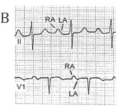

Figure 7. (A) Left and (B) Right Atrial Enlargement ECG Tracing
Adapted from Dr. F. Yanowitz, 1999

Hypertrophy and Chamber Enlargement
- **Left ventricular hypertrophy (LVH):**
  - Leads I, aVL, V5 and V6 show taller R waves
  - Leads V1 and V2 show deeper than normal S waves
  - Criteria for the diagnosis of LVH:
    - S wave in V1 or V2 >25 mm
    - R wave in V5 or V6 >25 mm
    - R wave in aVL >11 mm
    - R wave in I and S wave in III >25 mm
    - S wave in V1 or V2 and R wave in V5 or V6 >35 mm
  - Associated features: left axis deviation, left atrial enlargement, intrinsicoid deflection (longer QR interval, >0.05 s), ventricular strain
- **Right ventricular hypertrophy (RVH):**
  - Results in a large R wave in V1 and a large S wave in V6
  - Criteria for the diagnosis of RVH:
    - R wave >7 mm in V1
    - R wave >S wave in V1
    - R/S ratio <1 in V5 or V6
    - Right axis deviation
- **Bundle branch blocks:**
  - Left bundle branch block (LBBB)
    - Because of the LBBB, the right ventricle depolarizes first
    - RS or QS in V1, broad-notched R wave in I, aVL, V5, V6
    - QRS > 0.12s
  - Right bundle branch block (RBBB)
    - QRS in V6, rSR' in V1, terminal S slurring in I, V5, V6
    - QRS >0.12 s
    - Use first 0.06 s of the QRS complex to determine the mean QRS axis

CARDIOVASCULAR

Ischemia/Infarction

Transmural MI
- Q waves are possible evidence of a prior transmural MI
- A significant Q wave must be either 0.04 s wide (1 small box or greater) or one-third the height of the R wave. If neither of these conditions is met, the Q waves are not diagnostic of infarction

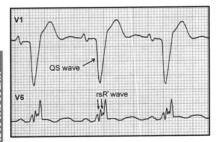

Figure 8. LBBB ECG Tracing
Adapted from Dr. GE Marquette, 2000

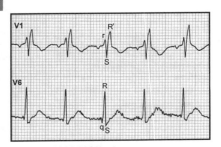

Figure 9. RBBB ECG Tracing
Adapted from Dr. GE Marquette, 2000

Table 13. Localization of the Acute MI

Anatomical Location	Leads with Abnormal ECG Complexes	Associated Coronary Artery
Posterior	V1, V2 (tall R, not Q)	RCA or CFX (distal
Inferior	II, III, aVF	RCA
Anterior septal	V1, V2	LAD
Anterior apical	V3, V4	LAD (distal)
Lateral	I, aVL, V5, V6	CFX
Anterior	V2-V5	LAD (proximal)
Right ventricle	R chest leads V3, V4	RCA

RCA = right coronary artery, CFX = circumflex artery, LAD = left anterior descending artery

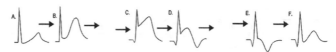

Figure 10. ECG Evolution during Acute Q-Wave MI

Adapted from Dr. F. Yanowitz, 1999

Table 14. Legend for Figure 10

Time Frame	ECG Changes
A. Normal	None
B. Acute	ST elevation
C. Hours	ST elevation, depressed R wave, Q wave begins
D. 1-2 Days	T wave inversion, increased Q wave
E. Days	ST normalizes, T wave inverted
F. Weeks	ST and T normal, Q wave remains

ST Segment and T Wave Abnormalities

- Non-Q wave MI involves only the subendocardial layers of the myocardium (not transmural)
- This results in ECG changes such as T wave inversions and ST segment depression
- Causes of ST segment depression:
  - Angina (ischemia)
  - Subendocardial infarction
  - Acute posterior wall MI (V1 and V2)
  - LVH strain
  - LBBB
- Causes of ST segment elevation:
  - Acute MI
  - Post MI
  - Acute pericarditis
  - Ventricular aneurysm
  - Early repolarization

Table 15. Metabolic Causes of ST Segment Changes

Cause	Feature of ECG Change	ECG Sample
Digoxin therapy	ST "scooped" depression, mild PR prolongation	
Hyperkalemia	Tall "peaked" T wave	
Severe hyperkalemia	Flattened P, widened QRS, long PR interval, "sine wave" appearance	
Hypokalemia	ST depression, flattened T, prominent U wave, prolonged QT interval	T U
Hypercalcemia	Shortened QT interval	
Hypocalcemia	Prolonged QT interval	

REFERENCES

Bickley LS, Szilagyi PG, Bates B. 2007. *Bates' Guide to Physical Examination and History Taking.* Philadelphia: Lippincott Williams & Wilkins.

Braunwald E, Zipes DP, Libby P. 2001. *Heart Disease: A Textbook of Cardiovascular Medicine.* Philadelphia: Saunders.

Dugani S, Lam D (eds.) 2009. *The Toronto Notes 2009: Comprehensive Medical Reference.* Toronto: Toronto Notes for Medical Students, Inc.

Etchells E, Bell C, Robb K. 1997. Does this patient have a systolic murmur? *JAMA* 277(7): 564-571.

Fauci AS. 2008. *Harrison's Principles of Internal Medicine.* New York: McGraw-Hill.

Huszar RJ. 1994. *Basic Dysrhythmias: Interpretation & Management.* St. Louis: Mosby Lifeline.

Lilly LS, Harvard Medical School. 2007. *Pathophysiology of Heart Disease: A Collaborative Project of Medical Students and Faculty.* Philadelphia: Wolters Kluwer/Lippincott Williams & Wilkins.

Swartz MH. 2006. *Textbook of Physical Diagnosis: History and Examination.* Philadelphia: Saunders Elsevier.

CARDIOVASCULAR

The Geriatric Exam

Editors:
Ali Okhowat & Roshan Razik

Faculty Reviewer:
Barry Goldlist, MD, FRCP(C)

TABLE OF CONTENTS

Approach to the Geriatric History and Physical Exam   79
Common Disorders   79
Focused History   80
Mental Examination   82
Focused Physical Exam   82
Common Clinical Scenarios   85
Elder Abuse   86
Driving Competency and Safety   88
Prescribing Opioids   89
Breaking Bad News: SPIKES Approach   90

APPROACH TO THE GERIATRIC HISTORY AND PHYSICAL EXAM

In addition to general history taking, important aspects of the geriatric history include:

- *Chief Complaint* – often a change in function or vague, often multiple complaints
- *History of Present Illness* – often nonorgan-specific or atypical presentation of disease; multiple pathologies (concurrence of disease) are very common
- *Medications* – polypharmacy is common; important to obtain full list of medications, including nonprescription and complementary medications
- *Psychological* – ask about depression
- *Social Data* – ask about supports, living arrangements, cultural background
- *Functional Assessment* – activities of daily living (ADLs); instrumental activities of daily living (IADLs); sensory function; geriatric giants
- *Review of Systems*

In addition to the general physical exam, include the following:

- Mental status (including cognition)
- Postural blood pressure
- Gait assessment
- Visual assessment

COMMON DISORDERS

Disorders marked with (✓) are discussed in **Common Clinical Scenarios**

- ✓ Falls
- ✓ Urinary incontinence
- Constipation
- Depression/Anxiety
- Dizziness
- Memory loss/Confusion
- Shortness of breath (dyspnea)
- Chest pain
- Joint pain
- Intermittent claudication
- Weight loss/Poor appetite
- Failure to thrive

GERIATRIC

FOCUSED HISTORY

When doing a geriatric history, remember to ask about the geriatric giants and the 5 Is:

Geriatric Giants	5 Is
Falls	Immobility
Confusion	Intellect
Incontinence	Incontinence
Polypharmacy	Iatrogenesis
	Impaired homeostasis

- As early as possible during the interview, evaluate the patient's ability to hear, see, understand and give an accurate historical account
- Due to communication difficulties or multiplicity of complaints, history taking can be lengthy. If the patient is medically stable, the history need not be completed at once and can be broken down into several sessions. Setting priorities is important for efficient management
- Underreporting of symptoms is a common occurrence in the elderly due to health beliefs, fear, depression, cognitive impairment or cultural barriers. Ask specific questions in a thorough review of systems to uncover medical problems
- A corroborative history, from a family member or caregiver, is often important

Chief Complaint

- Illness often presents as a change in function with atypical symptomatology

History of Present Illness

- Patients usually present with multiple issues and nonspecific symptoms without a definite organ system involved
- Making a comprehensive problem list is helpful in addressing all complaints in order of functional importance

Medications

- Polypharmacy is prevalent in the elderly and you must ask, in detail, about drugs they are taking, drugs they may have recently stopped taking and over-the-counter (OTC) medications, herbal remedies/teas and vitamins. It may be useful to have the patient or a caregiver bring in all medications that the patient is taking
- Note that polypharmacy is one of the risk factors of noncompliance
- The risk of drug-drug interactions and adverse drug reactions increases with the number of prescriptions
- Ask about pneumococcal, influenza and tetanus immunization status

Psychological Data

- Investigate recent lifestyle change, cognitive function, emotional function (depression, paranoia, anxiety, hallucinations, personality, coping skills)
- Geriatric Depression Scale (**Table 1**)

Table 1. Geriatric Depression Scale (Shortened Version)

1. Are you basically satisfied with your life?

2. Have you dropped many of your activities and interests?

3. Do you feel that your life is empty?

4. Do you often get bored?

5. Are you in good spirits most of the time?

6. Are you afraid that something bad is going to happen to you?

7. Do you feel happy most of the time?

8. Do you often feel helpless?

9. Do you prefer to stay at home rather than going out and doing a few things?

10. Do you feel you have more problems with your memory than most?

11. Do you think it is wonderful to be alive now?

12. Do you feel pretty worthless the way you are now?

13. Do you feel full of energy?

14. Do you feel that your situation is hopeless?

15. Do you think that most people are better off than you are?

Score 1 point for each depressed answer (1, 5, 7, 11, 13 = no, others = yes).

Normal = 0-4, Mildly depressed = 5-8, Moderately depressed = 9-11
Very depressed = 12-15

Adapted from Yesavage JA et al. 1983. *J Psychiatr Res* 17(1):37-49.

GERIATRIC

Social Data
- Determine living arrangements, marital status, willingness to accept help, family support and community resources available. Document existence of directives such as power of attorney or a living will
- Ask about the content of a typical day for the patient, extent of social relationships, suitability and safety of home, substance abuse (includes smoking, alcohol intake and daily caffeine consumption), occupational history, cultural background, interests
- Ask if plans exist for times of illness or functional decline
  - Ask caregivers whether a back-up plan of care exists for the patient in case of caregiver misfortune or ill-health
- Enquire about availability and attitude of caregivers and neighbours, availability of emergency help
- For inpatients, enquire about their discharge plans

Nutrition History
- Malnutrition is common in older adults, especially in the frail
- Ask about typical daily diet and fluid intake, pattern of weight during recent years, shopping and food preparation habits, sites of eating, skipped meals

The Functional Assessment
- Used as a screen to identify any impairments and dependence on others

Activities of Daily Living (ADLs) (**TEACHD**: *Toileting, Eating, Ambulating, Cleaning, Hygeine, Dressing*)
- Are you able to get out of bed by yourself in the morning?
- Can you use the bathroom by yourself?
- Do you bathe yourself and do your own grooming?
- Are you able to dress yourself?
- Are you able to walk without any assistance (person, cane, walker)?
- Do you experience difficulty going up or down stairs?

Instrumental Activities of Daily Living (IADLs) (**SHAFT**: *Shopping, Housework, Accounting, Food preparation, Transport, Telephoning, Taking medications*)
- Do you do the cooking, cleaning, laundry or shopping?
- Are you able to take care of banking, paying the bills and making financial decisions?
- Does anyone help you to make appointments?
- Are you driving at the moment? If yes, are you experiencing any difficulties with your driving? (see **Driving Competency and Safety** p. 88)

Review of Systems
Remember to ask about these systems in particular:
- *General*: appetite, weight change, fatigue, sleep patterns
- *Head and Neck*: visual changes, hearing loss
- *GI*: constipation
- *GU*: incontinence, frequency, nocturia, sexual function
- *CNS/MSK*: gait, balance, memory impairment, falls

MENTAL EXAMINATION
- The Folstein Mini-Mental State Exam (MMSE) is a screen for documenting dementia or delirium (see *Psychiatric Exam* p. 322)
  - Some patients may be upset or offended by the nature of the questions. Avoid using the word "test" or "exam". One approach is to introduce the MMSE by saying, "I have a few questions and tasks that will allow me to see how your memory and concentration are functioning today."
  - If the score is <24/30, suspect disturbed cognitive function
  - Note that MMSE scores may also be low in patients with sensory impairment, dysphasia, depression, poor English or low education level
- The MoCA (Montreal Cognitive Assessment) is a more sensitive tool for mild cognitive problems

FOCUSED PHYSICAL EXAM

Vital Signs
- *Weight*: acute weight loss (>3%) is the most specific sign of dehydration in the elderly
- *Height*: reduction may indicate osteoporosis, vertebral compression fractures
- Orthostatic hypotension (see *General History and Physical Exam* p. 21)
  - Could be a normal consequence of aging, medication side effect, or a disease state

- Check supine vs. standing (recommended); if unable, check supine vs. sitting or sitting vs. standing
- Do not miss auscultatory gap in elderly hypertensive patients (see *General History and Physical Exam* p. 21)

Head and Neck
- *Eyes* (see *Ophthalmological Exam*)
  - Visual acuity and fields
  - Screen for cataracts, macular degeneration, glaucoma
  - Note: previous cataract surgery can cause unequal and less reactive pupil
- *Ears* (see *Head and Neck Exam*)
  - Hearing impairment can be caused by wax impaction (can result in a 30% conductive hearing loss)
  - High frequency hearing loss is common with aging
  - Assess for presbycusis and tinnitus
- *Dentition*
  - Ask patient to remove dentures when examining the mouth
  - Check for dryness, dental and periodontal problems
  - Lack of dental work and ill-fitting dentures may lead to difficulty eating, weight loss and malnutrition
  - Look for signs of oral cancers
- *Neck* (see *Head and Neck Exam*)
  - Auscultate for carotid bruits as the prevalence of atherosclerosis is high in the elderly (carotid bruits can indicate diffuse vascular disease and should lead to detailed questioning about symptoms of CAD and past TIAs/strokes)
  - Thyroid exam (note: patients can have subclinical hypothyroidism)
  - Assess for neck masses (malignancy, infection, inflammation)
- *Lymph Nodes* (see *Lymphatic System and Lymph Node Exam*)
  - With advanced age, lymph nodes usually become smaller, decrease in number and become more fibrotic and fatty

Chest
- Examine for arrhythmias, cyanosis (see *Cardiovascular Exam* p. 64)
  - Murmurs and extra heart sounds should be assessed thoroughly
  - Although irregular rhythms are common, they should not be considered "normal"
  - A fourth heart sound is often associated with hypertension
- Examine for signs of pneumonia, COPD exacerbation, airway pathology (see *Respiratory Exam*)
- *Posterior Chest*
  - Dorsal kyphosis may indicate vertebral compression fractures and osteoporosis

PVS
- Peripheral pulses, edema (see *Peripheral Vascular Exam* p. 303)
- Arterial or venous insufficiency and complications (especially in diabetics)

GI
- Auscultate and palpate for abdominal aortic aneurysm (see *Peripheral Vascular Exam* p. 309)
- Hernial orifices (abdominal, umbilical) (see *Urological Exam* p. 359)

GERIATRIC

GU
- Examine for the following in particular: cystocele, rectocele, atrophic vaginitis (see *Gynecological Exam* p. 94 and *Urological Exam* p. 366)
- Urinary retention
- Hernial orifices (inguinal, femoral) (see *Urological Exam* p. 358)
- Rectal examination (see *Urological Exam* p. 359)

Dermatological
- Cancers are common, especially on the hands and face where sun exposure is greatest; actinic (solar) keratoses are precursor lesions and should be treated
- Investigate for any pressure sores, especially in immobile patients (e.g. sacrum, heel, bony occipital prominence)
- Ulcerations/edema in the lower extremities signal vascular or neuropathic impairments which must be investigated further

Musculoskeletal
- Determine range of motion of all joints
- Pay special attention to the hip and shoulder; impairment in the upper extremities could interfere with ADLs
- Check foot hygiene, deformity and assess need for chiropody
  - If appropriate, check footwear
- Joint abnormalities in the hips, knees and feet may lead to gait abnormalities

Neurological
- Diminished vibration sense and an absent ankle jerk reflex are common in elderly patients

Gait Assessment
- Observe the patient:
  - Rising from the bed or chair (note use of arms and foot stance)
    - Parkinsonian patients do not tuck their feet under chair when rising to stand and require several attempts to stand
  - Note posture, ataxia and use of hands while walking
    - Kyphosis may indicate osteoporosis
    - Sway and/or use of walking aid may indicate cerebellar dysfunction
  - Step height and step length usually decreased in elderly
    - Asymmetry in step height or length may result from stroke
  - Turning (one step turn vs. multi-step) and balance
    - Parkinsonian patients exhibit a multi-step turn
  - Double-stance time increase (where both feet are on the ground for prolonged time)
    - Parkinsonian shuffle: patient's feet never leave the ground

COMMON CLINICAL SCENARIOS

Falls

History
- Location and activity at time of fall, witnesses
- Associated symptoms: dizziness, palpitations, dyspnea, chest pain, weakness, confusion, loss of consciousness
- Previous falls, weight loss (malnutrition)
- Past medical history and medications

Physical Exam
- Complete physical exam with emphasis on:
  - *CVS*: orthostatic changes in blood pressure and pulse, arrhythmias, murmurs, carotid bruits
  - *MSK*: injury secondary to fall, degenerative joint disease, podiatric problems, poorly fitting shoes
  - *CNS*: vision, hearing, muscle power and symmetry, sensation, gait and balance, turning, getting in/out of a chair, Romberg test and sternal push, cognitive screen (if appropriate)

Urinary Incontinence
- Transient incontinence
  - Due to factors outside urinary tract
  - Among all elderly patients admitted to hospital who are incontinent of urine, 30% are transiently incontinent
  - Etiology of transient incontinence (**DIAPPERS**):
    - **D** elirium or confusional state
    - **I** nfection, urinary (symptomatic)
    - **A** trophic urethritis, vaginitis
    - **P** harmaceuticals (drugs)
    - **P** sychological disorder, depression
    - **E** xcessive urine output (e.g. due to hypercalcemia)
    - **R** estricted mobility
    - **S** tool impaction
- Established incontinence
  - If leakage persists after transient causes of incontinence have been addressed, lower urinary tract causes must be considered
- Overactive bladder (OAB or urge incontinence) and stress incontinence are common in the elderly
  - For details on classification and pathogenesis, see *Urological Exam*

History
- Characterize the voiding pattern and determine whether the patient has symptoms of abnormal voiding
  - Voiding record: record of volume and time of each void or incontinent episode; kept by the patient or caregiver during a 48 to 72 h period
  - Type: urge, reflex, stress, overflow or mixed
  - Frequency, hesitancy, duration
  - Pattern: diurnal, nocturnal or both; after taking medications
  - Precipitants
  - Palliating features
  - Associated symptoms, e.g. straining to void, incomplete emptying, dysuria, hematuria, suprapubic or perineal discomfort, prolonged voiding
  - Alteration in bowel habit or sexual function

- Medications, including nonprescription drugs
- Assess fluid intake (excessive volume or diuretics e.g. caffeine)
- "Irritative" symptoms – ask about **FUND**
  - **F** requency
  - **U** rgency
  - **N** octuria
  - **D** ysuria
- Note: the effects of the incontinence should be ascertained (e.g. emotional and social factors)

Physical Exam
- Identify other medical conditions, e.g. heart failure, peripheral edema
- Test for stress-induced leakage when bladder is full
- Observe or listen to voiding
- *Pelvic exam* – look for atrophic vaginitis, pelvic muscle laxity, pelvic mass
- *Rectal exam* – look for irritation, resting tone and voluntary control of anal sphincter, prostate nodules, fecal impaction
- *Neurological exam* – mental status and sensory/motor examination, including sacral reflexes and perineal sensation

Other Clinical Scenarios
- Delirium, dementia – see *Psychiatric Exam* p. 331
- Depression – see *Psychiatric Exam* p. 325
- Heart diseases – see *Cardiovascular Exam* p. 67

ELDER ABUSE

Definition
- Mistreatment or neglect that a senior experiences at the hands of their spouses, children, other family members, caregivers, service providers or other individuals in positions of power or trust; elder abuse is violence
- Abuse and neglect of older adults occur in both domestic and institutional settings
- Abused elderly have a significantly increased risk of death

Types of Elder Abuse
- Physical abuse
- Sexual abuse
- Psychological/emotional abuse
- Social isolation
- Financial exploitation
- Neglect

Prevalence
- An estimated 7% of people over age 65 experience some form of elder abuse (Statistics Canada, 2000)
- Almost 2% of older Canadians have experienced more than one type of abuse

Risk Factors
- Family history of violence
- Caregiver stress

Common Chief Complaints
- Patients are often reluctant to report abuse and rarely identify abuse as their initial problem
- Multiple visits for specific and often stress-related complaints
- Unexplained traumatic injuries
- Headache, insomnia, anxiety, depression
- Suicidal ideation, suicide attempts
- Pain in chest, GI, pelvis, back

Approach to the History
- Try to interview the patient alone (document if not possible)
- Ensure confidentiality
- Consider abuse in your differential diagnosis
- Screening questions:
  - Do you need help taking care of yourself?
  - What is a typical day like?
  - Who manages your finances?
  - Who gives you your medications?
- Specific questions:
  - Do you feel safe where you live?
  - Do you know someone you can turn to in a crisis?
  - What happens when you disagree with a family member?
  - Are you yelled at or punished in any way?
  - Has anyone threatened to hurt you?

Signs of Elder Abuse
- Difficult to detect unless obvious signs of physical injury
- Overall appearance and signs of neglect
- Injuries inconsistent with explanation
- Discrepancies between patient and caregiver account of illness or injury
- Behaviour – withdrawn, depressed, fearful, anxious
- Malnourishment
- Pressure ulcers
- Welts, scars, abrasions, lacerations, burns
- Alopecia
- Fractures and bruises
- Multiple injuries in varied stages of healing
- Recurrent injuries
- Signs of sexual abuse

Safety Planning
- Provide patient with emergency contact numbers
- Follow the provincial and hospital reporting policy
- Options may include temporary admission to hospital or respite homecare

The Medical Record
- Detailed history – report cause of injury in patient's own words; include chronic stress-related complaints
- Physical findings – body map of bruises and tender areas
- Include your own suspicions of abuse

GERIATRIC

DRIVING COMPETENCY AND SAFETY

Assessing an elderly patient's ability to operate a motor vehicle is a common task in many geriatric settings. In Ontario, the Ministry of Transportation requires everyone over the age of 80 to pass certain written tests as well as a medical examination by their primary care provider.

Some points to keep in mind when assessing such patients are as follows:

Alcohol
- Alcohol dependence: should not be allowed to drive, must complete a rehabilitation program and remain abstinent and seizure free for 12 months before driving
- Drinking and driving: must not drive for 12 months

Blood Pressure Abnormalities
- Hypertension: sustained BP >170/110 should be evaluated carefully
- Hypotension: if syncopal, discontinue until attacks are treated and preventable

Cardiovascular Disease
- Suspected asymptomatic CAD: no restrictions
- Acute MI, unstable angina pectoris, coronary bypass surgery: wait one month
- Angioplasty, stenting: wait 48 hours

Cerebrovascular conditions
- TIA: should not be allowed to drive until a medical assessment is completed
- Stroke: should not drive for at least one month, may resume driving if functionally able, if no obvious risk of sudden recurrence and if on medication

Chronic obstructive pulmonary disease (COPD)
- Mild/moderate impairment: no restrictions
- Moderate impairment requiring supplemental oxygen: road test with supplemental oxygen

Cognitive Impairment
- MMSE <24: ineligible for license pending complete neurologic assessment
- MMSE >24: should be evaluated if suspected of showing poor judgement, poor reasoning ability, poor abstract thinking and poor insight

Diabetes
- Diet controlled, oral hypoglycemics: no restrictions
- Insulin use: may drive if no history of impairment due to alcohol or drug abuse and no severe hypoglycemic episode in the last 6 months

Drugs
- Be aware of: analgesics, anticholinergics, anticonvulsants, antidepressants antipsychotics, opiates, sedatives, stimulants
- Degree of impairment varies: patients should be warned about the effect of the medication on driving

Hearing Loss
- Effect of impaired hearing on ability to drive safely is controversial
- Acute labyrinthitis, positional vertigo with horizontal head movement, recurrent vertigo: advise not to drive until condition resolves

Musculoskeletal Disorders
- Physician's role is to report etiology, prognosis and extent of disability (pain, range of motion, coordination, muscle strength)
- Post-operative
- Outpatient, conscious sedation: no driving up to 24 hours
- Outpatient, general anesthesia: no driving for >24 hours

Seizures
- First, single, unprovoked: no driving for 3 months until complete neurologic assessment, EEG, CT head
- Epilepsy: can drive if seizure-free on medication and compliant for 12 months

Visual Impairment
- Acuity: should not be <20/50 with adequate continuous field of vision when both eyes are examined simultaneously

Summary: Evaluate SAFE DRIVE:
- **S** afety and record (from DMV)
- **A** ttention skills
- **F** amily report
- **E** thanol use
- **D** rugs
- **R** eaction time
- **I** ntellectual impairement
- **V** ision and visuospatial ability
- **E** xecutive functions

Adapted from: Determining medical fitness to operate motor vehicles. 2006. *CMA Driver's Guide*, 7th ed.

PRESCRIBING OPIOIDS
When prescribing narcotics, remember NBAL:
- **N** arcotic (e.g. morphine 5 mg PO q4h)
- **B** reakthrough (e.g. morphine 2.5 mg PO q1h prn)
- **A** nti-emetic (e.g. dimenhydrinate 12.5 mg PO q4h)
- **L** axative (e.g. senokot 2 tabs PO qhs)

Opioid Equivalent Doses
- When converting from one opioid to another, use 50-75% of the equivalent dose to allow for incomplete cross-tolerance
- Rapid titration and prn use may be required to ensure effective analgesia for the first 24 hours
- The opioids often used to manage mild to moderate pain include codeine, hydrocodone and oxycodone
- Moderate to severe pain is often managed using morphine, hydromorphone, oxycodone, fentanyl, methadone or levorphanol
- See *Pain Management* p. 520 for opioid analgesic equivalencies

Serum creatinine does not reflect creatinine clearance in the elderly
Instead, use Cockcroft-Gault equation:
CrCl (mL/min) = $\frac{\text{(weight in kg)}(140 - \text{age}) \times 1.23}{\text{(serum creatinine in } \mu\text{mol/L)}}$

Multiply by 0.85 for females

BREAKING BAD NEWS: SPIKES Approach)

- See *General History and Physical Exam* p. 7

> **Clinical Pearl**
> 1. Blood pressure: Rely on home BP monitoring more as white coat hypertension is more prevalent in the elderly.
> 2. Fecal or urinary retention: rule outfecal impaction.
> 3. Driving: Always consider assessment of fitness to drive in management of any condition in the elderly.
> 4. Renal function: Creatinine clearance is a more accurate way to assess renal function than serum creatinine level due to the decline in renal clearance and lean muscle mass that may make serum creatinine normal in the elderly.
> 5. Advanced care directives: Make sure these are known to the team during routine visits. Such discussions are preferably held during normal outpatient visits rather than when an acute life-threatening event is imminent or occurring.

REFERENCES

Canadian Medical Association. 2006. Determining medical fitness to operate motor vehicles. *CMA Driver's Guide*, 7th Ed. Ottawa, ON: Canadian Medical Association.

Crum RM, Anthony JC, Bassett SS, Folstein MF. 1993. Population-based norms for the Mini-Mental State Examination by age and educational level. *JAMA* 269(18):2386-2391.

Ham RJ. 2007. *Primary Care Geriatrics: A Case-Based Approach*. Philadelphia: Mosby Elsevier.

McDonald L, Collins A. 2000. *Abuse and Neglect of Older Adults: A Discussion Paper*. Ottawa: Family Violence Prevention Unit, Health Canada.

Yesavage JA, Brink TL, Rose TL, Lum O, Huang V, Adey MB, Leirer VO. 1983. Development and validation of a geriatric depression screening scale: A preliminary report. *J Psychiatr Res* 17(1): 37-49.

GERIATRIC

The Gynecological Exam

Editors:
Sarah Erdman & Joanna Lazier

Faculty Reviewers:
Heather Shapiro, MD, FRCS(C)
Janet Bodley, MEd, MD, FRCS(C)
Richard Pittini, MEd, MD, FRCS(C)

TABLE OF CONTENTS

Essential Anatomy   91
Approach to the Gynecological History and Physical Exam   92
Common Chief Complaints   92
Common Disorders   93
Focused Gynecological History   93
Focused Gynecological Exam   94
Common Investigations   98
Common Clinical Scenarios   99

ESSENTIAL ANATOMY

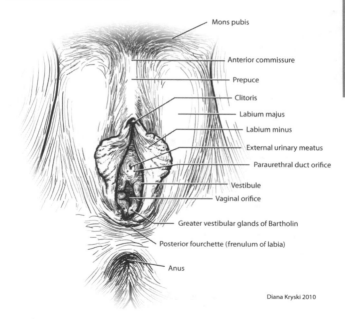

Mons pubis
Anterior commissure
Prepuce
Clitoris
Labium majus
Labium minus
External urinary meatus
Paraurethral duct orifice
Vestibule
Vaginal orifice
Greater vestibular glands of Bartholin
Posterior fourchette (frenulum of labia)
Anus

Diana Kryski 2010

Figure 1. External Female Genitalia

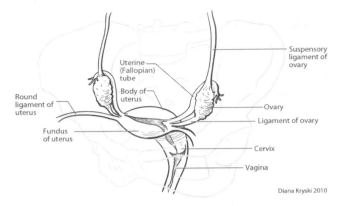

Suspensory ligament of ovary

Uterine (Fallopian) tube

Round ligament of uterus

Body of uterus

Ovary

Ligament of ovary

Fundus of uterus

Cervix

Vagina

Diana Kryski 2010

Figure 2. Female Reproductive Tract

APPROACH TO THE GYNECOLOGICAL HISTORY AND PHYSICAL EXAM

In addition to general history taking, important aspects of the gynecological history include:
- Menstrual history
- Sexual and contraceptive history
- Medications and substance use
- Gynecological history (e.g. Pap smears, surgeries, infections, infertility)
- Breast disease history (see **Breast Exam**)
- Obstetrical history (see **Obstetric Exam**)
- Family history (e.g. breast cancer, ovarian cancer)
- Past medical history of osteoporosis

Overview of the physical exam:
- Pelvic exam
  - Speculum examination
  - Bimanual exam
  - Rectovaginal examination

COMMON CHIEF COMPLAINTS
- Abdominal or pelvic pain
- Abnormal vaginal bleeding (between or during menses, postmenopausal)
- Absence/cessation of menses (amenorrhea)
- Painful menses (dysmenorrhea)
- Decreased libido
- Difficulty getting pregnant
- Painful intercourse (dyspareunia)
- Pelvic mass
- Symptoms of menopause
- Vaginal discharge
- Vulvovaginal itchiness

COMMON DISORDERS

Disorders marked with (✓) are discussed in **Common Clinical Scenarios**

- ✓ Endometriosis
- ✓ STIs
- ✓ Infertility
- ✓ Pelvic inflammatory disease (PID)
- ✓ Polycystic ovarian syndrome (PCOS)
- Ectopic pregnancy
- Ovarian cysts
- Miscarriage/abortion
- Endometrial/ovarian/cervical cancer
- Vaginitis/vulvitis
- Uterine fibroids (leiomyomata)

FOCUSED GYNECOLOGICAL HISTORY

Menstrual History

- Last menstrual period (LMP) – specify first day of menses
- Onset of menarche (normally between 9 to 16 years, mean 12.5 years)
- Onset of menopause (normally between 44 to 55 years, mean 51.2 years)
- Duration of menses (normally 3 to 7 days)
- Cycle regularity
- Cycle length (measured as interval between first day of menses to first day of menses in subsequent month; normally 21 to 35 days)
- Flow: normal = dark red discharge; bright red blood ± clots is excessive
  - Pad/tampon count and saturation can help quantify
- Symptoms of premenstrual syndrome (PMS) (4-10 days before menses): anxiety, nervousness, mood swings, irritability, food cravings, change in libido, difficulty sleeping, breast tenderness, headaches and fluid retention
- Dysmenorrhea: age of onset, severity, amount of disability (PQRST), current treatment
- Abnormal menstrual bleeding
  - Amenorrhea – absence of periods (primary vs. secondary)
  - Polymenorrhea – increased frequency
  - Oligomenorrhea – decreased frequency (>35 d)
  - Menorrhagia – increased duration or flow
  - Metrorrhagia – intermenstrual bleeding
  - Contact bleeding – post-coital, post-douching
- Menopause
  - Symptoms: hot flashes, flushing, sweating, sleep disturbances, vaginal dryness, vulvovaginal atrophy
  - Hormonal therapy
  - Postmenopausal bleeding (bleeding after 6 months without periods warrants further investigation)

Sexual and Contraceptive History

- Age at first intercourse
- Dyspareunia or bleeding with intercourse
- Number and gender of partners
- Type of sexual practices (vaginal, oral, anal sex)
- Satisfaction (desire, arousal, orgasm)
- Date and duration of marriage(s)/significant relationship(s)
- History of sexual assault or abuse
- Type and duration of each contraceptive method
- Compliance, reasons for any discontinuation
- Side effects, contraceptive failure
- Future conception plans

GYNECOLOGICAL

Medications and Substance Use
- Use of prescription/over-the-counter (OTC) medications and herbal remedies
  - Note exogenous hormones
- Use of cigarettes, alcohol, or recreational drugs

Gynecological History
- Infection history
  - STIs, PID, vaginitis, vulvitis, urinary tract infection (UTI); include treatment and complications
- Endometriosis
  - Dysmenorrhea, deep dyspareunia, infertility, chronic pelvic pain, menstrual irregularities, hematochezia/hematuria, dyschezia/dysuria
- Vulvovaginal symptoms
  - Sores, lumps, itching, discharge quantity, colour, consistency, odour, and presence of blood
- Personal hygiene
  - Use of douche, vaginal sprays, deodorants, or self-medications
- Micturition
  - Day/night frequency, pain, urge/stress incontinence, hematuria
- Bowel movements
  - Regularity, laxative use, history of pain or bleeding
- History of infertility
  - Duration, cause (if known), treatments sought
- Investigations
  - Last Pap smear, history/follow-up/treatment of abnormal smear
  - Gynecological or abdominal surgery (e.g. laparoscopy, hysteroscopy, hysterectomy)

Breast Disease History – see *Breast Exam*

Obstetrical History – see *Obstetric Exam*

Family History
- History of breast cancer, ovarian cancer, endometrial cancer, or colon cancer

FOCUSED GYNECOLOGICAL EXAM

Breast Examination – see *Breast Exam*

Pelvic Examination
- No student is to perform a pelvic examination without appropriate supervision
- Explain each step in advance
- Monitor comfort of examination by watching patient's face
- Warn patient to avoid intercourse, douching or use of vaginal suppositories for 24 to 48 hours prior to examination
- Patient to empty bladder and remove all clothing below waist
- Encourage questions and feedback about comfort and pain
- Avoid terminology which can be mistaken as sexual
  - "Let your knees fall apart" not "spread your legs"
  - "Removing the speculum" not "withdrawing the blade"

Lithotomy Positioning
- Drape cover sheet from lower abdomen to knees; depress drape between knees to provide eye contact
- Patient lies supine, with head and shoulders elevated, arms at sides or folded across chest to enhance eye contact and reduce tightening of abdominal muscles
- Place heels in foot rests and slide down table until buttocks flush with table edge
- Hips flexed, abducted and externally rotated

Inspection of External Genitalia
- Inspect mons pubis, labia, perineum and perianal area for masses, nodules, pubic lice, lesions, scars, fistulas, hemorrhoids, inflammation, discharge, pigmentation
- Inspection of vagina very important to pick up vaginal carcinoma
- Note any asymmetry

Speculum Examination
- *Preparation*
  - Place smear and culture material within reach (Pap smear kit, endo-cervical brush; vaginal culture medium, glass slide gonococcal, or chlamydia: sterile cotton swab and collection tube)
  - Warm speculum under running water, test temperature on inside of patient's thigh
  - Use water to lubricate if necessary, not gel (interferes with Pap smear and cultures)
- *Insertion of speculum*
  - Use index and middle finger to separate labia and expose vaginal opening
  - Insert speculum aiming for posterior fornix, avoiding contact with urethra
  - Slide speculum inward along posterior wall of vagina, applying downward pressure to keep the vaginal introitus relaxed
  - Open blades slowly
  - Locate cervix by sweeping speculum upward; lock speculum in open position once it is well exposed
- *Inspection of cervix*
  - Note cervical colour, shape of os, discharge, polyps, lesions, ulcerations, or inflammation
  - Deviation of cervix from midline may indicate pelvic mass, uterine adhesions or pregnancy
  - Note position of cervix
    - Anterior cervix – retroverted uterus
    - Posterior cervix – anteverted uterus
- ± *Gonococcal (GC) or chlamydial culture*
  - Introduce sterile cotton swab through open speculum and insert into os
  - Hold in place for 10-30 seconds (45 seconds for chlamydia)
  - Remove swab and insert into collection tube (charcoal transport media for GC, PCR media for chlamydia)
- ± *Pap smear*
  - For best results, patient should not be menstruating
  - Inform patient she may feel an uncomfortable scraping sensation

- *Pap smear*: obtain exocervical sample
  - Most centres use new liquid based technology (ThinPrep® System) which provide an improvement in detection over traditional methods
    - Insert tapered portion of brush into cervical os
    - Rotate 360° and remove
    - Twirl brush in ThinPrep® solution to loosen cells from brush and discard brush
  - Some centres still use the traditional method
    - Insert bifid end of spatula through open speculum until it reaches cervical os
    - Rotate it 360° against cervical tissue; remove spatula
    - Spread specimen on lower half of slide
- *Pap smear*: obtain endocervical sample
  - Insert endocervical brush through open speculum into os until virtually all bristles are inside
  - Rotate brush 90° and remove
  - Smear specimen over upper half of slide, spray with fixative and label
- ± *Vaginal culture*
  - Introduce sterile cotton swab through open speculum
  - Collect any obvious secretions
  - Remove swab and insert into collection container
- *Removal of speculum and inspection of vaginal walls*
  - Unlock speculum and remove slowly, rotating to inspect vaginal walls (careful not to pinch mucosa)
  - Gradually bring blades together while simultaneously withdrawing speculum; blades should be completely closed by the time the tip of the speculum is removed
  - Maintain downward pressure of speculum to avoid injuring urethra
  - Assess support of vaginal walls. Separate labia with middle and index fingers, ask patient to bear down. Look for any bulging of vaginal walls (cystocele or rectocele)
    - Cystocele – bulging of upper two-thirds of anterior vaginal wall
    - Rectocele – herniation of rectum into posterior wall of vagina

Palpation of External Genitalia
- *Labia*
  - Spread labia majora laterally to see labia minora, introitus and outer vagina
  - Palpate labia majora between thumb and second finger to feel for masses or tenderness
  - Separate labia minora and palpate as above; palpate introitus and perineum
  - Note any fusion of minora to majora or other distortion of anatomy
- *Vagina*
  - Place forefinger 2-3 cm into vagina, gently milk urethra and Skene's glands with upward pressure (warn patient about sensation of having to urinate)
  - Rotate forefinger posteriorly, palpate Bartholin's glands between finger and thumb
  - Note colour, consistency, and odour of any gland discharge, obtain culture
  - Assess vaginal muscles by asking patient to squeeze vaginal opening around your finger (usually better in nulliparous women)

Palpation of Internal Genitalia (bimanual examination)

- Lubricate index and middle finger of gloved examining hand
- Separate labia with non-examining hand and insert examining fingers into vaginal opening, pressing downward against perineum to help muscles relax
- Keep fourth and fifth fingers flexed into palm, thumb extended
- Palpate vaginal walls and fornices as you insert fingers
  - Normally smooth, homogenous and non-tender with no masses/growths
- *Examination of the cervix*
  - Locate cervix with palmar surface of fingers
  - Feel its end and circumference for size, length and shape
  - Consistency: hard suggests nonpregnant, soft suggests pregnant
  - Position: anterior/posterior as discussed in speculum exam
  - Gently move cervix side-to-side between fingers
    - Should move 1-2 cm each way without discomfort (watch for grimace)
    - Cervical motion tenderness suggests inflammatory process
  - Evaluate os patency by trying to insert fingertip 0.5 cm

Table 1. Methods for Examination of the Uterus – Different Positions

Position	Examination Method
Anteverted (most common)	Press down with palmar surface of free hand on abdomen, between umbilicus and pubic symphysis
	Place intravaginal fingers in posterior fornix and elevate cervix and uterus to abdominal wall
	If fundus felt by abdominal hand, uterus is anteverted
Retroverted	As above; if fundus best felt by intravaginal fingers, uterus is retroverted
Midposition	As above; if fundus not felt well by either hand, uterus is midposition

- *Examination of the uterus*
  - Slide fingers of pelvic hand into anterior fornix and palpate body of uterus between your hands. In this position, your intravaginal fingers can feel anterior surface and abdominal hand can feel posterior surface
  - Once position established, assess:
    - Size (larger in multiparous women and with fibroids)
    - Shape (usually pear-shaped; globular with adenomyosis)
    - Contour (rounded and smooth if nulliparous; irregular with fibroids)
    - Mobility in AP plane (absence indicates adhesions)
    - Mobility tenderness (pelvic inflammatory process, ruptured tubal pregnancy)
- *Examination of the adnexa*
  - Shift abdominal hand to RLQ and press inward and obliquely downward towards pubic symphysis
  - With intravaginal fingers in the right lateral fornix, elevate lateral fornix up to abdominal hand
  - Assess if ovaries are palpable (see p. 98)

- If ovaries palpable, assess:
  - Size (normally 3 x 2 x 1 cm)
  - Shape (normally ovoid)
  - Consistency (normally firm, smooth)
  - Tenderness (moderately sensitive to compression)
- Normal fallopian tube not palpable
- Repeat on left – exam more difficult due to sigmoid colon

Rectovaginal Examination
- Never do rectovaginal exam before vaginal exam
- Inspect anus for lesions, hemorrhoids, or inflammation
- Warn patient of possible sensation of having a bowel movement
- Insert lubricated index finger in vagina and lubricated middle finger of same hand against anus (insert fingertip into rectum just past sphincter)
- Note sphincter tone
  - Tight – anxiety, scarring, fissures, lesions, inflammation
  - Lax – neurological deficit
  - Absent – improper repair of childbirth tear or trauma
- Slide both fingers forward; rotate rectal finger to assess rectovaginal septum and posterior vaginal wall
  - Note any tenderness, thickening, nodules, polyps, or masses
- Body of a retroflexed uterus may be palpable with rectal finger
  - Assess with intravaginal finger in posterior fornix; push up against cervix and press down with abdominal hand just above pubic symphysis
- Assess cul-de-sac and uterosacral ligaments for nodularity or tenderness
  - Possible endometriosis, PID, or metastatic carcinoma
- Repeat adnexal exam (using same maneuvers as above) if palpation difficult or questionable on bimanual examination
- Gently withdraw fingers and note any blood, secretions, or stool

Conclusion
- Tell patient exam is complete
- Help her to sit up if necessary
- Provide towel for her to wipe herself; offer pad and tell patient to expect spotting after exam
- Leave room to allow patient to re-dress
- Return to discuss the findings

COMMON INVESTIGATIONS

Blood Work
- CBC: pre-op, or to evaluate abnormal uterine bleeding, anemia, or infection
- β-hCG: to investigate possible pregnancy/ectopic pregnancy
- LH, FSH, TSH, PRL, DHEAS, testosterone, estradiol: to investigate menstrual irregularities, menopause, infertility

Imaging
- Ultrasound: transvaginal and transabdominal – examination of pelvic structures
- Hysterosalpingography (HSG): x-ray of contrast-injected uterus and tubes
- Sonohysterogram: U/S of saline-infused, expanded uterus; visualizes uterine mass, abnormalities

Colposcopy
- Endoscopic exam of vagina and cervix
- Acetic acid allows visualization of areas to biopsy for identification of dysplasia and/or neoplasia

Genital Tract Biopsy
- Vulvar, vaginal, cervical, endometrial

COMMON CLINICAL SCENARIOS

1. Physiological

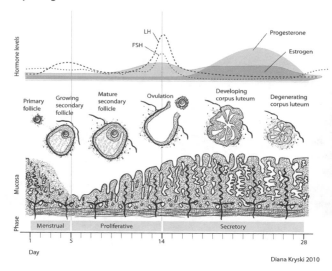

Figure 3. Normal Menstrual Cycle

Menarche

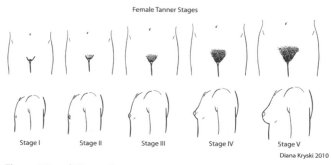

Figure 4. Female Tanner Stages

Table 2. Contraceptive Methods

Type	Effectiveness* (%)	Side Effects
Barrier	Condom alone: 90.0	Spermicide: vaginal irritation, may promote HIV transmission, messy, tastes bad, costly
	Condom with spermicide: 95.0	Diaphragm: UTI, vaginal irritation
	Spermicide alone: 82.0 Sponge: 90.0	
	Diaphragm with spermicide: 90.0	
	Lea's Shield® with spermicide: 95.0	
	Female condom: 75.0 Cervical cap: 64.0 (parous); 82.0 (nulliparous)	
Hormonal	Oral contraceptive pill (OCP): 98.0-99.5	OCP: breakthrough bleeding, nausea, headache, depression, bloating, decreased libido, increased venous thromboembolism (VTE) risk, increased stroke or MI risk in smokers and those with other risk factors
	Depo-Provera® injections: 99.0	Depo-Provera®: irregular bleeding, weight gain, mood changes, decreased bone density, delay in return of fertility (avg 9 months)
Implant	Intra-uterine device (IUD): 95.0-97.0	All: intermenstrual bleeding, expulsion, uterine wall perforation, greater chance of ectopic if pregnancy does occur, increased chance of PID in first 10 days
		Mirena®: bloating, headache
		Copper IUD: increased blood loss and duration of menses, dysmenorrhea
Surgical	Tubal ligation: 99.6	Invasive, generally permanent, surgical risks
	Essure™ System: 99.6	
	Vasectomy: 99.8	

Table 2. Contraceptive Methods (continued)

Type	Effectiveness (%)	Side Effects
Physiological	Abstinence of all sexual activity: 100.0	
	Withdrawal/Coitus interruptus: 77.0	
	Rhythm method/Calendar/Mucus/Symptothermal: 76.0	
	No method used: 10.0	
Emergency contraception	Yuzpe method: 98.0	Nausea, spotting
	"Plan B" ® Levonorgestrel only: 98.0	
	Postcoital IUD: 99.9	

*Effectiveness: percentage of women reporting no pregnancy after 1 year of use
Adapted from Dugani S, Lam D. *The Toronto Notes 2009*.

Menopause
- Retrospective diagnosis based on the lack of menses for 12 months, > age 40
- Average age for menopause is 51, with 95% of women experiencing it between the ages of 44 and 55
- 60% of menopausal women are relatively asymptomatic, while 15% experience moderate or severe symptoms
- Symptoms (mainly associated with estrogen deficiency)
  - Menstrual cycle alteration: cessation of menses for >12 months due to ovarian failure
  - Hot flushes and vasomotor instability
  - Sleep disturbances (night sweats)
  - Dyspareunia, vaginal dryness/pruritis, genital tract atrophy, vaginal bleeding
  - Increased frequency of urination, urgency, incontinence
  - Fatigue, irritability, mood changes, memory loss, decreased libido
- *Signs*
  - Skin thinning, decreased elasticity, increased facial hair, thin and brittle nails
  - Bone demineralization: osteoporosis, joint, muscle and back pain
- *Diagnosis*
  - Increased levels of FSH (>40 IU/L)
  - Decreased levels of estradiol
- *Treatment*
  - Hormone therapy (HT)
  - Selective estrogen receptor modulators (SERMs)
  - Calcium, vitamin D supplements (to decrease bone loss)
  - Bisphosphonates (if osteoporotic or osteopenic)
  - Local estrogen cream/vaginal suppository/ring, lubricants (for vaginal atrophy)
  - Non-medical (complementary medicine, exercise, counselling, healthy diet, other lifestyle modifications)

2. Pathological

Infectious

Sexually Transmitted Infections
- See **Infectious Diseases** p. 454

> **Clinical Pearl**
> If one STI is detected, other pathology or diseases may co-exist. Both
> partners must be treated for an STI to prevent recurrence.

> **Evidence-Based Medicine: HPV Vaccination**
>
>
>
> An RCT comparing the quadrivalent vaccine (HPV-6, 11, 16, 18) vs.
> placebo in young women found significantly less infection (efficacy
> 93.5% [95% CI 82.5%-98.3%]) and disease (efficacy 100% [95% CI
> 55.3%-100%]) with these strains at 5 years.
> Currently the HPV vaccine is licensed for females aged 9 to 26. Use in males is
> being studied. So far, no severe side effects have been noted.
>
> 1. Villa LL, Costa RLR, Petta CA, et al. 2005. *Lancet Oncol* 6:271–278.
> 2. Villa LL, Costa RLR, Petta CA, et al. 2006. *BJC* 95:1459-1466.

Pelvic Inflammatory Disease
- Inflammatory disorder of the uterus, fallopian tubes, and adjacent pelvic
  structures caused by direct spread of microorganisms ascending from the
  vagina and cervix
- Common organisms: *N. Gonorrhea*, *Chlamydia*, Genital Mycoplasmas
- Risk factors: young age at first intercourse, multiple partners, uterine
  instrumentation, smoking
- Complications: infertility, ectopic pregnancy, chronic pain
- *Symptoms*
  - Low abdominal or pelvic pain of recent onset that may be bilateral
  - Vaginal discharge
  - Irregular bleeding
  - Deep dyspareunia
- *Signs*
  - Fever
  - Abdominal tenderness; signs of peritoneal irritation
  - Cervical motion tenderness
  - Cervical discharge
  - Adnexal mass and/or tenderness on bimanual examination
- *Physical exam and investigations*
  - On abdo exam: look for focal tenderness/periotoneal signs
  - On speculum: look for mucopurulent dicharge
  - On pelvic exam: look for adnexal masses, cervical motion tenderness,
    adnexal tenderness

GYNECOLOGICAL

Common Neoplasms

- **BENIGN**
  - *Vulva: Lichen sclerosus*
    - Most common in post-menopausal women
    - Symptoms: pruritis, dyspareunia, burning
    - Treatment: topical steroids
  - *Cervix: Endocervical polyps*
    - Treatment: polypectomy
    - Uterus: leiomyomata (fibroids)
    - Growth from smooth muscle (monoclonal)
    - Can be submucosal, intramural, subserosal or pedunculated
    - Diagnosed in 40-50% of women >35 yrs, tend to regress after menopause
    - Clinical features: asymptomatic (60%), abnormal uterine bleeding (30%; most often from submucosal fibroid), pressure/bulk symptoms (20-50%), acute pelvic pain, infertility
    - Diagnosis: bimanual exam, CBC (anemia), ultrasound, sonohystero-gram/saline infusion hysterography
    - Treatment:
      - Conservative: useful if minimal symptoms, size <8 cm or stable
      - Medical: ibuprofen, tranexamic acid, OCP/Depo-Provera, GnRH agonists
      - Interventional radiology: uterine artery embolization
      - Surgical: myomectomy, hysterectomy
  - *Benign ovarian tumours:*
    - Mostly asymptomatic
    - May present as pain due to rupture or torsion
  - *Gestational trophoblastic neoplasms: Hydatidiform mole*
    - 80% of GTNs
    - Complete mole: 2 sperm fertilize empty egg or 1 sperm with redu-plication
      - Risk factors: maternal age >40 years, low beta carotene diet, vitamin A deficiency
      - Symptoms: vaginal bleeding, excessive uterine size, theca-lutein cysts >6 cm, pre-eclampsia, hyperemesis gravidum, hyperthyroid-ism, β-hCG >100,000, no fetal heart detected
    - Partial mole: single ovum fertilized by 2 sperm
      - Often associated with fetus that is growth restricted and has mul-tiple congenital malformations
      - Symptoms: similar to spontaneous abortion. Diagnosis often based on pathology from dilatation and curettage (D&C)
      - Diagnosis: ultrasound, β-hCG
      - Treatment: D&C with sharp curettage and oxytocin, hysterectomy if future fertility not desired, prophylactic chemotherapy (contro-versial). Rhogam if patient is Rh negative
- **MALIGNANT**
  - *Vulva*
    - 90% squamous cell carcinoma
    - 79% 5-year survival
    - Risk factors: HPV (types 16, 18), vulvar intraepithelial neoplasia (VIN)
    - Symptoms: asymptomatic, localized pruritis, lump, or mass, raised red, white or pigmented plaque, ulcer, bleeding, discharge, pain, dysuria

- *Cervix*
  - 95% squamous carcinoma
  - Mean age 52 years
  - Risk factors: HPV infection (high risk types 16, 18), smoking, high risk sexual behaviour
  - Symptoms:
    - Early: asymptomatic, discharge (watery, becoming brown or red), post-coital bleeding
    - Late: bleeding (post-coital, post-menopausal, irregular), pelvic or back pain, bladder/bowel symptoms
  - Prevention: regular Pap smears
  - Diagnosis: Pap screening, colposcopy, endocervical curettage, cervical biopsy, cone biopsy
- *Uterus: Endometrial carcinoma*
  - Most common gynecological malignancy
  - Mean age 60
  - 60-70% 5-year survival
  - Symptoms: post-menopausal bleeding, abnormal uterine bleeding
  - Diagnosis: endometrial biopsy, D&C ± hysteroscopy
  - Treatment:
    - Stage 1: total abdominal hysterectomy (TAH)/bilateral salpingo-oophorectomy (BSO) and washings
    - Stages 2 and 3: TAH/BSO, washings, and nodal dissection
    - Stage 4: Non-surgical
    - Adjuvant radiotherapy: based on myometrial penetration, tumour grade, lymph node involvement
    - Hormonal therapy: progestins for distant or recurrent disease
    - Adjuvant chemotherapy: based on disease progression

Clinical Pearl
Vaginal bleeding in post-menopausal women is endometrial cancer until proven otherwise.

- *Ovary*
  - 4th leading cause of cancer death in women. Overall 5 yr survival 15% if >50 yrs due to late diagnosis
  - Symptoms: usually asymptomatic until advanced (Stage III)
    - Early: vague abdominal symptoms (nausea, bloating, dyspepsia, anorexia, early satiety), postmenopausal or irregular bleeding (rare)
    - Late: increased abdominal girth, urinary frequency, constipation, ascites
  - Investigation: bimanual exam, CBC, LFTs, electrolytes, creatinine, CA-125, CXR, abdominal/pelvic U/S ± transvaginal U/S
- *Gestational trophoblastic neoplasms*
  - 15% locally invasive, 5% metastatic
  - Invasive mole or persistent GTN
    - Diagnosis: increase or plateau in β-hCG following treatment of molar pregnancy, molar tissue on histology
  - Choriocarcinoma: May follow any type of pregnancy, highly anaplastic
    - Diagnosis: CBC, electrolytes, creatinine, β-hCG, TSH, LFTs, CXR, pelvic U/S, CT abdomen/pelvis, CT head
    - Treatment: chemotherapy

Inflammatory

Endometriosis
- Affects 5-10% of reproductive-age women and 25-35% of women with infertility
- History of cyclic pelvic pain and dysmenorrhea supports the diagnosis but needs to be distinguished from chronic pelvic pain
- Symptoms: pelvic pain, dysmenorrhea (worsens with age), infertility, deep dyspareunia, premenstrual and postmenstrual spotting, increased frequency of urination, dysuria, hematuria, diarrhea, constipation, hematochezia
- Signs: tender nodularity of uterine ligaments and cul-de-sac, fixed retroversion of the uterus, firm, fixed adnexal mass (endometrioma)
- Diagnosis: responds to medical treatment (presumptive), laparoscopy ± histology (definitive)
- Treatment:
  - Medical: 1st line – NSAIDs, OCP (cyclic/continuous), progestin therapy (oral or injection), 2nd line – anti-estrogen agents (e.g. Danazol), gonadotropin releasing hormone agonists
  - Surgical: laparoscopic resection/vaporization/ablation of implants, removal of adhesions

Infertility
- A couple's failure to conceive after 1 year of unprotected sexual intercourse
- Approximately 40% due to a male factor, 40% due to a female factor, and 20% due to both male and female contributing causes, 10-15% unexplained
- Symptoms/signs: often asymptomatic; not recognized until pregnancy attempts unsuccessful
- Etiology and diagnosis
  - Ovulatory dysfunction (20-40% of cases)
    - Includes: hyperprolactinemia, thyroid disease, PCOS, luteal phase defects, certain systemic diseases, congenital diseases, poor nutrition, stress, excessive exercise, premature ovarian failure
    - Diagnosis: serum PRL, TSH, LH, FSH; history of cycle patterns, basal body temperature, mucus quality, endometrial biopsy for luteal phase defect, serum progesterone level, karyotype, liver and renal function
  - Tubal factors (20-30% of cases)
    - Includes: PID, adhesions, tubal ligation, previous gynecological surgery
    - Diagnosis: hysterosalpingogram, sonohysterogram, laparoscopy with dye
  - Cervical factors (<5% of cases)
    - Includes: structural abnormalities, anti-sperm antibodies, hostile acidic cervical mucous, glands unresponsive to estrogen
    - Diagnosis: post-coital test
  - Uterine factors (<5% of cases)
    - Includes: polyps, infection, intrauterine adhesions, congenital anomalies, leiomyomata
    - Diagnosis: hysterosalpingogram, sonohysterogram, hysteroscopy

GYNECOLOGICAL

Other Infectious Diseases

Candidiasis
- Overgrowth of yeast in the vagina
- Common organisms: *Candida albicans* (90%), *Candida tropicalis*, *Candida glabrata*
- Predisposing factors: immunosuppression, antibiotic use, pregnancy
- Symptoms
  - Asymptomatic (20%)
  - Itching, burning
  - White, curdy, "cottage cheese" discharge
- Investigations
  - pH test: pH ≤4.5
  - Wet mount: 50-60% sensitive; can see budding yeast, hyphae, pseudo-hyphae
  - Culture: higher sensitivity than wet mount; can identify species of yeast
- Treatment
  - Topical azole drugs most effective
    - Available as ovules and creams for 1, 3, or 7 days
  - Oral therapy also available
  - Treat male partner only if yeast balanitis present

Bacterial Vaginosis
- Replacement of normal vaginal flora with other organisms
- Common organisms: *Gardnerella vaginalis*, *Mycoplasma hominis*, certain anaerobes
- Symptoms
  - Malodourous
  - Thin, white/grey adherent discharge
  - Possible itching
- Investigations
  - pH test: pH >4.5
  - Wet mount: clue cells with adherent coccoid bacteria
  - KOH whiff test: fishy odour
- Treatment
  - Metronidazole
  - No treatment for male partner

GYNECOLOGICAL

REFERENCES

Dawson AE. 2004. Can we change the way we screen?: the ThinPrep Imaging System. Cancer 102(6):340-344.

Dugani S, Lam D (eds.) 2009. *The Toronto Notes 2009: Comprehensive Medical Reference*. Toronto: Toronto Notes for Medical Students, Inc.

Manson JE, Hsia J, Johnson KC, Rossouw JE, Assaf AR, Lasser NL, Trevisan M, Black HR, Heckbert SR, Detrano R, Strickland OL, Wong ND, Crouse JR, Stein E, Cushman M. 2003. Estrogen plus progestin and the risk of coronary heart disease. *N Engl J Med* 349(6):523-534.

McLachlin CM, Mai V, Murphy J, Fung-Kee-Fung M, Chambers A, Oliver TK. 2007. Ontario cervical cancer screening clinical practice guidelines. *J Obstet Gynaecol Can* 29(4):344-353.

Nanda K, McCrory DC, Myers ER, Bastian LA, Hasselblad V, Hickey JD, Matchar DB. 2000. Accuracy of the Papanicolaou test in screening for and follow-up of cervical cytologic abnormalities: a systematic review. *Ann Intern Med* 132(10):810-819.

Villa LL, Costa RL, Petta CA, Andrade RP, Ault KA, Giuliano AR, Wheeler CM, Koutsky LA, Malm C, Lehtinen M, Skjeldestad FE, Olsson SE, Steinwall M, Brown DR, Kurman RJ, Ronnett BM, Stoler MH, Ferenczy A, Harper DM, Tamms GM, Yu J, Lupinacci L, Railkar R, Taddeo FJ, Jansen KU, Esser MT, Sings HL, Saah AJ, Barr E. 2005. Prophylactic quadrivalent human papillomavirus (types 6, 11, 16, and 18) L1 virus-like particle vaccine in young women: a randomised double-blind placebo-controlled multicentre phase II efficacy trial. *Lancet Oncol* 6(5): 271-278.

Villa LL, Costa RL, Petta CA, Andrade RP, Paavonen J, Iversen OE, Olsson SE, Høye J, Steinwall M, Riis-Johannessen G, Andersson-Ellstrom A, Elfgren K, Krogh G, Lehtinen M, Malm C, Tamms GM, Giacoletti K, Lupinacci L, Railkar R, Taddeo FJ, Bryan J, Esser MT, Sings HL, Saah AJ, Barr E. 2006. High sustained efficacy of a prophylactic quadrivalent human papillomavirus types 6/11/16/18 L1 virus-like particle vaccine through 5 years of follow-up. *BJC* 95(11):1459-1466.

The Head and Neck Exam

Editors:
Vinay Fernandes, Modupe Oyewumi, & Jenny Wang

Faculty Reviewers:
Kevin M. Higgins, MD, FRCS(C)
Allan D. Vescan, MD, FRCS(C)

TABLE OF CONTENTS

Approach to the History and Physical Exam of the Head and Neck   107
Ear   108
Nose   114
Oral Cavity and Pharynx   116
Neck   120
Thyroid   123
Common Clinical Scenarios   125

APPROACH TO THE HISTORY AND PHYSICAL EXAM OF THE HEAD AND NECK

A consistent systemic approach to the clinical examination of the head and neck is essential to ensure completeness. In addition to general history taking, important aspects of the head and neck exam include:

EAR

History
- Subjective hearing loss
- Ear infection (acute, chronic)
- Recent URTI
- Discharge from ear (otorrhea)
- Pain (otalgia)
- Dizziness (± true vertigo)
- Ringing in the ear (tinnitus)
- Aural fullness

Physical
- External ear exam: inspection, palpation
- Auditory acuity testing: Whisper test, Rinne test, Weber test
- Otoscopic examination: tympanic membrane
- Cranial nerve testing I-XII
- Romberg's test
- Gait analysis
- Dix-Hallpike test

NOSE

History
- Sinus infection (acute, chronic)
- Nasal obstruction (unilateral, bilateral)
- Characterize discharge from nose
- Associated symptoms (e.g. facial pain, anosmia, postnasal drip)
- Environmental/occupational exposures including smoking

Physical
- External and internal exams
- Nasal speculum
- CN I (if indicated)

HEAD & NECK

THROAT (NECK, ORAL CAVITY AND PHARYNX)

History
- Neck mass (lateral vs. midline)
- Neck stiffness (nuchal rigidity)
- Oral cavity mass or ulcer
- Features of hyper/hypothyroidism
- Cough
- Hoarseness
- Respiratory obstruction
- Environmental/occupational exposures

Physical
- Inspection (oral cavity, pharynx, larynx)
- Palpation (lymph nodes, oral cavity, tongue, thyroid, salivary glands)
- Auscultation (carotid and thyroid bruits)
- CN VII, IX, X

EAR

Essential Anatomy

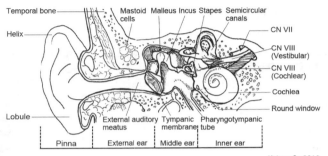

Kaiyan Su 2010

Figure 1. Cross Section of the Right Ear

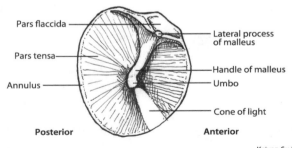

Kaiyan Su 2010

Figure 2. Tympanic Membrane of the Right Ear

Common Chief Complaints

Disorders marked with (✓) are discussed in **Common Clinical Scenarios**

- Ear pain (otalgia)
- Ear discharge (otorrhea)
- Ringing, whistling, blowing or humming in the ears (tinnitus)
✓ Dizziness
- Hearing loss

Focused History

For all otological complaints:

- See **Table 1** below
- Unilateral vs. bilateral (Note: always be cautious of anything unilateral)
- Onset, duration, progression, frequency
- Accompanying vestibular symptoms
- Previous surgery
- Recent or past head/ear trauma
- Noise exposure
- Family history
- Medications (especially ototoxic meds, e.g. aminoglycosides)
- Systemic diseases (e.g. multiple sclerosis, SLE, diabetes)
- Infection (local, systemic)

Table 1. Focused History for Specific Otological Complaints

Complaint	Focused History	Differential Diagnosis
Otalgia	OPQRSTUVW Hyperacusis (painful sensitivity to ordinary sound levels) Otorrhea (see below) Dizziness/Imbalance (see below)	**Local causes:** Acute otitis media (recent history of URTI) Acute mastoiditis (>2 wks after untreated AOM) Otitis externa (Swimmer's ear) Foreign body or impacted cerumen in canal **Referred from CN V, VII, IX, X (Ten Ts+2):** Eustachian **T**ube **T**MJ syndrome (pain in front of the ears) **T**rismus (spasm of masticator muscles, early symptom of tetanus) **T**eeth **T**ongue **T**onsils (tonsillitis, tonsillar cancer, posttonsillectomy) **T**ic (glossopharyngeal neuralgia) **T**hroat (cancer of larynx) **T**rachea (foreign body, tracheitis) **T**hyroiditis Geniculate herpes and Ramsay Hunt syndrome type 2 ± CN VII palsy (Bell's Palsy)

HEAD & NECK

Table 1. Focused History for Specific Otological Complaints (continued)

Complaint	Focused History	Differential Diagnosis
Otorrhea	Quality (colour, smell, quantity, consistency) Diabetes, elderly, immunocompromized (suspect necrotizing otitis externa) Recent ear or throat infection Recent otalgia Headache ± fever Pruritis in the ear Hearing loss Duration of symptoms Any recent above-shoulder body trauma Swimming injury	**Purulent discharge**: mastoiditis with tympanic membrane perforation, otitis externa with tympanic membrane perforation, cholesteatoma with tympanic membrane, acute and chronic suppurative otitis media, necrotizing otitis externa (Note: medical emergency) **Non-purulent discharge**: CSF leakage (head trauma), foreign body, invasive otitis externa **Bloody discharge**: hemorrhage (head trauma), barotrauma, foreign body, external trauma
Tinnitus (ear ringing)	Subjective vs. objective ear ringing Characteristic of ear sound (ringing, buzzing or hissing) Constant vs. intermittent Duration Unilateral vs. bilateral Hx of head trauma Hx of anxiety Medication Hx Presence/absence of vertigo Presence/absence of hearing loss Presence/absence of other neurological signs/ symptoms	**SUBJECTIVE (heard by patient; common)** **Otologic**: OME, otosclerosis, presbycusis, Meniere's disease, cerumen, noise-induced hearing loss **Drugs**: aminoglycosides, NSAIDs, antimalarials, heavy metals, antidepressants, loop diuretics, cisplatin-based chemotherapy, erythromycin **Metabolic**: hyperlipidemia, vitamin A deficiency, vitamin B deficiency **Neurologic**: head trauma, multiple sclerosis, meningitis, temporal lobe tumour, acoustic neuroma **Psychiatric**: anxiety, depression **OBJECTIVE (heard by others; rare)** **Muscular**: stapedius spasm, palatal myoclonus **Vascular**: arterial bruits, venous hums, ateriovenous malformation
Hearing loss	See **Table 2** (Conductive) and **Table 3** (Sensorineural)	
Dizziness/ Imbalance	See **Common Clinical Scenarios** p. 125	

Table 2. Conductive Hearing Loss

Differential Diagnosis	History	Otoscopic Examination
Physical obstruction (wax, foreign body)	Sudden (foreign body) or gradual (wax) painless loss	Obstruction visible in canal
Congenital (atresia of auditory canal, ossicular abnormalities)	Hearing loss present since birth	Various abnormalities
Tympanic membrane perforation (cholesteatoma, trauma, untreated infection)	Painless hearing loss (± pain prior to membrane perforation) History of ear infections/trauma Chronic drainage	Perforation is usually visible (check periphery)
Otitis externa (bacterial or fungal infection of the external auditory canal)	Sudden painful loss Moisture (swimming) Trauma (foreign bodies)	Narrow canal with debris Canal erythema Variable discharge Note: pain on moving pinna (vs. OM)
Otitis media (OME, AOM – viral, bacterial infection)	Sudden painful loss	Tympanic membrane: decreased mobility, red or yellow, bulging, injected or cloudy
Otosclerosis	Gradual painless loss	Normal otoscopy Audiogram: Carhart's notch (sensorineural loss at 2 kHz)
Glomus tumour/ Vascular abnormality	Gradual painless loss	Intact tympanic membrane Red-blue, pulsating mass behind tympanic membrane

Table 3. Sensorineural Hearing Loss

Differential Diagnosis	History/Physical Findings	Audiogram
Acoustic neuroma (CN VIII schwannoma)	Gradual unilateral hearing loss Tinnitus is common Unsteadiness (vertigo uncommon) Facial nerve palsy (late finding)	Gradual, asymmetric, sensorineural loss Unilateral
Congenital causes: genetic, ischemia, prenatal infection – TORCH, toxins	Present at birth	U-shaped or "cookie-bite" audiogram (hearing is better in low and high frequencies than in the middle frequencies)
Meniere's disease (idiopathic endolymphatic hydrops)	Unilateral, sudden, fluctuating, progressive loss Episodic tinnitus Episodic aural fullness Episodic vertigo ± nausea, vomiting	Low-frequency loss "peaking" (tent-shaped) or flat audiogram Unilateral

Table 3. Sensorineural Hearing Loss (continued)

Differential Diagnosis	History/Physical Findings	Audiogram
Noise-induced	Gradual onset Tinnitus common History of noise exposure (occupational, recreational)	Boiler maker's notch (loss centered at 4 kHz) Bilateral and symmetric
Ototoxic medications (e.g. aminoglycosides)	± tinnitus ± vertigo	High frequency loss Typically bilateral
Presbycusis (age-related hearing loss)	Gradual onset Noise exposure Tobacco use	High frequency loss Bilateral
Sudden sensorineural hearing loss* (e.g. idiopathic, viral, autoimmune, vascular, trauma)	Sudden onset <3 days 65% of patients recover hearing spontaneously	Loss >30 dB in three contiguous frequencies

*Medical emergency
TORCH = toxoplasmosis, others (e.g. HIV), rubella, cytomegalovirus, herpes simplex

Focused Physical Exam

External Exam

Inspection
- Pinna for size, position, deformity, inflammation, symmetry, nodules, scars or lesions
  - e.g. microtia, macrotia, cauliflower ear
- External auditory canal
- Look for presence of ear discharge: colour, consistency, clarity, presence or absence of an odour

Palpation
- Pinna, periauricular area and mastoid process for tenderness, nodules or inflammation
  - Pain elicited by tugging on pinna/tragus
  - Pain over the mastoid associated with an outward and inferior protrusion of the pinna and discharge

Auditory Acuity Testing
For Weber and Rinne testing, strike a 512Hz tuning fork on bony prominence (e.g. patella/styloid process of radius). Do not place tuning fork over hair.

Whisper Test
- Lightly rub your fingers together next to the ear NOT being tested and ask the patient to repeat what you whisper into tested ear
- If the patient cannot hear, continue to increase the volume of your voice until it is heard by the patient
- Repeat on other ear

Weber Test: tests sound lateralization
- Place the base of the tuning fork on the centre of the patient's forehead
- Ask the patient if they hear the sound louder on one side OR if it is equal on both sides
- Normal hearing = no sound lateralization (patient hears sound or feels vibration in middle)
- Conductive hearing loss = sound lateralization to AFFECTED ear
- Sensorineural hearing loss = sound lateralization to NON-AFFECTED ear

Rinne Test: compares air vs. bone conduction
- Apply tuning fork against the patient's mastoid process, then place it still vibrating next to the patient's ear (abbreviated version)
- Ask the patient to identify which placement sounds louder
- Repeat with opposite ear
- Rinne positive (normal) = air > bone conduction
- Rinne negative* (conductive hearing loss) = bone > air conduction
- Partial sensorineural hearing loss = air > bone conduction (but both decreased)

* Complete hearing loss in one ear in which patient may still process bone conduction that is picked up by contralateral cochlea is known as "false-negative Rinne"

Otoscopic Exam
- Examine:
  - External auditory meatus (foreign body, wax, inflammatory, discharge)
  - Tympanic membrane (see **Table 4** below)
- Techniques:
  - Use largest speculum that can be comfortably inserted to maximize visual field and to avoid irritation of bony canal
  - *Adults*: gently pull the pinna backwards and upwards
  - *Children*: gently pull the pinna backwards and slightly downwards
  - Stabilize otoscope by placing fifth digit against patient's cheek to protect against sudden movements

Table 4. Otoscopic Examination of the Tympanic Membrane

Inspect	Normal	Abnormal
Colour	Translucent and pearly grey	Red (hyperemia due to inflammation, fever, valsalva/crying/screaming) Yellow (pus in middle ear, suggests OME) Blue (glomus jugulare, glomus tympanicum)
Light reflex	Cone of light directed anteriorly and inferiorly	Absent/distorted (abnormal geometry due to bulging or retraction, perforation, thickening)
Landmarks	Pars flaccida Malleus (near centre) Incus (posterior to malleus)	Obscured landmarks may indicate inflammation, fluid/pus in middle ear or membrane thickening
Abnormal margins	Clear and tense margins	Perforation (untreated ear infection, cholesteatoma, trauma – e.g. cotton swab use)
Mobility	Brisk, equal movement with positive and negative pressure using pneumatic otoscopy	Reduced/absent mobility: increased middle ear pressure (mucoid, serous or purulent effusion) Increased mobility: negative middle ear pressure (Eustachian tube dysfunction)
Shape	Drawn inwards slightly at centre by handle of malleus	Bulging: suggests pus/fluid in middle ear Retraction: Eustachian tube dysfunction resulting in negative middle ear pressure

HEAD & NECK

NOSE

Essential Anatomy

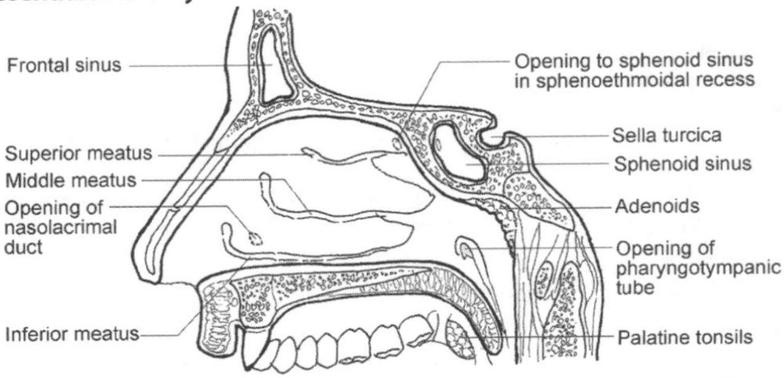

Labels (clockwise from left):
- Frontal sinus
- Superior meatus
- Middle meatus
- Opening of nasolacrimal duct
- Inferior meatus
- Opening to sphenoid sinus in sphenoethmoidal recess
- Sella turcica
- Sphenoid sinus
- Adenoids
- Opening of pharyngotympanic tube
- Palatine tonsils

Kaiyan Su 2010

Figure 3. Anatomy of the Right Nasal Cavity (lateral aspect)

Common Chief Complaints

Disorders marked with (✓) are discussed in **Common Clinical Scenarios**
- ✓ Nosebleeds (epistaxis)
- Stuffy nose (congestion)
- Loss of smell (anosmia)
- Facial pain
- Nasal discharge (rhinorrhea)

Focused History

- A focused history should be based on the chief complaint (see **Table 5**)

Table 5. Focused History for Nose and Sinuses

Chief Complaint	Focused History	Differential Diagnosis
Nasal obstruction	Congestion or stuffiness Nasal discharge, "runny nose" Facial tenderness/pain Noisy breathing, snoring Pruritus of nose, eyes (allergies)	**Common:** Acute/chronic allergic or vasomotor rhinitis (rhinitis medicamentosa) Septal deviation Adenoid/Inferior turbinate hypertrophy **Less Common:** Polyps, foreign bodies, trauma, enlarged turbinates **Rare:** Neoplasm (nasopharynx, nasal cavity) Septal hematoma or abscess
Rhinorrhea	Duration Exacerbating and alleviating factors Allergies Character and colour Associated facial pain	**Watery/mucoid (most common):** Allergic, viral or vasomotor rhinitis CSF (fracture of cribriform plate) **Mucopurulent (less common):** Bacterial infection, foreign body **Serosanguinous (rare):** Neoplasm, infectious (e.g. mucormycosis) **Bloody (rare):** Trauma, coagulopathy, hypertension/vascular disease, neoplasm

Table 5. Focused History for Nose and Sinuses (continued)

Chief Complaint	Focused History	Differential Diagnosis
Sinus/Facial pain	Rhinorrhea, purulent discoloured nasal discharge Post-nasal drip, cough Hyposmia/Anosmia Fever Diabetic, immuno-compromised, bone marrow recipient	Acute rhinosinusitis (commonly maxillary and anterior ethmoid sinuses) Chronic Sinusitis (>12 w, bacterial/fungal) Frontal, ethmoid, sphenoid acute bacterial rhinosinusitis* Mucormycosis** (invasive fungal infection common in diabetic, immunocompromised, and bone marrow recipients; rare in normal population)
Anosmia	Unilateral vs. bilateral Onset Associated neurological symptoms Recent head trauma, clear fluid on pillow Rhinorrhea	Nasal obstruction/congestion (URTI, polyps, enlarged turbinates, ethmoid tumour, rhinosinusitis) Head trauma (fracture of cribriform plate) Kallman's syndrome (congenital anosmia) Intracranial pathology (meningitis, hydrocephalus, frontal lobe tumour, meningioma of olfactory groove)
Epistaxis	See **Common Clinical Scenarios** p. 126	

*Requires aggressive management
**Medical emergency

> **Clinical Pearl**
> The allergic salute is a horizontal nasal crease below the bridge of the nose in children that results from persistent upward rubbing of the nose secondary to allergic rhinitis.

Focused Physical Exam

External Exam

Inspection
- Note any swelling, trauma, deviation and congenital abnormalities
- Extend patient's neck and examine the symmetry of the nares

Palpation
- Test airway patency: occlude one nostril and ask the patient to sniff then exhale and look for mirror fogging or movement of cotton wisp

Internal Exam: Nasal Speculum
- Hold speculum in nondominant hand and introduce horizontally, 1 cm into the vestibule. Place index finger of nondominant hand atop nose to anchor speculum
- Note any swelling, trauma, deviation, masses, discharge or congenital abnormalities
- Olfactory exam: UPSIT test (standardized scratch and sniff test)

HEAD & NECK

Inspection
- Septum for deviation or perforation
- Mucous membranes: normally pink, moist and smooth; blue/grey with allergies; red with inflammation
- Little's area for vascular engorgement or crusting (indicates recent epistaxis)
- Turbinates for size and colour (black turbinates may indicate mucormycosis)
- Presence of nasal polyps (greyish colour)
- Turbinates are rarely symmetric; asymmetry on inspection is frequently normal

ORAL CAVITY AND PHARYNX

Common Chief Complaints
Disorders marked with (✓) are discussed in **Common Clinical Scenarios**
- Cough
- Sore throat (pharyngitis)
- Difficulty swallowing (dysphagia)
- Painful swallowing (odynophagia)
- Lump (globus hystericus)
- ✓ Hoarseness

Focused History
- For all oral cavity and pharynx complaints, ask about hemoptysis, constitutional symptoms, and lifestyle habits (smoking, alcohol) (see **Table 6**)

Table 6. Focused History for Oral Cavity and Pharynx

Chief Complaint	Focused History	Differential Diagnosis
Cough	Onset and duration Worse day or night Dry or productive (volume, colour, odour, consistency, pus) Dyspnea and/or chest pain Environmental/ Occupational exposures (asbestos, radiation)	URTI (e.g. pharyngitis, bronchitis) Pneumonia COPD Tuberculosis Rhinosinusitis, post-nasal drip Neoplasms (e.g. primary or secondary lung, breast, laryngeal)
Pharyngitis	OPQRSTUVW Signs of infection (e.g. fever, malaise, anorexia, halitosis) Cough, acute or chronic Referred otalgia Neck lymphadenopathy Splenomegaly (EBV) Trismus, "hot potato" voice (peritonsillar abscess)	Otitis media Viral pharyngitis (EBV, HSV) Bacterial pharyngitis (strep throat) Tonsillitis Peritonsillar abscess (quinsy) Radiation-induced

Table 6. Focused History for Oral Cavity and Pharynx (continued)

Chief Complaint	Focused History	Differential Diagnosis
Dysphagia	Mass (painful, painless) Fluctuating pain with meals Regurgitation Aspiration Hoarseness Noisy breathing, drooling (suspect epiglottitis)	**Pharyngeal Causes:** Oro/Naso/Hypopharyngeal neoplasm Ranula (salivary pseudocyst from blocked sublingual gland) Epiglottitis*/Supraglottitis Retropharyngeal or peritonsillar abscess Ludwig's angina* Foreign body **Esophageal Causes:** See *Abdominal Exam*
Globus hystericus	Dysphagia (± odynophagia) Nocturnal cough Hoarseness Referred otalgia	Reflux laryngitis/ Laryngopharyngeal reflux Naso/Oro/Hypopharyngeal neoplasm Thyroid mass Functional Rhinosinusitis post-nasal drip (associated with nocturnal cough)

*Medical emergencies – must first ensure secure airway before examination

Focused Physical Exam
- Routine examination of the oral cavity is important as 30% of patients with oral carcinoma are asymptomatic

Inspection (see **Table 7**)
- Adequate lighting is required
- Ask patient to remove dentures if present
- If discharge present, note volume, colour, odour, consistency and presence of blood

HEAD & NECK

Table 7. Inspection of the Oral Cavity and Pharynx

Anatomical Region	Method of Inspection	Features to Assess
Oral cavity (lips, tongue, inside cheek, teeth, floor of mouth, gingivae, palate)	Inspect entire oral cavity visually using two tongue depressors	General (lesions, lumps, ulcers, purulence, blood, gum disease, xerostomia = dry mouth) Lips (colour, pigmentation, symmetry, lesions, edema, ulcers, sores, lumps, fissures) Tongue (lesions, size, lumps, atrophy, fasciculations, symmetry) Teeth (number, size, wasting, pitting) Palate (perforation, edema, petechiae) Buccal mucosa (white lesions)
Palatine tonsils (between anterior and posterior pillars)	Inspect visually using tongue depressor	Enlargement, injection, exudate, ulcerations, crypts
Salivary apparatus (parotid gland, submandibular gland)	Direct – bimanual with two tongue depressors	Gland enlargement Lumps, masses, lesions Painful or painless mass Discharge, salivary production Salivary stones Ranula
Posterior nasopharynx (posterior nasal choanae, posterior nasopharyngeal wall, Eustachian tube orifices)	Indirect laryngoscopy and tongue depressor or flexible nasopharyngoscopy	Nasal polyps Lesions Ulceration Inflammation, edema Purulence, blood
Hypopharynx/larynx (posterior tongue, epiglottis, piriform fossa, vocal cords, false cords, posterior and lateral pharyngeal walls)	Indirect laryngoscopy and tongue depressor or flexible nasopharyngoscopy	Lesions, nodules Inflammation Ulceration Leukoplakia

Palpation
- With a gloved hand, palpate inside the mouth using one finger and use the opposite hand to follow alongside on the surface of the face
- Examine for texture, tenderness, masses and lesions including plaques, vesicles, nodules and ulcerations
- Follow a systemic approach: palpate the vermilion of the lips, the inner mucosa of lips, mandible, cheeks, roof of mouth, floor of mouth, top of tongue, floor of mandible as far as the angle of the jaw, tonsils (ask patient not to bite)
- Salivary apparatus
  - Parotid and submandibular glands (enlargement, masses, tenderness, salivary stones)
  - Examine the orifice of each gland:
    - Stenson's duct (parotid duct orifice) opposite upper second molar on buccal mucosa
    - Wharton's duct (submandibular duct orifice) lateral to frenulum of tongue on floor of mouth

- Massage the gland and observe the discharge from each orifice:
  - Clear vs. cloudy
  - Pain on palpation of the gland
- The most common salivary tumour is of the parotid gland and typically presents as a firm, nontender mass anterior to the ear with normal overlying skin

Motor Exam (see **Neurological Exam** p. 186)
- Gag reflex (CN IX/X)
- Equal palatal elevation (CN X)
- Central tongue protrusion (CN XII)

Common Investigations of the Oropharynx
- See **Table 8**

Table 8. Investigations for Mouth and Throat Pathology

Indication	Test
Infection	CBC and differential
Sore throat with fever >38°C Swollen, red tonsils with exudate Peritonsillar abscess	Throat swab and culture (sensitivity for GAS 80-90%)
Suspected neoplasm (neck mass, salivary gland, thyroid) Note: diagnosis of follicular adenoma (thyroid) not possible with FNAB	Fine needle aspiration biopsy (FNAB)
Salivary stone >90% submandibular calculi are radiopaque >90% parotid calculi are radiolucent	Plain Film Ultrasound CT
Neoplasm (Hx smoking, smokeless tobacco, alcohol), salivary stone, abscess, branchial cleft cyst/sinus	CT/MRI Bone scan if mandible involved

Evidence-Based Medicine: Strep Throat
McIsaac modification of the Centor Strep Score (prospectively validated in a mixed population of adults and children and compared to throat swab culture)

Symptom or Sign	Points
• History of fever or measured temperature >38°C	1
• Absence of cough	1
• Swollen, tender, anterior cervical adenopathy	1
• Tonsillar swelling or exudate	1
• Age 3-14 years	1
• Age ≥45 years	−1

Total Points	Likelihood Ratio	Management
-1 or 0	0.05	No further testing or antibiotic required
1	0.52	
2	0.95	Culture ALL; antibiotics only for positive results
3	2.5	
4 or 5	4.9	Treat empirically with antibiotics

McIsaac WJ et al. 2004. *JAMA* 291(13): 1587-1595.

NECK

Essential Anatomy

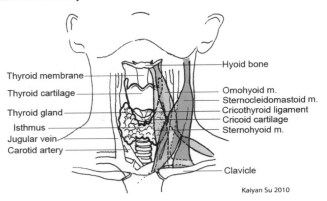

Thyroid membrane
Thyroid cartilage
Thyroid gland
Isthmus
Jugular vein
Carotid artery

Hyoid bone
Omohyoid m.
Sternocleidomastoid m.
Cricothyroid ligament
Cricoid cartilage
Sternohyoid m.
Clavicle

Kaiyan Su 2010

Figure 4. Anatomy of the Neck

Table 9. Lymph Node Groups and Levels of the Head and Neck (see **Figure 5**)

Nodal Group/Level	Location	Drainage
Occipital	Base of skull, posterior	Posterior scalp
Posterior auricular	Superficial to mastoid process	Scalp, temporal region, external auditory meatus, posterior pinna
Preauricular	In front of ear	External auditory meatus, anterior pinna, soft tissues of frontal and temporal regions, root of nose, eyelids, palpebral conjunctiva
Submental (Level IA)	(Midline) Anterior bellies of digastric muscles, tip of mandible and hyoid bone	Floor of mouth, anterior oral tongue, anterior mandibular alveolar ridge, lower lip
Submandibular (Level IB)	Anterior belly of digastric muscle, stylohyoid muscle, body of mandible	Oral cavity, anterior nasal cavity, soft tissues of the mid-face, submandibular gland
Upper jugular (Levels IIA and IIB)	Skull base to inferior border of hyoid bone along sternocleidomastoid (SCM) muscle	Oral cavity, nasal cavity, naso/oro/hypopharynx, larynx, parotid glands
Middle jugular (Level III)	Inferior border of hyoid bone to inferior border of cricoid cartilage along SCM muscle	Oral cavity, naso/oro/hypopharynx, larynx
Lower jugular (Level IV)	Inferior border of cricoid cartilage to clavicle along SCM muscle	Hypopharynx, thyroid, cervical esophagus, larynx
Posterior triangle* (Levels VA and VB)	Posterior border of SCM, anterior border of trapezius, from skull base to clavicle	Nasopharynx and oropharynx, cutaneous structures of the posterior scalp and neck
Anterior compartment** (Levels VI)	(Midline) Hyoid bone to suprasternal notch between the common carotid arteries	Thyroid gland, glottic and subglottic larynx, apex of piriform sinus, cervical esophagus

* Includes some supraclavicular nodes
**Contains Virchow, pretracheal, precricoid paratracheal and perithyroidal nodes

HEAD & NECK

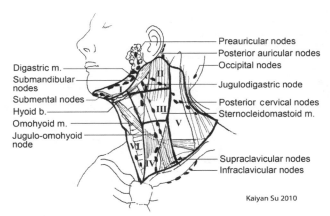

Preauricular nodes
Posterior auricular nodes
Occipital nodes
Jugulodigastric node
Posterior cervical nodes
Sternocleidomastoid m.
Supraclavicular nodes
Infraclavicular nodes

Digastric m.
Submandibular nodes
Submental nodes
Hyoid b.
Omohyoid m.
Jugulo-omohyoid node

Kaiyan Su 2010

Figure 5. Lymph Node Groups and Levels of the Head and Neck

Common Chief Complaints

- Stiff neck (nuchal rigidity)
- Neck lump
- Neck swelling
- Neck pain

Focused History

Neck Stiffness

- Headache (if no other signs/symptoms, suspect tension headache)
- Fever (if present, assess for meningitis, see ***Essentials of Infectious Diseases*** p. 463)
- Cardiovascular history (referred pain from angina or myocardial infarct)
- If associated with focal neurological symptoms, suspect CVA

Neck Mass

- Location: lateral vs. midline (see **Table 10**)
- Age of patient
    - Young (<40): congenital or inflammatory, neoplasms rare
    - Adult: neck mass malignant until proven otherwise
- Onset, tenderness and rate of growth
    - A tender mass with rapid onset of swelling is suggestive of an inflammatory, acute infectious etiology or metastasis
    - A nontender, slow-growing mass is suggestive of a malignancy
- Constitutional symptoms (fever, chills, night sweats, weight loss)
- Risk factors for cancer (e.g. tobacco use, alcohol, radiation)
- Presence of recurrent head and neck infection (e.g. HPV, EBV)
- Cough, hemoptysis, bone pain
- See ***Essentials of Endocrinology*** p. 422 for thyroid disorders

Table 10. Differential Diagnosis of Neck Mass

Chief Complaint	Focused History	Differential Diagnosis
Lateral neck mass	Unilateral/bilateral Delimitation (borders) Epistaxis/nasal obstruction Oral ulcers, persistent sore throat (>3 weeks) Otalgia (referred) Dysphagia, odynophagia hoarseness, dyspnea Environmental/ Occupational exposures (e.g. radiation, asbestos) Travel history	**Congenital:** Branchial cleft cyst Laryngocele Lymphatic malformation **Benign Neoplastic:** Salivary gland neoplasm (pleomorphic adenoma, Warthin's tumour) Vascular lesions (carotid body tumour, aneurysm) Hemangioma Lipoma Fibroma Nerve or nerve sheath tumour **Malignant Neoplastic:** Primary: Hodgkin's or non-Hodgkin's lymphoma, salivary gland neoplasm (parotid, submandibular), thyroid, sarcoma Metastatic: head and neck (usually squamous cell carcinoma), thoracic, abdominal, leukemia **Inflammatory/ Infections:** Reactive adenopathy (abscess, tonsillitis, viral URTI, mononucleosis, HIV, Kawasaki's) Granulomatous disease (TB, sarcoidosis, syphilis, toxoplasmosis, cat scratch disease) Salivary glands (sialadentitis, sialolithiasis)
Midline neck mass	Features of hyper/ hypothyroidism Hoarseness Environmental/ Occupational exposures	Thyroglossal duct cyst* Thyroid tumour, goitre or pyramidal lobe Ranula Dermoid cyst
Diffuse neck swelling	Signs and symptoms of infection, inflammation	Ludwig's angina (neck space infection)** Lymphangioma, hemangioma

* A thyroglossal duct cyst is the most common anterior midline neck mass in children
** Medical emergency – associated swelling may obstruct airway

---

Clinical Pearl
90% of pediatric neck masses are inflammatory whereas 90% of adult neck masses are malignant.

Focused Physical Exam

Head and Neck

Inspection
- Position of head, symmetry
- Hair quantity, quality, distribution
- Skin texture, colour, moisture, scars
- Skin lesions (location, arrangement, colour, size, type)
- Signs of muscle weakness/paralysis of CN VII, X, XII (e.g. facial drooping, flattened nasolabial fold)
- Neck masses (size, location, symmetry)
- Enlarged parotid or submandibular glands
- Trachea (should be in midline)

Palpation
- See *Lymphatic System and Lymph Node Exam* p. 134
- Have the patient sit with head slightly flexed forward and neck relaxed
- Use a consistent order when palpating lymph nodes (e.g. start with occipital nodes, move to post-auricular and pre-auricular nodes and then palpate the levels of the neck in order)
- Use bimanual approach to examine Level I (submandibular and submental nodes) with one gloved finger in the floor of the mouth and fingers of other hand following along skin externally
- Note tenderness, size, consistency, mobility, level
- Palpate salivary glands

> **Clinical Pearl**
> Left-sided enlargement of a supraclavicular node (Virchow's node) may indicate an abdominal malignancy; right-sided enlargement may indicate malignancy of lungs, mediastinum or esophagus.
> Enlargement of occipital nodes may be a sign of rubella.

THYROID

Inspection
- Identify the thyroid and cricoid cartilages and the trachea (note any tracheal deviation)
- Visible thyroid probably indicates enlargement (goiter)
- Look for systemic signs of thyroid disease (see *Essentials of Endocrinology* p. 422)

Palpation
- Patient's neck should be slightly flexed
- *Anterior Approach*: position yourself in front and to the side of the patient
- *Posterior Approach*: position yourself behind the patient's chair
- Examine one side at a time:
  - Relax the right sternocleidomastoid by turning patient's head slightly to right
  - Landmark using thyroid and cricoid cartilages
  - Displace trachea to right while palpating right side
  - Ask patient to swallow some water and feel for glandular tissue on right side rising under fingers
  - Repeat for left side

- The thyroid isthmus is often palpable
- Describe gland:
  - Shape/Size: normal ~ size of an adult distal phalanx of thumb
  - Consistency:
    - Rubbery (normal)
    - Hard (associated with cancer or scarring)
    - Soft (associated with toxic goiter)
  - Nodules: size, consistency, number, tenderness (suggests thyroiditis)
- *Pemberton's sign*: a large goiter extending retrosternally may block the thoracic inlet and compress jugular veins, causing facial plethora when both arms are raised

Auscultation
- Auscultate over the lateral lobes to detect any bruits
- A localized systolic or continuous bruit may be heard in thyrotoxicosis (e.g. Graves' disease)

> **Clinical Pearl**
> A thyroglossal duct cyst will elevate with tongue protrusion while a thyroid nodule will not.

Common Investigations of the Neck & Thyroid
- See **Table 11**

Table 11. Investigations for Head and Neck Pathology

Test	Indication/Finding
CBC and differential	Infection (acute, chronic) Tumour
T4 and TSH levels	Suspected thyroid disease
Indirect laryngoscopy, laryngoscopy and/or flexible nasopharyngoscopy	Hoarseness >14 days of unknown etiology Persistent neck mass of unknown etiology Visualize naso/oro/hypopharynx for neoplasm Suspected laryngocele
CT/MRI	Lateral or midline mass (tumours, cysts, salivary stones, abscess) Enhancing wall, contents of mass
Ultrasound	Branchial cleft cyst, ranula, multinodular goiter, thyroid goiter, thyroid nodule
Fine needle aspiration biopsy (FNAB)	Persistent neck mass (>4 wks) unknown etiology
Endoscopy with biopsy	Suspicious neck mass/primary, difficult biopsy sites

COMMON CLINICAL SCENARIOS

Dizziness

- *Dizziness*: a term used to describe any of a variety of sensations that produce spatial disorientation
- *Vertigo*: illusion that the body or environment is spinning or tumbling (rotational, linear or tilting movement)
- *Lightheadedness*: sense of impending faint, presyncope
- *Oscillopsia*: inability to focus on objects with motion
- *Disequilibrium*: sensation of instability of body positions, "off-balance"
- Differential diagnosis of dizziness complaint:
  - Peripheral: BPPV, Meniere's disease, vestibular neuronitis, cerebellopontine angle tumour (e.g. acoustic neuroma)
  - Central: MS, other neurologic disorders (stroke, seizure, cerebellar lesion)
  - Systemic: metabolic (e.g. hypo/hyperthyroidism, diabetes)
  - Medications and intoxicants
  - Vascular: basilar migraine syndrome, vertebrobasilar insufficiency

Focused History

- ± of illusion of rotary motion (true vertigo)
- Exacerbating and alleviating factors (postural changes, head movement, closing eyes)
- Changes in hearing and/or presence of tinnitus
- Changes in taste, swallowing or speech (suspect central cause)
- Cardiovascular history
- Alcohol consumption and anxiety
- Associated neurological symptoms (facial paralysis, sensorineural hearing loss)

Focused Physical

- Vital signs
- Orthostatic blood pressure measurement
- Evaluation of the cardiovascular and neurological systems
- Otologic examination
- *Vestibular system function:*
  - Test extraocular eye movements for spontaneous and/or positional nystagmus
  - Dix-Hallpike maneuver (test for benign paroxysmal positioning vertigo)
    - Start in sitting position, turn and support head at 45 degrees to right
    - Swiftly move patient into supine position with head overhanging bed
    - Maintain the head at 45 degrees and watch eyes (i.e. keep them open)
    - Can have latency up to 30 seconds before nystagmus occurs
    - Crescendo-decrescendo rotatory geotropic nystagmus (subsides within minutes)
    - When present, indicates disease in the ear closest to the ground
    - Upon sitting back up, look for nystagmus (if present, could reverse in direction or in an oblique upbeat direction)
- *Dizziness stimulation tests*: positional vertigo, orthostatic hypotension, hyperventilation

Investigations and Management

- Management dependent on the underlying cause
  - Benign paroxysmal positioning vertigo: Canalith repositioning maneuver (Epley Maneuver, Brandt's exercises)

Acute Otitis Media
- Acute inflammation of the middle ear
- 60% to 70% of children have at least 1 episode before 3 years of age

Focused History
- Presence of triad: otalgia (ear pain), fever and conductive hearing loss
- Tinnitus, vertigo and facial nerve paralysis are rare
- Hx of irritability, poor sleeping, often presents only with fever
- Hx of vomiting and diarrhea
- May be associated with ear tugging

Focused Physical
- ± fever
- Otoscopic examination of the tympanic membrane
  - Hyperemia
  - Bulging
  - Loss of landmarks (short process of the malleus is not visible)

Investigations and Management
- No investigations needed if history and physical findings suggest acute otitis media
- Positive otoscopic exam is definitive
- 10-day antibiotic treatment:
  - 1st line: amoxicillin
  - 2nd line (if amoxicillin fails): amoxicillin-clavulanate or cephalosporins
- Symptomatic therapy:
  - Antipyretics/analgesics (acetaminophen)
  - Decongestants
- Disease prevention:
  - Antibiotic prophylaxis
  - Pneumococcal and influenza vaccines

Epistaxis
- Anterior epistaxis (from Kiesselbach's plexus in Little's area) is most common (80%) and more often in children
- Posterior epistaxis is less common (20%) and more often in patients over 50 years old

> **Clinical Pearl**
> Severe, unilateral epistaxis with no history of trauma in an adolescent male is **juvenile nasopharyngeal angiofibroma** until proven otherwise. Recurrent epistaxis in older males of south-eastern Asian or southern Chinese descent is **nasopharyngeal carcinoma** until proven otherwise.

Focused History
- Onset/duration of bleeding
- Frequency and past episodes
- Taste of blood in throat
- Medications and street drugs (cocaine)
- Symptoms of local problems and systemic diseases (see **Table 12**)

Focused Physical
- Vitals
- Volume assessment
- Nasal speculum exam (use suction, gloves, face mask and eye protection)
- Posterior bleeds often reveal little bleeding from the nostrils and more blood along the posterior pharynx
- Flexible nasopharyngoscope for suspicion of posterior epistaxis

Management
- Anterior epistaxis
  - Have the patient pinch their nose over cartilaginous portion (not nasal bones)
  - Most bleeds will respond to local finger compression within 10-12 min
  - If bleeding persists and the patient has no history of heart disease, consider application of topical vasoconstrictor (oxymetazoline, cocaine hydrochloride)
  - If bleeding persists, attempt silver nitrate chemical cautery or anterior pack
  - If bleeding still persists, suspect hypertension, inadequate exterior packing, coagulopathy or posterior epistaxis
- Posterior epistaxis
  - Requires a posterior pack
  - Treat hypertension if present
  - If bleeding persists after 3-5 days, consider endoscopic arterial ligation or embolization
- Correct hypovolemia if present
- If indicated, discontinue NSAIDs, adjust anticoagulant dose, replace clotting factors

Investigations
- If bleeding is minor and does not recur, no investigations needed
- If bleeding is recurrent and/or heavy:
  - Blood type and cross-match
  - CBC, hematocrit
  - aPTT, INR, LFTs (anticoagulant use, suspected liver disease)
  - CT and/or MRI and/or nasopharyngoscopy if foreign body or neoplasm suspected

HEAD & NECK

Table 12. Differential Diagnosis of Epistaxis

Category	Differential Diagnosis
Local factors	Trauma (nose-picking, accidental injury) Mucosal drying secondary to nasal septal deviation, spurs, perforations causing turbulent air flow Foreign body (unilateral, foul discharge, occasional epistaxis) Iatrogenic (septal, orbital, turbinate, sinus surgery) Inflammation (URTI, sinusitis, allergies, chemical irritation) Chemicals (cocaine, nasal sprays, ammonia, gasoline, phosphorus, chromium salts, sulphuric acid, mercury)
Environmental	Barotrauma; cold, dry air
Neoplasms	Adults: melanoma, squamous cell carcinoma, inverted papillomas, adenoid cystic carcinoma Children: polyps, encephaloceles, gliomas, meningoceles
Systemic	Coagulopathies: anticoagulant use (coumadin, heparin), liver disease, hemophilia, thrombocytopenia, von Willebrand's disease, NSAIDs, chemotherapy Vascular disorders: hypertension, arteriosclerosis, Osler-Weber-Rendu disease (hereditary hemorrhagic telangiectasia) Malignant tumours Granulomatous diseases: Wegener's, SLE, TB, rhinoscleroma, sarcoidosis, leprosy

Hoarseness (Dysphonia)
- Abnormality of the voice affecting one or more of: pitch, volume, resonance, quality
- Often associated with URTI of viral origin in otherwise healthy patients
- Hoarseness lasting more than 14 days must be investigated with a complete head and neck exam including indirect laryngoscopy and/or nasopharyngoscopy to rule out laryngeal cancer
- See **Table 13** for differential diagnosis

Focused History
- Onset and progression, past occurrences
- Timing (a.m. or p.m. or continuous)
- Associated pharyngitis and/or otalgia (referred via CN IX and X)
- Cough, hemoptysis, constitutional symptoms
- Associated dysphagia, odynophagia
- Habits (smoking, alcohol)
- Past history of radiation exposure (treatment of scars, occupational exposure)
- Previous surgery and/or intubations
- History of GERD, past or present lung or breast cancer or lymphoma

Focused Physical
- Palpation of head and neck lymph nodes
- Laryngeal crepitus:
  - Normal: crepitus is felt when larynx is gently moved laterally
  - Absence of crepitus suggests mass in retropharyngeal space or hypopharynx
- Examination of oral and nasal cavities
- Indirect laryngoscopy and/or flexible nasolaryngoscopy:
  - Have the patient say 'EEEEE' to assess vocal cord mobility

Table 13. Hoarseness: Differential Diagnosis, Historical and Physical Findings

Differential Diagnosis	Historical Findings	Physical Findings
Acute viral laryngitis	Viral URTI preceding aphonia ± history of pharyngitis	Bilateral vocal cord edema and erythema
GERD-associated laryngitis	History of GERD and its precipitating factors	Erythema and edema of the mucosa lining the arytenoids ± ulcers or granulomas in same region
Vocal cord nodules	Singers, females and children Aggravated by URTI, sinusitis, smoke and alcohol	Acute: soft, red Chronic: fibrotic, hard, white Bilateral (paired) on anterior 1/3 of cords
Vocal cord polyp	Males, smokers, vocal misuse or abuse or irritant exposure ± dyspnea, cough	Unilateral or bilateral, asymmetric, broad-based and pedunculated with a smooth, soft appearance
Squamous papillomas	HPV infection Past episodes	Anterior commissure and true vocal cord most common location; subglottic and supraglottic areas may be involved White to reddish verrucous mass
Laryngeal carcinoma	Risk factors: alcohol, smoking, exposure to radiation, juvenile papillomatosis (HPV), nickel exposure, laryngocele Dysphagia, odynophagia Otalgia (referred from CN IX, X) Hemoptysis Cough	Dysplasia or carcinoma in-situ may appear as leukoplakia Tumour appears as ulcerated growth on vocal cord membrane ± neck mass Paralyzed vocal cord
Spasmodic dysphonia	Strained, strangled voice associated with facial grimacing Voice is normal during singing, crying or laughing	Hyperadduction of the true and false cords

Table 13. Hoarseness: Differential Diagnosis, Historical and Physical Findings (continued)

Differential Diagnosis	Historical Findings	Physical Findings
Cord paralysis	Dramatic "breathy" voice due to air escape Bilateral paralysis may lead to airway compromise History of recurrent laryngeal nerve damage (surgical, endotracheal tube, breech birth in neonates) Lung, breast cancer (infiltration of recurrent laryngeal nerve as it loops through thorax)	Unilateral: cord abducted in resting position and unable to adduct during phonation Bilateral: cords adducted, unable to abduct with little space between
Trauma	History of trauma to the larynx Trauma-induced lesions of the vocal cord (screaming, singing)	Severe trauma can result in fracture or dislocation of arytenoids Vocal abuse results in benign vocal cord polyps, nodules or contact granulomas

Investigations
- Indirect laryngoscopy and/or nasopharyngoscopy
- Pneumatic otoscopy
- CXR, CT with contrast
- TSH, CBC, ESR, RF and biopsy

REFERENCES

Cummings CW. 2005. *Otolaryngology – Head & Neck Surgery.* Philadelphia: Elsevier Mosby.
Dhillon RS, East CA. 2006. *Ear, Nose, and Throat and Head and Neck Surgery: An Illustrated Colour Text.* Edinburgh; New York: Churchill Livingstone/Elsevier.
Dugani S, Lam D (eds.) 2009. *The Toronto Notes 2009: Comprehensive Medical Reference.* Toronto: Toronto Notes for Medical Students, Inc.
Jafek BW, Murrow BW. 2005. *ENT Secrets.* Philadelphia: Elsevier/Mosby.
McIsaac WJ, Kellner JD, Aufricht P, Vanjaka A, Low DE. 2004. Empirical validation of guidelines for the management of pharyngitis in children and adults. *JAMA* 291(13):1587-1595.
Robbins KT, Clayman G, Levine PA, Medina J, Sessions R, Shaha A, Som P, Wolf GT. 2002. Neck dissection classification update: revisions proposed by the American Head and Neck Society and the American Academy of Otolaryngology-Head and Neck Surgery. *Arch Otolaryngol Head Neck Surg* 128(7):751-758.

The Lymphatic System and Lymph Node Exam

Editors:
Kimberly Bremer &
Varinder Randhawa

Faculty Reviewers:
Blake C. Papsin, MD, MSc, FRCS, FACS, FAAP
Howard B. Abrams, MD, FRCP(C)

TABLE OF CONTENTS

Essential Anatomy   131
Approach to Lymphatic History and Physical Exam   133
Common Chief Complaints   133
Common Disorders   133
Focused History   133
Focused Physical Exam   134
Common Investigations   136
Common Clinical Scenarios   137

ESSENTIAL ANATOMY

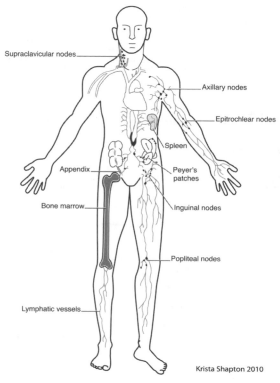

Supraclavicular nodes

Axillary nodes

Epitrochlear nodes

Spleen

Appendix

Peyer's patches

Bone marrow

Inguinal nodes

Popliteal nodes

Lymphatic vessels

Krista Shapton 2010

Figure 1. Overview of Lymphatic System

LYMPHATIC

Table 1. Functional Overview of Lymph Tissues

Lymphoid Tissue	Function	Site
Lymph nodes	Lymphatic drainage of various body areas	Located throughout body (see **Table 2** for details)
Tonsils (lingual, palatine, tubal, adenoids making up Waldeyer's ring)	Protects entrance to respiratory passage	Base of tongue, pharyngeal and nasopharyngeal walls
Spleen	RBC and platelet storage, defective RBC disposal, antibody formation by intrinsic B-cells	Left upper quadrant of abdomen
Peyer's patch	IgA antibody formation by intrinsic B-lymphocytes	Ileal walls
Appendix	IgA immune response to ingested antigens	Lower cecal outpouching

Table 2. Overview of Lymph Node Drainage

Lymph Node Group	Location	Drainage
Head & Neck Nodes – refer to *Head & Neck Exam,* **Table 9** (p. 120)		
Supraclavicular	Superior to clavicle	H&N and axillary nodes
Infraclavicular	Inferior to clavicle	H&N and axillary nodes
Scalene	Posterior to clavicle	H&N and axillary nodes
Upper Extremities – Axillary		
Apical group	At apex of axilla	All other axillary nodes
Central group	High in axilla, deep to pectoralis minor (often palpable)	Pectoral, lateral and subscapular nodes
Pectoral (anterior) group	Inside anterior axillary fold, along lower border of pectoralis major	Anterior chest wall and breast
Subscapular (posterior) group	Deep in posterior axillary fold, along lateral border of scapula	Anterior chest wall and breast
Lateral group	Along upper humerus	Most of arm
Epitrochlear or cubital	Above medial epicondyle	Ulnar aspect of hand and forearm
Lower Extremities – Superficial inguinal		
Vertical group	Near upper portion of leg along great saphenous vein	Superficial tissue of upper leg
Horizontal group	Just below inguinal ligament	Skin of lower abdominal wall, external genitalia (except testes), anal canal, lower third of vagina, gluteal region
Deep inguinal	Deep medial aspect of femoral vein	Popliteal and superficial inguinal regions
Superficial popliteal	Popliteal fossa (one node)	Heel and outer aspect of foot

LYMPHATIC

APPROACH TO LYMPHATIC HISTORY AND PHYSICAL

The lymphatic system focused history should include questions on:
- Location of enlarged lymph node(s), and whether localized or generalized
- Nature of swollen extremities
- Family history of malignancy and/or infection
- Social or past history of sexual behaviours, occupation, travel, infections and/or trauma

The lymphatic system physical exam approach should include:
- *Inspection*: **SEADS** = **S**welling, **E**rythema, **A**trophy/Hypertrophy, **D**eformity, **S**ymmetry
- *Palpation*: note pain or pitting edema
  - Head and neck, upper extremities (axillary, epitrochlear, supraclavicular), and lower extremities (inguinal, popliteal)

- In primary care, over two-thirds have lymphadenopathy resulting from non-specific or upper respiratory causes (<1% due to malignancy)
- Of patients referred for evaluation of lymphadenopathy, 84% have a benign course (16% due to malignancy, either lymphoma or metastatic adenocarcinoma)

COMMON CHIEF COMPLAINTS
- Enlarged lymph node (e.g. lump or bump with or without pain)
- Swollen extremity (e.g. arm, leg or ankle as in lymphedema)

COMMON DISORDERS
Disorders marked with (✓) are discussed in **Common Clinical Scenarios**

✓ Acute suppurative lymphadenitis
✓ Epstein-Barr Virus mononucleosis
✓ HIV sero-positivity
✓ Acute lymphangitis
✓ Lymphedema

✓ Elephantiasis
✓ Systemic lupus erythematosus
✓ Mycoplasma infection
✓ Drugs causing generalized lymphadenopathy

The following disorders are discussed in the *Essentials of Oncology* chapter
- Metastatic carcinoma
- Non-Hodgkin's lymphoma
- Hodgkin's lymphoma

FOCUSED HISTORY

History of Present Illness
- Enlarged lymph node: "Do you have any abnormal lumps or bumps?"
  - Character: onset, location, duration, tenderness, number
  - Associated symptoms: pain, fever, erythema, warmth, itchiness, red streaks
  - Predisposing factors: infection, surgery, trauma
- Swollen extremity: "Do you have any swelling?"
  - Character: unilateral/bilateral, intermittent/continuous, duration
  - Associated symptoms: warmth, erythema, discoloration, ulceration
  - Predisposing factors: cardiac and/or renal disorder, malignancy, surgery, infection, trauma, venous insufficiency
  - Alleviating factors: support stockings, elevation
- Constitutional symptoms: fever, night sweats, weight loss, fatigue

LYMPHATIC

Past Medical History
- Past surgeries/injuries (e.g. trauma to regional lymph nodes), medications (e.g. phenytoin, chemo-radiation), malignancy, recurrent infections, chronic inflammatory diseases (e.g. SLE, RA), immunosuppression

Family History
- Malignancy, recurrent infections, TB

Social History
- Sexual behaviour, STIs (e.g. syphilis, chlamydia, HIV), occupation/travel (e.g. infectious or carcinogenic exposures)

FOCUSED PHYSICAL EXAM
Often the lymphatic system is examined along with other body systems, and consists primarily of inspection and palpation of lymph nodes. Consider the regional drainage patterns of these lymph nodes, and look for any signs of infection or malignancy in those areas. Distinguish between regional and generalized lymphadenopathy by assessing for lymph nodes elsewhere.

Screening Exam
- In a patient who is otherwise asymptomatic or presenting with an un-related chief complaint: inspect and palpate H&N, axillary and inguinal nodes, liver and spleen

Inspection
- In each region, look for visible node enlargement, edema, muscle bulk/symmetry, color changes (e.g. erythema or red streaks) or ulceration

Palpation
- In each area, using the pads of the index and middle fingers, move in circular motions over the underlying tissues first by applying light pressure, then gradually increasing the pressure
- Note that excess pressure from the start may displace or obscure the nodes into deeper soft tissues before they are recognized
- For comparison, palpate right and left lymph nodes simultaneously and note:
  - Location
  - Size (<1 cm or >1 cm)
  - Shape (regular or irregular borders)
  - Delimitation (discrete or malted together)
  - Mobility (fixed or mobile/tethered to skin or deeper tissue)
  - Consistency (soft, hard or firm)
  - Tenderness (tender or non-tender)
- A normal lymph node should be <1 cm in size, feel soft and non-tender, and have regular and discrete borders

> **Clinical Pearl**
> Lymph nodes that increase rapidly in size, fixate to skin or soft tissues, or become confluent may indicate malignancy.

- If edema is noted, check for pitting edema to rule out lymphedema, which does not have characteristic pitting associated with other causes of edema
- Approach an unexplained enlarged lymph node by examining **PALS**: **P**rimary site, **A**ll associated nodes, **L**iver, **S**pleen

> **Clinical Pearl**
> A firm, deliberate, gentle touch will feel less ticklish to the patient.

> **Clinical Pearl**
> Distinguishing a Lymph Node from other structures:
>
> | Character | Lymph Node | Artery | Cyst | Muscle |
> |---|:---:|:---:|:---:|:---:|
> | Rolls in 2 directions | ✓ | × | × | × |
> | Pulsates | × | ✓ | × | × |
> | Transilluminates with direct light | × | × | ✓ | × |

Head & Neck

- *Supraclavicular*: ask patient to turn head towards side of palpation, raise same shoulder and bend head forward to relax the SCM, then hook fingers over clavicle and rotate them over entire supraclavicular area
- *Infraclavicular*: rotate fingers below clavicle over entire infraclavicular area
- *Scalene*: roll fingers gently behind clavicles and instruct patient to Valsalva (e.g. cough or bear down)

Upper Extremities

- *Axillary*: to examine the right axilla, support and slightly abduct the patient's flexed right arm with your right hand and palpate 5 regions with left hand including:
    - *Anteriorly*: pectoral muscles
    - *Posteriorly*: latissimus dorsi and subscapularis
    - *Medially*: rib cage
    - *Laterally*: upper arm
    - *Apically*: axilla
- Vice versa for the left axilla
- *Epitrochlear*: support patient's flexed elbow in one hand, and palpate using the other hand in the depression above and posterior to the medial condyle of the humerus

Lower Extremities

- *Inguinal*: ask patient to lie supine with knee slightly flexed, roll fingers above and below inguinal ligament to access only the superficial nodes (small nodes of 0.5 cm are often found; deeper abdominal, pelvic and para-aortic nodes that drain the testes and internal female genitalia are inaccessible by palpation)
- *Popliteal*: with both hands hooked around knee, place thumbs on tibial tuberosity and palpate deeply in popliteal fossa with 3-4 fingers from each hand (one node is occasionally palpable)

Table 3. Significance of Lymph Node Character and Location

Character	Indication
Hard (often asymmetry with unremarkable contralateral node), size >2 cm, non-tender, fixed	Carcinoma
Firm, rubbery, non-tender	Lymphoma
Tender	Inflammation
Non-pitting edema (pitting edema more often associated with other causes)	Lymphedema
Location of Enlarged Nodes	
Occipital	Scalp infection, rubella
Pre-auricular	Conjunctival infection, cat-scratch disease
Cervical	URTI, oral and dental lesion, infectious mononucleosis (posterior) or other viral illness, metastases from H&N, lung, breast or thyroid
Supraclavicular and scalene (always abnormal)	Metastases: Left-sided Virchow's: from lung, breast, testes, ovaries Right-sided Virchow's: from thoracic regions (mediastinal, lung, esophageal)
	Non-neoplastic causes: TB, sarcoidosis, toxoplasmosis
Axillary	Infection/injury of ipsilateral upper extremity, metastases from breast, melanoma of upper extremity
Epitrochlear	Syphilis, non-Hodgkin's lymphoma
Inguinal	Infection/injury of ipsilateral lower extremity, metastases from rectum/genitalia (penile/scrotal or vulval/lower third of vaginal areas), melanoma of lower extremity, certain STIs (primarily syphilis)

Note: A normal palpable lymph node is <1 cm in size, soft and non-tender, with regular and discrete borders

COMMON INVESTIGATIONS

- Laboratory tests should be used to confirm a diagnosis suspected on the basis of history and physical exam findings (e.g. infectious or malignant). If this initial evaluation is non-confirmatory, diagnostic work-up should consider if the adenopathy is localized or generalized
- *Generalized*: CBC, electrolytes, CXR (AP and lateral views), urine R&M/C&S, throat and genital swabs
  - If normal, consider infections: PPD, HIV antibody, RPR, ANA, heterophile test
  - If uncertain, then: excisional biopsy of most abnormal node (or supraclavicular, neck, axilla or groin in this order if a single node is unattainable) for abnormal cells and architecture using local anesthesia

- *Localized*: observe for 3-4 weeks if history is not suggestive of malignancy, but if adenopathy is non-resolving then consider an open biopsy
  - Fine needle aspiration for cytology (especially in HIV+ patients)
  - Core needle biopsy for special studies and architecture
  - Lymphangiography for adenopathy in the abdomen and thorax (not in the periphery)
- *Imaging*: CT, U/S, Doppler or MRI are all modalities to distinguish enlarged lymph nodes from other structures, to define pathological processes, to stage malignancy and to help guide fine needle aspiration

---

Clinical Pearl
Incision and drainage of a fluctuant node is useful to help relieve pain and reduce infection, but not useful for diagnosis.

COMMON CLINICAL SCENARIOS

Disorders caused by Disease Spread to Lymph Nodes

Acute suppurative lymphadenitis
- *Etiology*: Group A beta-hemolytic *Streptococci* or coagulase-positive *Staphylococci* (often young children) causing one-sided pus-forming inflammation of lymph nodes
- *Character*: firm and tender swollen nodes on palpation, possible erythema on overlying skin and tissue
- *Associated with*: sudden onset fever, anorexia, and irritability

Epstein-Barr Virus mononucleosis
- *Etiology*: viral infection producing abnormally large number of mononuclear leukocytes (mostly B cells) in blood, and leading to bilateral inflammation of any lymph node chains (especially cervical)
- *Character*: generally discrete and sometimes tender nodes with varying firmness on palpation (especially if anterior and posterior cervical chain lymph nodes)
- *Associated with*: pharyngitis, often fever, fatigue, malaise, nausea only, and splenomegaly

HIV sero-positivity – refer to **Infectious Diseases** (p. 451) for more detail
- *Etiology*: HIV virus causing persistent generalized lymphadenopathy for >3 months and involving 2 or more extra-inguinal sites (may be first sign of initial infection and is part of the asymptomatic phase)
- *Character*: generally tender, discrete and freely mobile nodes on palpation
  - Presence of small, ill-defined nodes may indicate disease progression and/or treatment failure
- *Associated with*: severe fatigue, malaise, fever, weight loss, weakness, arthralgias, and persistent diarrhea

Disorders of the Lymphatic Vessels

Acute lymphangitis
- *Etiology*: infection at a site distal to the lymph vessel resulting in inflammation of the lymphatic vessels
- *Character*: fine red streaks along the course of lymphatic collecting ducts
  - Tubules may be slightly indurated and palpable by gentle touch
  - Inspect distally for sites of infection, especially in the interdigital spaces for cracks
- *Associated with*: pain in affected extremity, malaise and possibly fever

Lymphedema

- *Etiology*: swelling of the subcutaneous tissue from accumulation of lymph fluid due to primary (congenital) or secondary (acquired) obstruction of lymph drainage
  - Primary lymphedema: hypoplasia or maldevelopment of the lymphatic system
  - Secondary lymphedema: lymph node dissection or radiation, malignant obstruction, and infection
- *Character*: painless, nonpitting swelling of an extremity, usually with involvement of the digits
  - Over time, the skin becomes dry, firm and fibrous to palpation
- *Associated with*: increased susceptibility to local inflammation from infection or limb injury; should evaluate for cellulitis from staphylococcal or streptococcal skin infections

Lymphatic filariasis (Elephantiasis)

- *Etiology*: infection with one of three nematodes, *Wuchereria bancrofti*, *Brugia malayi*, or *Brugia timori* causing lymphatic obstruction through host immune response, direct actions of the parasite or its products
- *Character*: initially similar to lymphedema, over time texture of the skin changes and becomes hyperkeratotic with verrucous and vesicular skin lesions
- *Associated with*: three distinct phases: asymptomatic microfilaremia, acute episodes of adenolymphangitis (ADL), and chronic disease (irreversible lymphedema), which is often superimposed upon repeated episodes of ADL
- Major cause of disfigurement and disability in endemic areas, leading to significant economic and psychosocial impact

Other Common Scenarios

Systemic lupus erythematosus

- *Etiology*: the exact etiology of SLE remains unknown; there is a role for genetic, hormonal, immunologic, and environmental factors. Clinical manifestations of this multisystem disorder are mediated directly or indirectly by antibody formation and the creation of chronic immune complexes
- *Character*: nodes are typically soft, nontender, discrete, variable in size, and usually detected in the cervical, axillary, and inguinal areas
- *Associated with*: the onset of disease or an exacerbation. Lymph node enlargement can also be the result of infection or a lymphoproliferative disease in SLE; when infections are present the enlarged nodes are more likely to be tender

Mycobacterium infection

- *Etiology*:
  - Adults: *M. tuberculosis*
  - Children: other mycobacteria (e.g. *M. avium* complex, *M. scrofulaceum*)
  - In patients with generalized lymphadenopathy, miliary tuberculosis should be considered
- *Character*: nodes are typically nontender, enlarge over weeks to months without prominent systemic symptoms, and can progress to matting and fluctuation
- *Associated with*: lymphadenopathy alone, especially in the neck

Drugs causing generalized lymphadenopathy

- Several medications may cause serum sickness that is characterized by fever, arthralgias, rash, and generalized lymphadenopathy
- Examples: allopurinol, atenolol, captopril, carbamazepine, cephalosporins, gold, hydralazine, penicillin, phenytoin (can cause generalized lymph-adenopathy in the absence of a serum sickness reaction), primidone, pyrimethamine, quinidine, sulfonamides, sulindac

REFERENCES

Bickley LS, Szilagyi PG, Bates B. 2007. *Bates' Guide to Physical Examination and History Taking.* Philadelphia: Lippincott Williams & Wilkins.

Fauci AS. 2008. *Harrison's Principles of Internal Medicine.* New York: McGraw-Hill.

Moore KL, Dalley AF, Agur AMR. 2006. *Clinically Oriented Anatomy.* Philadelphia: Lippincott Williams & Wilkins.

Porter RS (ed.) 2006. *The Merck Manual of Diagnosis and Therapy.* Whitehouse Station: Merck Research Laboratories.

Seidel HM. 2006. *Mosby's Guide to Physical Examination.* St. Louis: Mosby Elsevier.

Swartz MH. 2006. *Textbook of Physical Diagnosis: History and Examination.* Philadelphia: Saunders Elsevier.

LYMPHATIC

The Essentials of Clinical Examination Handbook, 6th ed.

The Musculoskeletal Exam

Editors:
Kevin Koo & Ian Mayne

Faculty Reviewers:
David Backstein, MD MEd FRCS(C)

TABLE OF CONTENTS

Approach, Focused History and Physical Exam   141
Common Clinical Scenarios   145
Upper Extremity Exam (Shoulder, Elbow, Wrist, Hand)   147
Spine Exam   159
Lower Extremity Exam (Hip, Knee, Ankle, Foot)   166

APPROACH TO THE MUSCULOSKELETAL HISTORY AND PHYSICAL EXAM

In addition to general history taking, important aspects of the musculoskeletal history include:

- Pain – **OPQRST** (see p. 142)
- Referred symptoms
- Inflammatory symptoms
- Mechanical/degenerative symptoms
- Neoplastic and infectious symptoms
- Neurological symptoms
- Vascular symptoms

Overview of the physical exam:

- Vitals
- LOOK/FEEL/MOVE
- Inspect – **SEADS** (see p. 143)
- Palpation
- Range of Motion (ROM) (active and passive)
- Power Assessment/Isometric Movements
- Functional Assessment
- Reflexes
- Special Tests
- Other: gait, PVS, neurological exam

COMMON DISORDERS

Disorders marked with (✓) are discussed in **Common Clinical Scenarios**

- ✓ Compartment Syndrome
- ✓ Rotator cuff tendonitis/rupture
- ✓ Fractures
- ✓ Joint dislocation
- ✓ Carpal tunnel syndrome
- ✓ Osteoporosis
- ✓ Osteoarthritis
- ✓ Sciatica
- ✓ Hip fracture

- ✓ Patello-femoral syndrome
- ✓ Bicipital tendonitis
- ✓ Epicondylitis
- ✓ Rheumatoid arthritis
- ✓ De Quervain's disease
- ✓ Cauda equina syndrome
- ✓ Avascular necrosis
- ✓ Meniscal/ligamentous injury

MUSCULOSKELETAL

FOCUSED HISTORY

Pain – OPQRST
- **O**nset (slow or sudden)
- **P**alliative factors, **P**rovocative factors (pain associated with rest, activity, certain postures, time of day)
- **Q**uality
    - Nerve pain: sharp, burning, run in distribution of nerve
    - Bone pain: deep, localized;
    - Vascular pain: diffuse, aching, poorly localized, may be referred to other areas
    - Muscle pain: dull and aching, hard to localize, may be referred to other areas
- **R**adiation, **R**eferred pain
- **S**ymptoms associated (joint locking, unlocking, instability; changes in colour of limb, pins and needles)
- **T**iming (onset, duration, frequency)

Referred Symptoms from other Joints/Organs
- Shoulder pain (from heart or diaphragm)
- Arm pain (from neck)
- Leg pain (from back)
- Knee pain (from hip or back)

Inflammatory Symptoms
- Pain, erythema, warmth, swelling, morning stiffness (>30 min)
- Improves with activity
- Important to differentiate from mechanical/degenerative manifestations

Mechanical/Degenerative Symptoms
- Pain is worse at end of day, better with rest, worse with use
- Ligament or meniscal symptoms (joint giving way, clicking, locking, instability)

Neoplastic and Infectious Symptoms
- Constant pain, night pain, fever, chills, weight loss, anorexia, fatigue, weakness
- History of prostate, thyroid, breast, lung or kidney cancer

Neurological Symptoms
- Paresthesia, tingling, bowel and bladder complaints, headaches, weakness

Vascular Symptoms
- Differentiate vascular from neurologic claudication

FOCUSED PHYSICAL EXAM
- Always examine the joint above and below the site of interest
- If lower extremity complaint: examine lower back and perform complete neurological exam of lower limbs
- If upper extremity complaint: examine neck and perform complete neurological exam of upper limbs
- Refer to anatomical sites for site specific tests

Inspection

In general, inspect each joint for the following: **SEADS**

- **S**welling
- **E**rythema
- **A**trophy of muscle
- **D**eformity (alterations in shape, bony alignment or posture)
- **S**kin changes (bruising, discolouration)

Also, inspect for the following:

- Symmetry of the bony contours, soft-tissues, limb positions
- Presence of scars to indicate recent injury/surgery
- Any crepitus or abnormal sound in joints when patient moves them
- Patient's attitude (apprehensiveness, restlessness)
- Patient's facial expression (indicating discomfort)
- Patient's willingness to move; normality of movements

Palpation

In general, palpate skin, soft tissues, bones and joints while patient is as relaxed as possible. Palpation must be carried out in a systematic fashion to ensure that all structures are examined and any asymmetry is noted.

The following should be noted when palpating:

- Identify shapes, structures, tissue type and detect any abnormalities
- Determine tissue thickness and texture and determine whether it is pliable, soft, or resilient
  - Specifically, feel for tenderness, nodules, warmth, crepitus, effusion
- Determine joint tenderness by applying firm pressure to the joint. The degree of tenderness can be graded as follows:
  - Grade I: Patient complains of pain
  - Grade II: Patient complains of pain and winces
  - Grade III: Patient winces and withdraws the joint
  - Grade IV: Patient will not allow palpation of the joint
- Feel for variation in temperature, pulses, tremors, and fasciculations
- Feel for dryness or excessive moisture of the skin

Range of Motion (ROM)

Active Movements

- Performed voluntarily by patient
- Abnormalities in active ROM result from either neurological problems or mechanical disruption of flexor/extensor mechanisms
- When testing active movements, note the following:
  - Any movements resulting in pain and quality/amount of pain
  - Amount of observable restriction
  - Any limitation and its nature
  - Willingness of patient to move the joint
  - Quality of movement
  - Crepitus

Passive Movements

- Joint is put through a range of motion by the examiner while the patient is relaxed
- Detect any limitation of movement (stiffness) or excessive range (hypermobility), and any associated pain
- Hypermobile joints: possibly a result of ligament sprains, joint effusion, chronic pain, tendinitis resulting from lack of control, rheumatoid arthritis
- Hypomobile joints: possibly a result of muscle strains, pinched nerve syndromes, and tendinitis resulting from overstress, osteoarthritis

End Feel
- Defined as the sensation felt in the joint as it reaches the end of its ROM
- In passive movement, the examiner should determine the quality of end feel
- Abnormal end feel indicates pathology
- 3 normal types of end feel:
  1. Bone to Bone: a "hard" unyielding compression that stops further movement (e.g. elbow extension)
  2. Soft Tissue Approximation: a yielding compression that stops further movement (e.g. elbow and knee flexion where movement is stopped by muscles)
  3. Tissue Stretch: hard or "springy" (firm) movement with a slight give. There is a feeling of elastic resistance towards the end of the ROM with a feeling of "rising tension". Feeling depends on thickness of tissue and may be very elastic (Achilles tendon stretch) or slightly elastic (wrist flexion) (e.g. lateral rotation of shoulder/knee, extension of metacarpophalangeal joint)

Power Assessment/Isometric Movements
- Type of movement that consists of strong, static, voluntary muscle contraction
- Examiner positions the joint in the resting position and asks the patient to maintain the position against an applied force
- Muscle weakness can be a result of:
  - Upper motor neuron lesion
  - Injury to peripheral nerve
  - Neuromuscular junction pathology
  - Pathology of muscles themselves
- In certain anatomic sites (lumbar spine, cervical spine), isometric contractions are used to test for myotome function

Functional Assessment
- Should always be performed on the joint during examination
- May involve task analysis or simply a history of patient's daily activities
- Assess limitations in activities of daily living (ADLs):
  - Getting up and sitting down, walking up stairs
  - Using bathroom, brushing teeth, combing hair
  - Transferring from shower or bathtub

Reflexes
- Test reflexes to assess the nerve or nerve roots that supply the reflex (see **Neurological Exam** p. 190)

Special Tests
- Refer to specific anatomic sites

Other Considerations
- Gait Assessment
  - *Walking*: normal, heel-to-toe, heels only, toes only
  - *Look for*: Trendelenburg gait in hip disorders, high stepping, circumduction, antalgic (due to pain)
- Peripheral vascular exam
  - Test peripheral pulses
  - See **Peripheral Vascular Exam** p. 303
- Neurological exam
  - Test sensation, power
  - See **Neurological Exam**

COMMON CLINICAL SCENARIOS

Fracture

- Establish the mechanism of injury, the activity at the time of the injury, the magnitude of the applied forces (i.e. fell from a height), point of impact and the direction of the applied force (i.e. fall on an outstretched hand)
- Inspect injury for bony deformation, instability, hematoma, loss of function, localized edema, localized pain and severity
- Note any parasthesia, loss of pulse or decrease in capillary refill below the fracture
- Fracture Description
    - Open/Closed
    - Involvement of Joint (intra-/extra-articular)
    - Part of Bone (epiphyseal, metaphyseal, diaphyseal – proximal, middle, distal)
    - Displacement
        - Angulation: distal fragment position relative to proximal fragment; orientation (degrees) of the distal bone fragment towards (valgus) or away (varus) from the midline
        - Translation: "sliding" (percentage) of the distal bone fragment in relation to proximal
        - Rotation: movement of distal fragment (longitudinal axis) in relation to proximal fragment
        - Impaction: bone ends are compressed together
    - Fracture Pattern (**Figure 1**)

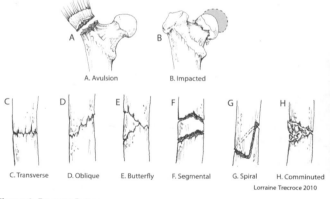

A. Avulsion   B. Impacted

C. Transverse   D. Oblique   E. Butterfly   F. Segmental   G. Spiral   H. Comminuted

Lorraine Trecroce 2010

Figure 1. Fracture Patterns

Compartment Syndrome

- Increased tissue pressure decreases the perfusion and function of the tissues and nerves within the compartment
- Establish underlying mechanism: trauma, hemorrhage, previous fracture or surgical procedure, external compression (cast, wound closure)
- Perform motor and sensory exams, note 5 **P's**:
    - **P**ain (early, increases with passive stretch)
    - **P**allor
    - **P**arathesia
    - **P**aralysis (late)
    - **P**ulselessness (very late, tissue damage likely)

Osteoporosis

- Affects 1 in 4 women and 1 in 8 men over the age of 50 in Canada
- Systemic disease characterized by low bone mass and micro-architectural deterioration of bone tissue
- Leads to increased risk of fragility fractures
- Areas of main concern are wrist, humerus, ribs, vertebral body, pelvis and hip
- May present with height loss and a history of fragility fractures
- Osteoporosis related history
    - Age (>65)
    - History of low trauma fractures
    - Family history of osteoporotic fracture
    - Height loss (4 cm historical or 2 cm prospective height loss)
    - Systemic glucocorticoid therapy of >3 months duration
    - Early menopause (before age 45)
    - Dietary calcium intake
    - Weight <57 kg

Osteoarthritis

- Joint wear that occurs with age; cartilaginous surfaces are worn down, causing bone to rub on bone
- Disease occurs most commonly in weight-bearing joints
- Patient complains of pain with movement and after prolonged rest (i.e. pain worse in the morning), pain on palpation
- Decreasing joint ROM, grinding (crepitus), swelling and stiffness, bony enlargement of joint, fixed flexion deformity, limb shortening, referred pain to the knee, generally worse with activity, better with rest

Rheumatoid Arthritis

- Systemic inflammatory disorder characterized by destructive hypertrophic synovitis
- Symptoms include:
    - Symmetrical peripheral polyarthritis causing pain and stiffness that is most prominent in the morning and lasts >30 min
    - Insidious onset with involvement of an increasing number of joints including wrists, elbows, shoulders, ankles, knees and hips
    - Systemic features such as malaise, weight loss and low-grade fever
    - Soft tissue problems such as carpal tunnel syndrome and flexor tenosynovitis
- Physical signs include:
    - Soft tissue swelling, tenderness, stiffness, erythema and increased temperature of affected synovial joints (often peripheral joints)
    - Synovial effusions
    - Raynaud's phenomenon, tenosynovitis, carpal tunnel syndrome
    - Swan-neck and boutonniere deformities of the fingers (see **Table 7** p. 156), volar and ulnar subluxation of the fingers at the metacarpophalangeal joints
- Diagnosis can be made if at least 4 of the American College of Rheumatology 1987 Criteria are met: morning stiffness (>1 h, >6 weeks), arthritis in at least three areas (>6 weeks), arthritis of hands or wrists (>6 weeks), symmetrical arthritis (>6 weeks), rheumatoid nodules, positive rheumatoid factor, radiographic changes in wrists/hands

Examination of Specific Joints

- Each joint should be inspected, palpated, put through the various range of motion maneuvers, reflex examination, and special tests if appropriate
- Look for the signs listed above

SHOULDER

Common Symptoms

- Pain – always consider possibility of referral from chest/abdomen or neck
- Weakness
- Muscle atrophy – may point to lesions in cervical nerves

Common Clinical Scenarios

- Rotator cuff tendinitis (impingement syndrome)
- Rotator cuff tear/rupture
- Bicipital tendinitis
- Dislocation (95% anterior, 5% posterior)
- Rheumatoid Arthritis
- Adhesive Capsulitis (frozen shoulder)
- Clavicular Fracture
- Acromioclavicular Joint Pathology

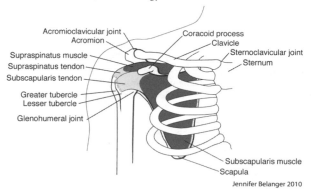

Jennifer Belanger 2010

Figure 2. Anatomy of the Right Shoulder

Physical Exam

Inspection

- Compare shoulder contours (anteriorly), alignment of the clavicles, symmetry of sternoclavicular and acromioclavicular joints, and scapulae (posteriorly)
- Note any scars, masses, lesions, abrasions, bruising and erythema of the skin at and around the shoulders
- Note any swelling, deformity, muscle atrophy and asymmetry of the soft tissues and bones
- Note biceps tendon rupture by asking the patient to flex their arm and observe for a bulge of tissue ("popeye sign")

MUSCULOSKELETAL

Palpation
- Palpate the sternoclavicular joint and along the clavicle to the acromioclavicular joint to feel for asymmetry and/or discontinuity
- Palpate the anterior and lateral aspects of the glenohumoral joint: feel the bicipital groove, subdeltoid bursa and rotator cuff insertion (for tenderness)
- Palpate the glenohumoral joint for crepitus by placing your hand over the subacromial bursa and passively circumduct the arm
- Palpate over the deltoids to test for touch sensation by the axillary nerve

Range of Motion
- Perform the following screening test, noting any crepitus by cupping your hand over the shoulder joint during these movements (see **Table 1** for normal values):
    - *Forward flexion* – "Raise both your arms in front of you until they are straight above your head"
    - *External rotation and abduction* – "Place both your hands behind your neck with your elbows out to the sides"
        - Hands should reach the neck base
    - *Abduction and adduction* – "Raise both arms from your sides straight over head, palms together; now bring them slowly down to your side again"
    - *Extension and internal rotation* – "Bring your arms towards your back and place your hands between the shoulder blades"
        - Hands should normally reach the inferior angle of the scapulae; record the level of the scapulae that can be reached
- Pain during motion can be localized
- Both shoulders can be assessed simultaneously
- If the screening tests above demonstrate any limitation of motion, assess the range of motion for passive movements as well

Table 1. Shoulder: Normal Ranges of Motion

Movement	Normal Range of Motion
Forward flexion	165°
Backward extension	60°
Abduction	170°
Adduction	50°
External rotation (with elbows at sides)	70°
Internal rotation (with shoulder abducted to 90° and elbow flexed)	70°

Special Tests

Tests for Anterior Shoulder Instability
- *Anterior Apprehension Test*: With patient sitting or standing, patient's arm is passively abducted to 90°, elbow is flexed to 90° and arm is externally rotated 90° (into a "throwing position"). Examiner applies pressure to posterior aspect of humerus
    - Expression of apprehension that the shoulder will dislocate or pain is a positive result
- *Relocation Test*: With patient supine, patient's arm is passively abducted to 90°, elbow is flexed to 90° and arm is externally rotated 90°. Examiner applies downward (posterior) pressure to humeral head
    - Relief of symptoms of apprehension or pain is a positive result

- *Anterior Release Test*: The relocation test is performed, and the examiner's hand is suddenly removed from the proximal humerus
  - Expression of apprehension or pain is a positive result

Test for Posterior Shoulder Instability (Posterior Apprehension Test)
- With the patient supine, the arm is abducted to 90° and the humerus is maximally internally rotated
- Examiner applies downward (posterior) pressure to humeral head
- Apprehension by the patient is a positive result and indicates posterior instability

Test for Inferior Shoulder Instability (Sulcus Sign)
- The patient stands or sits with the arm by the side and shoulder muscles relaxed
- Arm is pulled vertically downward
- Presence of a sulcus sign (indentation between acromion and humeral head) is suggestive of inferior shoulder instability

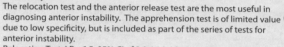

> **Evidence-Based Medicine: Shoulder Instability or Labrum Lesion Instability:**
> The relocation test and the anterior release test are the most useful in diagnosing anterior instability. The apprehension test is of limited value due to low specificity, but is included as part of the series of tests for anterior instability.
> Relocation Test: LR+ 6.5, 95% CI of 3.0-14.0; LR- 0.18, 95% CI of 0.07-0.45
> Anterior Release Test: LR+ 8.3, 95% CI of 3.6-19; LR- 0.09, 95% CI of 0.03-0.27
> The sulcus sign for inferior instability has a sensitivity of 31% and a specificity 89%.
>
> Luime JJ et al. 2004. *JAMA* 292(16):1989-1999.

Test for Glenoid Labral Pathology
- *O'Brien's Sign*: The patient's arm is flexed to 90° with the elbow in full extension and then adduct the arm 15° medial to sagittal plane. The arm is then internally rotated (thumb pointing downwards) and the patient resists the examiner's downward force
- Procedure is then repeated in supination
- If pain is elicited by the first maneuvre and it is reduced by the second maneuvre, this indicates a positive test
- A false positive result may occur with rotator cuff of AC joint pathology

Test for Impingement Syndrome (Rotator Cuff Tendinitis)
- *Neer's Test*: With patient sitting or standing, the examiner stabilizes the patient's scapula and maximally forward flexes the patient's shoulder with the other hand. Reproduction of patient's pain at maximal forward flexion is a positive test. This test can be repeated with the patient's elbow flexed and humerus internally rotated to increase the discomfort if no pain is felt on first test (**Figure 3**)
- *Hawkin's-Kennedy Test*: With patient standing, the examiner will raise the patient's arm to 90° forward flexion and then gently internally rotate the arm so that the thumb is turning downwards
  - Reproduction of patient's pain with internal rotation and shoulder flexion is a positive test
- *Swim Stroke Test*: With patient sitting or standing, the examiner will instruct the patient to circumduct their arm so that they are imitating free-style swimming stroke
  - Pain with active abduction between 60-120° is a positive test

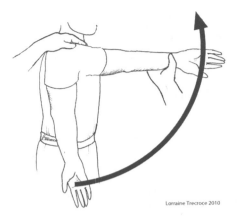

Lorraine Trecroce 2010

Figure 3. Neer's Test for Shoulder Impingement

Tests for Rotator Cuff Tears

- *Drop Arm Test*: The patient's arm is passively abducted to 90° with the elbow in full extension. The patient is then asked to slowly lower his/her arm back to the side. If arm drops suddenly or if patient has severe pain, this indicates rotator cuff tear
- *Empty Can (Jobe's) Test*: The patient's shoulder is abducted to 45° and with their hands turned downwards so that the thumbs are pointing down (i.e. emptying a can). The patient is then asked to move their arm upwards as you apply a downward resistance. If the patient has severe pain, this indicates a tear in the supraspinatus muscle (**Figure 4**)

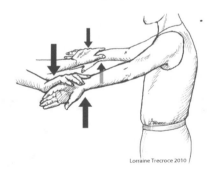

Lorraine Trecroce 2010

Figure 4. Empty Can (Jobe's) Test for Supraspinatus Tear

- *Infraspinatus and Teres Minor Strength Test*: The patient's shoulder is abducted to 25° with elbows bent at 90°. The patient is then asked to rotate their shoulders externally as you apply a resistance on their arms towards the midline of their body. If the patient has severe pain, this indicates a tear in the infraspinatus and/or teres minor muscle (**Figure 5**)

MUSCULOSKELETAL

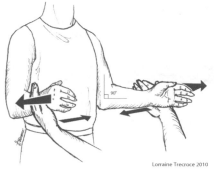

Lorraine Trecroce 2010

Figure 5. Infraspinatus and Teres Minor Strength Test

- *Gerber's Lift Off Test*: The patient's hands are placed behind their back with palms facing out, with forearms almost 90° to the length of the spine. The patient is then asked to lift their hands away from their back as you apply a resistance towards their body. If the patient has severe pain, this indicates a tear in the subscapularis muscle (**Figure 6**)

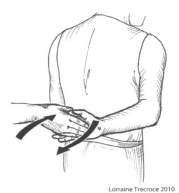

Lorraine Trecroce 2010

Figure 6. Gerber's Lift-Off Test for Subscapularis Tear

> **Clinical Pearl**
> Shoulder pain (radiating down the arm to the elbow) when combing one's hair, putting on a coat or reaching into a back pocket indicates supraspinatus inflammation.
>
> Diffuse shoulder pain upon moving the humerus posteriorly (without radiation to the arm) indicates infraspinatus inflammation.
>
> Discomfort and weakness of the upper extremity and "winging" of the ipsilateral scapula indicates a dysfunction of the serratus anterior or trapezius muscles, often secondary to long thoracic or accessory nerve palsies.

MUSCULOSKELETAL

Common Clinical Scenarios

Shoulder pain can be acute or chronic in nature and is commonly caused by soft tissue trauma/inflammation (**Table 2**)

Table 2. Common Clinical Conditions of the Shoulder

Condition	Clinical Features
Rotator cuff tendinitis	Shoulder pain on activity Sharp pain on elevation of arm into overhead position History of chronic usage (e.g. throwing, swimming) or trauma
Rotator cuff tear/rupture	Sharp pain after trauma Pain over greater tuberosity Characteristic shoulder shrug and pain on attempted abduction Weakness on external rotation
Bicipital tendinitis	Generalized anterior tenderness over long head of biceps Associated with pain, especially at night Hallmark is reproduction of anterior shoulder pain during resistance to forearm supination

ELBOW

Common Symptoms
- Pain (well-localized)
- Swelling
- Stiffness

Common Clinical Scenarios
✓ Arthritis
✓ Lateral epicondylitis (tennis elbow)
✓ Medial epicondylitis (golfer's elbow)
✓ Olecranon bursitis

Physical Exam

Inspection
- Inspect for swelling or masses (e.g. olecranon bursitis or rheumatic nodules)
- Ask the patient: "With your palms facing up, bend and then extend your elbow"
- Note differences in carrying angles, flexion contractures, hyperextension

Palpation
- Palpate olecranon process, medial and lateral epicondyles, and extensor surface of forearm (3-4 cm distal to olecranon) for swelling, masses, tenderness and nodules
- Grasp the elbow with your fingers under the olecranon and your thumb next to the biceps tendon
- Passively flex and extend the elbow; note any crepitus, tenderness or restricted movement
- Feel for masses on each side of the biceps tendon

Range of Motion

- Ask the patient: "Bend your elbows until you can touch your shoulders (flexion) and then place your arms back down (extension)"
- With the patient's arms at sides and elbows flexed, ask the patient to turn his/her palms up (supination) and down (pronation); having patients hold a pencil in their fist may help with estimating the range of motion in degrees
- Note any limitation of motion (see **Table 3**) or pain

Table 3. Elbow: Normal Ranges of Motion

Movement	Normal Range of Motion
Flexion	145°
Extension	0°
Supination	80° from vertical (with pencil grasped in hand)
Pronation	75° from vertical (with pencil grasped in hand)

Interpretation of Findings

Table 4. Clinical Features Differentiating Diseases Affecting the Elbow

Clinical Feature	Rheumatoid Arthritis	Psoriatic Arthritis	Acute Gout	Osteo-arthritis	Lateral Epicondylitis
Age	3-80	10-60	30-80	50-80	20-60
Pain onset	Gradual	Gradual	Abrupt	Gradual	Gradual
Stiffness	Very Common	Common	Absent	Common	Occasional
Swelling	Common	Common	Common	Common	Absent
Redness	Absent	Uncommon	Common	Absent	Absent
Deformity	Flexion contractures, usually bilaterally	Flexion contractures, usually bilaterally	Flexion contractures, only in chronic state	Flexion contractures	None

Adapted from Swartz M.H. 2002. *Textbook of Physical Diagnosis: History and Examination,* 4th edition. W.B. Saunders Co. Philadelphia.

Common Clinical Scenarios

Epicondylitis

- Characterized by pain in the region of the epicondyle(s) of the humerus, radiating down the surface of the forearm
- Patients often experience pain when attempting to open a door or when lifting a glass

Test For Tennis Elbow (lateral epicondylitis)

- While palpating the lateral epicondyle, pronate the patient's forearm, flex the wrist fully, and extend the elbow
- Pain over the lateral epicondyle is diagnostic

Test For Golfer's Elbow (medial epicondylitis)

- While palpating the medial epicondyle, the patient's forearm is supinated and the elbow and wrist are extended
- Pain over the medial epicondyle is diagnostic

MUSCULOSKELETAL

WRIST

Common Symptoms
- Pain in the wrist or hand
- Numbness or tingling (paresthesia) in the wrist or fingers
- Loss of movement and stiffness
- Deformities

Common Clinical Scenarios
✓ Carpal tunnel syndrome
✓ Rheumatoid arthritis

Physical Exam

Inspection
- Inspect the palmar and dorsal surfaces of the wrist for swelling over the joints or deformities

Palpation
- Palpate the distal radius and ulna on the lateral and medial surfaces
- Palpate the groove of each wrist joint with your thumbs on the dorsum of the wrist, your fingers beneath it
- Note any tenderness, swelling, warmth or redness
- Palpate the anatomical snuffbox (a hollowed depression just distal to the radial styloid process formed by the abductor and extensor muscles of the thumb)
  - Tenderness over the snuffbox suggests a scaphoid fracture or carpal arthritis

Range of Motion
- *Extension*: ask the patient to press the palms of the hands together in the vertical plane and to bring the forearms into the horizontal plane
- *Flexion*: ask the patient to put the backs of the hands in contact and then to bring the forearms into the horizontal plane
- Note any asymmetry and limitation of motion (see **Table 5**)
- Test active ulnar and radial deviation
- Test active pronation and supination (having patients hold a pencil in their fist may help with estimating the range of motion in degrees)

Table 5. Wrist: Normal Ranges of Motion

Movement	Normal Range of Motion
Flexion	75°
Extension	75°
Radial deviation	20°
Ulnar deviation	35°
Supination	80° from vertical (with pencil grasped in hand)
Pronation	75° from vertical (with pencil grasped in hand)

MUSCULOSKELETAL

Common Clinical Scenarios

Carpal Tunnel Syndrome
- *Carpal tunnel*: A bony trough covered by the flexor retinaculum through which the median nerve and wrist flexors pass
- Usually diagnosed in patients 20-40 yrs old; ratio of women to men is 3:1
- Entrapment of the nerve produces symptoms of burning, tingling, pins and needles, and numbness in the median nerve distribution (generally worse at night)
- Common causes: fluid retention (common in pregnancy), hypothyroidism, diabetes mellitus and overuse of the tendons from repeated forceful movements of the wrist (either at work or recreation)

Tests for Carpal Tunnel Syndrome
- *Tinel's Sign*: A sharp tap is given with the fingers directly over the median nerve (located medial to the flexor carpi radialis tendon at the most proximal aspect of the palm)
    - Tingling, paresthesia or pain in the area of the thumb, index finger, middle finger and radial half of the ring finger is a positive test
- *Phalen's Sign*: The patient is asked to put the dorsal aspects of their hands in contact so that their wrists are maximally flexed
    - Test is positive if the patient notes paresthesia or numbness in the area of the thumb, index finger, middle finger and radial half of the ring finger after holding this position for 60 seconds or less
- *Katz hand diagram*: Ask patient to indicate location of sensory symptoms on a diagram of hand and arm
    - Classic pattern or probable pattern (**Table 6**) suggests diagnosis
- Compare ability to perceive painful stimuli applied along the palmar aspect of the index finger compared with the ipsilateral little finger
    - Decreased sensitivity to pain (hypalgesia) in the index finger suggests diagnosis
- Test strength in abductor pollicis brevis (thumb abduction)
    - Weakness suggests diagnosis

Table 6. Katz Hand Diagram

Pattern	Description
Classic pattern	At least two of the thumb, index finger or middle finger are affected. This pattern permits symptoms in the ring finger and small finger, wrist pain, and radiation of pain proximal to wrist. Symptoms on palm or dorsum of hand are not allowed
Probable pattern	Same as classic but palmar symptoms allowed unless solely confined to ulnar aspect
Possible pattern	Symptoms involve only one of thumb, index finger or middle finger
Unlikely pattern	No symptoms are present in thumb, index finger or middle finger

HAND

Common Symptoms
- Pain and swelling of joints

Common Clinical Scenarios
✓ De Quervain's Stenosing Tenosynovitis (De Quervain's Disease)
✓ Rheumatoid arthritis

Physical Exam

Inspection
- Carefully inspect for deformities, cuts, scars and wounds, with special emphasis on possible damage to nerves and tendons (see **Table 7**)
- Note any tenderness, redness, or swelling

Table 7. Common Deformities of the Hand

Name of Deformity	Description	Interpretation
Mallet finger/thumb	Flexed DIP caused by damage to the extensor tendon	Trauma or RA
Swan neck deformity	Flexed DIP and hyperextended PIP	RA, but has many other causes
Boutonniere deformity	Hyperextended DIP and flexed PIP Occurs when the central slip of the extensor tendon detaches from the middle phalanx	Trauma or RA
Dupuytren's contracture	Flexion deformity of the fingers at the MCP and IPs, associated with nodular thickening in the palm and fingers	Associated with diabetes, epilepsy, alcoholism and hereditary tendencies
Heberden's nodes	Hard dorsolateral nodules of DIPs, often associated with a deviation of the distal phalanx	OA
Bouchard's nodes	Similar to Heberden's nodes, but affects the PIPs	OA

DIP=distal interphalangeal joint, RA=rheumatoid arthritis, PIP=proximal interphalangeal joint, OA=osteoarthritis, MCP=metacarpophalangeal joint, IP=interphalangeal joint

MUSCULOSKELETAL

Palpation
- Compress the MCP joints by squeezing the patient's hand between your thumb and index finger
  - If this causes pain, use your thumb to palpate the dorsal side of each MCP joint while using your index finger to feel the heads of the MCPs on the palmar side
- Palpate the medial and lateral aspects of each PIP and DIP joint (dorsal and volar surfaces) with your index finger and thumb

Range of Motion
- Check for smooth, coordinated and easily performed movements
- See **Table 9** for sensory and motor distribution of the radial, ulnar and median nerves
- Ask the patient: "Make a fist with each hand with your thumb across the knuckles, and then open your hand and spread your fingers"
- During flexion:
  - Normal fingers should flex to the distal palmar crease
  - Thumb should oppose the DIP joint
- During extension:
  - Each finger should extend to the zero position in relation to its metacarpal upon opening
- Assess motion of the thumb: flexion, extension, abduction, adduction, opposition (movement of the thumb across the palm)

Table 8. Hand: Normal Ranges of Motion

Digit	Joint	Range of Motion
Fingers	MCPs	0-90°
	PIPs	0-100°
	DIPs	0-80°
Thumb	MCP	5° extension; 55° flexion
	IP	20° extension; 80° flexion

Special Tests
- For intact flexor digitorum superficialis: restrict motion of 3 out of 4 fingers by holding down distal phalanges with the dorsum of the patient's hand (palm up) rested on a table; ask the patient to flex the free finger and look for PIP flexion
- For intact flexor digitorum profundus: hold down both the proximal and middle phalanges and ask the patient to flex fingers; look for DIP flexion

MUSCULOSKELETAL

Interpretation of Findings

Table 9. Nerves Supplying the Hand

Nerve	Sensory	Motor
Radial	Dorsum of first webspace	Extension of fingers, thumb, and wrist
Posterior interosseous branch	None	Thumb extension
Ulnar	Tip of small finger (dorsum) Small finger/medial ring finger (palmar)	Finger abduction and adduction, ring and small finger DIP flexion, opposition of small finger, wrist flexion
Median	Tip of index/middle/lateral half of ring finger (dorsum) Index/middle/lateral half of ring finger (palmar)	Thumb IP flexion, index/middle finger flexion, wrist flexion
Anterior interosseous branch	None	Flexion of index/middle finger
Lateral terminal branch	None	Thumb opposition

Table 10. Arthritis in the Hand and Wrist

Joint	Osteoarthritis	Rheumatoid Arthritis
DIP	Very common	Rare
PIP	Common	Very common
MCP	Rare	Very common
Wrist	Rare*	Very common

*Osteoarthritis will sometimes affect only the carpometacarpal joint of the thumb

Common Clinical Scenarios

De Quervain's Disease

- Tenosynovitis involving abductor pollicis longus and extensor pollicis brevis
- Patient complains of weakness of grip and pain at the base of the thumb which is aggravated by certain movements of the wrist
- *Finkelstein Test*: ask the patient to flex thumb and close the fingers over it; then attempt to move the hand into ulnar deviation
    - Excruciating pain with this maneuver occurs in De Quervain's tenosynovitis

SPINE

Common Symptoms
- Pain (most common symptom with characteristic patterns)

Table 11. Common Patterns of Back Pain

Etiology	Clinical Features
Intervertebral discs or adjacent ligament involvement	Back dominant (back, buttock, trochanter, groin) Pain: worse with flexion Pattern: constant or intermittent
Posterior joint complex involvement	Back dominant Pain: worse with extension (never worse with flexion) Pattern: intermittent
Sciatica-L4, L5, S1, S2	Leg dominant (below buttock) Pain: worse with back movement Pattern: previously or currently constant
Neurogenic Claudication due to nerve compression	Leg dominant Pain: worse with acitivity and better with rest Pattern: intermittent (short duration)

Common Clinical Scenarios
- ✓ Cervical spondylosis
- ✓ Whiplash and extension injuries of the neck
- ✓ Scoliosis
- ✓ Kyphosis
- ✓ Ankylosing Spondylitis
- ✓ Spina Bifida
- ✓ Prolapsed Intervertebral Disc
- ✓ Spinal stenosis
- ✓ Spondylolisthesis
- ✓ Degenerative disc disease

Differential Diagnosis of Back Pain (Age-Dependent)
- Degenerative (90% of all back pain)
  - Mechanical problem (degenerative, facet)
  - Spinal stenosis (congenital, osteophyte, central disc)
  - Peripheral nerve compression (disc herniation)
- Other
  - Infection
  - Cauda equina syndrome
  - Neoplastic: primary or metastatic
  - Trauma: fracture (compression, distraction, translation, rotation)
  - Spondyloarthropathies (e.g. ankylosing spondylitis)
  - Referred: aorta, renal, ureter, pancreas

Physical Exam for Cervical Spine

Inspection
- May be examined with the patient seated; in general, check for deformity, unusual posture, physical asymmetries, and guarding
- In normal sitting posture, nose should be in line with manubrium and xyphoid process of sternum; from side, ear lobe should be in line with acromion process

- Check for the head tilting or rotation to one side; indicates possible torticollis
- Check for Klippel-Feil syndrome (fusion of the cervical vertebrae resulting in a short and relatively immobile neck; congenital)
- Check for venous obstruction in the upper limbs
  - Note any temperature changes, sensory changes, altered colouration of the skin, ulcers, or vein distension

Palpation
- Palpate for any tenderness, trigger points, muscle spasms, skin texture and bony/soft tissue abnormalities on the posterior, lateral and anterior aspects of the neck
- Posterior aspect: external occipital protuberance, spinous processes and facet joints of cervical vertebrae, mastoid processes
- Lateral aspect: transverse processes of cervical vertebrae, lymph nodes and carotid arteries, temporomandibular joints, mandible, and parotid glands
- Anterior aspect: hyoid bone, thyroid cartilage, supraclavicular fossa

Range of Motion – Active Movements
- Ask the patient to perform the movements in **Table 12**

Table 12. Active Movements of the Cervical Spine and Their Normal Ranges of Motion

Maneuver	Normal Range of Motion
Flexion ("Touch your chin to your chest")	80-90°
Extension ("Put your head back")	70°
Side Flexion* ("Touch each shoulder with your ear without raising your shoulders")	20-45°
Rotation* ("Turn your head to the left and right")	70-90°

*Look for symmetrical movements

Range of Motion – Passive Movements
- Flexion, extension, side flexion and rotation should all be tested with passive movements to test the "end feel" of each movement
- For each movement, the end feel should be tissue stretch

Power Assessment/Isometric Movements
- Flexion, extension, side flexion and rotation should all be tested with isometric movements
- Determine muscle power and possible neurological weakness originating from the nerve roots in the cervical spine by testing the myotomes with isometric movements. Each contraction should be held for at least 5 seconds. The movements and their myotomes are given in **Table 13**

Table 13. Cervical Spine Movements and Their Respective Myotomes

Movement	Myotome
Neck flexion	C1-C2
Neck side flexion	C3
Shoulder elevation	C4
Shoulder abduction	C5
Elbow flexion and/or wrist extension	C5-C6
Elbow extension and/or wrist flexion	C7
Thumb extension and/or ulnar deviation	C8
Abduction and/or adduction of hand intrinsics	T1

MUSCULOSKELETAL

Reflexes
- Biceps (C5, C6), triceps (C7, C8), brachioradialis (C5-C6) need assessment
- See **Neurological Exam** p. 190

Special Tests

Tests for Thoracic Outlet Syndrome
- Look for evidence of ischemia in one hand (coldness, discolouration, trophic changes)
    - Bilateral changes are more suggestive of Raynaud's disease
- Palpate radial pulse and apply traction to arm; obliteration of pulse is not diagnostic, but a normal pulse present on opposite arm may suggest thoracic outlet syndrome
- Paresthesia in the hand is usually severe
- May have hypothenar wasting; thenar wasting less common

Physical Exam for Thoracic Spine

Inspection
- Examine with the patient standing
- SEADS
- Inspect for
    - Kyphosis, scoliosis (an imaginary line drawn down from T1 should fall through the gluteal cleft)
    - Adam's Forward Bend Test – have the patient bend over and see if there is a rib prominence (rib hump) on one side. This is an indication of scoliosis
- Check breathing – children tend to breathe abdominally, women are upper thoracic breathers, men tend to be upper and lower thoracic breathers, elderly are lower thoracic and abdomen breathers
- Inspect for chest deformities
    - e.g. pectus carinatum, pectus excavatum, barrel chest
- Note asymmetry
    - Look for symmetrical folds of skin on either side of the spine
- Look for differences in height of shoulders and iliac crests
- Inspect for any cutaneous manifestations, hairy patches (evidence of congenital anomalies e.g. diastematomyelia), café au lait spots (evidence of neurofibromatosis), scars

Palpation
- Palpate for tenderness, muscle spasm, altered temperature, swelling
    - Usually done with patient sitting
- Anterior aspect – sternum, ribs and costal cartilages, clavicles, abdomen
- Posterior aspect – scapulae, spinous processes of the thoracic spine

Percussion
- Percussion of spine is performed routinely to examine for tenderness and irritability
- Ask patient to stand and bend forward
- Lightly percuss spine with fist in an orderly progression from root of neck to sacrum
- Significant pain is a feature of TB and other infections, trauma (especially fractures) and neoplasms

MUSCULOSKELETAL

Range of Motion – Active Movements
- Ask the patient to perform the movements in **Table 14**

Table 14. Active Movements for the Thoracic and Lumbar Spine and their Normal ROM

Maneuver	Normal Range of Motion	
	Thoracic Spine	**Lumbar Spine**
Forward flexion: "Bend forward and touch your toes"*	20-45°	40-60°
Extension: Standing behind the patient at an arm's length, stabilize pelvis to prevent him/her from falling; then ask: "Arch your back"	25-45°	20-35°
Side flexion: For each side, ask patient to: "Slide your hand down your leg"**	20-40°	15-20°
Rotation: With the patient seated, ask the patient to: "Rotate toward each side"	35-50°	3-18°
Chest expansion: Place a tape measure around patient's chest; note difference between rest and full inspiration	Normal is >5 cm	N/A

*With forward flexion, the distance from the fingers to the ground is measured; the majority of patients can reach the ground within 7 cm. Other methods are: 1) The examiner first measures the length of the spine from the C7 spinous process to the T12 spinous process with the patient standing. The patient is then asked to bend forward, and the spine is measured again – a 2-7 cm difference in tape measure length is considered normal; and 2) The examiner compares the length of the spine from the C7 spinous process to the S1 spinous process with the patient standing and with the patient bent forward – a 10 cm difference in tape measure length is considered normal. This measures thoracic and lumbar movement, but with most movement, 7.5 cm occurs between T12 and S1
**With side flexion, distance from fingertips to floor is measured and compared with other side – should be same

Range of Motion – Passive Movements
- Flexion, extension, side flexion, and rotation should all be tested with passive movements to test the "end feel" (tissue stretch) of each movement

Power Assessment/Isometric Movements
- Performed with patient sitting
- The examiner is positioned behind the patient. Instruction of "Don't let me move you" is given, and the movements of forward flexion, extension, side flexion, and rotation of the spine are tested

Reflexes
- Patellar (L3-L4), medial hamstring (L5-S1), and Achilles reflex (S1-S2) need assessment since pathology of thoracic spine can affect these reflexes
- Abdominal reflexes should also be tested to assess the mid-thoracic cord
- See ***Neurological Exam*** p. 190

Special Tests

Slump Test (Sitting Dural Stretch Test)
- The patients sits and is asked to "slump" – spine flexes and shoulders sag while head and chin are held erect by examiner
  - If no symptoms (pain) are produced, examiner flexes the neck and applies a small amount of pressure
  - If no symptoms are produced, one knee is extended passively
  - If no symptoms are produced, the foot on the same side is dorsiflexed

MUSCULOSKELETAL

- Process is repeated with other leg
- Positive Test: reproduction of patient's symptoms (pain) may indicate possible impingement of the dura, spinal cord or nerve roots

Physical Exam for Lumbar Spine

Inspection
- Deformities or swelling
- Inspect for scoliosis, lumbar lordosis (see thoracic spine)
- Check body type of patient (ectomorphic, mesomorphic or endomorphic)
- Inspect gait
- Inspect total spinal posture (waist angles should be equal, "high" points on iliac crest should be the same height, leg length should be equal)
- Inspect for skin markings: a "faun's beard" (tuft of hair) may indicate a spina bifida occulta or diastematomyelia. Café-au-lait spots may indicate neurofibromatosis or collagen disease
- Check for dimples, scars

Palpation
- Tenderness, altered temperature, muscle spasm
- Palpate the paravertebral muscles
- Anterior Aspect: with patient supine, palpate umbilicus, inguinal areas (look for hernia, abscess, infection), iliac crests, symphysis pubis
- Posterior Aspect: with patient prone, palpate spinous processes of lumbar vertebrae and at the lumbosacral junction, sacrum, sacroiliac joints, coccyx, iliac crests, ischial tuberosities

Percussion
- Same procedure as percussion for thoracic spine (p. 161)

Range of Motion
- See **Table 14** for directions and normal ROM

Power Assessment/Isometric Movements
- As described in thoracic spine isometric movement exam (p. 162)
- Myotomes are tested with the examiner placing the test joint or joints in a neutral or resting position and then applying a resisted isometric pressure that is held for at least 5 seconds (see **Table 15**)

Table 15. Lower Limb Movements and Their Respective Myotomes

Lower Limb Movement	Myotome
Hip flexion	L2
Knee extension	L3
Ankle dorsiflexion	L4
Great toe extension	L5
Ankle plantar flexion, ankle eversion, hip extension	S1
Knee flexion	S2

Reflexes
- Patellar (L3-L4), medial hamstring (L5-S1), lateral hamstring (S1-S2), posterior tibial (L4-L5) and Achilles (S1-S2) reflexes should be assessed
- See *Neurological Exam* p. 190

MUSCULOSKELETAL

Special Tests

Straight Leg Raise (Lasegue) Test (see **Figure 7**)

- The patient is in the supine position with the hips in a neutral position
- The examiner, ensuring the patient's knee remains extended, supports and raises the leg until radicular pain (back or leg) is felt
- This maneuver stretches the sciatic nerve
- Note the degree of elevation (pain usually occurs less than 60° only if there is an abnormality). Also note quality and distribution of the pain
- Back pain suggests a central disc prolapse while leg pain suggests a lateral protrusion (ensure that pain is not due to hamstring tightness)
- The leg is lowered in increments until pain is relieved
- If dorsiflexion of the ankle results in a return of the pain, it is an indication of nerve root irritation (positive Lasegue Sign)
- Paresthesia or radiating pain in the distribution of the sciatic nerve (L4 - S3) suggests nerve root irritation/tension
    - Note: The pain must be below the knee if the roots of the sciatic nerve are involved
- Compare with the other leg (with central disc protrusions, cross-over pain may occur (e.g. straight leg raising on one side may cause pain down the opposite leg)

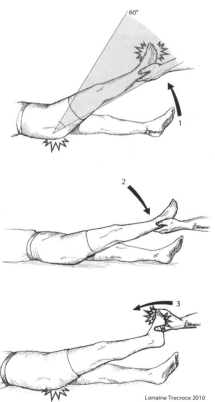

Lorraine Trecroce 2010

Figure 7. Straight Leg Raise (Lasegue) Test for Nerve Root Irritation

Femoral Stretch Test (Reverse Lasegue)

- With the patient lying prone; stretch the femoral nerve roots (L2-L4) by extending the hip (lift the thigh with one hand and use the other hand to maintain full extension of the knee)
- Limited hip extension due to pain radiating into the thigh suggests nerve root irritation

Rib-Pelvis Distance

- Assesses height loss (due to vertebral compression fractures)
- Examiner's hands are inserted into the space between inferior margin of the ribs and superior surface of pelvis in the midaxillary line while the patient is standing
- The rib-pelvis distance is determined in fingerbreadths to the closest whole value

Screen the Hips

- Both osteoarthritis of the hip and a prolapsed intervertebral disc (at L2-3 or L3-4) are often confused with spinal stenosis

Peripheral Vascular System

- Crucial to obtain a thorough history to distinguish between claudication due to vascular insufficiency versus due to spinal stenosis
  - i.e. vascular claudication versus neurogenic claudication
- Claudication due to vascular insufficiency: constant pain, worse with walking, occurs after walking a very consistent distance; involves a stocking type of sensory loss; peripheral pulses usually absent; is rapidly relieved by rest
- Claudication due to spinal stenosis: relieved by changes in posture (sitting, bending, flexing spine) and rest; slower to be relieved by pain than claudication due to vascular insufficiency

MUSCULOSKELETAL

Common Clinical Scenarios

Sciatica
- Pain due to entrapment of sciatic nerve
- Patients complain of pain, burning, or aching in buttocks radiating down posterior thigh to the posterolateral aspect of calf
- Pain is worsened by sneezing, laughing or straining during bowel movement
- Use Straight Leg Raising Test to help in diagnosis (see **Figure 7**)

Cauda Equina Syndrome
- Most frequent cause is large central disc herniation (do *not* miss this diagnosis!)
- Progressive neurological deficit presenting with:
  - Saddle anesthesia
  - Decreased anal tone and reflex
  - Fecal incontinence
  - Urinary retention (overflow incontinence)
  - Bilateral lower leg weakness
  - **Surgical emergency!** Will cause permanent urinary/bowel incontinence

Thoracic Outlet Syndrome
- Compression of the lower trunk of the brachial plexus and the subclavian artery
- May be due to fibrous bands or abnormalities in the scalene attachments at the root of the neck or by a Pancoast tumour
- May also be due to a cervical rib (rare)

HIP

Common Symptoms
- Pain
- Stiffness

Common Clinical Scenarios

Hip Fracture
- May be due to trauma or fragility fracture due to osteoporosis
- Injured leg is unable to bear weight, is shorter and may be internally or externally rotated
- Patient experiences sharp pain in groin and down thigh

Avascular Necrosis
- Bone cell death due to decreased blood flow to the head of the femur
- Causes include hip fracture, prolonged steroid use, idiopathic, alcoholism, diving to depth

> **Clinical Pearl**
> Pain referred to groin and thigh is HIP pain.
> Pain referred to buttocks is BACK pain.

Physical Exam

Inspection
- With patient standing
  - Inspect from the front and from behind for any pelvic tilting or rotational deformity
  - Note any abnormalities of bony or soft tissue contours
  - From the side, note presence of lumbar lordosis that may indicate a fixed flexion deformity
  - Observe the contour of the buttock for any abnormality (gluteus maximus atrophy or atonia)
- Examine gait
  - Note antalgic gait (to avoid pain, time spent on injured limb during stance phase is minimized)
  - Note Trendelenberg gait (dropping of the pelvis on the unaffected side during the stance phase of the affected side)
- Trendelenburg Test
  - Ask the patient to stand on one leg
  - Pelvis on non-weight bearing side should not drop, indicating functioning abductors on the weight bearing leg
  - If the pelvis drops, it is a positive test
    - Can be caused by gluteal muscle weakness (mainly gluteus medius), inhibition from pain, or a hip deformity
- Measurement of Leg Length
  - True leg length – pelvis must first be set square and feet placed 15-20 cm apart; measure each leg from anterior superior iliac spine to the medial malleolus
  - Apparent length – apparent shortening (e.g. uncorrectable pelvic tilting) may also be assessed by comparing the distances between the umbilicus and each medial malleolus

Palpation
- Anterior Aspect
  - Palpate the iliac crest, greater trochanter and trochanteric bursa, anterior superior iliac spine, inguinal ligament, femoral triangle and symphysis pubis
  - Palpate the hip flexors, adductor and abductor muscles for signs of pathology
  - Palpate for crepitations by placing your fingers over the femoral head (which is just lateral to the femoral artery below the inguinal ligament)
  - Roll the relaxed leg medially and laterally to detect any crepitations
- Posterior Aspect
  - Palpate the iliac crest, posterior superior iliac spine, ischial tuberosity, greater trochanter, sacroiliac, lumbosacral, and sacrococcygeal joints

Range of Motion
- See **Table 17** for maneuvers and normal ROM

Table 17. Maneuvers for the Hip and Normal Range of Motion

Maneuver	Normal Range of Motion
Flexion – with patient lying supine, have patient pull knee to chest; knee is also flexed	~120°
Extension – with patient lying on side, palpate the ASIS and PSIS and have patient fully extend the leg until pelvis shifts	~15°
Abduction – place one hand on the contralateral ASIS and with the other hand, grasp the heel and abduct the patient's leg until the pelvis shifts	~40°
Adduction – place one hand on the ipsilateral ASIS and with the other hand, grasp the heel and adduct the patient's leg until the pelvis shifts	~25°
Rotation – flex knee and hip to 90°, grasp the lower leg and move medially (external rotation) and laterally (internal rotation) OR with patient lying supine with the leg fully extended, roll the leg medially and laterally	External Rotation in ext: ~35° External Rotation at 90° flex ~45° Internal Rotation in ext: ~45° Internal Rotation at 90° flex ~45°

Power Assessment/Isometric Movements
- Performed with patient in supine position (except for hip extension), noting which movements cause pain or show weakness
- Since hip muscles are strong, instruction of "Don't let me move your leg" ensures that the movement is isometric
- All active movements performed should be tested isometrically

Special Tests

Patrick's Test (Fabere or Figure Four Test)
- Patient lies supine, with both knees flexed
- The foot of the test leg is placed on top of the knee of the opposite leg
- Gently press down on the knee of the test leg, lowering it towards the examining table
- Test is negative when test leg is at least parallel with the opposite leg
- Test is positive when the leg remains above the opposite leg
- Positive test indicates an affected hip or sacroiliac joint, or that iliopsoas spasms exist
- Pain indicates early osteoarthritic changes

Thomas Test
- Used to assess hip flexion contracture (fixed flexion deformity), the most common contracture of the hip
- With the patient supine, place your hand under the lumbar spine
- Reduce lumbar lordosis by passively flexing the hip by bringing the patient's knee to his/her abdomen (or ask the patient to hold their leg against their abdomen)
- Elevation of the opposite thigh suggests a loss of extension in that hip (tight hip flexors) and a fixed flexion deformity
- Useful observations to accompany this test:
  - Note the degree of knee flexion in the free leg (knee flexion <90° suggests tight quadriceps)
  - Note the degree of leg abduction in the free leg (abduction of the leg suggests tight abductors and/or tight ITB)

MUSCULOSKELETAL

KNEE

Common Symptoms
- Pain
- Instability
- Swelling
- Locking

Common Clinical Scenarios

Patello-femoral Syndrome
- May be due to misalignment in the articulation between the femur and the patella
- Pain is a dull ache at the anterior surface of the knee
- Pain is normally worse when going downstairs, squatting and getting up after sitting for prolonged periods
- Examination may reveal atrophic quadriceps muscles and mild knee swelling

Meniscal Injury
- Tear of the fibrocartilage cushioning the joint
- Knee may lock and/or click
- Tell tale sign is tenderness of the joint line over the involved meniscus

Ligamentous Injury
- Tear of a ligament due to trauma
- Pain is acute and severe
- Examination will reveal effusion (possibly hemarthrosis if rapid in onset), instability, bruising, limited ROM due to muscle spasm
- ACL injuries are commonly accompanied with MCL and medial meniscus injuries (O'Donoghue's triad)

Physical Exam

Inspection
- SEADS
  - *Swelling*: note any swelling in knees; specifically, look at the medial fossa and any bulging on the sides of the patellar ligament (indicative of small effusion)
  - *Atrophy*: inspect quadriceps for muscle atrophy (vastus medialis)
  - *Deformity*: ask the patient to stand with his/her feet together; inspect for genu valgum (knock-knee), genu varum (bow-leg), genu recurvatum (hyper-extended knee) or flexion contracture
- Inspect the patient's gait
  - Patient will limit extension and flexion of a painful knee and minimize time spent on the injured knee while walking (antalgic gait)

Palpation
- Anterior palpation with knee extended
  - With the back of the hand, palpate the knee for temperature; compare both sides proximal to the joint, over the patella and distal to the joint; normally, the patella is the coolest area of the knee

MUSCULOSKELETAL

- Palpate the anatomical structures noting tenderness, swelling or nodules; patellar tendon, tibial tuberosity, suprapatellar pouch (feel for thickening or swelling of the suprapatellar pouch starting 10 cm proximal to the superior border of the patella), quadriceps muscles, medial collateral ligament
- Anterior palpation with knee flexed
  - Using thumbs, palpate the tibiofemoral joint line; noting the lateral aspect for swelling (meniscal cysts), tibial condyles, femoral condyles
- Posterior palpation with knee flexed
  - Palpate the popliteal fossa (for a Baker's cyst), hamstrings and gastrocnemius muscles
- Range of Motion – Active Movement (see **Table 18**)

Table 18. Knee: Normal Ranges of Motion

Maneuver	Normal Range of Motion
Flexion	135°
Extension	0°

Range of Motion
- While patient is lying prone, have him/her actively flex and extend knee
- With the patient supine, passively flex and extend the patient's knee by placing one hand over the joint and one hand on the lower leg
  - Note any crepitus, clicking, as well as the end-feel of the motion
- Passive, medial and lateral movement of patella is also tested for mobility, symmetry:
  - Normally, patella should move half of its width laterally and medially
  - Note whether patella tilts, rotates, or stays parallel to femoral condyles

Special Tests

Tests for Effusion

Patellar Tap Test
- Place hand on the top of the femur, about 15 cm proximal to the patella, with index finger and thumb placed on either side
- Displace fluid from the suprapatellar pouch by sliding hand distally to just above the patella
- While maintaining pressure with the left hand, push down quickly on the patella with the tips of your thumb and 3 fingers of free hand
- In the presence of an effusion, a palpable tap (click) will be transmitted and felt by index finger and thumb on either side of the patella
- If the effusion is slight, the exam will be negative

Fluctuation/Ballotment Test
- Compress suprapatellar pouch back against the femur with your left hand as above
- With your right hand placed just below the patella, feel for fluid entering the patellar fossae spaces next to the patella with your right thumb and index finger
- If you feel fluid, confirm its presence by pushing the fluid between the medical and lateral fossae
  - Note: do not move the patella itself back and forth
- Press the patella backward against the femur with your right hand and feel fluid returning to the suprapatellar pouch

Fluid Displacement / "Milk" Bulge Test (for detecting small effusions)
- Place hand on the top of the femur, about 15 cm proximal to the patella, with index finger and thumb placed on either side
- Squeeze fluid out of the suprapatellar pouch as above
- With the back of the hand, stroke upwards on the medial side of the knee to milk fluid into the lateral compartment
- Stroke downwards on the lateral side of the knee and observe for fluid returning to the medial compartment, distending the medial fossa
- The wave of fluid may take up to 2 seconds to appear
- Normally, the knee contains 1 to 7 mL of synovial fluid
- This test shows as little as 4 to 8 mL of extra fluid in knee
- This test is positive if the effusion is small and negative if the effusion is large

Ligament Tests

Anterior Drawer Test for Anterior Cruciate Ligament (ACL) Tear
- With the patient supine, flex the hips to 45° and flex both knees to 90°
- Inspect the joint lines of both knees; a false positive can occur if the tibia was initially subluxed posteriorly due to a torn posterior cruciate ligament (PCL) (see **Posterior Sag Sign** p.172)
- Sit close to the foot to steady it, grasp the leg just below the knee with both hands, ensure the hamstrings are relaxed and pull the tibia forward (see **Figure 8**)
- Compare both knees, noting any abnormal forward displacement of the tibia
- Movement ≥1.5 cm is indicative of an ACL tear (sensitivity 62%)

Lachman Test for ACL Tear
- Relax the knee in 15° of flexion
- Grasp the distal femur with one hand and the upper tibia with the other
- With the thumb of the tibial hand resting on the joint line to detect movement, simultaneously pull the tibia forward and push the femur back
- A positive test shows anterior tibial movement and a spongy end point
- This exam is the most sensitive test (84%) for ACL insufficiency

Posterior Drawer Test for Posterior Cruciate Ligament (PCL) Tear
- Perform the same maneuver as the anterior drawer test, including inspection for subluxed tibia, but push the tibia backwards instead (see **Figure 8**)
- Sensitivity of this exam is 55%

MUSCULOSKELETAL

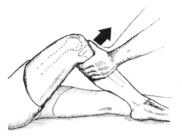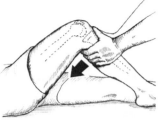

Anterior Drawer Test	Posterior Drawer Test

Figure 8. Anterior and Posterior Drawer Tests for ACL and PCL Tears

Posterior Sag Sign
- Patient is supine with hips flexed to 45° and test knee flexed to 90°
- If the PCL is torn, the tibia drops back or sags on the femur; compare to the other knee
- Positive result can produce a false positive for the anterior drawer test

Medial Collateral Ligament (MCL)
- With knee extended, place one hand on the lateral aspect of the knee at the level of the joint
- Pull the lower leg laterally with the other hand, applying a valgus force
- This test opens up the MCL

Lateral Collateral Ligament (LCL)
- Place one hand on the medial aspect of the knee at the level of the joint
- Push the lower leg medially with the other hand applying a varus force
- This test opens up the LCL

Menisci Tests

General Examination of the Meniscus
- Examine the joint for tenderness along the joint line
- Discern if there is a springy block to full extension
- These two signs in association with quadriceps wasting are the most consistent and reliable signs of a meniscus tear

McMurray Maneuver for Medial Meniscus
- Fully flex the knee and place the thumb and index finger along the joint line with the palm of the hand resting on the patella
- Externally rotate the foot and extend the knee joint smoothly with the other hand
- A meniscal tear is suggested if the patient's pain is reproduced or if a click accompanies the pain
- Symptomless, non-pathological clicks may be caused by tendons or other soft tissues snapping over bony prominences

McMurray Maneuver for Lateral Meniscus
- Similar to the test above, but with the foot internally rotated

MUSCULOSKELETAL

Thessaly Test for Medial or Lateral Meniscus

- This test is completed first on the normal (unaffected) leg and then on the injured leg
- The examiner supports the patient while they stand flatfooted on the normal leg
- The patient slightly flexes the knee (5°) and internally and externally rotates their knee and body three times
- The same process is completed with the knee flexed at 20°
- A meniscal tear is suggested if the patient experiences medial or lateral joint line discomfort
- The patient may also experience the sensation of locking or catching of the knee joint

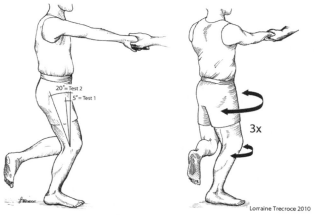

Figure 9. Thessaly Test for Medial and Lateral Meniscus Tears

Evidence-Based Medicine: Torn Meniscus		
The gold standard for the diagnosis of a torn meniscus of the knee is arthroscopy		
Test	**Sensitivity**	**Specificity**
Joint Line Tenderness[†]	63%	71%
McMurray Maneuver[†]	71%	71%
Thessaly Test (5°)[‡]	66% Med / 81% Lat	96% Med / 91% Lat
Thessaly Test (20°)[‡]	89% Med / 92% Lat	97% Med / 96% Lat

[†] Hegedus EJ et al. 2007. *J Orthop Sports Phys Ther* 37(9):541-550.
[‡] Karachalios T et al. 2005. *J Bone Joint Surg Am* 87(5):955-962.

MUSCULOSKELETAL

ANKLE AND FOOT

Common Symptoms
- Pain
- Instability
- Swelling

Common Clinical Scenarios

Ankle Sprain
- Ligaments supporting ankle joint are torn due to trauma
- Pain is acute and localized, accompanied by swelling, hematoma, loss of ROM and inability to bear weight
- Tenderness over the bony prominences should be examined more closely for fracture

Bunion (Hallux valgus)
- Proximal phalanx of the great toe begins to drift producing a valgus deformity
- A protective bursa forms over the deformed MTP joint
- On examination, gross deformity associated with localized pain and stiffness is observed

Physical Exam

Inspection
- SEADS
  - Inspect the feet and ankles with and without weight bearing
  - Inspect bony or soft tissue prominences, noting any deformities or asymmetries, edema, scars, bruising, toe alignment, skin or nail changes
  - Inspect the plantar surface of the foot for ulcerations, fungal infection, excess callous formation
- With the patient weight bearing
  - Inspect the posture of the ankle and foot anteriorly, posteriorly and laterally, noting any splaying of the forefoot
  - With the patient standing, assess, from behind, for pronation (valgus) deformity of subtalar joint
  - Slip fingers under the arch to detect pes cavus (high arch) or pes planus (flat foot)
  - Have patient stand on toes to differentiate between a flexible and fixed flat foot
- Assess gait with and without shoes
  - Note the posture of the foot during walking (i.e. pronation of the ankle during the stance phase)

Palpation
- Palpate the feet and ankles
  - Palpate the bony prominences for tenderness and swelling
  - Note any temperature differences that exist between the feet
  - Place one hand over the anterior surface of the ankle and passively plantar and dorsiflex the ankle, noting any crepitus
  - Examine the pedal pulses and the more proximal pulses if required
  - Screen for tenderness of the MTP joints by compressing the forefoot between thumb and fingers
  - To evaluate joints individually, firmly palpate the metatarsal heads and grooves between them with thumbs and index fingers

Range of Motion – Active Movements
- Ankle (Tibiotalar) joint
  - Dorsiflex and plantar flex the foot
  - Invert and evert the feet; note that these motions involve several joints
- Metatarsophalangeal joints
  - Ask the patient to flex and extend the toes
  - See **Table 19** for the complete list of active movements to be examined

Range of Motion – Passive Movements
- Ankle (Tibiotalar) joint
  - Test passive dorsiflexion and plantar flexion by grasping the foot proximally to the subtalar joint (or lock the subtalar joint in inversion) as subtalar dorsiflexion may be confused with ankle dorsiflexion
- Subtalar joint
  - Stabilize the ankle with one hand, grasp the calcaneus with the other and invert and evert the forefoot
  - This should be done with the ankle in dorsiflexion to lock the ankle joint
- Metatarsophalangeal joints
  - Steady the heel with one hand and flex and extend the MTP and IP joints of the great toe and lesser toes

Table 19. Ankle: Normal Ranges of Motion

Maneuver	Normal Range of Motion
Plantar flexion	55°
Dorsiflexion	15°
Inversion of heel	20°
Eversion of heel	10°
Supination of the forefoot	35°
Pronation of the forefoot	20°
Toe extension	Lateral Toes: (MTP: 40°, PIP: 0°, DIP: 30°) Great Toe: (MTP: 65°, IP: 0°)
Toe flexion	Lateral Toes: (MTP: 40°, PIP: 0°, DIP: 60°) Great Toe: (MTP: 40°, IP: 60°)

MUSCULOSKELETAL

Special Tests

Anterior Drawer for Ankle Stability
- With the knee at 90° and the foot flat on the table, stabilize the tibia and pull the foot forward to detect abnormal movement
- Alternatively, immobilize the foot and shift the tibia backwards

Ligament Tests
- When testing the integrity of each ligament, it is important to stabilize the lower leg
- Each ligament is preferentially stressed passively as follows:
  - Anterior talofibular ligament (ATFL): plantarflexion and inversion
  - Calcanofibular ligament (CFL): inversion at 90°
  - Posterior talofibular ligament (PTFL): dorsi-flexion and inversion
  - Deltoid ligament: eversion

Ottawa Ankle Rules

- The purpose is to discern the need for an x-ray
- Rules do not apply to patients less than 16 years old
- Palpation must be done of the bone only, not the soft tissue
- An ankle x-ray is indicated if a patient suffers an inversion injury and has any one of the following:
  - Tenderness at the tip of either malleolus or 6 cm proximally to malleolus
  - Tenderness at the base of the fifth metatarsal
  - Tenderness over the navicular
  - Inability to walk four steps
  - Age >50
- An x-ray is indicated in the presence or absence of bone pain if the patient cannot walk
- During palpation, note the presence of isolated medial tenderness. Palpate the proximal fibula to rule out a Maisonneuve's fracture (fracture of the fibular head and disruption of the interosseous membrane secondary to an ankle fracture)
- Sensitivity is 100%, negative predictive value is 1 (i.e. by applying the rules, no significant ankle fractures are missed)

REFERENCES

Bickley LS, Szilagyi PG, Bates B. 2007. *Bates' Guide to Physical Examination and History Taking.* Philadelphia: Lippincott Williams & Wilkins.

Dandy DJ, Edwards DJ. 2009. *Essential Orthopaedics and Trauma.* Edinburgh; New York: Churchill Livingstone/Elsevier.

D'Arcy CA, McGee S. 2000. The rational clinical examination. Does this patient have carpal tunnel syndrome? *JAMA* 284(11): 1384.

Hegedus EJ, Cook C, Hasselblad V, Goode A, McCrory DC. 2007. Physical examination tests for assessing a torn meniscus in the knee: a systematic review with meta-analysis. *J Orthop Sports Phys Ther* 37(9):541-550.

Karachalios T, Hantes M, Zibis AH, Zachos V, Karantanas AH, Malizos KN. 2005. Diagnostic accuracy of a new clinical test (the Thessaly test) for early detection of meniscal tears. *J Bone Joint Surg Am* 87(5):955-962.

Luime JJ, Verhagen AP, Miedema HS, Kuiper JI, Burdorf A, Verhaar JA, Koes BW. 2004. Does this patient have an instability of the shoulder or a labrum lesion? *JAMA* 292(16):1989-1999.

Magee DJ. 2008. *Orthopedic Physical Assessment.* St. Louis: Saunders Elsevier.

McRae R. 2004. *Clinical Orthopaedic Examination.* Edinburgh; New York: Churchill Livingstone.

Post M. 1987. *Physical Examination of the Musculoskeletal System.* Chicago: Year Book Medical Publishers.

Siminoski K, Warshawski RS, Jen H, Lee KC. 2003. Accuracy of physical examination using the rib-pelvis distance for detection of lumbar vertebral fractures. *Am J Med* 15(3):233-236.

Swartz MH. 2006. *Textbook of Physical Diagnosis: History and Examination.* Philadelphia: Saunders Elsevier.

Vroomen PC, de Krom MC, Knottnerus JA. 1999. Diagnostic value of history and physical examination in patients suspected of sciatica due to disc herniation: a systematic review. *J Neurol* 246(10):899-906.

The Neurological Exam

Editors:
Allison Kwan &
Vincent Leung

Faculty Reviewers:
Marika Hohol, MD, FRCP(C)
Todd Mainprize, MD, FRCP(C)

TABLE OF CONTENTS

Essential Anatomy	177
Approach to the Neurological History and Physical Exam	177
Common Chief Complaints	179
Common Disorders	179
Focused History	180
Focused Physical Examination	182
Common Investigations	196
Common Clinical Scenarios	197

ESSENTIAL ANATOMY

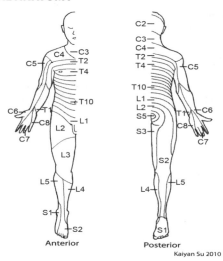

Kaiyan Su 2010

Figure 1. Map of Dermatomes

APPROACH TO THE NEUROLOGICAL HISTORY AND PHYSICAL EXAM

In addition to general history, important aspects of the neurological history are:

- Neurological symptoms – see **Table 3**
- Focal vs. diffuse symptoms
- Onset, timing, distribution
- Precipitating events (e.g. trauma, medications)
- Past neurological history (e.g. TIA, stroke)

NEUROLOGICAL

Overview of the physical exam:

- Two important questions:
    - *Where is the lesion?* (anatomic diagnosis)
        - Cerebrum, basal ganglia, brainstem, cerebellum, spinal cord, motor neuron, nerve, neuromuscular junction, muscle – see **Table 1**
        - Clues from history and physical
    - *What is the lesion?* (pathological diagnosis)
        - Vascular, infectious, congenital, traumatic, neoplastic, auto-immune, nutritional/toxic, metabolic, degenerative – see **Table 2**
        - Is the disease process focal or diffuse?
            - focal/asymmetrical – traumatic, neoplastic, vascular, degenerative
            - diffuse/symmetrical – infectious, auto-immune, nutritional/toxic, metabolic, degenerative
        - Use investigative tests
- Cranial nerves (I-XII)
    - CN I: smell
    - CN II: visual acuity; visual fields; colour test; fundoscopy; pupillary light reflex
    - CN III, IV, VI: extraocular movements; pupillary light reflex
    - CN V: motor (mastication); sensory (V1-V3); corneal reflex, jaw jerk reflex
    - CN VII: motor (facial expression); sensory (taste); corneal reflex
    - CN VIII: hearing; vestibular function
    - CN IX, X: motor (palatal elevation, swallowing, articulation); taste; gag reflex
    - CN XI: motor (trapezius and sternocleidomastoid)
    - CN XII: motor (tongue)
- Sensory
    - Primary (e.g. light touch, pain, temperature, vibration, proprioception)
    - Secondary (e.g. two-point discrimination, stereognosis, graphaesthesia, point localization)
- Motor
    - Inspection: bulk, involuntary movements, posture
    - Tone
    - Power
    - Reflexes: deep tendon, primitive, superficial
- Coordination/Cerebellar Function
    - Gross
    - Fine
    - Gait
    - Balance
- Mental Status Examination (MSE)
    - Folstein's Mini-Mental State Examination – see *Psychiatric Exam* p. 322

Table 1. Where is the Lesion?

Level of Lesion	Signs and Symptoms
Cerebrum	Seizures, confusion, hemianopsia, aphasia, hemiparesis Defects on contralateral side of head and body
Basal ganglia	Tremor, rigidity, involuntary movements
Brainstem	Diplopia, vertigo, alternating hemiparesis Defects on ipsilateral side of head, contralateral side of body below neck
Cerebellum	Ataxia, intention tremor, dysarthria, hypotonia Defects on ipsilateral side of head and body

NEUROLOGICAL

Table 1. Where is the Lesion? (continued)

Level of Lesion	Signs and Symptoms
Spinal cord	Paraparesis, sensory level, incontinence Defects frequently bilateral at and below level of lesion
Motor neuron	Diffuse weakness, fasiculations, atrophy
Peripheral nerve	Glove/stocking paraesthesia, areflexia
Neuromuscular junction	Ptosis, diplopia, dysarthria, dysphagia
Muscle	Proximal weakness

Table 2. What is the Lesion?

Type of Lesion	Signs and Symptoms, DDx
Vascular	Acute, focal, hypertension, fibrillation, bruit *e.g. TIA, infarction, SAH, ICH*
Infectious	Acute, diffuse, headache, fever, nuchal rigidity, back pain *e.g. Meningitis, encephalitis, osteomyelitis, discitis*
Congenital	Early onset, static, suggestive habitus *e.g. Hydrocephalus, cerebral palsy*
Traumatic	Focal, pain, tenderness *e.g. SDH, vertebral fracture, sciatica, carpal tunnel, DIA*
Neoplastic	Progressive, accelerating, focal, headache, back pain *e.g. Primary, metastatic*
Autoimmune	Subacute, relapsing, multifocal/diffuse *e.g. Polymyositis, myasthenia gravis, GBS, MS*
Nutritional/ toxic	Acute/chronic, diffuse *e.g. Medications, substance abuse, pernicious anemia*
Metabolic	Acute/chronic, diffuse *e.g. DM, electrolytes, uremia, cirrhosis, myxedema, sepsis*
Degenerative	Chronic, diffuse, familial *e.g. DMD, CMT, ALS, Parkinson's, Alzheimer's*

COMMON CHIEF COMPLAINTS

- Weakness
- Paralysis
- Change in consciousness
- "Dizziness" or sensation of movement
- Difficulty swallowing (dysphagia)
- Frequent tripping or falls
- Loss of coordination
- Headache
- Numbness or tingling (paraesthesia)

- Pain
- Visual disturbances (e.g. transient scotoma, flashing lights)
- Visual loss
- Loss of taste and/or smell
- Difficulties sleeping
- Memory problems
- Personality change
- Speech difficulties
- Involuntary movements (e.g. tremors, seizures, restless leg syndrome)

NEUROLOGICAL

COMMON DISORDERS

Disorders marked with (✓) are discussed in **Common Clinical Scenarios**

- ✓ Stroke
- ✓ Headache
- ✓ Brain Tumours
- ✓ Diabetic Neuropathy
- ✓ Alzheimer's Disease
- ✓ Seizures
- ✓ Parkinson's Disease (PD)
- ✓ Multiple Sclerosis (MS)

- ✓ Herpes Simplex Encephalitis
- ✓ Lumbar Disc Prolapse
- ✓ Spinal Cord Disorders
- ▪ Huntington's Disease
- ▪ Bell's (CN VII) Palsy
- ▪ Guillain-Barré Syndrome (GBS)
- ▪ Amyotrophic Lateral Sclerosis (ALS)

FOCUSED HISTORY

- **OPQRSTUVW** questions regarding each complaint
- Complaint-specific questions – see **Table 3**
- Associated risk factors for diseases (e.g. stroke – hypercholesterolemia, hyperlipidemia, hypertension, family history of stroke, etc.)

Table 3. Chief Complaints and Specific Queries to Elicit History

Chief Complaint	Signs and Symptoms
Headache	Onset (e.g. thunderclap)
	Pattern (e.g. worse in the morning = increased ICP)
	Differences from previous headaches
	Associated symptoms (e.g. nausea and/or vomiting, neck stiffness)
	Preceding symptoms/aura
	Systemic conditions (e.g. infections)
	Current medications/addictions
Loss of consciousness	Complete vs. partial, syncope vs. seizure
	Duration
	Changes in body position (e.g. loss of balance, fetal position, prone)
	Associated symptoms (e.g. tongue-biting, body movements, incontinence)
	Preceding symptoms (e.g. lightheadedness)
	Post-attack symptoms (e.g. confusion, drowsiness)
	Previous diagnosis of systemic disorders (e.g. cardiovascular problems)
	Current medications
	Collateral/corollary information (e.g. bystanders)
Dizziness	Vertigo vs. presyncope vs. ataxia
	Associated symptoms:
	- Inner ear (nausea, vomiting, nystagmus, tinnitus, hearing loss)
	- Brainstem/cerebellar (ataxia, diplopia, dysarthria)
	- Migraine aura
	- Changes in sensation between eyes open vs. closed, or with head positioning
	Current medications
Visual disturbances	Duration
	Diplopia (vertical, horizontal, or skew)
	Associated symptoms (e.g. eye pain, headache)
	Positive symptoms (e.g. flashing lights)
	Negative symptoms (e.g. monocular vs. binocular scotoma)

Chief Complaint	Signs and Symptoms
Numbness	Paraesthesia vs. dysaesthesia Distribution (hemi body vs. radicular vs. peripheral nerve) Course (e.g. worse on exertion, worse in the morning)
Pain	Onset, timing (acute/transient vs. chronic/permanent) Distribution (dermatome vs. diffuse) Associated symptoms Previous trauma, surgery, family history
Weakness	Nerve vs. neuromuscular junction vs. muscle Associated activities (one activity vs. all activities) Pattern: - proximal vs. distal - unilateral vs. bilateral - hemiparesis vs. para/quadriplegia Course, especially fatigability
Tremor	Character (e.g. worse at rest, with posture, with movement) Activity-specific vs. general Associated symptoms (e.g. postural instability, bradykinesia) Medications and food: - alcohol, tea, coffee, chocolate, medication, drugs - symptom-alleviating vs. symptom-enhancing effects
Speech disturbance	Dysphasia vs. dysarthria Impaired naming, mixing up words (paraphasia) Reading problems vs. writing problems vs. comprehension problems Onset
Gait	Weakness vs. ataxia Onset (e.g. on exertion) Course Associated symptoms (sensory impairment, muscle fatigability) Associated signs: - loss of position sense, postural stability - weakness, fatigability, spasticity

FOCUSED PHYSICAL EXAMINATION

Cranial Nerves

- Cranial nerves may have sensory function, motor function, or both – see **Table 4**

Table 4. The Cranial Nerves

Nerve	Name	Function	S/M/B
CN I	Olfactory	Smell	S
CN II	Optic	Vision Afferent limb of the pupillary light reflex	S
CN III	Oculomotor	Innervates medial/superior/inferior rectus, inferior oblique, levator palpebrae Efferent limb of the pupillary light reflex Involved in the accommodation reflex	M
CN IV	Trochlear	Innervates superior oblique	M
CN V	Trigeminal		
	V1 = ophthalmic	Forehead and tip of nose Afferent limb of the corneal reflex	S
	V2 = maxillary	Medial aspect of cheek Afferent limb of jaw jerk reflex	S
	V3 = mandibular	Chin, except angle of the jaw (C2) Innervates jaw muscles Efferent limb of jaw jerk reflex	B
CN VI	Abducens	Innervates lateral rectus	M
CN VII	Facial	Innervates facial expression muscles Taste to anterior 2/3 tongue Sensory from skin posterior to ear, external acoustic meatus Efferent limb of corneal reflex Phonation	B
CN VIII	Vestibulocochlear (Acoustic)	Hearing and balance	S
CN IX	Glossopharyngeal	Taste for posterior 1/3 tongue Phonation	B
CN X	Vagus	Swallowing Phonation Sensory from skin posterior to ear, external acoustic meatus, dura in posterior cranial fossa	B
CN XI	Spinal Accessory	Innervates sternocleidomastoid, trapezius	M
CN XII	Hypoglossal	Innervates tongue muscles	M

S/M/B = Sensory/Motor/Both, CN = Cranial Nerve

Clinical Pearl
The common cold is the most common cause of CN I dysfunction

CN I
- *Smell Test:* test each nostril separately using cloves, coffee, mint (a familiar, non-irritating scent retained over long storage); patient closes eyes and occludes one nostril; note unilateral vs. bilateral loss
- *Pathology:* nasal disease, head trauma, smoking, aging, cocaine use, congenital

NEUROLOGICAL

CN II

- *Visual Acuity* (tests central acuity)
  - Test each eye separately using a Snellen chart or near card; patient covers other eye with palm of hand (no pressure on covered eye); estimate best corrected vision; use pinhole card if patient's glasses not available
  - Snellen chart: numerator = distance patient can read chart, denominator = distance normal eye can read chart (e.g. 20/200: what the normal eye can see at 200 ft, this patient reads at 20 ft)
- *Visual Fields by Confrontation:*
  - Face patient; patient closes left eye and looks into the examiner's left eye (examiner closes right eye)
  - Test using "counting" or "object" method in each of 4 quadrants (upper and lower temporal, upper and lower nasal)
    - Counting method – hold up fingers in quadrant being tested and ask patient, "How many fingers?"
    - Object method – bring finger or a pen tip slowly towards the quadrant being tested; ask patient to "Tell me when you first notice the object"
  - Repeat for other three quadrants and then for other eye
  - Test for extinction: patient looks with both eyes uncovered into examiner's eyes; hold up fingers on both hands and ask patient "How many fingers?"
  - Location of visual field defect can suggest diagnosis – see **Table 5**

Table 5. Visual Field Defects (CN II)

Lesion Location	Anatomy	Differential diagnosis
Single eye	Anterior to optic chiasm	Glaucoma, retinal hemorrhage, optic neuropathy Central retinal artery occlusion leads to potential monocular blindness (amaurosis fugax)
Both eyes (bitemporal hemianopsia)	At optic chiasm	Upper > lower – inferior chiasmal compression (pituitary adenoma) Lower > upper – superior chiasmal compression
Both eyes (homonymous hemianopsia)	Behind optic chiasm	Cerebral infarcts, hemorrhages, tumours

- *Pupillary Light Reflex:* see **CN III/CN IV/CN VI exam**
- *Colour Test:* have patient read Ishihara plates
- *Fundoscopic Exam* (both eyes for symmetry) – see *Ophthalmological Exam* p. 239
- *Pathology:* optic atrophy, papilloedema

CN III/CN IV/CN VI

- *Inspect:* ptosis, pupil size/shape/asymmetry, eye position, resting nystagmus; defects may help localize lesions – see **Table 6**

Table 6. Defects of CN III, IV, VI

Defect	Location of Lesion
Eye position down and out, ptosis, mydriasis	CN III palsy (complete)
Ptosis, miosis, anhydrosis (Horner's syndrome)	Sympathetic pathway
Difficulty looking down and in (e.g. walking down stairs)	CN IV palsy
Difficulty looking laterally	CN VI palsy
Slow adduction of ipsilateral eye and nystagmus in abduction of contralateral eye	Medial Longitudinal Fasciculus (MLF) Internuclear ophthalmoplegia (suggests Multiple Sclerosis)

Note: Outer CN III fibers control papillary constriction. Inner CN III fibers control ocular movements and upper eyelids.

- *Eye Alignment:* hold penlight in front of patient; patient looks straight ahead into the distance; normal – location of light in centre of both pupils

> **Clinical Pearl**
> RAPD is an important finding in optic neuritis, which is common in multiple sclerosis

- *Ocular Movements*
  - Test smooth pursuit of both eyes at same time; patient tracks target without moving head through "H" pattern; normal – absence of end-point nystagmus and diplopia (monocular vs. binocular)
  - Test for saccadic eye movements: ask patient to shift gaze quickly between two closely placed targets (e.g. examiner's nose and index finger)
  - Test for accommodation reflex: ask patient to alternate between focusing on distant object and object held 5 inches from nose; normal – presence of eye convergence and pupil constriction
- *Pupillary Light Reflex:* dim lights; ask patient to look into the distance, shine light obliquely into pupils; normal – presence of direct and consensual responses
- *Swinging Light Test*
  - Shine light in eye "B," then swing light to eye "A." If CN II of "A" is damaged, "A" and "B" will paradoxically dilate when light swung to "A"
  - CN II damage causes "A" to have more consensual response (when light is at "B") than direct response (when light is at "A") – i.e. a relative afferent pupillary defect (RAPD) in that eye (or a "Marcus Gunn pupil")
  - If CN II is damaged in "A", light directed to "A" will cause no change in either pupil. However, light directed to "B" will elicit both a direct and consensual response (intact CN III of "A" and CN II, III of "B")
  - If CN III of "A" is damaged but CN II of "A" is intact, will see a consensual response in "B" but no direct response in "A." Additionally, no consensual response will occur in "A" when light is directed to "B"

CN V
- *Inspect:* temporal wasting, jaw alignment with open mouth (jaw deviates towards affected side)

NEUROLOGICAL

- *Motor – Ask patient to:*
  - "Clench teeth" (palpate masseter and temporalis muscles)
  - "Open mouth" – pterygoids and masseter
  - "Open mouth against resistance" – masseter and temporalis
  - "Divert jaw to side against resistance" – pterygoids
- *Sensory:*
  - Test light touch; patient closes eyes; apply tip of cotton wool at single point and have patient respond with "yes" when contact is made; compare both sides of forehead (V1), upper lip/cheeks (V2), and lower lip/chin (V3); avoid nose (V1) and angle of jaw (C2)
  - Test pain; patient closes eyes; vary application of end of broken tongue depressor vs rounded end in same distribution as for light touch; have patient respond with "sharp" or "dull"
- *Reflexes:*
  - Corneal – patient looks up and away as examiner approaches with a piece of cotton/tissue from side; avoid eyelashes and touch cornea (not conjunctiva or sclera); normal – presence of direct and consensual responses
  - Jaw jerk – patient opens mouth slightly; place finger over patient's chin and tap downwards with reflex hammer; normal – minimal elevation (increased reflex = pseudobulbar palsy)

CN VII
- *Inspect:* nasolabial fold (e.g. flattened), palpebral fissure (e.g. eyelid retracted), mouth (e.g. drooping), involuntary facial movements

> **Clinical Pearl**
> With a LMN lesion you lose entire ipsilateral function including frontalis muscle; with a UMN lesion you lose contralateral function with sparing of the forehead (frontalis) bilaterally.

- *Motor - Ask the patient to:*
  - "Raise your eyebrows" – frontalis
  - "Close your eyes tight and don't let me open them" – orbicularis oculi
  - "Show me your teeth" – buccinator
  - "Puff your cheeks out and don't let me pop them" – orbicularis oris
  - "Show me your bottom teeth only" – platysma
  - Distribution of paralysis differs between LMN and UMN lesions – see **Table 7**
- *Sensory:* test taste; patient sticks out tongue; touch each side of tongue on anterior 2/3 (CN VII) and posterior 1/3 (CN IX) with 4 primary tastes (sweet = sugar, salty = salt, sour=vinegar, bitter=quinine); keeping tongue protruded, ask patient to point to taste perceived on card displaying taste options; provide sip of water between tests
- *Corneal Reflex:* see **CN V exam**

NEUROLOGICAL

Table 7. Defects of CN VII

Type of Lesion	Distribution of Paralysis
LMN lesion (e.g. Bell's palsy)	Facial paralysis on same side as lesion, including forehead
UMN lesion (cortex, corticospinal tract)	Partial facial paralysis; forehead relatively spared

CN VIII
- **Hearing Test** – Test each ear separately:
  - *Whisper test:* mask sounds entering one ear by rubbing tragus or snapping fingers; whisper numbers/letters into other ear and ask patient to repeat

> **Clinical Pearl**
> Wax is the most common cause of conductive deafness.

  - *Rinné test:* strike 512 Hz tuning fork and place on patient's mastoid process; ask patient to indicate when sound disappears; immediately place tines of fork in front of auditory canal without touching ear; normal – patient will note 'reappearance' of sound (air > bone conduction)
  - *Weber test:* strike 512 Hz tuning fork and place on patient's forehead in midline; normal – absence of sound lateralization (equal on both sides)
  - Rinné and Weber tests can be used to differentiate between conductive and sensorineural hearing loss – see **Table 8**
- **Vestibular Function** – Not usually tested in office setting except:
  - Romberg test – see **Sensory Exam**
  - Positional nystagmus (induced with changes in head position)
  - Gaze-evoked nystagmus (induced at extreme eccentricities of gaze – see **CN III/CN IV/CN VI exam**)

Table 8. Defects of CN VIII

Loss	Rinné (affected ear)	Weber
Conductive	Bone > Air Conduction	Lateralization to affected ear
Sensorineural	Air > Bone Conduction	Lateralization to non-affected ear

CN IX + CN X
- **Motor:**
  - Palatal elevation: depress patient's tongue with depressor; ask patient to "Say Ahh"; normal – symmetrical elevation of soft palate and uvula (uvula deviates to non-affected side)
  - Swallowing: ask patient to swallow sip of water; normal – no retrograde passage of water through nose after nasopharynx closed off
  - Articulation: ask patient to "Say PaTaKa"
    - Pa = CN VII; Ta = CN IX, X, XII; Ka = CN IX, X
- **Sensory:** see **CN VII exam**
- **Gag Reflex:** touch posterior wall of pharynx with tongue depressor; normal – palate moves up; pharyngeal muscles contract; uvula remains midline; palatal arches do not droop
- **Note:** An absent gag reflex can be normal

> **Clinical Pearl**
> Uvula deviates to the strong side; jaw and tongue deviate to the weak side.

CN XI
- **Inspect:** neck and shoulder; look for fasciculations, atrophy, asymmetry
- **Motor** – Ask patient to:
  - "Shrug your shoulders" (with and without resistance) – trapezius
  - "Turn your head to the side" (with and without resistance) – sterno-cleidomastoid

NEUROLOGICAL

- *Pathology:*
  - Weak trapezius – shrugging of shoulders on the ipsilateral side is impaired
  - Weak sternocleidomastoid – turning head to the contralateral side is impaired

CN XII
- *Inspect:* tongue at rest in the floor of the mouth; look for fasciculations, atrophy, asymmetry
- *Motor* – Ask patient to:
  - "Stick your tongue out and move it side to side"; normal – symmetrical protrusion of tongue (tongue deviates to affected side)
  - "Push your tongue into your cheek" (with and without resistance)
- **Note:** Correct facial weakness by supporting patient's upper lip on side of weakness to differentiate between CN VII and CN XII dysfunction

Table 9. Multiple CN Abnormalities

CN Combination	Likely Cause
Unilateral III, IV, V1, VI	Cavernous sinus lesion
Unilateral V, VII, VIII	Cerebellopontine angle lesion
Unilateral IX, X, XI	Jugular foramen syndrome
Bilateral X, XI, XII	Bulbar palsy (LMN), pseudobulbar palsy (UMN)

The Motor Examination
- Considerations for pathology:
  - UMN vs. LMN pattern – see **Table 10**
  - Pyramidal (corticospinal tract) vs. extrapyramidal tract lesion
  - Localization to specific root or peripheral nerve

Table 10. Pattern of Upper and Lower Motor Neuron Lesions

	UMN Lesion	LMN Lesion
Appearance	Atrophy of disuse, arms flexed, legs extended	Atrophy, fasciculations
Power	Weak/absent	Weak/absent
Tone	Increased/spastic	Decreased
Coordination	Impaired due to weakness	Impaired due to weakness
Reflexes		
Superficial	Absent	Absent
Deep	Increased/clonus	Decreased
Plantar	Upgoing	Downgoing

Inspection
- Muscle bulk (atrophy, hypertrophy, abnormal bulging/depression) – distribution of muscle wasting can suggest possible causes – see **Table 11**
- Symmetry
- Fasciculations – quivering of the muscle under skin. Typically benign, may be associated with LMN lesion (e.g. ALS)

NEUROLOGICAL

- Abnormal movements and positioning:
  - Asterixis – brief, jerky downward movements of the wrist when patient extends both arms with wrists dorsiflexed, palms forward and eyes closed
  - Tics – involuntary contractions of single muscles or groups of muscles (e.g. Tourette Syndrome)
  - Myoclonus – brief (<0.25 s), generalized muscle jerk
  - Dystonia – muscle contraction that is more prolonged than myoclonus and results in spasms
  - Athetosis – slow, writhing spasms– patient may assume peculiar postures
  - Chorea – "dance" – somewhat purposeful movements affecting multiple joints
  - Hemiballismus – violent flinging movement of half of the body (lesions of subthalamic nucleus)
  - Seizure automatisms – repeated eye blinks, tonic or clonic motor activity

Table 11. Distribution of Muscle Wasting or Weakness

Pattern	Possible Causes
Focal (one limb)	Nerve root or peripheral nerve pathology
Proximal (bilateral)	Myopathy (no sensory loss)
Distal (bilateral)	Peripheral neuropathy (distal sensory loss)

Muscle Tone
- Slight residual tension in a normal muscle when it is relaxed voluntarily - test by flexion/extension, pronation/supination of joint through its range of motion
- Hypotonia (decreased tone) – seen in LMN lesions, acute stroke, spinal shock, some cerebellar lesions
- Hypertonia (increased tone) – may manifest as spasticity or rigidity
- Patterns of tone – characteristic of abnormal tone suggests possible causes – see **Table 12**
  - Spasticity – velocity-dependent: limb moves, then catches, and then goes past catch (spastic, clasp-knife); best appreciated during rapid supination of forearm or flexion of knee; pyramidal lesion
  - Rigidity – velocity-independent: increased tone through range of movement (cog-wheeling, lead-pipe); best detected with circumduction of the wrist; extrapyramidal lesion

Table 12. Causes of Abnormal Tone

Characteristic	Possible Causes
Decreased tone: flaccidity	LMN lesion, cerebellar; rarely myopathies, "spinal shock" (e.g. early response after a spinal cord trauma), chorea
Increased tone: spasticity ("clasp-knife")	UMN lesion: corticospinal tract (commonly late or chronic stage after a stroke)
Increased tone: rigidity ("lead-pipe", "cog-wheeling")	Extrapyramidal tract lesion – parkinsonism, phenothiazines

Power

- Measure active motion of the patient against resistance; compare both sides; graded on a standard scale – see **Table 13**
- Ensure all muscle groups are tested – see **Table 14**

Table 13. Grading Power

Grade		Assessment
0	Absent	No contraction detected
1	Trace	Slight contraction detected but cannot move joint
2	Weak	Movement with gravity eliminated only
3	Fair	Movement against gravity only
4	Good	Movement against gravity with some resistance
5	Normal	Movement against gravity with full resistance

Note: since this rating scale is skewed towards weakness, many clinicians further subclassify their finding by adding a (+) or a (-), e.g. 4- or 4+

Weakness vs. Paralysis
Impaired strength is weakness (paresis). Absence of strength is paralysis (plegia).

Table 14. Muscle Groups to Test (Myotomal Distribution)

Muscle	Movement	Nerve	Spinal
Deltoid	Arm abduction	Axillary	**C5**, C6
Triceps	Elbow extension	Radial	C6, **C7**, C8
Biceps	Elbow flexion	Musculocutaneous	C5, C6
Wrist extensors	Wrist extension	Radial	**C7**, C8
Flexor pollicis longus	Thumb IP flexion	Median	C7, **C8**
Interossei of hand	Fingers ab/adduction	Ulnar	C8, **T1**
Iliopsoas	Hip flexion	Femoral	**L1, L2**, L3
Hip adductors	Hip adduction	Obturator	**L2, L3**, L4
Hip abductors	Hip abduction	Superior gluteal	**L4, L5**, S1
Quadriceps	Knee extension	Femoral	L2, **L3, L4**
Hamstrings	Knee flexion	Sciatic	L5, **S1**, S2
Tibialis anterior	Ankle dorsiflexion	Deep peroneal	**L4**, L5
Gastrocnemius, soleus	Ankle plantar flexion	Tibial	S1, S2
Extensor hallucis longus	Great toe dorsiflexion	Deep peroneal	**L5**, S1
Tibialis	Posterior foot inversion	Posterior tibial	**L4**, L5
Peroneus longus, brevis	Foot eversion	Superficial peroneal	L5, S1

Pronator Drift
- Have the patient stand or sit with their eyes closed and arms held straight out from their body with hands in supine positions
- Pronator drift positive if patient cannot maintain position; may be due to:
  - Muscle weakness (may see pronation and outward drift of arm and hand)
  - UMN lesion (may see pronation and downward drift)

Deep Tendon Reflexes
- Monosynaptic spinal segmental reflexes
- Patient should be relaxed with muscle mildly stretched
- Strike tendon briskly and compare both sides
- Make sure that you watch or feel muscle for contraction
- If reflexes appear to be hyperactive, examine for clonus at the ankle and knee
- If reflexes are absent, have patient use reinforcement:
  - For upper body reflexes: clench teeth or push down on bed with thighs
  - For lower body reflexes: lock fingers and try to pull hands apart (Jendrassik's maneuver)
- Graded on a standard scale – see **Table 15**
- Characteristic of deep tendon reflex can suggest possible causes – see **Table 16**

Table 15. Grading Reflexes

Grade	Response	
0	Absent	
1+	Diminished	
2+	Normal	
3+	Increased (no clonus)	
4+	Hyperactive (associated with clonus)	

- *Biceps tendon reflex (C5, C6)*
  - Have patient relax arm and pronate forearm midway between flexion or extension
  - Place your thumb on the tendon and strike the hammer on your thumb
  - Observe for contraction of the biceps followed by flexion at the elbow
- *Brachioradialis tendon reflex (C5, C6)*
  - Have patient rest forearm on the knee in semiflexed, semipronated position
  - Strike hammer on stylus process of radius about 1-2 inches above wrist
  - Observe for flexion at elbow and simultaneous supination of the forearm
- *Triceps tendon reflex (C6, C7, C8)*
  - Have patient partially flex their arm at the elbow and pull towards patient's chest
  - Alternatively, allow patient's arm to hang relaxed while supporting anterior arm
  - Strike hammer on tendon above insertion of the ulnar olecranon process (1-2 in. above the elbow)
  - Observe for contraction of triceps with extension at the elbow
- *Patellar tendon reflex = knee jerk (L2, L3, L4)*
  - Bend the knee to relax the quadriceps muscle
  - With your hand on the quadriceps, strike the patellar tendon firmly
  - Observe for extension at the knee and contraction of the quadriceps

- *Achilles tendon reflex = ankle jerk (S1, S2)*
  - Place your hand under the foot to dorsiflex the ankle; strike the tendon
  - Observe for plantar flexion at the ankle and contraction of the calf muscle

Clonus
- *Ankle* – with knee flexed, quickly dorsiflex foot and maintain flexed position
- *Knee* – with knee extended, grasp quadriceps muscle just proximal to patella and exert sudden downward force
- Clonus is present if sudden movements elicit rhythmic involuntary muscle contractions; suggests UMN lesion

Table 16. Interpreting Deep Tendon Reflexes

Characteristic	Possible Causes
Increased reflex or clonus	UMN lesion above root at that level
Absent	Generalized – peripheral neuropathy Isolated – peripheral nerve or root lesion
Reduced (insensitive)	Peripheral neuropathy, cerebellar syndrome (may be absent in early phases of UMN lesion e.g. "spinal shock")
Inverted (reflex tested is absent e.g. biceps but there is spread to lower or higher level e.g. produces a triceps response)	LMN lesion at level of the absent reflex, with UMN below (spinal cord involvement at the level of the absent reflex)
Pendular (reflex continues to swing for several beats)	Cerebellar disease
"Hung" (slow to relax, especially at ankle)	Hypothyroidism

Primitive Reflexes
- Generally not present in adults – when present, signifies diffuse cerebral damage, particularly of the frontal lobes (e.g. "frontal lobe release")
- *Glabellar* – tap forehead and watch if eyes blink. Abnormal if individual cannot overcome the reflex and continues blinking as long as the tapping continues
- *Snout and Pout* – tap filum (above upper lip) and watch for protrusion of lips
- *Palmo-Mental* – scrape palm over thenar muscles and watch for chin muscle contraction
- *Grasp* – place fingers in palm to see if grasp reflex elicited

Superficial Reflexes
- *Abdominal reflex* – stroke abdomen towards umbilicus along the diagonals of the four abdominal quadrants
  - Normal: ipsilateral muscles contract, umbilicus deviates towards the stimulus
  - Above umbilicus tests T8, T9, T10
  - Below umbilicus tests T10, T11, T12
- *Cremasteric reflex* – draw line along medial thigh
  - Normal: elevation of ipsilateral testis in the scrotum
  - Abdominal and cremasteric reflexes may be absent on the side of a corticospinal tract lesion

- *Corneal reflex* (see **CN V and VII exam**)
- *Plantar response (Babinski's sign) (L5-S1)* – stroke the sole from the heel to the ball of the foot curving medially across the heads of the metatarsal bones
  - Normal (downgoing): plantar flexion of big toe, curling of the other toes
  - Abnormal (upgoing): dorsiflexion of the big toe, fanning of the other toes; associated with UMN lesion
  - Stroking the lateral aspect of the foot (Chaddock's sign) and downward pressure along the shin (Oppenheim's sign) can elicit the same reflex
- *Anal reflex (anal wink)* – stroke perianal skin
  - Normal: contraction of the muscles around the rectal orifice
  - Loss or reflex signifies lesion in S2-3-4 reflex arc (e.g. cauda equina lesion)

The Sensory Exam

- Primary sensory exam: peripheral sensory nerve tests (light touch, pain, temperature, vibration, proprioception)
- Secondary sensory exam: test cortical functions regarding sensation (two-point discrimination, stereognosis, graphesthesia, point localization); test fails if spinal/peripheral nerves are severely impaired
- Always 'program' patients before starting a test so that they know exactly how to respond (i.e. run a sample test with the patient's eyes open, and ask him/her to say whether sensation is 'sharp', 'dull', etc.)
- Have the patient close his/her eyes before testing
- Test both sides of the body and ask the patient to compare sensation on each side
- Start each test distally with fingers and toes; if normal, proceed to next test; if abnormal, proceed proximally until the abnormality is mapped out
- Compare sensory function: right to left; distal to proximal; peripheral nerve to spinal nerve dermatomes (see **Figure 1**, for dermatomal distribution)
- Note the location, magnitude, and quality of each sensory deficit found
- There is considerable overlap and variation in peripheral nerve distribution; therefore, a deficit in one area may be compensated for by another area
- Distribution of sensory loss can suggest location of lesion – see **Table 17**

Primary Sensory Exam
- *Light touch:* posterior column and spinothalamic tract function
  - Use cotton or tissue paper tip to touch skin; ask patient to say "yes" if touch is felt
  - **Note:** light touch is not a useful test to distinguish between lesions in the spinothalamic tract or the posterior columns, but light touch can be used to determine gross abnormalities within the PNS and CNS
- *Pain:* spinothalamic tract function
  - Alternate between sharp and dull touches (and false touches to see if the patient is using other cues)
  - Ask the patient to identify sensation as sharp or dull
- *Temperature:* spinothalamic tract function (often not done if pain sensation normal)
  - Run your tuning fork under cold water
  - Ask the patient to identify whether the tuning fork feels cold, and compare to the other side
- *Vibration:* posterior column function
  - Place a 128 Hz tuning fork on joint (e.g. DIP) and ask the patient when the 'buzzing' stops

- *Proprioception* (position sense): posterior column function
  - Hold the patient's joint (e.g. DIP) from the sides so he/she does not get cues from the pressure of your hand
  - Begin with the joint in the neutral position; raise or lower the digit and ask the patient to state the direction of movement
  - Return the digit to the neutral position before moving it in another direction
- *Romberg Test* (tests proprioception)
  - Have the patient stand in front of you with his/her feet together; be prepared to catch or support patient if he/she falls
  - Ask the patient to close both eyes and stand still for one minute
  - Positive Romberg sign if the patient falls in any direction without being aware of the fall
  - If the patient sways, ask him/her to stand perfectly still – this is NOT a positive Romberg sign
  - This test has low specificity because a positive test may be present in peripheral sensory denervation, vestibular dysfunction, or cerebellar disease

Table 17. Lesions Involving Sensory Modalities

Location of Lesion	Distribution of Sensory Loss	Examples
Single nerve	Within distribution of single nerve; commonly median, ulnar, peroneal, lateral cutaneous nerve to the thigh	Entrapment, most commonly in diabetes mellitus, carpal tunnel syndrome, rheumatoid arthritis, and hypothyroidism; multiple (mononeuritis multiplex) = vasculitis
Root or roots	Confined to single root or roots in close proximity; commonly C5, 6, 7 in arm and L4, 5, S1 in leg	Compression by disc prolapse
Peripheral nerve	Distal glove and stocking deficit	Diabetes mellitus, alcohol-related B_{12} deficiency, drugs
Spinal Cord	Depends on level of lesion and complete vs. partial lesion	Trauma, spinal cord compression by tumour, cervical spondylitis, MS
Brainstem	Pain and Temperature: ipsilateral face, contralateral body	Demyelination (young), brainstem stroke (older)
Thalamic sensory loss	All modalities; contralateral hemisensory loss (face, body) and pain – dysesthesia (e.g. burning feeling)	Stroke, cerebral tumour, MS, trauma
Cortical (parietal)	Able to recognize all primary modalities but localizes them poorly; loss of secondary modalities	Stroke, cerebral tumour, trauma

Secondary Sensory Exam
- Must first confirm that primary modalities are intact
- Inability to perform these tests suggests a lesion in sensory cortex

- *Neglect and extinction* (parietal lobe)
  - Touch right side, left side, and then both sides
  - Patients with parietal lobe lesions can identify when each side is touched independently, but will neglect the side contralateral to the lesion when both sides are touched
  - Start with light stimulus and increase stimulus intensity if extinction occurs
  - Can also test extinction using visual and auditory stimuli
- *Two-point discrimination* (parietal lobe)
  - Ask patient if they feel two stimuli or one (use an untwisted paper clip)
  - Normal minimum values for discrimination are 2 mm on fingertips, 3-8 mm on toes, 8-12 mm on palms, 40-60 mm on back
- *Stereognosis* (integration between parietal and occipital lobes)
  - Place objects in the patient's hand one at a time and ask the patient to recognize them by feeling the object (e.g. a coin, pen, key, paperclip)
  - Patient must only use one hand to feel object
  - Tactile agnosia: inability to recognize objects by touch; suggests a parietal cortex lesion
- *Graphaesthesia* (parietal lobe)
  - Use a blunt object to write numbers on a patient's hand in the correct orientation to the patient; patient tries to identify the numbers
- *Point localization* (sensory cortex)
  - Touch the patient and ask them to point to the area touched

Coordination/Cerebellar Function
- Assess speech, nystagmus, tremor
- Inspect for stiff, slowed, non-rhythmic movements; movements should normally be rapid, smooth and accurate

Gross Motor Coordination
- *Finger-To-Nose Test*
  - Ask the patient to alternate between touching his/her nose and your finger (held at an arm's length from the patient)
  - Make sure that your finger is far enough away from the patient in order to stress the system; keeping your finger too close makes the test too easy
  - Watch for:
    - 'Past pointing' where patient persistently overshoots target
    - Tremor as the finger approaches the target
  - inability to perform test (dysmetria) may indicate cerebellar disease
- *Heel-To-Knee Test*
  - Have patient slide the heel of one foot down the opposite shin, starting at knee
  - Watch for wobbling of the heel from side to side

Fine Motor Coordination
- *Rapid alternating movements (RAM)*
  - Dysdiadochokinesia – an abnormality in doing RAM (may be due to cerebellar lesion)
  - Upper extremities:
    - Pronate and supinate one hand on the other hand rapidly
    - Touch the thumb to each finger as quickly as possible
  - Lower extremities:
    - Tap toes of foot and then heel of foot to floor in rapid alternation

Gait

- Ask patient to:
  - "Walk straight ahead"
  - "Stop and return to me, now on tiptoe" (also tests strength of plantar flexors)
  - "Walk away again but this time on your heels" (also tests strength of dorsiflexors)
  - "Stop, return by walking in tandem gait with one foot placed in front of the other (like walking on a tightrope)"
- Pathologic pattern of gait may suggest possible causes – see **Table 18**

Table 18. Pathologic Patterns of Gait

Gait Pattern	Possible Causes
Hemiplegia	Unilateral UMN lesion due to stroke, MS
Parkinsonian (shuffling)	Parkinson's, extrapyramidal effects of anti-psychotics, major tranquilizers
Spastic or scissor (legs held in adduction at the hip, thighs rub together, knees slide over each other)	Cerebral Palsy, MS
Cerebellar ataxia (spreads legs wide apart to provide wider base of support – veers towards side of lesion)	Drugs (e.g. phenytoin), alcohol, MS, cerebrovascular disease
Foot drop/steppage (takes high steps as if climbing a flight of stairs)	Unilateral: common peroneal palsy, corticospinal tract lesion, L5 radiculopathy Bilateral: peripheral neuropathy
Sensory ataxia	Joint position sense (see **Romberg Test**) due to peripheral neuropathy, posterior column loss

Balance

- Observe the patient while standing; look for swaying from side to side
  - **Note:** this is not the Romberg test. The Romberg Test is part of the sensory examination to assess the posterior columns, not cerebellar function
- *Pull Test*
  - Stand behind the patient and give a sudden but gentle pull backward
  - Normally, the patient remains steady or takes one step back
  - A posturally unstable patient falls backward or festinates (takes multiple small rapid steps), e.g. in Parkinson's

Glasgow Coma Scale

- Used to assess the patient's level of consciousness
- Scored as a total between 3 and 15, but it is best to report each of the three components separately (e.g. E3 V2 M4 instead of a total of 9)

Table 19. Glasgow Coma Scale

Best Eye Response (E)	Best Verbal Response (V)	Best Motor Response (M)
1. No eye opening	1. No verbal response	1. No motor response
2. Eye opening to pain	2. Incomprehensible sounds	2. Extension to pain
3. Eye opening to verbal command	3. Inappropriate words	3. Flexion to pain
4. Eyes open spontaneously	4. Confused	4. Withdrawal from pain
	5. Orientated	5. Localizing pain
		6. Obeys Commands

- Coma is defined as 1) not opening eyes, 2) not obeying commands, and 3) not uttering understandable words
- As a general rule, 90% of patients with a score of ≤ 8 will be in a coma
- When testing response to pain, apply central pain to the supraorbital region (deep pinching of the skin) or the sternum (firm twisting pressure applied with the examiner's knuckles) because spinal reflexes may occur with peripheral stimulation

COMMON INVESTIGATIONS
- See *Essentials of Medical Imaging* for a detailed approach to neuroimaging
- *Lumbar Puncture* – laboratory assessment of CSF fluid for infection, blood content
- *CT* – blood vessels, hemorrhage (e.g. trauma) and neoplasm with injected contrast
- *MRI* – high resolution imaging using magnetic field distortions
- *Functional MRI (fMRI)* – functional imaging to map language, motor and sensory areas (e.g. post-stroke)
- *X-Ray* – imaging of bony deviation or fracture, calcified pineal gland used to determine mid-line deviation
- *Positron Emission Tomography (PET)* – functionally activated brain regions
- *Angiography* – aneurysm, arterial thrombosis, arteriovenous (AV) malformation
- *CT angiogram/MRI angiogram* – useful especially for carotid stenosis
- *EEG* - graphic record of the electrical activity of the brain over time-characteristic patterns in disease – useful especially for seizures/epilepsy
- *EMG/EOG* - graphic record of the electric currents associated with muscular action in the muscles of the body (EMG) or eye (EOG) over time – useful especially for myasthenia gravis (EMG), eye movement disorders/saccades/nystagmus (EOG)
- EEG + EMG + EOG = sleep studies
- *Nerve Conduction* – multiple electrodes placed along known course of a specific nerve – one electrode stimulates nerve and a second electrode picks up this stimulation → time between stimulation and recording determines nerve conduction velocity (compared to known standards) - useful especially for nerve entrapment syndromes (e.g. carpal tunnel syndrome)

COMMON CLINICAL SCENARIOS

Stroke

- Classification
  - Ischemic (80%) – thrombosis, embolism, and systemic hypoperfusion
  - Hemorrhagic (20%) – intracerebral, subarachnoid, subdural/extradural bleeds
- History
  - Onset of the symptoms
  - Temporal progression of the symptoms – maximal at onset vs. progressive
  - Activity during the onset of the symptom
  - Past history of strokes and TIAs
  - History of seizures, migraines, tumours, aneurysms, head trauma, MS
- Risk factors
  - Hypertension
  - Hyperlipidemia
  - Age
  - Cardiac disease – angina, MI, palpitations, valvular heart disease, atrial fibrillation, CHF
  - Peripheral vascular disease
  - Smoking
  - Diabetes
  - Family history
  - Clotting disorders
  - Medications, illicit drug use
- Physical Exam
  - Head and Neck
    - Signs of trauma
    - Retinal changes – hypertensive changes, cholesterol crystals, papilloedema
  - PVS
    - Bruits over the carotid, common iliac and femoral arteries
    - Decreased pulses
    - Signs of ischemic skin changes
  - CVS
    - Murmurs
  - Neurological findings can help localize location of occlusion – see **Table 20**
- Imaging
  - CT Scan - imaging of choice in acute stroke to determine if hemorrhagic
  - MRI - used to follow patient over time

Table 20. Common Stroke Syndromes

Location of Artery Occlusion	Clinical Significance
Left sided	Aphasia
Right sided	Neglect of left space, lack of awareness of deficit, apathy, impersistence
Anterior cerebral artery (ACA)	Contralateral weakness of the lower limb and shoulder shrug
Middle cerebral artery (MCA)	Contralateral motor, sensory and visual loss
Posterior cerebral artery (PCA)	Contralateral hemianopia and hemisensory loss
Internal carotid artery (ICA)	Contralateral MCA and ACA signs May also have ipsilateral transient monocular blindness (amaurosis fugax)
Basilar artery	Bilateral motor weakness, ophthalmoplegia and diplopia
Lacunar	Pure contralateral motor weakness, pure sensory loss, clumsy hand + dysarthria, ataxia, or mixed symptoms

Headache
- Different types of headaches have characteristic symptoms – see **Table 21**

Table 21. Common Headache Syndromes

Type	Characteristics
Tension	Lasts 30 min-7 days Non-pulsating, mild-moderate in intensity, bilateral Not aggravated by exertion, not associated with nausea/vomiting or sensitivity to light, sound, or smell
Migraine	Lasts 4-72 h Throbbing, moderate to severe intensity, unilateral (not always same side) Worse with exertion Associated with photophobia, phonophobia, nausea/vomiting May be preceded by short prodromal period of depression, irritability, restlessness, or anorexia; 10-20% occurrences associated with an aura – transient, reversible visual, somatosensory, motor, and/or language deficit – usually precedes headache by no >1 h, can be concurrent
Cluster	Lasts 15-180 min, occurs up to 8 times per day Severe, unilateral, located periorbitally and/or temporally Associated with at least one of: tearing, red eye, stuffy nose, facial sweating, ptosis, miosis
Subarachnoid hemorrhage	Acute, severe, "thunderclap" May have neurologic deficits or changes in level of consciousness

Brain Tumours
- Commonly present with:
  - Progressive focal neurological deficit
  - Headache: worse in the morning, improves during the day, worse when lying down or with Valsalva maneuver, may be associated with signs of increased intracranial pressure (nausea/vomiting, blurring of vision, papilloedema, transient visual obscuration)

- Seizures
- Cognitive deficits
- Most often metastases from other locations, spread hematogenously
- Benign tumours are still significant due to mass effect within fixed space

Diabetic Neuropathy
- Peripheral nerve damage from poor glucose control
- More common and more severe with increasing age
- Signs of diabetic neuropathy:
  - Peripheral polyneuropathy
  - Autonomic neuropathy – e.g. orthostatic hypotension, gastroparesis
  - Ataxia (large fibre involvement)
  - Motor weakness (starts distally)
  - Paresthesia/hyperesthesia (small fibre involvement)
  - Loss of deep tendon reflexes
  - Impotence
  - Pupil abnormalities

Alzheimer's Disease
- Gait, reflexes, sensation, hearing, visual fields, ocular movement; other brainstem functions mostly preserved
- Early stages
  - Anterograde amnesia (impairment of ability to make new memories)
  - Speech becomes halting, with grasping for words
  - Slower comprehension
  - Errors in calculation
  - Defective visuospatial orientation
- Middle stages
  - Disorientation
  - Amnesia
  - Aphasia
  - Apraxia
  - Agnosia
- Later stages
  - Involuntary primitive reflexes
  - Shortened step
  - Mild rigidity
  - Slowness of movement

Seizures
- Simple partial seizures
  - Motor, sensory, or psychomotor phenomena without loss of consciousness
  - Seizures can begin in one part of the body and spread to other parts
- Complex partial seizures
  - May be preceded by an aura (sensory or psychic manifestations that represent seizure onset)
  - Staring, performing of automatic purposeless movements, uttering of unintelligible sounds, resisting aid
  - Motor, sensory, or psychomotor phenomena
  - Post-ictal confusion
- Tonic-clonic seizures (formerly known as grand-mal)
  - Tonic phase – stiffening of limbs
  - Clonic phase – jerking of limbs

- Respiration may decrease during tonic phase but usually returns during clonic phase, although it may be irregular
- Incontinence may occur
- Post-ictal confusion
- Atonic seizures
  - Brief, primarily generalized seizures in children
  - Complete loss of muscle tone, resulting in falling or pitching to the ground
  - Risk of serious trauma, particularly head injury
- Absence seizures (formerly known as petit-mal)
  - Brief, primarily generalized attacks manifested by a 10 to 30-second loss of consciousness
  - Eyelid flutterings at a rate of 3 Hz
  - No loss of axial muscle tone
  - No falling or convulsing
  - No post-ictal symptoms
- *Status epilepticus* – a medical emergency!
  - Repeated seizures with no intervening periods of normal neurologic function
  - Generalized convulsive status epilepticus may be fatal
  - With complex partial or absence seizures, an EEG may be needed to diagnose seizure activity

Parkinson's Disease
- Extrapyramidal neurodegenerative disorder of unknown origin
- Neuronal loss in the substantia nigra (especially pars compacta) with Lewy bodies in the substantia nigra and other brainstem nuclei
- **TRAP** mnemonic:
  T remor (pill-rolling)
  R igidity (cog-wheeling)
  A kinesia/dyskinesia
  P ostural instability (stooped)
- Other findings
  - fixed, immobile facial expression
  - festinating gait
  - progressive dementia
  - excessive salivation
  - dysarthria

Multiple Sclerosis (MS)
- A demyelinating disease characterized by focal disturbances of function and a relapsing and remitting course, later becoming progressive. A minority of cases are primary progressive
- Women are affected more than men
- Most common presenting symptom is optic neuritis characterized by partial/total loss of vision associated with eye pain
- Neurologic dysfunction in different parts of the nervous system at different times
- Diagnosis, requires dissemination in both space and time (different parts of the body affected on at least two separate occasions)
- Other symptoms/signs include:
  - Brainstem: diplopia, internuclear ophthalmoplegia, tic douloureux, Bell's Palsy
  - Cerebellum: nystagmus, ataxia, intention tremor, gait disturbances

- Spinal cord: weakness, spasticity, hyperreflexia/clonus, upgoing toe(s), bladder or bowel dysfunction/incontinence, sexual dysfunction, paraparesis, Lhermitte's sign (sensation of electric shock down the back and into the limbs with forward flexion of neck)

Herpes Simplex Encephalitis
- 1/3 cases due to primary HSV cases, 2/3 due to reactivation of latent HSV
- Rapidly progressive disease with profound neurologic derangement
- Mortality if untreated is 70%; 50% of treated individuals are left with significant morbidity
- Alteration of consciousness
- Fever
- Headache
- Dysphasia
- Psychiatric symptoms
- Ataxia
- Seizures
- Vomiting
- Focal weakness or hemiparesis
- Cranial nerve defects
- Memory loss
- Visual field defects
- Papilloedema
- Less common findings: photophobia, movement disorders

Lumbar Disc Prolapse
- Due to the strength of the posterior longitudinal ligament in the midline, most herniated discs occur slightly off to one side and compress the nerve root exiting through the foramen below the affected level
- Often a history of falling or of lifting heavy weights
- Other findings:
  - Pain in the distribution of irritated/compressed root
  - Restricted spinal movement
  - Decreased straight leg raising with exacerbation of pain by dorsiflexing foot
- Motor, sensory, and reflex abnormalities can help localize level of disc prolapse – see **Table 22**

Table 22. Compression of Lumbar Discs and Physical Findings

Disc	Root	Motor Weakness	Sensory Loss	Reflex Affected
L4/L5	L5	Dorsiflexors, EDL, EHL	Lateral calf and dorsum of foot	Medial hamstring None
L5/S1	S1	Plantar flexors	Lateral foot and sole	Ankle jerk

EDL = extensor digitorum longus, EHL = extensor hallucis longus

Spinal Cord Disorders

- Paraplegia or quadriplegia due to complete transverse lesions
- Effect depends on level (e.g. C1-C3: death from respiratory paralysis)
- Two stages:
  - Spinal shock
    - Loss of all reflex activity below level of lesion
    - Atonic bladder/bowel with overflow incontinence
    - Gastric dilatation
    - Loss of vasomotor control
  - Heightened reflex activity
    - Hyperactive tendon reflexes
    - Frequency and urgency of urination, automatic emptying of bladder
    - Hyperactive vasomotor and sweating reactions
- *Central Cord Syndrome*
  - Occurs more often in older people or in patients with cervical spondylosis
  - Weakened hands with impaired pain sensation (most prominent symptom)
  - Relatively few long tract signs
- *Anterior Cord Syndrome*
  - Caused by infarction in anterior spinal artery territory or tumour invasion or inflammatory myelitis in similar region
  - Paraplegia or quadriplegia
  - Urinary retention
  - Bilateral loss of pain and temperature sensation below the lesion
  - Sparing of posterior column (joint position and vibration) sense
- *Conus Medullaris* and *Cauda Equina Syndromes*
  - Pain localized to the low back with radiation to legs
  - Loss of bladder and bowel control
  - Laxity of the anal sphincter
  - Erectile dysfunction
  - Loss of sensation in sacral segments (saddle paresthesia)
  - Often asymmetric leg weakness with upper and lower motor neuron signs

REFERENCES

Agur AMR, Dalley AF. 2009. *Grant's Atlas of Anatomy*. Philadelphia: Wolters Kluwer Health/Lippincott Williams & Wilkins.

Benarroch EE. 1999. *Medical Neurosciences: An Approach to Anatomy, Pathology, and Physiology by Systems and Levels*. Philadelphia: Lippincott Williams & Wilkins.

Bickley LS, Szilagyi PG, Bates B. 2007. *Bates' Guide to Physical Examination and History Taking*. Philadelphia: Lippincott Williams & Wilkins.

Carter LP, Spetzler RF, Hamilton MG. 1994. *Neurovascular Surgery*. New York: McGraw-Hill, Inc., Health Professions Division.

Goldstein LB, Matchar DB. 1994. The rational clinical examination. Clinical assessment of stroke. *JAMA* 271(14):1114-1120.

Greenberg MS. 2001. *Handbook of Neurosurgery*. Lakeland: Thieme Medical Publishers.

Kandel ER, Schwartz JH, Jessell TM. 2000. *Principles of Neural Science*. New York: McGraw-Hill, Health Professions Division.

Levine AM. 1998. *Spine Trauma*. Philadelphia: Saunders.

Ross RT. 2006. *How to Examine the Nervous System*. Totowa, N.J.: Humana Press.

Snell RS. 2000. *Clinical Anatomy for Medical Students*. Philadelphia: Lippincott Williams & Wilkins.

Zigmond MJ. 1999. *Fundamental Neuroscience*. San Diego: Academic Press.

NEUROLOGICAL

The Obstetric Exam

Editors:
Sarah Blissett, Homan Cheng &
Amanda Cipolla

Faculty Reviewers:
Paul Bernstein, MD, FRCS(C)
Mathew Sermer MD, FRCS(C)
Rory Windrim, MD, FRCS(C)

TABLE OF CONTENTS

Essential Anatomy   203
Approach to the Obstetrical History and Physical Exam   203
Common Chief Complaints   205
Common Disorders   206
Preconception Counselling   209
Diagnosis of Pregnancy   209
Initial Prenatal Assessment   209
Subsequent Prenatal Assessment   213
Labour   217
Puerperium and Post-partum Period   224

ESSENTIAL ANATOMY

Refer to the *Gynecological Exam* p. 91 for a diagram of the external and internal genitalia

APPROACH TO THE OBSTETRICAL HISTORY AND PHYSICAL EXAM

In addition to general history taking, important aspects of the obstetrical history and physical include:

- Diagnosis of Pregnancy
  - May present with amenorrhea, nausea/vomiting, urinary frequency, breast tenderness
- Stage of Pregnancy and Frequency of Visits
  - 1st trimester (weeks 0 to 12): usually 1 visit before 12 weeks
  - 2nd trimester (weeks 13 to 27): monthly
  - 3rd trimester (week 28 to 42): every 2 weeks until week 36; every week thereafter
- Initial Prenatal Assessment
  - Pregnancy Summary
    - Menstrual History (see *Gynecological Exam* p. 93)
    - History of Current Pregnancy
    - Contraception
    - **GPA status**: **G**ravida – number of pregnancies (including current pregnancy); **P**arity/para – number of deliveries after 20 wks; **A**bortion – any pregnancy loss prior to 20 wks
    - **EDB**: Estimated Date of Birth (estimated due date)
      - Also referred to as EDC – estimated date of confinement
  - Obstetrical History
  - Nutritional Assessment
  - Discussion Topics: work, lifestyle, coitus, prenatal classes, genetic testing, avoiding cat litter
  - Complete Physical Exam (see **Table 4**)

OBSTETRIC

- Subsequent Prenatal Assessment
  - **ABCDE: A**citivity of fetus, **B**leeding, **C**ontractions, **D**ripping, EDB
  - BP, weight gain
- Stage-dependent Physical Exam
  - At diagnosis: Goodell's Sign, Chadwick's Sign, Hegar's Sign (p. 209)
  - 1st trimester: complete physical exam
  - 2nd and 3rd trimesters: Vitals (BP, weight gain), Symphysis-Fundal Height (SFH), fetal heart assessment
  - 3rd trimester: Leopold Maneuvers (see **Figure 2**)

Table 1. Physiological Changes During Pregnancy

Parameter	Changes	Comments
General		
Weight	↑ 25% (~12.5 kg)	0.5 kg/wk in second 1/2 of pregnancy
Energy needs	↑ 15%	
Respiratory		
ABG	pCO_2 98% (28-32 mmHg)	pCO_2 in maternal blood facilitates placental pCO_2 transfer
Tidal volume	↑ 40%	
Cardiovascular		
Cardiac Output	↑ 30-50% (6.0 L/min)	CO peaks at 24 wks due to ↑ stroke volume
HR	↑ 15-20 bpm (85 bpm)	
Plasma volume	↑ 45%	
BP	systolic: ↓ 5-10 mmHg diastolic: ↓ 10-15 mmHg	BP lowest at 20-24 wks and then gradually
Hematologic		
Hemoglobin (Hb)	↓ 15-20 g/L	Hb starts ↓ by 12 wks lowest at 30-34 wks (~120 g/L) 1.8x ↑ risk thromboembolism (#1 cause of maternal death)
WBC	↑ 3.5 x 10⁹/L	
Coagulation	↑ Factors VII to X ↑ venous stasis	
Renal		
GFR	↑ 50%	No change in urine output due to tubular reabsorption

COMMON CHIEF COMPLAINTS

Table 2. Common Chief Complaints

Chief Complaints secondary to physiologic changes		
Common Complaint	**Trimester (T)**	**Possible Causes**
Breast tenderness/heaviness	1	Growth of breast tissue ↑ blood flow to breast
Fatigue	1	Unknown
Nausea/vomiting	1	↑ estrogen and hCG ↑ gastric motility
Weight loss	1	Decreased appetite from nausea and vomiting
Heartburn	1, 2, 3	Relaxation of lower esophageal sphincter allows reflux from stomach
Backache	1, 2, 3	Relaxation of joints and ligaments Growth of uterus Weight of fetus
Amenorrhea	1, 2, 3	↑ estrogen, progesterone, ß-hCG
Constipation	1, 2, 3	Decreased peristalsis
Urinary frequency	1, 2, 3	1 – ↓ plasma osmolality 2, 3 – ↑ vascularity, pressure of enlarged uterus Term – pressure of fetal head on bladder
Leukorrhea	1, 2, 3	Hormonal effects of pregnancy lead to increased blood flow to vagina
Chief Complaints secondary to pathological processes		
Bleeding	1, 2, 3	1, 2 – Spontaneous abortion, abnormal pregnancy (ectopic, molar), trauma 2, 3 – placenta previa, abruptio placentae 3 – Bloody show (effacement of cervix prior to delivery)
Decreased fetal movements	2, 3	Fetal distress, fetal demise
Contractions	2, 3	Pre-term labour, normal labour Braxton-Hicks 'contractions' are not true contractions; they are non painful uterine activity
Leaking	3	Premature rupture of membranes, onset of labour Yeast or other infection, normal secretions, urine

OBSTETRIC

COMMON DISORDERS

Disorders marked with (✓) are discussed in further detail

Pregnancy-Induced Conditions

✓ Hypertensive disorders: Pregnancy-induced hypertension, pre-eclampsia, eclampsia
✓ Gestational Diabetes Mellitus (GDM)
- Rhesus discrepancies
- Urinary tract infection (UTI)
- Anemia
- Hyperemesis gravidarum
- Infections (e.g. TORCH)

Antenatal Complications

✓ Miscarriage
✓ Ectopic pregnancy
✓ Abruptio placentae
✓ Placenta previa
✓ Premature rupture of the membranes (PROM)
- Intra-uterine growth restriction (IUGR)

Labour and Post-partum

✓ Breech Presentation
✓ Post-partum Depression

1. Pregnancy-Induced Conditions

Hypertensive Disorders

- Pregnancy-induced hypertension (PIH)
  - Hypertension (>140/90 mmHg, or an increase from baseline of 30 systolic or 15 diastolic) that develops during pregnancy and regresses postpartum (usually within 10 days)
- **Pre-eclampsia**
  - Presence of both hypertension and proteinuria
  - Mild vs. severe
- **Eclampsia**
  - Pre-eclampsia with seizures or coma
  - History:
    - Swelling: face, hands, feet
    - Excessive weight gain
    - Headache
    - Visual disturbances
    - Seizures
    - Dyspnea
    - RUQ or epigastric abdominal pain
  - Physical exam:
    - HEENT: facial edema, scotomas, loss of peripheral vision
    - Respiratory: crackles (pulmonary edema)
    - Cardiovascular: S3, S4, murmurs (CHF)
    - Abdominal: RUQ tenderness
    - Neurological: hyperreflexia, clonus
    - Fetal evaluation: abnormal FHR, non-stress test, biophysical profile

Gestational Diabetes Mellitus (GDM)
- Glucose intolerance present only in pregnancy
- Occurs in about 3% of pregnancies
- Asymptomatic, therefore must screen
- Screening (at 24-28 wks):
  - Oral glucose challenge test (OGCT): 50 g oral glucose
- Confirmation (if OGCT abnormal)
  - Oral glucose tolerance test (OGTT): 2 h 100 g OGTT
- Effects of diabetes on pregnancy
  - Increased perinatal loss
  - Increased incidence of fetal abnormalities
  - Macrosomia (large fetus size)
  - Delayed lung maturation
  - Increased risk of other complications (pre-eclampsia, polyhydramnios, UTI)
  - Pregnant women with IDDM should be considered at high-risk of complications and cared for by a team of endocrinologists and high-risk obstetricians

- Rhesus Discrepancies: 10% deliveries; with treatment only affects 0.5%
  - Sensitization of Rh negative mother to Rh positive blood from fetus
- Urinary tract infection (UTI): 4% pregnancies
- Anemia: 3/4 of cases due to iron deficiency; deficient RBC production due to increased iron and folate demands
- Hyperemesis gravidarum: intractable nausea and vomiting in T1, T2; in 3.5 of 1000 pregnancies

2. Antenatal Complications
Miscarriage
- 40% caused by fetal abnormality: e.g. structural, chromosomal, genetic
- 60% due to other causes including abnormalities of implantation, multiple pregnancy, endocrine deficiency, uterine abnormalities, trauma, maternal disease, infections, poisons, immunological factors, cervical incompetence, and autoimmune diseases (e.g. SLE)
Ectopic pregnancy
- Most commonly occurs in fallopian tube, especially ampulla (80%)
- Variable presentation
  - Vague lower abdominal pain (95% of cases)
  - Minimal vaginal bleeding (50-80% of cases)
  - Catastrophic shock if ruptured
Abruptio placenta (see **Table 3**)
- Premature separation of normally implanted placenta
- Presents with bleeding in 80% of cases, internal/concealed in 20%
- Hemorrhage from decidual spiral arteries
Placenta previa (see **Table 3**)
- Occurs in 1 in 150-250 births in T3
- Abnormal location of placenta at or near the cervical os
  - Low-lying (NOT a previa)
  - Marginal
  - Partial
  - Total
- More than 90% resolve by T3
- Repeat U/S at 30-32 wks
- **DO NOT PERFORM VAGINAL EXAMINATIONS** and counsel against coitus
- Common presentation: painless bleeding at 30 wks
- Fetus is at risk of prematurity, growth retardation and cerebral palsy
- Patient should be delivered by Cesarean section

Table 3. Placenta Previa vs. Abruptio Placentae

Feature	Placenta Previa	Abruptio Placentae
Onset of symptoms	Depends on degree of previa Mean: 30 wks GA 1/3 present before 30 wks GA	After 20 wks GA
Vaginal bleeding	Painless and recurrent Bright red blood	Painful Dark, bright or clotted blood
Uterus	Soft and non-tender	Tender, increased tone
Diagnosis	U/S	Clinical

Premature rupture of membranes (PROM)
- Rupture of fetal membranes prior to onset of labour
- Diagnosis
    - Sterile speculum exam (no digital vaginal exam to decrease risk of infection)
    - Pooling of fluid in vaginal vault
    - Valsalva fluid leakage from cervical os
    - Nitrazine paper indicator: turns blue with amniotic fluid (also with blood, urine, and semen)
    - Ferning: allow fluid to evaporate on slide; with amniotic fluid, pattern visible on microscopy
        - Gold standard test

3. Labour and Post-partum
Breech Presentation
- Presentation of fetal buttocks or lower extremities into the maternal pelvis
- Occurs in about 3-4% of term pregnancies vs. 30% at 30 wks
- 3 types
    - Complete (5-10%)
        - Thighs and knees flexed, feet above buttocks
    - Frank (50-75%)
        - Thighs flexed, knees extended
    - Footling (20%)
        - Single: one thigh extended; foot is presenting part
        - Double: both thighs extended
- Diagnosis
    - Leopold maneuvers
    - U/S
- May be avoided with successful external cephalic version (attempted after 34 weeks)
- Delivery
    - Best done by Cesarean section

Post-partum Depression (see section 6)

PRECONCEPTION COUNSELING

- Genetic history
- Proper nutrition
- Supplementation of vitamin D, iron, folic acid (0.4-1 mg/d, 4-5 mg if neural tube defect in previous pregnancy)
- Risk factors
  - Alcohol, tobacco, drugs (prescription, over-the-counter and illicit)
  - Maternal age greater than 35
  - Certain occupational hazards (e.g. chemical or radiation exposure)
- Rubella immunity
- Medical conditions that may impact fertility (see *Gynecological Exam* p. 105)
- Mental health
- Maternity/paternity leave

DIAGNOSIS OF PREGNANCY

- Symptoms
  - Amenorrhea
  - Nausea/vomiting
  - Breast tenderness
  - Urinary frequency
  - Fatigue
- Signs on pelvic examination
  - *Goodell's Sign* – softening of the cervix and vagina (4-6 wks)
  - *Chadwick's Sign* – bluish discoloration of cervix and vagina (6 wks)
  - *Hegar's Sign* – softening/compressibility of uterine lower segment (6-8 wks)
  - Uterine enlargement
- Investigations: serum – definitive test for pregnancy diagnosis

INITIAL PRENATAL ASSESSMENT

- Usually done by 12th week post-LMP

A. Focused History

Patient Identification
- Age, occupation, marital status

Fertility Summary
- *Menstrual history* (see *Gynecological Exam* p. 93)
  - Date of LMP, cycle frequency
  - Estimated Date of Birth (EDB)
    - ◆ (1) by date of LMP using Nagele's Rule: 1st day of LMP + 7 days – 3 months (if cycle is not 28 days, add number of additional days, e.g. add 4 if 32-day cycle)
    - ◆ (2) By ultrasound (most accurate before 20 weeks GA). Once established by U/S, EDB does not change
- *Contraception*
  - Type, duration of use, date of last use
- *History of current pregnancy*
  - Physiologic symptoms: vomiting, fatigue, urinary frequency, etc. (see **Table 1** and **Table 2**)
  - Potentially harmful exposures: smoking, alcohol, radiation, occupational

OBSTETRIC

- Nutritional assessment: balanced diet, adequate calcium intake, folate supplementation; avoid unpasturized milk products, raw meats and sushi
- Red flags: bleeding (duration, amount, any clots), discharge/leaking fluid, cramping/contractions/abdominal pain
- **GTPALM** status
  - **Gravida**   # of pregnancies
  - **Term**   # of deliveries at 37-42 wks gestation
  - ***Premature**   # of deliveries <37 wks gestation
  - **Abortion**   # of abortions (spontaneous and therapeutic)
  - **Live**   # of live deliveries
  - **Multiples**   # of multiple pregnancies
  - *Note: some physicians prefer to use P to indicate 'Parity' or births >20 wk GA

Obstetrical History of All Previous Pregnancies
- Year, place of birth
- Sex, gestational age, birth weight of baby
- Abortion (medical vs. surgical dilatation/curettage)
- Labour duration, type of delivery (vaginal, forceps, vacuum, Cesarean section)
  - Type of Cesarean section, if applicable (classical vs. lower segment)
- Pregnancy/delivery/perinatal/post-partum complications (e.g. pulmonary embolism, gestational DM, post-partum depression)
- Health status of previous children (alive, well, illnesses)

Medical History
- Kidney disease
- Cardiac/pulmonary disease
- GI/liver disease
- Endocrine disease: thyroid disease, diabetes
- Hypertension
- Infections (e.g. TORCH, HIV, STDs/HSV/BV, varicella status, TB risk)
- Psychiatric history
- Transfusion history
- Surgical history
- Anesthesia complications
- Allergies and Medications

Family History
- Diabetes, hypertension, DVT/PE, thyroid disease, post-partum depression
- Developmental delay, congenital abnormalities, chromosomal disorders, genetic disorders
- At risk population: Ashkenazi Jewish (Tay-Sachs disease, Canavan, Niemann-Pick, Gaucher, CF), Mediterranean and Asian (thalassemia), African (sickle cell anemia)

Social History
- Social supports
- Smoking, alcohol, recreational drugs (prior to and during pregnancy)
- Relationship with partner/father of baby or single parent
- Family violence (see **Clinical Pearl** p. 211)

OBSTETRIC

Other Discussion Topics
- Exercise: encourage regular low-moderate physical activity as routinely done prior to pregnancy, target HR should be 3/4 of non-pregnant target HR; discourage participation in high impact activities (scuba diving, horseback riding)
- Coitus: safe during pregnancy (except placenta previa)
- Prenatal classes
- Avoiding cat litter boxes (risk of toxoplasmosis)
- Screening test schedule

Clinical Pearl

Intimate partner violence is a serious and surprisingly common problem, affecting around 7% of pregnant women (Violence against Women Survey, Stewart & Cecutti, 1993). Physical abuse during pregnancy is associated with increased risk of antepartum hemorrhage, IUGR, and perinatal death (Janssen et al., 2003). Routine screening questions addressing personal safety and violence should be included during the prenatal period.

B. Focused Physical
- Baseline physical assessment:
  - Height
  - Pre-pregnancy weight and current weight
  - BP (important for detection of present/future hypertensive disorders)
  - Pelvic exam
- Systematic assessment (**Table 4**)

Table 4. Physical Exam by System

Systems	Common Observations	Abnormalities
Thyroid	Symmetrical enlargement	Marked or asymmetrical enlargement
Cardiovascular		
Palpation	PMI slightly higher than normal (dextro-rotation of heart)	
Auscultation	Soft, blowing, systolic ejection murmurs often reflect increase blood flow in vessels	All diastolic murmurs are abnormal. All murmurs ≥3/6 are abnormal
Breasts		
Inspection	Marked venous pattern	
Palpation	Tender and nodular	Pathological masses (see **Breast Exam**)
Nipple compression	Colostrum may be expressed	Bloody/purulent discharge

Table 4. Physical Exam by System (continued)

Systems	Common Observations	Abnormalities
Abdominal		
Inspect	Scars due to previous surgeries (e.g. C-section), striae (shiny, purple)	
Palpate	Organs, masses, fetal size, Leopold maneuvers (in third trimester)	
Measure	Symphysis-Fundal Height (see **Table 7** and **Figure 1**)	If >2 cm greater than expected: multiple gestations, large baby, polyhydramnios, uterine myomata If >2 cm less than expected: missed abortion, transverse lie, growth retardation, false pregnancy, oligohydramnios
Auscultate	Fetal heart: doptone (after 12 wks)	Not audible: GA less than expected, fetal demise, false pregnancy, technical difficulties
	Fetoscope (after 24 wks)	Drop with fetal movement: poor placental circulation Lack of variability: fetal compromise
Pelvic, Genital, and Anal		
Inspect	External genitalia: should appear normal; look for scars (previous episiotomy or tear) Anus: hemorrhoids	Vaginal irritation/itching with discharge: infection
Speculum exam	Pap smears, vaginal/cervical swabs Vaginal wall: bluish/violet colour deep rugae, leukorrhea	Purulent discharge, lesions, etc.
Bimanual exam	Cervix: length (1.5-2 cm before 34-36 wks), consistency, dilatation (smooth and closed in nulliparous; irregular with small opening in parous), friable cervix	Adnexal mass: ectopic pregnancy, ovarian cyst Uterine fibroids

PMI = point of maximal impulse, GA = gestational age
* Fetal movements are felt by mother at 18-20 wks

C. Common Investigations

Diagnosis of Pregnancy
- *Serum β-hCG*: positive 9 days post-conception
- *Urine β-hCG*: positive 28 days after LMP (i.e. within 1 day of first missed period)
- *U/S*: should detect uterine sac by 4wks; fetal heart beat by 6 wks

Initial Prenatal Assessment
- *Bloodwork*:
  - CBC (Hb, MCV)
  - Blood group and type, Rh status and other antibody screen
  - Rubella titre
  - VDRL (syphilis)
  - Hep B surface antigen
  - HIV (offer to all patients)
- *Urinalysis*: routine and microscopy (R&M), culture and sensitivity (C&S)
- *Cervix*: PAP, culture for chlamydia and gonorrhea, culture for bacterial vaginosis if history of preterm labour

4. SUBSEQUENT PRENATAL ASSESSMENT
- Recommended frequency of prenatal visits is outlined in **Table 5**

Table 5. Schedule for Uncomplicated Pregnancies

Gestational Age	Usual Frequency of Visit
Up to 32 wks	Monthly
32 - 36 wks	Every 2 weeks
36 wks to delivery	Every week

A. Focused History
- Note any changes to information on initial assessment
- **A**ctivity of fetus
- **B**leeding
- **C**ontractions
- **D**ripping (discharge, fluid)
- **E**DB

Table 6. Essential Aspects of History Taking for Acute Presentations

Presenting Complaints	Questions Asked
Pain	Onset, duration, quality, quantity, temporal profile, aggravating/alleviating factors
Contractions	Location (abdomen/back), onset, frequency, duration, radiation
Vaginal discharge	Colour, consistency, quantity, presence of mucus, blood
Edema	Location (hands, face)
Absence of fetal movement	Instruct patient to sit in a quiet room and count 6 movements in two hours every 24 hours; to return to doctor if movements not felt

*With all complaints, ask about associated symptoms, which may include: paresthesia, scotoma, blurry vision, epigastric pain, pruritus, dysuria, severe headache, fever

- Discussion topics
  - Diet/nutrition, rest
  - Signs of labour, premature labour
  - Prenatal education classes
  - Review labour and delivery plans (e.g. supports, pain relief)
  - Circumcision
  - Breast feeding

OBSTETRIC

B. Focused Physical

General and Vitals
- Gestational age
- HR
- BP (during T1-T2 normally lower than non-pregnant state)
- Weight
  - T1 weight loss common due to nausea and vomiting
  - Hyperemesis gravidarum if loss >5 lbs due to vomiting
  - Ideal total gain 25 lbs; average total weight gain 35 lbs
    - T1: 5 lbs, T2: 10 lbs, T3: 10 lbs
    - Weight gain >25 lbs is common – physiologic increase in interstitial fluid due to increased estrogen; not associated with adverse pregnancy outcomes

Abdominal Exam – see **Table 4**
- Symphysis-Fundal Height (SFH) (see **Table 7** and **Figure 1**)
  - At 20-37 wks, SFH = GA ± 2cm e.g. 30 weeks = 30 cm

Table 7. Symphysis-Fundal Height Reference Chart

Gestational Age (wks)	Location of Fundus
12	Pubic symphysis
20	Umbilicus
36	Palpable just below xyphoid
Term	No longer reliable due to engagement and descent

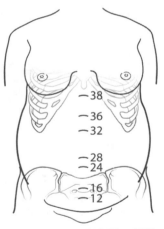

Caitlin O'Connell 2010

Figure 1. Expected Symphysis Fundal Height by Gestational Age Weeks

OBSTETRIC

Fetal Heart Rate Assessment
- Every visit beginning at 12 wks with doptone (Doppler U/S or fetoscope)

Leopold Maneuvers (see **Figure 2**)
- Done in T3
- Determines fetal location within the uterus
- Carried out to identify lie, presentation, and position of the fetus
- *First maneuver* – distinguishes which part of the fetus occupies the fundus
  - Face patient's head and stand to one side of patient while supine
  - Palpate the fundal area
    - Buttocks at fundus/vertex: soft or irregular
    - Head at fundus/breech: round, hard, ballotable
- *Second maneuver* – determines side on which fetal back lies
  - Place hands on lateral sides of the abdomen and palpate
    - Back: linear and firm
    - Extremities: multiple parts ("small parts")
- *Third maneuver* – determines the presenting part
  - Place one hand just above the symphysis
  - Grasp the presenting part between the thumb and third finger
    - Unengaged head/vertex: round, firm, and ballotable
    - Breech: irregular and nodular
- *Fourth maneuver* – determines head flexion or extension
  - Face patient's feet and place hands on either side of lower abdomen just above inlet
  - Exert pressure in direction of inlet; one hand will usually descend further than the other
    - Head flexed: cephalic prominence prevents descent of one hand which is on the same side as the small parts (suggests occiput presentation)
    - Head extended: occiput is felt prominently on the same side as the back (suggests face presentation)

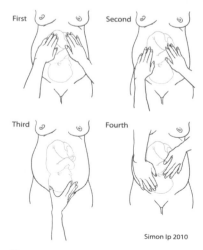

First   Second

Third   Fourth

Simon Ip 2010

Figure 2. Leopold Maneuvers

C. Common Investigations

- Routine urine dip: glucose and protein
  - Done at each visit

First Trimester Screening (FTS)

- Done between 11-14 wks GA
- Measures nuchal translucency (NT), β-hCG, pregnancy-associated plasma protein A (PAPP-A)
- Estimates risk of Down syndrome (Trisomy 21)

Maternal Serum Screen (MSS)

- Done at 16 wks GA
- Measures maternal serum α-fetoprotein (MSAFP), β-hCG, estriol (µE3)
- Estimates risk of Trisomy 21, Trisomy 18 and neural tube defects (NTDs)

Integrated Prenatal Screen (IPS)

- Integrates parts of FTS and MSS to yield a more specific screening test for Trisomy 21, Trisomy 18 and NTDs
- Part 1 done at 10-14 wks: NT by US and PAPP-A
- Part 2 done at 15-18 wks: MSS markers

Chorionic Villus Sampling

- Done at 10-13 wks
- Placental biopsy (transabdominal or transcervical)
- Additional miscarriage risk <1%
- Available to all patients; indicated if high risk population for chromosomal abnormalities (e.g. Ashkenazi Jewish, increased maternal age, family history of chromosomal abnormality)

Amniocentesis

- Sample of amniotic fluid aspirated transabdominally with ultrasound guidance
- Additional miscarriage risk of 0.5% or less
- Available to all patients; indicated if high risk population for chromosomal abnormalities

Ultrasound (U/S)

- Done at 18 wks for anatomical scan or when indicated (e.g. assess presentation, confirm interuterine pregnancy)
- Transabdominal or transvaginal

Other tests as indicated

- TB skin test, sickle cell/thalassemia screen (Hb electrophoresis)
- Other genetic screens as indicated by family history/ethnicity

OBSTETRIC

Table 8. Gestational Age-Dependent Tests

Gestational Age (wks)	Tests
All visits	Urine dip for proteinuria, glucosuria, ketones
12-14	CVS, U/S (nuchal translucency and dates), blood work
15-16	Amniocentesis
16	MSS
18-20	U/S (anatomical scan)
24-28	Oral glucose challenge test (50 g load)
26	Screen for Rh and give RhoGAM at 28 wk to Rh negative women
28-32	Repeat CBC to determine need for iron supplementation
36-37	Group B Strep culture (anovaginal)

CVS = chorionic villus sampling, U/S = ultrasound, MSS = maternal serum screen, Rh = Rhesus factor

Antenatal Monitoring

Non-Stress Test (NST)
- Assess fetal heart rate in relation to fetal movement using an external Doppler
- Indicated if suspect uteroplacental insufficiency or fetal distress

Biophysical Profile (BPP)
- U/S assessment of fetus ± NST
- Indicated if non-reassuring NST, post-term pregnancy, decreased fetal movement, any suggestion of fetal distress
- Each of the following four parameters are given a score of 2 (reassuring) or 0 (non-reassuring)
    - Amniotic fluid volume (most important parameter)
    - Fetal tone
    - Fetal movement
    - Fetal breathing

5. LABOUR
- *Labour* – regular painful uterine contractions leading to cervical dilatation and effacement and resulting in the expulsion of the products of conception (fetus, membranes and placenta)
- *Preterm labour* – 20-37 weeks GA
- *Term labour* – 37-42 weeks GA
- *Postterm labour* – >42 weeks GA
- *Braxton-Hicks contractions* ("false labour") – irregular, occur throughout pregnancy and do not result in cervical dilatation, effacement or fetal descent (see **Table 9**)

OBSTETRIC

Table 9. True vs. False Labour

	True Labour	**False Labour**
Contraction intervals	Regular	Irregular
Duration of intervals	Gradually shorten	Remains long
Intensity of contractions	Gradually increases	Remains unchanged
Discomfort	Back and abdomen	Lower abdomen
Relief by sedation	Not relieved by sedation	Often relieved by sedation
Cervix	Effacement and dilatation	No effacement and dilatation

Cervical Changes
- Effacement
  - Thinning of cervical walls caused by pressure of fetal head
  - Expressed in % of total effacement
    - 0% – none, 100% – complete thinning
  - May result in release of mucous plug within cervical canal ("bloody show")
- Dilatation
  - Opening of cervical canal
  - Expressed in cm: 0 cm – no dilatation, 10 cm – full dilatation

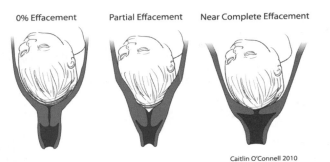

0% Effacement   Partial Effacement   Near Complete Effacement

Caitlin O'Connell 2010

Figure 3. Stages of Cervical Effacement and Dilatation

Stages of Labour
- *First Stage*: onset of true labour to full dilatation of the cervix (10 cm)
  - Latent phase: cervical effacement and dilatation (0-3 cm)
  - Active phase: rapid cervical dilation (3 cm – full dilatation)
    - Nulliparous: 1.2 cm/h
    - Multiparous: 1.5 cm/h
- *Second Stage*: delivery of fetus
- *Third Stage*: delivery of placenta
- *Fourth Stage*: from placental delivery until patient is stable; e.g. 1st postpartum hour

Table 10. Duration of Normal Labour

Stage	Nulliparous	Multiparous
First	6 - 18 h	2 - 10 h
Second	30 min - 3 h	5 - 30 min
Third	5 - 30 min	5 - 30 min
Fourth	Until postpartum condition of patient has stabilized (usually 1 h)	

Physical Exam and Investigations During Labour and Delivery

On Admission
- Vital signs and fluid status
- Abdominal examination
  - Determine fetal lie, position and station of presenting part
- If placenta previa known/suspected, do *not* attempt vaginal exam
- Urine for protein, glucose and ketone bodies

First Stage of Labour
- Vaginal examination
  - Repeated every 2 hours or as clinically indicated
  - Separate vulva and labia with left hand and use right index and middle fingers to examine
  - Assess position of cervix: anterior vs. posterior
  - Assess degree of dilatation and effacement of cervix
    - Softness of cervix increases with increased effacement
    - Cervical dilatation:
      - 1 finger ~ 2 cm
      - 2 fingers ~ 3.5 cm (1/3 dilated)
      - 3 fingers ~ 5.5 cm (1/2 dilated)
      - 4 fingers ~ 7.5 cm (3/4 dilated)
- Assess if membranes have ruptured
  - Pooling of fluid in speculum exam
  - ↑ pH of vaginal fluid
  - Ferning of fluid under light microscopy
  - ↓ AFV on U/S
- After membranes have ruptured, examine the amniotic fluid, noting any meconium
- Determine the position of the presenting part by palpating suture lines and fontanelles in relation to pelvic diameters
  - Feel for sagittal and coronal sutures which come together to form the anterior fontanelle (λ shape)
  - Follow the sagittal suture to the posterior fontanelle and occiput
  - Determine the position of the occiput in relation to the maternal pelvis
    - Occiput anterior (OA)
    - Occiput posterior (OP)
    - Occiput transverse (OT)
  - Determine position of the occiput in relation to maternal left or right side
- Find the level of the presenting part in relation to the pelvic brim or ischial spines (**Figure 4**)
  - 0 = level of ischial spines
  - Using index and middle fingers, palpate the ischial spines

OBSTETRIC

- Locate most inferior aspect of presenting part determine whether it is above, at or below level of ischial spines
- Estimate level in thirds or fifths above (+) or below (-) zero

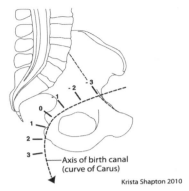

Krista Shapton 2010

Figure 4. Level of Head in Thirds Above or Below Ischial Spines

Electronic Fetal Heart Rate (FHR) Monitoring
- Assess baseline FHR, variability, and periodicity (decelerations and accelerations)

Table 11. Intrapartum FHR Monitoring (see also **Figure 5**)

	Normal	Atypical	Abnormal
Baseline FHR (bpm)	110-160	Slow 100-110 Fast >160 for 30-80 min Rising baseline	Slow <100 Fast >160 for >80 min Erratic baseline
Variability (bpm)	6-25 <5 for <40 min	<5 for 40-80 min	<5 for >80 min >25 for >10 min Sinusoidal
Deceleration	None or occasional Early of variable decels	Repetitive (>3) variable decels Occasional late decels Single prolonged decel for 2-3 min	Repetitive (>3) variable decels Late decels >50% of contractions Single prolonged decel for 3-10 min Slow to return to baseline
Acceleration	Spontaneous Occurs with fetal scalp stimulation	Absence of accel. with fetal scalp stimulation	Absent
Action	Routine intrapartum monitoring	Frequent reassessment and further management as indicated clinically	Confirm fetal well-being Fetal scalp blood sample Consider operative delivery Intrauterine resuscitation

OBSTETRIC

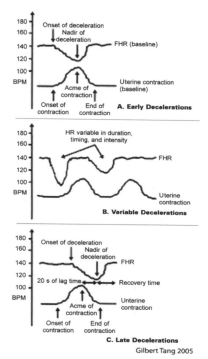

Figure 5. Fetal Heart Monitoring Strips

SECOND STAGE OF LABOUR

Cardinal Movements of the Fetus During Delivery (see **Figure 6**)
1. Descent
   - Begins before onset of labour or during first stage
   - Continues until fetus is delivered
2. Flexion
   - Fetal head flexes chin to chest
   - Reduces diameter of presenting part
3. Internal Rotation
   - Fetal head rotates laterally during descent through the pelvis
4. Extension
   - Fetal neck extends to negotiate under the symphysis pubis
   - Crowning: largest diameter of fetal head is encircled by vulvar ring (station +3 or +5 if measuring station by thirds or fifths respectively)
5. Restitution/External Rotation
   - Fetal head returns to the position at the time of engagement
   - Fetal back and shoulders align
6. Expulsion
   - Delivery of anterior shoulder, posterior shoulder, then the rest of the body

OBSTETRIC

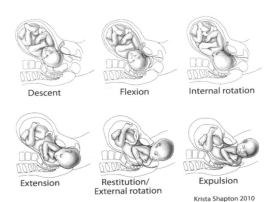

Descent   Flexion   Internal rotation

Extension   Restitution/   Expulsion
             External rotation

Krista Shapton 2010

Figure 6. Cardinal Movements of the Fetus During Delivery

Delivery of the Fetus
- Mother is positioned left lateral or supine
- Episiotomy (incision in perineum) only if necessary
- Delivery of fetal head
  - Ritgen maneuver: exert forward pressure on the chin of the fetus through the perineum just in front of coccyx with left hand, while exerting pressure superiorly against occiput with right hand
- Check for nuchal cord
- Clear fetal airway using suction bulb: oral cavity first, then nares
- Delivery of anterior shoulder
  - Hold sides of the head with two hands and apply gentle downward pressure
- Delivery of posterior shoulder
  - Gently elevate the head and apply upward pressure
- Delivery of rest of body
- Check fetal APGAR scores 1 and 5 minutes after birth (**Table 12**)

Table 12. APGAR Scores

Sign	0	1	2
Appearance: colour	Blue, pale	Body pink, extremities blue	Completely pink
Pulse: heart rate	Absent	<100 bpm	>100 bpm
Grimace: irritability	No response	Grimace	Sneeze or cough
Activity: muscle tone	Flaccid	Some flexion of extremities	Good flexion
Respiratory effort	Absent	Weak, irregular	Good, crying

OBSTETRIC

Third Stage of Labour

- Signs of placental separation
  - Uterus becomes firm and globular
  - Gush of blood
  - Umbilical cord visibly lengthens
  - Uterine fundus rises in abdomen
- Patient is positioned supine
- Place left hand on abdomen over the uterine fundus
- Exert gentle pressure on uterine fundus while keeping the umbilical cord slightly taut with right hand
- Do NOT pull on umbilical cord!

Fourth Stage of Labour

- Monitor vital signs and ensure patient is stabilized
- Inspect placenta for completeness (i.e. no retained products) and blood vessels (2 arteries and 1 vein)
- Send samples of umbilical artery and umbilical vein cord gasses to lab after every delivery
- Palpate to ensure uterine contraction and check for uterine bleeding
- Repair episiotomies or tears

Operative Delivery

- Use of forceps, vacuum extraction or surgery to deliver the fetus
- Common indications for Cesarean section
  - Maternal:
    - Obstruction of birth canal
    - Active herpetic lesions on vulva
    - Underlying maternal illness (eclampsia, HELLP)
    - Previous Cesarean section
    - Elective
  - Maternal-fetal:
    - Failure to progress
    - Cephalopelvic disproportion (CPD)
    - Multiple gestations
    - Placenta previa
    - Placental abruption
  - Fetus:
    - Malpresentation – breech (3-4% of deliveries), transverse lie (3-4/1000 births)
    - Fetal distress, non-reassuring fetal heart rate (1-2% of cases)
    - Low-birth weight infant
    - Macrosomic infant (>4 kg)

OBSTETRIC

Examination of the Newborn
- Full head-to-toe examination within 24 hours of delivery (see *Pediatric Exam* p. 253)

6. PUERPERIUM AND POST-PARTUM PERIOD
- 6-week period after pregnancy when pregnancy-related anatomic and physiologic changes are reversed

PHYSIOLOGIC CHANGES
- Uterus
  - Uterus decreases in size and cervix regains firmness
  - Uterus should involute 1 cm (1 finger breadth) below umbilicus per day for first 4-5 days
  - Uterine spasms can cause pain 4-7 days postpartum
  - Returns to non-pregnant state in 4-6 weeks
- Resumption of ovarian function
  - Ovuation resumes in 45 days in non-lactating patients, and 3-6 months in lactating women
  - Breastfeeding is NOT a method of contraception – unless patient wishes to conceive, use a barrier method
- Lochia: normal vaginal discharge postpartum
  - Decreases and changes colour from red (lochia rubra) to yellow (lochia serosa) to white (lochia alba)
- Breast changes
  - Engorgement in late pregnancy
  - Colostrum expression can occur in late pregnancy up to 72 h postpartum
  - Full milk production by 3-7 days
  - Mature milk by 15-45 days

Postpartum Disorders

Postpartum Hemorrhage (PPH)
- Loss of >500 mL of blood at time of vaginal delivery or >1000 mL in C/S
- Early (within 24 hours of delivery) or delayed (24 hours to 6 weeks post-delivery)
- Incidence 5-15%, significant cause of maternal mortality
- Causes: 4T's
  - Tone: uterine atony
  - Tissue: retained products
  - Trauma
  - Thrombosis: coagulopathy

Endometritis
- Entry of normal GI or gynecological bacteria into the usually sterile uterus
- Higher risk following Cesarean compared to vaginal delivery
- Suspect if foul smelling lochia

Postpartum Depression
- Spectrum of mood conditions ranging from "baby blues" to psychotic depression
- Predictors: stressful life events, past history of depression, family history of mood disorders
- Screening: postpartum visits, well baby visits

- *Postpartum "baby" blues*
  - Occurs in 85% of new mothers, onset day 3-10
  - Presentation: weeping, sadness, irritability, anxiety, confusion, extreme elation
  - Symptoms peak around 4th day after delivery and resolve within 2 weeks
- *Postpartum depression (PPD)*
  - Major depression occurring within 6 months of delivery
  - Incidence 10-20%, 50% recurrence
  - Presentation: despondent mood, feelings of inadequacy as a parent, impaired concentration, changes in appetite and sleep, thoughts of harming the infant
  - Long term adverse effects for mother and child if untreated
- *Postpartum psychosis*
  - Acute psychotic episode or abrupt onset of depressive symptoms over 24-72 hours within first postpartum month
  - Occurs in approximately 1-2 in 1000 women after delivery
  - Presentation: psychosis with delusions, hallucinations, or both, plus mood disorder
  - Symptoms may appear to resolve then reoccur acutely and severely
  - More likely to act on thoughts of harming their infants if untreated

Breastfeeding
- Breast milk is the optimal food for infants. Canadian Paediatric Society recommends exclusive breastfeeding for the first 6 months of life for healthy, term infants, up to 2 years and beyond
- Benefits of breastfeeding for baby:
  - Optimal nutrition: easily digested and low renal solute
  - Immunologic: immune protection, less allergenic
  - Better outcomes in later life
- Benefits of breastfeeding for mother:
  - Decreased risk of breast, ovarian and endometrial cancer
  - Helps prevent postpartum hemorrhage
  - Decreased insulin requirements in diabetic mothers
  - Decreased risk of osteoperosis
- Other benefits of breastfeeding
  - Bonding between mother and child
  - Lower cost
- Early mother-baby interaction after delivery is key to initiating breastfeeding
- Latching:
  - Mother and baby should be positioned comfortably with the infant's mouth fully open
  - Aim nipple for the upper lip, such that the entire areola (not just nipple) should be in infant's mouth
  - Breastfeeding should be pain-free if infant is properly latched
- Common maternal concerns:
  - Sore breasts, cracked or bleeding nipples
  - Breast engorgement
  - Mastitis
- No evidence to support need for first feed to occur immediately after delivery

OBSTETRIC

REFERENCES

Enkin M. 2000. *A Guide to Effective Care in Pregnancy and Childbirth*. Oxford; New York: Oxford University Press.

Janssen PA, Holt VL, Sugg NK, Emanuel I, Critchlow CM, Henderson AD. 2003. Intimate partner violence and adverse pregnancy outcomes: a population-based study. *Am J Obstet Gynecol* 188(5):1341-1347.

Miller LJ. 2002. Postpartum depression. *JAMA* 287(6):762-765.

Robohm JS, Buttenheim M. 1996. The gynecological care experience of adult survivors of childhood sexual abuse: a preliminary investigation. *Women Health* 24(3):59-75.

Schmidt B, Kirpalani H, Rosenbaum P, Cadman D. 1988. Strengths and limitations of the Apgar score: a critical appraisal. *J Clin Epidemiol* 41:843-850.

Stewart DE, Cecutti A. 1993. Physical abuse in pregnancy. *CMAJ* 149(9):1257-1263.

The Ophthalmological Exam

Editors:
Henry Becker,
Yingming Chen &
Christine Law

Faculty Reviewers:
Alan Berger, MD, FRCS(C)
Kenneth Eng, MD, FRCS(C)
Baseer Khan, MD, FRCS(C)

TABLE OF CONTENTS

The Essentials	227
Approach to the Ophthalmological History and Physical Exam	227
Common Chief Complaints	228
Common Disorders	228
Essential Anatomy	229
Definition of Refractive Error	229
Focused History	229
Summary of Focused History	232
Focused Physical Exam	233
Summary of Focused Physical Exam	241
Common Clinical Scenarios	241

THE ESSENTIALS

- Ocular history: pay special attention to related symptoms (e.g. pain, vision loss, redness, unilateral vs. bilateral, associated symptoms)
- Ophthalmic examination: visual acuity, confrontation visual fields, external examination, pupils, motility/alignment, slit lamp, intraocular pressure (tonometry), and fundoscopy
- Common abbreviations: OD (Oculus Dexter) = right eye; OS (Oculus Sinister) = left eye; OU (Oculus Uterque) = both eyes
- Common prefixes and suffixes: *presby-* = old; *core-* = pupil; *blepharo-* = eyelid; *kerato-* = cornea; *dacryo-* = tear; *-phakos* = lens; *-opsia* = vision

APPROACH TO THE OPHTHALMOLOGICAL HISTORY AND PHYSICAL EXAM

In addition to general history taking, aspects of the ophthalmological history include:

- Ocular symptoms (see **Common Chief Complaints**)
- Past ocular history (e.g. corrective lens use, prior trauma, surgery, infections, eye diseases)
- Past medical history (for ocular effects of systemic diseases)
- Family history of eye disease
- Ocular and systemic medications

Overview of the physical exam

- Measure visual acuity
- Examine pupils
- Check visual fields
- Evaluate extraocular muscles and eye alignment
- Inspect external aspects of the eye such as the lids, lacrimal apparatus, and lashes
- Examine the anterior segment
- Measure intraocular pressure by indentation or applanation tonometry
- Perform fundoscopy

COMMON CHIEF COMPLAINTS

- Loss of vision: sudden vs. gradual, transient vs. prolonged, central vs. peripheral field loss
- Pain
- Redness
- Double vision (diplopia)
- Tearing
- Dryness (sicca)
- Foreign body sensation
- Itchy (pruritis)
- Discharge
- Eyelild crusting
- Eyelid swelling
- Drooping eyelid (ptosis)
- Floaters
- Flashes (photopsia)
- Haloes
- Sensitivity to light (photophobia)
- Headache

COMMON DISORDERS

Disorders marked with (✓) are discussed in **Common Clinical Scenarios**

Acute Diseases

- Acute conjunctivitis: inflammation of the conjunctiva (bacterial, viral or allergic)
- Acute iritis: inflammation of the iris
- Blepharitis: inflammation of the eyelid
- Corneal abrasions (CA): self-limited loss of the corneal epithelium
- Corneal ulcers: infection of the cornea (bacterial or viral); deeper and more opaque lesion than CA, with less defined contours
- ✓ Acute Angle-closure glaucoma
- Anterior Ischemic Optic Neuropathy (AION): sudden, usually unilateral loss of vision
- Optic Neuritis (ON): inflammation of the optic nerve; isolated or in Multiple Sclerosis
- Papilloedema: optic disc swelling secondary to elevated intracranial pressure
- ✓ Retinal Detachment
- Retinal Vascular Occlusions: common cause of sudden unilateral visual loss

Note: Amaurosis fugax is the transient loss of unilateral vision due to an arterial occlusion; an important sign of carotid atheroma

Chronic Diseases

- Strabismus: ocular misalignment
- Amblyopia: decrease in vision in an eye that is otherwise anatomically normal
- ✓ Cataract
- ✓ Diabetic retinopathy
- ✓ Age-Related Macular Degeneration (ARMD)
- ✓ Glaucoma

ESSENTIAL ANATOMY

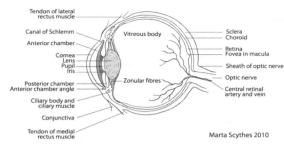

Figure 1. Anatomy of the Eye

Marta Scythes 2010

DEFINITION OF REFRACTIVE ERROR

- Emmetropia: no refractive error
- Myopia: nearsightedness
    - **LMN** = **L**ong eyeball, **M**yopic (nearsighted), corrected with a **N**egative lens
- Hyperopia: farsightedness
    - Light rays focused beyond retina; correct with a positive lens or accommodation
- Presbyopia: decreased accommodation with aging (not a true refractive problem)
    - Correct with a positive lens for reading
- Astigmatism: non-spherical cornea or lens; light rays not refracted uniformly
    - Correct with a cylindrical lens

FOCUSED HISTORY

Reasons for visit or referral are usually for loss or disturbance of vision, pain/irritation or redness

Pain

Associated with:

- Blinking (e.g. corneal abrasions, foreign bodies, keratitis)
- Eye movement (e.g. optic neuritis)
- Headache and nausea (e.g. acute angle-closure glaucoma)
- Brow or temporal pain (e.g. may indicate temporal arteritis)
- Photophobia (e.g. iritis, corneal irritation)
- Irritation or "gritty sensation" (e.g. conjunctivitis, corneal abrasion)

Table 1. Location of Pain and Possible Interpretation

	Acute Conjunctivitis	Acute Iritis	Angle Closure Glaucoma	Corneal Abrasion
History	Sudden onset conjunctivitis	Fairly sudden onset, often recurrent	Rapid onset, possible previous attack	Trauma, pain

Table 1. Location of Pain and Possible Interpretation (continued)

	Acute Conjunctivitis	Acute Iritis	Angle Closure Glaucoma	Corneal Abrasion
Vision	Normal: discharge may mildly obscure	Impaired if untreated	Impaired and permanently lost if untreated	Can be affected if central
Pain	Gritty feeling	Photophobia	Severe	Sharp
Bilateral	Frequent	Occasional	Rarely	Not usually
Vomiting	Absent	Absent	Common	Absent
Cornea	Clear	Variable	Cloudy/edematous	Irregular light reflex
Pupil	Normal, reactive	Sluggishly reactive, may be irregular shape, usually miotic	Partially dilated, nonreactive, oval	Normal, reactive
Iris	Normal (NL)	NL or Various changes possible	Hard to see due to corneal edema	Defect shadow often detected on iris
Ocular Discharge	Mucopurulent or watery	Watery	Watery	Watery or Mucopurulent
Prognosis	Self-limited	Poor (untreated)	Poor (untreated)	Good

Red Eye

Some questions to ask:

- Injury to the eye?
- Associated eye pain or discharge?
- Contact with anyone with a red eye?

Diplopia (Double Vision)

- Due to misalignment of the eyes (compensatory head postures may be used)
- Occurs in ocular motor palsies (cranial nerves III, IV, VI), thyroid abnormalities, trauma ("blow out fracture"), myasthenia gravis, brain stem lesions, MS, myasthenia gravis, circle of willis aneurysms, diabetes (pupil-sparing), and neoplasm
- Occurs in one or multiple fields of gaze when cranial nerves are affected
- Third nerve palsy can be caused by cavernous sinus thrombosis (e.g. AIDS or other infectious, inflammatory and post-traumatic causes): ask about risk factors
- Myasthenia gravis: diplopia occurs later in the day as muscles begin to tire

Loss of Vision

- Monocular or binocular
- Transient (amaurosis fugax): "like a curtain closing over the eye"
  - e.g. retinal vascular occlusion (emboli), artery spasm, acute papilloedema

- Acute:
  - *Painless:* retinal detachment, retinal vascular occlusion, vitreous hemorrhage, optic neuropathy, cortical blindness (e.g. stroke)
  - *Painful:* acute angle-closure glaucoma, optic neuritis, acute iritis
- Gradual:
  - Cataract
  - Open-angle glaucoma
  - Macular degeneration (primary, usually age related)
  - Refractive error (i.e. myopia/hyperopia/presbyopia)
  - Intracranial or intraorbital tumour
  - Diabetic retinopathy
  - Macular edema from uveitis or retinal venous occlusive disease
  - Changes secondary to medications (e.g. cataracts, macular degeneration)

Table 2. Other Common Visual Eye Symptoms and Disease States

Visual Symptom	Possible Causes
Coloured haloes around light	Acute angle closure glaucoma, opacities in lens or cornea
Colour vision changes	Cataracts (rarely noticed by patient), drugs (e.g. digitalis increases yellow vision, viagra can cause a blue hue)
Difficulty seeing in dim light	Myopia, vitamin A deficiency, retinal degeneration, cataract, diabetic retinopathy
Distortion of vision	Wet age-related macular degeneration, macular pucker, central serous retinopathy
Flashes (photopsias) and floaters	Migraine, retinal tear/detachment, posterior vitreous detachment, retinal tear, vitritis, vitreous hemorrhage
Glare, photophobia	Iritis, cataracts
Loss of visual field or presence of shadow or curtain	Retinal detachment or hemorrhage, branch retinal vein or arterial occlusion, AION, chronic glaucoma, stroke

Table 3. Common non-painful ocular symptoms with potential causes

Non-Visual / Non-Painful Symptom	Possible Causes
Discharge	Watery: allergy/viral infection Mucoid (yellow): allergy/viral infection Purulent (creamy white/yellow): bacterial infection
Dryness	Decreased secretion due to aging, corneal abrasion, damage to lacrimal apparatus, dry-eye syndrome, Grave's disease, Bell's palsy, Sjögren's syndrome, anti-cholinergic drugs
Eyelid swelling	Chalazion, stye, conjunctivitis, cellulitis, dermatitis, systemic edema, dacryocystitis, endophthalmitis
Protrusion of eyes	Graves proptosis, aging changes in the lid, retrobulbar tumour
Itching	Dry eyes, eye fatigue, allergies
Sandiness, grittiness	Conjunctivitis
Tearing	Hypersecretion of tears, blockage of drainage, cholinergic drugs, ocular inflammation, abnormal lid positions, corneal abrasion/keratitis, normal emotion

OPHTHALMOLOGICAL

Past Ocular History
- Use of eyeglasses and/or contact lenses: duration, frequency, cleaning practice
- Previous eye surgery, laser treatment, infections, trauma, foreign body presence (e.g. metal workers)
- Presence of chronic eye disease such as amblyopia, glaucoma, cataracts, macular degeneration, diabetic retinopathy

Past Medical History
- *Systemic diseases:* many have ocular sequelae (e.g. diabetes, hypertension, thyroid, autoimmune, systemic infections like HIV, MS, connective tissue disorders)
  - Lung disease and kidney stones are possible contraindications for the prescription of beta-blockers and carbonic anhydrase inhibitors, respectively
- Allergies: rhinoconjunctivitis (hay fever)

Family History
- Corneal disease, glaucoma, cataracts, retinal disease, strabismus, amblyopia
- Family history giving risk for systemic diseases that can affect eyes (see **Past Medical History,** above)

Medications
- Ocular meds, current and prior use
- Common topical ocular medications include the following:
  - NSAIDs
  - Miotics (pupillary constriction)
  - Mydriatics/cycloplegics (pupillary dilation)
  - Steroidal anti-inflammatories
  - Adrenergic agonists
  - Carbonic anhydrase inhibitor (used for glaucoma)
  - Anti-infectives
  - Prostaglandin analogues
  - Anti-infectives, steroidal anti-inflammatories, artificial tears, prostaglandin analogs
  - Beta-blockers
- Many systemic medications have ocular side effects (e.g. corticosteroids can cause glaucoma, cataracts, and central serous retinopathy)

SUMMARY OF FOCUSED HISTORY
Reason for visit usually visual changes, pain/irritation or red eye
1. Loss of vision:
   - Binocular vs. Monocular
   - Acute vs. Gradual
   - Painless vs. Painful
2. Ask about common symptomatology
3. Past ocular history
4. Past medical history and family history are important as many systemic diseases affect the eye
5. Review all medications as many systemic medications can affect the eye

FOCUSED PHYSICAL EXAM
Visual Acuity (VA)
- Tests the integrity of the macula, optic nerve, optic tract and visual cortex
- Test distance and near vision for best corrected visual acuity (BCVA, i.e. with glasses/contacts); one eye at a time (right eye first) with the other eye occluded
- A pinhole occluder improves vision in an eye with uncorrected refractive error but NOT neural lesion or media opacity (e.g. cataract)
- Legal blindness = 20/200 BCVA in better eye or <20° of binocular visual field
- Driving in Ontario requires 20/50 BCVA with both eyes open, and a continuous visual field of 120° horizontally plus 15° both above and below fixation. Regulations vary by province/state

Distance Visual Acuity Testing
- Snellen chart – test at 20 ft (6 m)
- Recorded as a ratio: the numerator is the testing distance for the patient; the denominator is the distance at which a normal eye can read the line of letters
  - e.g. 20/100 = the patient can read at 20 feet what a "normal" eye can read at 100 feet
- If the patient cannot see the largest letters, do the following in this sequence:
  - Bring chart closer and record a new numerator as the new distance (e.g. 5/70)
  - *Count Fingers (CF):* if unable to see the largest letter at 3 ft, ask the patient to count your fingers and record best distance (e.g. CF 1ft)
  - *Hand Motion (HM):* wave your hand at a moderate speed and record best distance (e.g. HM 2 ft)
  - *Light Perception (LP):* with a penlight, record as LP, LP with projection (can locate the light) or NLP (No Light Perception)

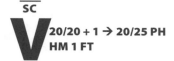

$$\overline{SC}$$

V **20/20 + 1 → 20/25 PH**
HM 1 FT

VA of R eye is recorded first.
CC = corrected acuity (i.e. with glasses); **SC** = uncorrected acuity
- **20/70+1** = All of 20/70 plus one letter of 20/50
- **20/25 PH** = improved VA with pinhole occluder
- **CF 3 ft** = counting fingers at 3 feet; **HM 1 ft** = hand motion at 1 feet; **LP (with projection)** = light perception (with projection); **NLP** = no light projection

---

Near Visual Acuity Testing
- Test if near vision complaint or if distance testing is difficult (e.g. no vision chart available)
- Use pocket vision chart (e.g. Rosenbaum Pocket Vision Screener)
- Test at 14 inches (30 cm) and record as Jaeger values (e.g. J2 at 14 inches), which can be converted to distance equivalent (e.g. 20/30)

Testing of Patients Who Cannot Read
- For children, illiterate patients, non-English speakers and dysphasics
- Use tumbling "E" chart or Landolt "C" chart with the patient describing/motioning the direction of the "E" or "C"
- Picture chart and the Sheridan-Gardiner matching test are often used for children between 2-4 years and adults with expressive aphasia

Colour Vision
- Ishihara Pseudoisochromatic Plates
- Assess macula/optic nerve function; often in pediatrics to screen for colorblindness.

Confrontational Visual Field Testing
- Approximates large field defects in the four quadrants of each eye
- Testing the patient's right eye:
    - Sit ~3 feet directly in front of the patient and close your right eye
    - Tell patient to cover left eye and focus right eye on your open left eye
    - Slowly bring in your left hand from the periphery from different directions, asking the patient to say "yes" when the moving hand becomes visible. Alternatively, flash one to three fingers in each quadrant and ask the patient to state the number of fingers they see
- Repeat for the patient's left eye by covering the patient's right eye
- Note any areas of field loss and record as below:

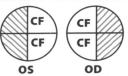

- Monocular visual field: 100° temporally, 60° nasally, 60° superiorly, and 75° inferiorly
- Blind spot: 15° temporal to fixation, below the horizontal meridian
- Amsler grid: tests central or paracentral scotomas
- Formal perimetry: Goldmann, Humphrey

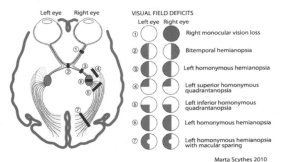

Marta Scythes 2010

Figure 2. Brain Lesions and the Resulting Visual Field Defects

Pupil Examination (see *The Neurological Exam* p. 184)
- Ask patient to fixate on distant target in dimmed room
- Shine a penlight obliquely to both pupils; assess pupil size, shape, and symmetry (measure using the pupil gauge found on the near vision card)

Pupillary Light Reflex
- Shine penlight directly into the right eye and observe symmetric pupillary constriction in the right eye (direct response) and the left eye (consensual response)
- 3+ to 4+ = pupil constricts rapidly and completely; 1+ to 2+ = slowly and incompletely; 0 = does not constrict

Table 4. Differential Diagnosis of Constricted, Dilated, and Asymmetrical Pupils

Constricted Pupil	Dilated Pupil
Horner's syndrome	CN III Palsy
Iritis	Acute Glaucoma
Drug-induced†	Drug-Induced‡ Adie's Pupil (mostly considered normal variant) Post-trauma

†Parasympathetic activation and/or sympathetic block
‡Sympathetic activation and/or parasympathetic block

Swinging Light Test (see *The Neurological Exam* p. 184)
- Swing light from one pupil to the other to assess relative afferent pupillary defect (RAPD)/Marcus Gunn pupil
- Pupil dilation in either eye as the light is shone on it indicate a RAPD, a sign of an optic nerve or retinal lesion

Accommodation Reflex
- Ask patient to look into the distance and then at an object (e.g. your finger) positioned 10 cm from the patient's nose
- Observe normal pupil constriction and eye convergence

OPHTHALMOLOGICAL

External Ocular Examination

- Inspect the orbits looking for exophthalmos (protruding eye) and enophthalmos (sunken eye)
- Inspect the four **L**'s:
  - **L**ymph nodes: preauricular, submandibular nodes
  - **L**ids:
    - ◆ Ptosis, swelling (allergy), crusting, xanthelasma (lipid deposits), smooth opening and closure, entropion/ectropion (inversion/eversion)
    - ◆ Chalazion: chronic inflammation of meibomian gland; localized painless swelling
    - ◆ Hordeolum/stye: acute inflammation of meibomian gland
    - ◆ Blepharitis: chronic inflammation of lid
  - **L**ashes:
    - ◆ Direction and condition
    - ◆ Trichiasis: corneal irritation due to inward turned lashes
  - **L**acrimal apparatus:
    - ◆ Tearing, obstruction, discharge, swelling
    - ◆ Dacryocystitis: infection of lacrimal sac
    - ◆ Keratoconjunctivitis sicca: dry eye syndrome
    - ◆ Epiphora: excessive tearing

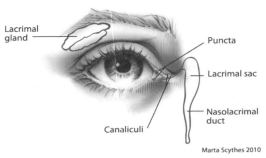

Marta Scythes 2010

Figure 3. Lacrimal Apparatus

Upper Lid Eversion

- To look for foreign bodies or other conjunctival lesions
- May require topical anesthetic
- As patient looks down, grasp eyelashes and upper lid between thumb and index finger; with other hand, place cotton tip applicator gently on the skin at the lid fold (8 mm above lid margin), and press down as the lid margin is pulled up by the lashes

Extraocular Muscle Evaluation (see *Neurological Exam* p. 184)
Motility

- Smooth pursuit: instruct patient to follow an object (e.g. tip of pen) in six cardinal positions of gaze; look for nystagmus (horizontal, vertical, or rotator) and ask patient to report diplopia (double vision) in any position of gaze
- Saccadic movement: instruct patient to rapidly shift their gaze from your index finger (positioned in the periphery) to your nose

- Strabismus – any type of ocular misalignment. Use the following tests:
  - *Hirschberg corneal reflex test:* ask patient to fixate on a distant object. Shine penlight into both eyes from ~14 inches (30 cm) away. Aligned eyes show symmetric light reflection near the center of both corneas. Misaligned eyes show displacement of corneal reflection in one eye
  - *Cover test:* Ask patient to fixate on a distant object. Cover the patient's right eye with a hand or an occluder, and observe for positional shift in the left eye. Rapidly change the cover to the patient's left eye, and observe for shift in the right eye. Positional shift in the non-covered eye indicates presence of a tropia (a manifest or apparent deviation)
  - *Cover-uncover test:* Ask patient to fixate on a distant object. Cover the patient's right eye and then uncover it. Repeat for the left eye. Positional shift in the testing eye upon uncovering indicates presence of a phoria (a latent deviation not apparent when both eyes are fixating)

Table 5. Possible Outcomes of Eye Alignment Tests

	Eye Movement*			
	Outward	**Inward**	**Up**	**Down**
Tropia	Esotropic	Exotropic	Hypotropic	Hypertropic
Phoria	Esophoric	Exophoric	Hypophoric	Hyperphoric

*Refers to eye movement in uncovered eye (tropia) and eye that was covered (phoria); eso/exo/hypo/hyper – describe movement of eye during the application of cover in each test

Pupillary Dilation (Mydriasis)

- Mydriatics provide significantly better viewing of the lens, vitreous, and retina
- Contraindications: narrow anterior chamber, acute angle-closure glaucoma
- Usually with tropicamide 1% and phenylephrine hydrochloride 2.5%
- Wait 15-20 minutes after instilling mydriatic to allow dilation to occur
- To instill eyedrop:
  - Seat patient, tilt head back, patient looks up, pull down on lower eyelid
  - Instill drop into sac made by lower eyelid and globe
  - Instruct patient to close eyes for a few seconds, provide a clean tissue

---

Common Causes of Motility/Alignment Defects
Congenital and late-onset strabismus, cranial nerve palsies, Grave's disease, myasthenia gravis, stroke, brain tumour and orbital trauma.

Slit Lamp Examination

- Provides binocular, stereotypic, and magnified views of all structures of the anterior segment of each eye, including eyelid, sclera, conjunctiva, cornea, iris, anterior chamber and lens
- Stereoscopic view of the fundus and vitreous can be obtained with special lenses (78 or 90 diopter)
- Using a cobalt blue filter, corneal abrasions can be visualized upon staining with fluorescein dye
- Best performed with pupils dilated

OPHTHALMOLOGICAL

Anterior Segment

- Examine the following structures of the anterior segment:
  - Lids and lashes (with lids everted if necessary)
  - Conjunctiva
    - Blood vessel dilatation, pigment, pallor, hemorrhage, redness (note pattern), swelling, nodules
    - Pinguecula – benign deposits of white-yellow hyaline/elastic tissue near the nasal or temporal limbus with aging
    - Pterygium – growth of fibrovascular tissue of the conjunctiva onto cornea
  - Sclera
    - Nodules, redness, discolouration (jaundice)
    - Episcleritis: self-limiting inflammation of the episclera, asymptomatic or with mild pain
    - Scleritis: bilateral, severely painful red eye with photophobia and decreased vision
  - Cornea
    - Abrasion, foreign body, smoothness, clarity/opacity, scarring, ulceration
    - Keratitis: inflammation of cornea with pain, redness, and tearing with blinking
    - Corneal edema: cornea with irregular reflection and haze
    - *Arcus senilis:* white ring of lipid deposits in peripheral cornea related to atherosclerosis
    - Kayser-Fleischer ring: Wilson's disease
    - AFTER examining corneal clarity, use fluorescein dye and cobalt blue filter to visualize corneal abrasions, ulcers and foreign bodies; Rose Bengal dye for dying corneal epithelium.
  - Anterior chamber
    - Examine for blood (hyphema), pus (hypopyon), cells (graded 1+ to 4+)
    - Depth measurement:
      - Slit lamp: direct narrow beam onto peripheral cornea at an oblique angle of 60°; chamber is shallow if distance between corneal endothelium and iris surface ≤¼ of corneal thickness
      - Penlight: shine light at an oblique angle from the temporal side of the head; chamber is shallow if ≥²/₃ of nasal iris is covered by the shadow

---

Clinical Pearl
To differentiate corneal ulcers from abrasions, view the cornea before staining with fluorescein. Ulcers have an opaque base, whereas abrasions have a clear base.

  - Iris
    - Cysts, nodules, colour differences between eyes (congenital Horner's), neovascularization, synechiae (adhesions to cornea or lens)
    - Iritis: unilateral, usually accompanied by concurrent inflammation of ciliary body, iridocyclitis
  - Lens: opacities (cataracts), dislocation, intraocular lens implant

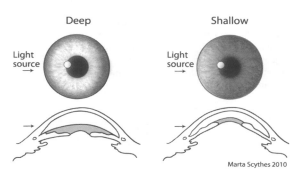

Figure 5. Anterior Chamber Depth Assessment

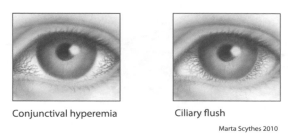

Conjunctival hyperemia   Ciliary flush

Marta Scythes 2010

Figure 6. Ciliary Flush vs. Conjunctival Hyperemia

Intraocular Pressure (IOP) Measurement
- Normal = 10-21 mmHg, mean = 15 mmHg
- Elevated IOP indicates glaucoma
- Measured by:
  - Applanation: Goldmann applanation tonometry (GAT) using slit lamp, gold standard
  - Indentation: Tono-pen or Schiotz; topical anaesthetic with patient supine
  - Non-contact applanation: air-puff tonometry

Direct Ophthalmoscopy/Fundoscopy
- Filters: red-free (visualize blood vessels and haemorrhages); polarizing (reduce corneal reflection); cobalt blue (corneal abrasions upon fluorescein stain)
- Red numbers = minus lenses for myopic eye; green numbers = plus lenses for hyperopic eye
- Technique:
  - Hold the ophthalmoscope in your R hand and use your R eye to examine the patient's R eye
  - Use large aperture for dilated pupil, small aperture for undilated pupil. Use low light intensity!
  - Set the focusing wheel at +5 and begin to look at the R eye at 1 foot away to detect the red reflex
  - Slowly come closer to the patient at 15° temporally until <2 inches from the eye (as close as possible!). Turn the focusing wheel in the negative direction until patient's retina comes into focus

- Follow a retinal vessel until it widens into the optic disc (nasal to the macula). Examine the following landmarks in order:
  - Optic disc: size, shape, colour, margin (normal sharp), symmetry, haemorrhages, elevation, cup-to-disc ratio (normal <0.5)
  - Retinal vessels: arteries are lighter, thinner and have a brighter reflex than veins. Follow arteries from the disc and veins back to the disc in each quadrant, noting arteriovenous (A/V) crossing patterns
  - Retinal background: colour (normal red-orange), pigmentation, lesions (diffuse flecks, flame-shaped, cotton wool spots)
  - Macula: ask patient to look directly into the light; usually appears darker than surrounding retina and produces the foveolar reflex
- Repeat for the left eye

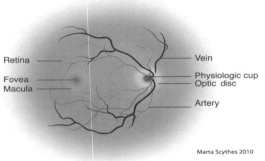

Retina

Fovea
Macula

Vein

Physiologic cup
Optic disc

Artery

Marta Scythes 2010

Figure 7. Retina

Red Reflex
- Shine ophthalmoscope light into the pupils from ~1 foot away and look through the viewer
- Observe for evenness of colour, presence of shadows/opacities
- An eye with clear ocular media (cornea, anterior chamber, lens, and vitreous) gives off bilateral even red reflexes

---

Common Causes of Abnormal Red Reflex (Absent or Dull)
Corneal scar, hyphema (blood in aqueous humour), cataract, vitreous hemorrhage, endophthalmitis, large refractive error, ocular misalignment.

Table 6. Findings on Ophthalmoscopy

Retinal Disease	Findings on Ophthalmology
Diabetic retinopathy	
▪ Non-proliferative	▪ Hemorrhages, microaneurysms, cotton wool spots, exudates
▪ Proliferative	▪ Neovascularization, vitreous hemorrhage
Central retinal artery occlusion (CRAO)	Whitened retina, cherry red spot in macula
Central retinal vein occlusion (CRVO)	Dilated, tortuous veins, flame-shaped hemorrhages, cotton wool spots, optic disc hyperemia/edema
Hypertensive retinopathy	Arteriolar narrowing, and straightening with areas of silver-wire appearance, changes in arteriovenous crossings, cotton wool spots, micro-aneurysms, flame-shaped hemorrhages, disc edema
Papilloedema	Optic disc edema, blurred elevated disc margins, ± flame-shaped hemorrhages
Glaucomatous optic neuropathy	Increased cup to disc ratio, asymmetric cup size between eyes, cup approaching disc margin, optic nerve pallor, vessel displacement in disc
Retinal detachment	Elevated retinal folds
Age-related macular degeneration	Drusen (yellow nodules), retinal pigment epithelium atrophy (depigmentation in macula), subretinal fluid, subretinal lipid (hard exudates, or subretinal hemorrhage

Application of an Eye Patch
- Can be used for corneal abrasions
- Contraindicated if suspicion of infection or corneal ulceration present
- With eye closed, apply two patches on the eye, tape patches to eye with moderate pressure using 3 strips of tape
- Instill antibiotic drops if necessary

SUMMARY OF FOCUSED PHYSICAL EXAM
1. Visual acuity (distance/near with correction)
2. Visual Fields (by confrontation)
3. Pupillary examination (with hand held light)
4. External exam (4L's, with upper lid eversion if indicated)
5. Extraocular muscle evaluation (motility, alignment)
6. Slit lamp (front to back – sclera/conjunctiva to back of lens)
7. IOP measurement (12-21 normal range)
8. Fundoscopy (direct covered here, indirect more advanced)

COMMON CLINICAL SCENARIOS

Retinal Detachment (RD)
- Neurosensory retina separates from the underlying retinal pigment epithelium
- Classification:
  - *Rhegmatogenous* – most common type; happens in the setting of detachment of the vitreous humor from the retina (posterior vitreous detachment), which is a normal phenomenon in older adults
  - *Tractional* – occurs via mechanical forces on the retina; usually mediated by fibrotic tissue resulting from previous hemorrhage, injury, surgery, infection, inflammation or diabetic retinopathy

OPHTHALMOLOGICAL

- *Exudative (or serous)* – results from accumulation of serous and/or hemorrhagic fluid in subretinal space due to hydrostatic factors (e.g. severe acute hypertension), inflammation, or neoplastic effusions
- Signs and symptoms:
  - Retinal tears may occur without symptoms, but often photopsia (light flashes in vision) and/or floaters are noted; if untreated, retinal tears can progress to retinal detachments
  - Acute floaters and acute vision loss; altered red reflex
  - Visual field loss usually in the periphery that progresses toward the central visual axis over hours to weeks
- Risk factors – aging, cataract surgery, myopia, family history, history of RD in the other eye, trauma, congenital, and diabetic retinopathy
- Treatment:
  - Retinal detachment is a true ophthalmic emergency
  - Prevention is best achieved by treating retinal breaks by laser or cryopexy burns before they progress to retinal detachments
  - Surgical correction usually required for repair
    - *Pneumatic Retinopexy* – injection of a gas bubble into the vitreous cavity done if there are few and localized retinal breaks within the superior 8 clock hours of retina
    - *Scleral Buckling* – affix a silicon band on outside surface of sclera
    - *Vitrectomy* (more difficult cases) – vitreous gel is removed and replaced with a large gas bubble

Glaucoma
- Progressive optic neuropathy often associated with elevated intraocular pressure (IOP)
- Categorized into open- and closed-angle forms; as well as primary and secondary forms
- Final common pathway of many disorders that affect the eye

Table 7. Characteristics of Major Types of Glaucoma

	Congenital Glaucoma	Primary Open Angle Glaucoma (POAG)	Normal-Tension Glaucoma (NTG)	Acute Angle-Closure Glaucoma
Definition/ Etiology	*Primary infantile:* abnormal development of anterior chamber *Secondary infantile:* linked with various ocular and systemic syndromes and surgical aphakia (removal of lens)	Progressive loss of optic nerve without occlusion of outflow tract	A variety of POAG with normal IOP	Iris apposition or adhesion to the trabecular meshwork causing a decrease in outflow and an increase in IOP and optic nerve damage
Epidemiology	Arises in children <2 years old; seen in 1:10000 to 1:15000 live births in U.S.	2% of general population; 55% of all glaucoma cases; leading cause of irreversible world blindness	A significant proportion of POAG cases	0.1% of general population; older individuals, especially those with hyperopia

Table 7. Characteristics of Major Types of Glaucoma (continued)

	Congenital Glaucoma	Primary Open Angle Glaucoma (POAG)	Normal-Tension Glaucoma (NTG)	Acute Angle-Closure Glaucoma
Symptoms	Photophobia	May be asymptomatic until patient presents with tunnel vision	May be associated with migraine	Sudden onset of blurred vision and eye pain, nausea and excessive sweating during attacks, prodrome of rainbow coloured halos around lights
Signs	Corneal edema/clouding, epiphoria and/or red eye, corneal enlargement	Elevated IOP >21, optic nerve cupping, visual field loss especially in the periphery	IOP within normal range, optic nerve cupping ± hemorrhage, peripheral vasospasm, visual field changes	Corneal edema resulting in blurring of red reflex, conjuctival injection, mid-dilated, non-reactive vertically oval pupil, IOP elevated often to shallow anterior chamber, flare and cells in anterior chamber
Risk Factors	Lensectomy, small cornea	IOP >25 mmHg, enlarged optic nerve cup (>0.5 cup-to-disc ratio), age >40, black race, family hx, myopia, vascular diseases	Similar to POAG	Family history, age >40, female, family hx of angle-closure symptoms, hyperopia, pseudoexfoliation race (Inuit>Asian>Caucasian =African)
Management	Surgical (not medical)	Directed at lowering IOP: medications, laser trabeculoplasty/trabeculectomy	Directed at lowering IOP: correction of circulatory deficiencies at optic nerve head (theoretical)	Directed at lowering IOP: laser iridotomy or trabeculectomy

Cataracts

- Clouding and opacification of the crystalline lens of the eye
- Opacity may occur in the cortex, nucleus of the lens, or posterior subcapsular region, but it is usually in a combination of areas
- Epidemiology – highest cause of treatable blindness; peak incidence is after 40 years of age (senile cataract) and in early life (heredity cataract)
- Etiology – Most are age-related but may be related to heredity, trauma, toxins, corticosteroid use (cause posterior subcapsular cataract), radiation, inflammation, diabetes mellitus, and many other systemic/congenital illnesses
- Signs and symptoms – blurred vision, decreased acuity and glare around lights at night; cloudiness and opacification of lens and altered red reflex on physical exam
- Treatment – surgery to remove the lens and replace with intraocular lens implant

OPHTHALMOLOGICAL

Age-Related Macular Degeneration (AMD or ARMD)

- A common, chronic degenerative disorder that affects older individuals; severe central visual loss as a result of geographical atrophy, serous detachment of the retinal pigment epithelium (Bruch's membrane) and choroidal neovascularization (CNV)
- Drusen (small yellowish, protein lipid deposits in the retina) are generally accepted to be precursor lesions when they are soft or indistinct
- Epidemiology – average age at onset of visual loss is about 75 years
- Risk factors – female, family history, smoking, age, sunlight exposure, obesity, elevated cholesterol level, hypertension
- Classification:
  - *Non-neovascular (dry)* – 90% of cases; geographical atrophy (depigmentation or hypopigmentation of RPE mainly involving the fovea) seen in dry AMD causes approximately 21% of all cases of legal blindness in NA
  - *Neovascular (wet)* – hallmark is ingrowth of CNV from choriocapillaries under the macular region; less prevalent but responsible for nearly 80% of significant visual disability associated with AMD; more rapid progression of visual loss compared to non-neovascular AMD
- Signs and symptoms:
  - Subacute onset except in some cases of neovascular AMD, where abrupt visual loss is noted
  - Blurred vision (metamorphopsia) usually bilateral but often asymmetric, may be asymptomatic
  - Decreased reading ability especially in dim light
  - Clinical exam findings may include drusen, subretinal fluid, macular edema, hemorrhage, retinal or subretinal lipid exudates, plaque-like membrane or grey or yellow-green discrete discoloration and, RPE detachment or tear
- Treatment:
  - *Dry AMD* – vitamin A, C, E and mineral supplementation (zinc and copper) in patients with stage 3 or 4 dry AMD decreases risk of progression to wet form
  - *Wet AMD with CNV* – laser photocoagulation for extrafoveal membranes; intravitreal injections of anti-VEGF for subfoveal membranes; CNIB and low vision aids

Eye Complications in Diabetes Mellitus

- Diabetic retinopathy
  - Progressive dysfunction of the retinal vasculature caused by chronic hyperglycemia
  - Microaneurysms, retinal hemorrhages, retinal lipid exudates, cotton-wool spots, capillary non-perfusion, macular edema and, neovascularization
  - Successful management via a combination of glucose control, laser therapy, and vitrectomy reduces the risk of severe visual loss to 10%
  - Best predictor for the disease is duration of DM (71–90% with DM type I for 10 years have diabetic retinopathy; incidence is slightly lower for type II)
- Cataracts
- Cornea
- Glaucoma
- Optic Neuropathy

REFERENCES

Age-Related Eye Disease Study Research Group. 2001. A randomized, placebo-controlled, clinical trial of high-dose supplementation with vitamins C and E, beta carotene, and zinc for age-related macular degeneration and vision loss: AREDS report no. 8. *Arch Ophthalmol* 119(10):1417-1436.

Bradford CA. 2004. *Basic Ophthalmology.* San Francisco, CA: American Academy of Ophthalmology.

OPHTHALMOLOGICAL

The Pediatric Exam

Editors:
Emily Baker, Amy Shafey &
Eric Tseng

Faculty Reviewers:
Sanjay Mehta, MD, FRCP(C)
Laura McAdam, MD, FRCS(C)

TABLE OF CONTENTS

APPROACH TO THE NEONATE, INFANT AND CHILD
Approach to the Pediatric History and Physical Exam   247
Common Disorders and Chief Complaints   248
General Pediatric History   249
Focused Physical Exam   253
Immediate Postnatal Assessment   253
The Screening Exam   254
General Survey and Vitals   254
Head and Neck   257
Respiratory   262
Cardiovascular   263
Gastrointestinal   267
Genitourinary and Reproductive System   268
Musculoskeletal   269
Neurological   271

APPROACH TO THE ADOLESCENT
Approach to the Adolescent History and Physical Exam   274
Common Chief Complaints   275
Focused History   275
Focused Physical   277

Common Investigations   283
Common Clinical Scenarios and Disorders   283
Genetic Disorders   292
Psychiatric and Behavioural Issues   292
Child Abuse   294
Growth and Development   297

APPROACH TO THE NEONATE, INFANT AND CHILD

APPROACH TO THE PEDIATRIC HISTORY AND PHYSICAL EXAM

History
- Often given by third party: identify relationship with child

Physical Exam
- A full physical exam should be done for every pediatric exam, except in emergency or walk-in situations where a more focused exam may be more appropriate
- Knowledge of adult exam is assumed for pediatric exam
  - *General:* state of well-being, presence or absence of signs of distress, e.g. colour, vitals, alertness, affect, speech, crying, physical and cognitive development

- *H&N:* shape and symmetry, fontanelles and sutures, auscultate temples and vertex
- *Ears:* hearing, otoscopic exam
- *Eyes:* visual acuity, fundoscopy, cover uncover test
- *Mouth:* mucous membranes, number of teeth, uvula, tonsils, tongue, frenulum
- *Neck:* glands, nodes, thyroid, stiffness
- *Resp:* respiratory distress, dyspnea, respiratory noises
- *CVS:* postural distress, cyanosis, femoral and radial pulse, auscultation over 4 valves, axilla, supraclavicular areas and back
- *GI:* umbilical and inguinal hernia; omit rectal exam unless disease suspected
- *GU:*
  - Male: circumcised or not, urethral orifice, testicular development/descent
  - Female: mons pubis, labia major and minor, hymen, vagina/cervix if indicated
- *MSK:* ROM, Barlow's test, Ortolani test, scoliosis, Trendelenberg test
- *CNS:* developmental milestones, mental status, motor function, cranial nerves, reflexes
- *Derm:* rashes, hemangiomas, signs of abuse

COMMON DISORDERS AND CHIEF COMPLAINTS

Disorders marked with (✓) are discussed in **Common Clinical Scenarios**

Head and Neck:
- ✓ Pharyngitis
- ✓ Oral thrush
- Nasal discharge
- ✓ Earache

Respiratory
- Cough
- ✓ Asthma
- ✓ Respiratory Distress in the Newborn

Cardiovascular:
- Breathing difficulties
- Cyanosis
- ✓ Dehydration

Gastrointestinal:
- Constipation/diarrhea
- Difficulty swallowing
- ✓ Jaundice
- Vomiting
- Abdominal pain
- ✓ Rectal bleeding

Genitourinary:
- ✓ Urinary changes
- ✓ Incontinence

Musculoskeletal:
- ✓ Limping
- Pain in joints, muscle or bone

Neurological:
- ✓ Falls
- ✓ Headache
- ✓ Seizure

Dermatological:
- ✓ Chicken pox
- ✓ Allergies
- ✓ Rashes

Genetic:
- ✓ Down's syndrome
- ✓ Edward's syndrome
- ✓ Turner's syndrome
- ✓ Kleinfelter's syndrome

Psychiatric and Behavioural:
- ✓ Anxiety
- ✓ Inattention
- ✓ Autism
- ✓ Depression
- ✓ Sleep problems
- ✓ Child abuse

GENERAL PEDIATRIC HISTORY

- Observe parent-child interaction for non-verbal cues and family dynamics
- Allow parent to discuss their feelings and acknowledge their concerns
- Ask parents about specific concerns (for hidden or unexpressed fears/agendas)

Neonate:

- Inquire about the family's adaptation to the newborn
- Inquire about the mother's emotional state (baby blues) and supports for the mother
- Ask about future follow-up visits: baby's pediatrician or family doctor

Chief Complaint (CC)

- There may be more than one CC, e.g. cough, runny nose, and earache
- Note duration and temporal sequence of complaints
- Child's CC may not be the main issue and child may not in fact be the real patient

History of Present Illness

- Establish timeline: "When was child last well?" In infants, "When was the child last feeding or sleeping well?"
- Similar problems in relatives/daycare contacts?
- Aggravating/alleviating factors including medications and alternative remedies

Past Medical History

- Prenatal
  - Mom's obstetrical history: previous pregnancies, miscarriages, abortions
  - Pregnancy: planned or not, number of weeks, single or multiple pregnancy, complications
  - Mom's health during pregnancy: age, hospitalizations, medications, bleeding, illnesses, accidents, vitamins, supplements, herbals, hypertension, diabetes
  - Tests: U/S, Amniocentesis, CVS (when and why), GBS
  - Both parents: alcohol, smoking, drug exposure
- Labour and Delivery
  - Spontaneous labour or induced? If induced, why?
  - Premature or prolonged rupture of membranes?
  - Labor duration and problems (maternal fever, non-reassuring FHR, meconium)
  - Vaginal, forceps, vacuum or caesarian delivery
  - Birth weight, APGAR scores (see *Obstetric Exam* p. 222)

Table 1a. Major Developmental Milestones (2-12 months)

	2 months	4 months	6 months	9 months	12 months
Gross Motor	Prone: lifts chin	Head Control Prone: raises head and chest Rolls from front to back	Tripod sitting	Pull to stand Crawling (optional)	First steps
Fine Motor	Pulls at clothes	Holds objects in midline Reaches	Transfers across midline	Finger-thumb grasp	Pincer grasp

Table 1a. Major Developmental Milestones (2-12 months) (continued)

	2 months	4 months	6 months	9 months	12 months
Speech and Language	Coos	Responds to voice	Babbles Responds to name		First word
Adaptive and Social Skills	Follows moving person with eyes	Laughs	Raises arms for up Stranger anxiety	Pat-a-cake Waves bye-bye Peek-a-boo Separation anxiety	Drinks from a cup

Table 1b. Major Developmental Milestones (18 months-5 years)

	18 months	2 years	3 years	4 years	5 years
Gross Motor	Runs stiffly	Runs well Climbs stairs 1 at a time	Rides a tricycle	Hops on one foot	Skips Rides Bicycle
Fine Motor	Draws a line and scribbles Stacks 2 cubes	Stacks 6 cubes Runs Kicks ball	Pulls on shoes	Copies squares	Copies triangles
Speech and Language	20+ words Follows simple commands with cues	2 words together 50-100 words	3-4 word sentences Colours	Nursery rhymes Alphabet	Future tense in speech
Adaptive and Social Skills	Uses spoon Points to body parts	Temper tantrum Parallel play	Counts to 10 Dresses (except buttons) Toilet training	Cooperative play Buttons clothes	Knows 4 colours

- Postnatal Period
  - Jaundice, cyanosis, breathing or feeding problems, seizures, other difficulties
  - Did the baby require NICU (e.g. for ventilation) or antibiotics after birth?
  - Was the baby kept in hospital for any reason?
- Feeding History
  - Breast feeding or formula
    - *Breast-fed:* frequency, duration, associated problems (difficulty latching, sleeping on breast)
    - Vitamin D 400 IU/day if breastfed or premature?
  - Formula: type, dilution, any formula changes, feeding frequency and amount
  - Age of introduction to solids and current diet composition
  - Problems with feeding, colic, vomiting
  - Supplements: including vitamins, fluoride, and natural products
  - Regurgitation: amount, frequency, bilious/nonbilious
  - Outputs: Urine output (number of diapers/day), stools
- Growth development (see **Tables 1a** and **1b**)
- Immunizations
  - Which and when? see **Table 2**
  - Adverse reactions: local, systemic, or allergic

- Allergies
  - Environment, food, and medication: reaction experienced, action taken, time to resolution of symptoms, presence of a viral illness, exercise, heat, cold
  - Family history of atopy (hypersensitivity to environmental allergens)
- Previous illnesses, hospitalizations or surgeries

Table 2. Publicly Funded Immunization Schedules (Ontario, 2009)

Age at Vaccination	DTaP-IPV	Hib	PCV7	MMR	Men C-C	VZV	Hep B	HPV (Girls)	dTaP	Td	Flu
2 mo	X	X	X								
4 mo	X	X	X								
6 mo	X	X	X								
12 mo				X	X						
15 mo			X			X					
18 mo	X	X		X							
4-6 yrs	X										
12 yrs (Gr. 7)							X				
13 yrs (Gr. 8)								X			
14-16 yrs									X		
Adult years (q10y after)										X	
Every autumn (6 mo onward)											X

DTaP   Diphtheria, tetanus, pertussis (acellular) vaccine
IPV   Inactivated polio vaccine
Hib   Haemophilus influenzae type b conjugate vaccine
PCV7   Pneumococcal 7-valent conjugate
MMR   Measles, mumps, and rubella vaccine
MenC-C   Meningococcal C conjugate
VZV   Varicella zoster
HepB   Hepatitis B vaccine
HPV   Human Papillomavirus Vaccine (Gardasil)
dTap   Diptheria, tetanus and acellular pertussis adult adolescent formulation
Td   Tetanus and diphtheria adult type formulation
Flu   Influenza vaccine

Family History
- Genogram may be helpful
- Ask about consanguinity
- Family history of disease: early onset MI, headaches, enuresis (bedwetting)
- Broader family: congenital abnormalities, allergies, recurrent illnesses, early deaths

Social History
- Family:
  - Extended/reconstituted family, birth parents, custody and access
  - Household: space, pets, occupants, frequency of moves
  - Family dynamics: who cares for child?
  - Support systems, stress/discord/violence
  - Recreation history "What does the family do as a group?"
  - Major life events (deaths, accidents, separations, divorce)

- Parents:
  - Occupational history (prolonged absences, exposures to toxins or infection)
  - Approach to discipline
  - Financial issues/problems (including any social assistance)
  - Substance abuse
- Child:
  - Interests and activities

Review of Systems

- General: Health, growth, activity level, weight, fatigue, sleep, school performance
- H&N:
  - Otalgia (earache may be manifested by rubbing of or pulling at ears), otorrhea (discharge), ear infections, hearing loss: does child turn up TV loud?
  - Vision: does he/she need to be very close to books, TV or blackboard?
  - Infections: number, fevers, sore throat, swallowing difficulties, swollen glands

  Neonate:
  - Head: any swelling of the head post-delivery? Has it decreased?
  - Eyes: conjunctivitis, scleral icterus
  - Throat/mouth: cleft lip/palate? Neck masses?
- Resp:
  - Respiratory difficulties (croup, wheeze, cough, stridor)
  - Allergic salute: child rubs nose with palm frequently
  - Allergic shiners: dark coloration surrounds the eye in allergy
  - Rhinorrhea
- CVS:
  - *Infant:* fatigue or sweating during feeding, does the baby pull away to breathe while feeding?
  - Cyanosis
  - *Older infant and child:* pre-/syncope, murmurs, inability to keep up with peers
- GI:
  - Appetite, weight gain, height, growth
  - Bowel movements: frequency, consistency, blood, mucous, pain associated with meals, diarrhea or bowel movements
  - Vomiting: onset, progression, frequency, amount, bilious, bloody, relation to meals
  - Abdominal pain: site, duration, radiation, effect on activity level, vomiting
- GU:
  - Number of wet diapers, haematuria
  - Frequency, dysuria, enuresis, UTIs
- CNS:
  - Headache, seizure, weakness, tingling, numbness
- Derm:
  - Rash, pruritus (itchiness), pigmented lesions (e.g. birthmarks), sun damage
  - *Neonate:* jaundiced skin: distribution, worsening or improving

FOCUSED PHYSICAL EXAM

Tips for Examining Pediatric Patients

1. *Use parent as a helper to soothe child.* With younger children/infants, do most of exam with infant sitting/lying in the caregiver's lap. Ensure cranky infants are well-fed
2. *Begin by observation:* much of the neurologic exam can be done by observing the child play, move and respond to outside stimuli
3. *Introduce yourself and your tools:* let child see and safely touch tools you will be using during the exam. You can also use toys as distractions
4. *Be flexible:* perform distressing manoevers towards the end of the exam. Give the child as much choice as possible: e.g. Which body part to examine first?
5. Make a game out of the exam:
   - *Head and neck exam* – often best saved for the end, as many children dislike having their ears and throats examined. "Let me see how big your tongue is!"
   - *Cardiac exam* – if the child is afraid of the stethoscope ask Mom or Dad if it would be OK to listen to their chest first. Make a show of listening to the heart "ba-boom"
   - *Resp exam* – to get the child to take a deep breath in and out, hold up your finger and tell them to practice blowing out the candle
   - *Abdomen exam* – Have them put their hands on top of yours while you palpate the abdomen – this may make them less ticklish
   - *MSK/Neuro exam* – to test upper body strength, have the child "show you how strong they are". For lower body strength, use descriptors like "push on the gas". For the cranial nerve exam "Simon Says" is a favourite

IMMEDIATE POSTNATAL ASSESSMENT

- Airway, Breathing, Circulation (ABC's) and overall evaluation of the child's well-being
- Ensure warmth, good oxygenation, appropriate ventilation
- APGAR Score (see **Obstetric Exam** p. 222)

Table 3. Gestational Age and Birth Weight

Birth Weight Classification	Weight
Extremely low birth weight	<1000 grams
Very low birth weight	<1500 grams
Low birth weight	<2500 grams
Normal birth weight	≥2500 grams
Gestational Age Classification	**Gestational Age**
Preterm	<37 weeks
Term	37-42 weeks
Postterm	≥42 weeks

- Also classify birth weight on an intrauterine growth curve
  - Small for gestational age (SGA) is <10th percentile
  - Appropriate for gestational age (AGA) is 10-90th percentile
  - Large for gestational age (LGA) is >90th percentile
- Preterm AGA infants are more prone to respiratory distress syndrome, apnea, hypoglycemia, hypocalcemia, hypothermia, anemia, retinopathy of prematurity, patent ductus arteriosus, and infection
- Preterm SGA infants are at higher risk of asphyxia, hypoglycemia, hypothermia, hypocalcemia, polycythemia

THE SCREENING EXAM

- Should be done during the first day of life, optimally within 8 hours of birth
- "Head to toe" exam, preferably when baby is in a quiet but alert state
- Normal full-term baby lies in a symmetrical position, with limbs semi-flexed and legs partially abducted at the hip
- To optimize the exam, keep the baby quiet by placing the tip of your gloved finger in a crying baby's mouth to sooth the baby. This also assesses the suck reflex and palate. Appropriate physical exam skills are found in separate physical exam sections below

GENERAL SURVEY AND VITALS

- Most important aspect of the general survey is to assess whether the patient is exhibiting any signs of distress, colour change, or abnormal vital signs
- Observe the child's chest and neck for signs of accessory muscle usage and respiratory distress any more intrusive steps are taken
- Assuming the patient is stable, note alertness, activity, facial expressions

Recordings for height, weight and head circumference:

- *Height:* measure infant supine up to 2 years, then standing >2 years
- *Weight:* loss of up to 10% of birth weight in first few days of life is normal
- *Head circumference:* all infants <2 years and those with misshapen heads
- Measure the greatest circumference around the occipital, parietal, and frontal prominences above the brows and ears
    - Average circumference at term is ~35 cm
- Plot data on growth charts to determine percentiles; focus on trend of growth longitudinally rather than individual values
- *Pay attention to crossing of percentile ranges*
- *Failure to thrive: when a child's weight for age falls below the fifth percentile of the standard growth chart or if it crosses two major percentile curves*
- Find out parents' sizes and appearance at their child's age before judging apparent abnormalities (e.g. macrocephaly)

Calculating Mid-Parental Height (MPH)
This formula can be used to estimate child's future adult height (in cm):
  MPH for girl = (father's height + mother's height - 12.5) / 2
  MPH for boy = (father's height + mother's height + 12.5) / 2

Temperature:

The recommended technique depends on the child's age.
How to take a rectal temperature:

- Use disposable slip covers where available
- Lubricate the thermometer prior to insertion. Spread the buttocks and insert a rectal thermometer slowly through the anal sphincter to 0.5-1 inch; read after 1 minute

Taking a Temperature: Recommended Techniques

Age	Recommended technique
Birth to 2 years	1. Rectal (definitive) 2. Axillary (screening low risk children)
2 years to 5 years	1. Rectal (definitive) 2. Axillary, Tympanic (or Temporal Artery if in hospital) (screening)
Older than 5 years	1. Oral (definitive) 2. Axillary, Tympanic (or Temporal Artery if in hospital) (screening)

Clinical Pearl

Normal rectal temperature > oral temperature > axillary temperature

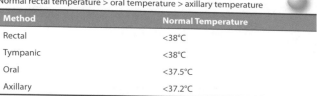

Method	Normal Temperature
Rectal	<38°C
Tympanic	<38°C
Oral	<37.5°C
Axillary	<37.2°C

Pulse:

- Palpate the radial, then femoral pulses
- A comparatively weak femoral pulse may indicate aortic coarctation
- For each 1°C rise, the pulse increases by ~10 beats/min
- Auscultate the heart; sinus arrhythmia is normal

Respiratory rate:

- Measure respiratory rate before more intrusive procedures are done
- Placing your hand just below the child's xiphoid process or listening to breath sounds through the stethoscope may help to get an accurate respiratory rate
- For each 1°C rise, the respiratory rate increases by ~3 breaths/min
- Abnormally fast or slow respiratory rates reflect a disturbance in the respiratory, cardiovascular or central nervous systems

Blood pressure:

- Systolic = 80 + 2 × age in years
- Diastolic ≈ 2/3 systolic
- Measurement is not indicated for those under 3 years, unless hospitalized or specific indication
  - For children <3 years of age: doppler ultrasound method
  - For children >3 years of age: auscultation method
- Use of proper sized cuff is essential
- Pressure should be taken in both arms and legs
- *Consistently high blood pressures may indicate hypertension; consistently low diastolic (relative to systolic) pressures may indicate a patent ductus arteriosus*
- *Large differences in mean arterial pressure between arms and legs may indicate aortic coarctation*

Table 4. Average Ranges for Pediatrics Vital Signs

Age	Resp Rate	Heart Rate	Systolic Blood Pressure	Weight (kg)
Infant	30-50	120-160	>60	3-4
6 mo – 1 yr	30-40	120-150	70-80	8-10
2 – 4 yrs	20-30	110-140	70-80	12-16
5-8 yrs	14-20	90-120	90-100	18-26
8-12 yrs	12-20	80-110	100-110	26-50
>12 yrs	12-16	60-100	100-120	>50

Adapted from Schafermeyer R. 1993. *Emerg Med Clin North Am* 11(1):187-205.

Clinical Evaluation of Dehydration/Volume Depletion

- Weight loss is the gold standard; however it is useful to examine capillary refill time, skin turgor, respiratory pattern, heart rate, urine output, blood pressure
- It is important to approximate the child's level of dehydration as mild, moderate or severe, as this affects the management strategy

Table 5. Signs of Dehydration/Volume Status

Sign/Symptom	Mild Dehydration (<3% body wt lost)	Moderate Dehydration (3-9% body wt lost)	Severe Dehydration (>9% body wt lost)
Mental status	Alert	Fatigued/irritable	Lethargic/obtunded
Thirst	Drinks well	Thirsty, eager to drink	Drinks poorly/unable to drink
Fontanelles/Eyes	Normal	Depressed	Sunken
Mucous Membranes	Moist	Dry	Parched
Heart Rate	Normal	Slightly tachycardic	Tachycardia → bradycardia
Blood Pressure	Normal	Normal/orthostatic change	Decreased
Respiratory Rate	Normal	Normal/tachypneic	Tachypneic
Capillary Refill	Normal	>2 s	>4 s
Skin Turgor	Warm, normal turgor	Cool, recoil <2 s	Cold, mottled, recoil >2 s
Peripheral Pulses	Normal	Normal to decreased	Weak, tready or impalpable
Urine Output	Normal to decreased	Decreased	Minimal

Adapted from "Gastroenteritis and Oral Rehydration". In Lalani A, Schneeweiss S (eds.) 2008. *Handbook of Pediatric Emergency Medicine*. Jones and Bartlett Publishers.

HEAD AND NECK

Head

Inspection
- Size, Shape (macrocephaly, microcephaly, dolicocephaly, brachiocephaly) and symmetry of head
  - Asymmetry of the cranial vault (plagiocephaly) may result from consistently placing the child supine; ask about child's sleeping or playing positions
- Sutures and fontanelles
  - An enlarged posterior fontanelle may be seen in congenital hypothyroidism
- Palpebral fissures
  - Angle from line drawn from inner and outer canthus (up slanting may indicate Down syndrome, down slanting may indicate Noonan's syndrome, short may indicate fetal alcohol syndrome)
- After vaginal vertex delivery/prolonged labour
  - Occipitally elongated head (for ~1 wk)
  - Overriding cranial bone sutures, harmless scalp swelling, caput succedaneum (subcutaneous edema in occipitoparietal region that resolves 1-2 days post-partum; does not respect suture lines) or cephalohematoma (subperiosteal hemorrhage that resolves in a few months; respects suture lines)
- After breech delivery or cesarean section
  - Head can be symmetrical and round

Palpation
- Sutures feel like ridges and usually flatten by 6 months
- Fontanelles feel like soft concavities: anterior fontanelle is 4-6 cm, and usually closes in 4-26 months, posterior fontanelle is 1-2 cm, and usually closes by 2 months
- Bulging, tense fontanelle suggests increased intracranial pressure and is seen when baby cries, vomits, or has underlying pathology (CNS infection, neoplasm, hydrocephalus, injury)

Auscultation
- Cranial bruit may be evident in older children with significant anemia or vascular abnormalites

Percussion
- Temples and vertex: large, harsh bruits suggest arteriovenous malformation (AVM)
- *Macewen's sign:* percuss the parietal bone on each side of the skull to produce a "cracked pot" sound (in normal infants before closure of cranial sutures)
- *Chvostek's sign:* percussion at top of cheek below zygomatic bone, in front of ear causing facial grimacing
  - Indication of hypocalcemia, tetanus, and tetany due to hyperventilation

Eye
- Small colourful toys are often useful as fixation devices for young children
- Young infants respond best to human faces, so place your face directly in front of theirs

Inspection

- Observe position of eyes, eyelids (ptosis), conjunctivae, sclerae, irises, pupils
- Examine the red retinal (fundus) reflex and optic disk (lighter in colour than adults, foveal light reflection may not be visible)

Visual Acuity

- <3 years old:
    - Visual acuity may not be possible if patient cannot identify pictures on eye chart
    - *Cover-uncover test* – assess fixation by alternately covering one eye and observing for strabismus (strabismus present if covered eye moves towards object after being uncovered)
    - Examine optic blink reflex: blinking in response to bright light, or quick movement of object toward eyes
- >3 years old: *use Snellen chart; average acuity is not 20/20 (6/6) until 2-4 years*

Visual Fields

- Bring toy in from periphery; child's eyes should conjugately deviate towards object when it is seen

Fundoscopy

- Examine the red retinal (fundus) reflex and optic disk (lighter in colour than adults, foveal light reflection may not be visible)
- Look for retinal hemorrhages, cataracts, corneal opacity
- A thorough ophthalmoscopic exam is difficult in infants, but may be needed if ocular or neurologic abnormalities are noted

Table 6. Differential Diagnosis of Findings on Observation of Eyes

Finding	Differential Diagnosis
Fixed eyes staring in one direction (doll's eye reflex), intermittent alternating convergence strabismus (crossed eyes), or intermittent alternating divergent strabismus (intermittent laterally deviated eyes)	Normal in newborns due to dysconjugate gaze. Abnormal after 6 months
Pendular nystagmus or roving eye movements	Highly suspicious for blindness after 6 weeks of age
Hypertelorism, Brushfield's spots	Down's Syndrome
Inner epicanthal folds	Normally found in Asian children, Down's
Appearance of sclera between upper lid and iris	Hydrocephalus, Grave's Disease
Drooping eyelid	Paralysis of oculomotor cranial nerve
Painful, red, swollen eyelid	Stye
Nodular, non-tender area	Cyst
Sunken area around eyelids	Dehydrated
Subconjunctival hemorrhages	Normal in newborn
Red conjunctivae	Bacterial or viral infection, allergy, irritation

Table 6. Differential Diagnosis of Findings on Observation of Eyes (continued)

Finding	Differential Diagnosis
Pale conjunctivae	Anemia
Yellow sclerae	Jaundice
Bluish sclerae	Premature baby, osteogenesis imperfecta, glaucoma, hyperbilirubinemia
Absence of colour in iris	Albinism
Notch at outer edge of iris	Visual field defect
Constriction of pupils (miosis)	Iritis, drug induced (morphine)
Fixed unilateral dilation of a pupil	Local eye injury or head injury
Dilation of pupils (mydriasis)	Acute glaucoma, drug induced, trauma, circulatory anesthesia, emotionally induced
White pupils (leukocoria)	Coloboma (failure of retinal development), Intraocular tumour (retinoblastoma), Cataract, Retinopathy of prematurity, Congenital infection (toxoplasmosis)

Ear

Inspection
- Position, shape and features of ears
- If an imaginary line is drawn from outer canthi of eyes, it should cross pinna or auricle
  - Low-set ears occur if pinna is below this line; may indicate congenital defect
- Look for absence of wax (over-cleaning or acute otitis media), foul-smelling discharge (rupture of tympanic membrane or recent insertion of myringotomy tubes), and bloody discharge (foreign body irritation or scratching)

Neonate
- A neonate's ears are flat against the head
- The tympanic membrane is obscured with accumulated vernix caseosa (white cheesy substance that covers baby's skin at time of birth) for the first few days of life

Infant
- Pull auricle gently downward rather than upward for best view, since ear canal will be directed downward from the outside
- Once tympanic membrane is visible, the light reflex may be diffuse and may not become cone-shaped for several months

Child
- Young children may sit in the parent's lap or may need to be restrained while lying down by parents to examine ears
- To restrain a child, have the parent hold the child's elbows firmly by the side of the child's head while you lean over the child's body
- Pull the auricle upward, outward and backward for best view

> **Evidence-Based Medicine: Acute Otitis Media**
> The most useful signs for detecting AOM are cloudiness, bulging and distinct immobility of the tympanic membrane (adjusted positive LR = 34, 51 and 31, respectively, all with 95% CI). Normal, as opposed to red colour, makes AOM less likely (adjusted positive LR = 0.2).
>
> Rothman R, Owens T, Simel DL. 2003. *JAMA* 290(12):1633-1640.

Hearing

Child

- Grossly test for hearing by whispering a command or question 8 feet away and not in the line of the child's vision
- Children >4 years should have a full-scale acoustic screening test
- Young children who fail screening maneuvers should have audiometric testing

Table 7. Neonate and Infant Signs of Hearing

Age	Sign of hearing
0-2 months	Startle and blink response to a sudden noise Calming down with soothing voice or music
2-3 months	Change in body movements in response to sounds Change in facial expression to familiar sounds
3-4 months	Turning eyes and head to sound
6-7 months	Turning to listen to voices and conversation

Nose and Paranasal Sinuses

Inspection

- Nasolabial folds: asymmetry indicates facial nerve impairment or Bell's palsy
- With otoscope, inspect nasal mucous membranes, noting colour and condition
- Look for nasal septal deviation and polyps

Palpation

- Test for patency of nasal passages by gently occluding each nostril alternately while holding the baby's mouth closed

Mouth and Pharynx

Inspection

All pediatric patients

- Look at lips, gingival and buccal mucosa for hydration and cyanosis
- Check hard and soft palate, uvula, and tonsils for exudates or infection
- Assess breath
  - Odour indicates oropharyngeal/gingival infection, dehydration, constipation or poor oral hygiene

Infant

- Epstein's pearls: tiny white or yellow rounded mucous retention cysts along the posterior midline of the hard palate; they disappear within months
- A prominent protruding tongue may signal congenital hypothyroidism or Down syndrome

Child
- Teeth – Examine for timing and sequence of eruption, number, character, condition and position
  - First teeth erupt at around 6 months; permanent teeth erupt at 6 years
  - Significant delay may be a sign of delayed skeletal development
  - Malformed teeth may indicate systemic insult
  - Look for maxillary protrusion (overbite) and mandibular protrusion (underbite) by asking the child to bite down hard and part the lips

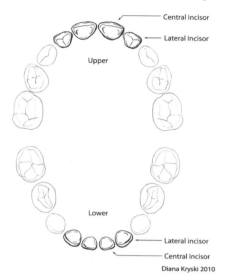

Central incisor

Lateral incisor

Upper

Lower

Lateral incisor

Central incisor

Diana Kryski 2010

Figure 1. Dentition in Children 5-12 Months Old

- Inspect tongue
  - Common abnormalities include coated tongue from viral infection, and strawberry tongue found in scarlet fever, streptococcal pharyngitis, or Kawasaki disease
- Tonsils – note size, position, symmetry and appearance
  - Size of tonsils is assessed from 1+ (easy visibility of gap between tonsils) to 4+ (tonsils which touch the midline with the mouth wide open)
  - A peritonsillar abscess is suggested by asymmetric enlargement of the tonsils and lateral displacement of the uvula
- Notching of the posterior margin of the hard palate or a bifid uvula are clues of a submucosal cleft palate

Palpation
Neonate
- Palpate the upper hard palate to make sure it is intact (especially important in newborns or children with frequent ear infections or delayed speech)

Neck
Inspection
- Webbing or extra neck folds may indicate Turner syndrome or Down syndrome
- Look for enlarged nodes/glands and the thyroid size, masses, and texture

Palpation
Neonate and Infant
- Best palpated while patient is supine since the neck is short

Child
- Best examined while sitting
- Neck mobility, either passive or active, depending on child's age
- Ensure the neck is supple and mobile in all directions
- *Congenital torticollis:* "wry neck", bleeding into the sternocleidomastoid leaving a firm fibrous mass (fibromatosis coli) during the stretching process of birth; disappears over months
- *Nuchal rigidity:* for suspected meningitis, ask child to touch chin to chest and note pain/restriction
- Clavicles, to look for evidence of fracture, i.e. tenderness or a lump
- Lymph nodes and presence of any additional masses (congenital cysts)
- The majority of enlarged lymph nodes in children are due to infection, not malignant disease
- Malignancy is more likely if node is >2 cm, hard, fixed, and accompanied by systemic signs such as weight loss

RESPIRATORY
- The pediatric respiratory exam should be completed using the same criteria as in the adult exam (see ***Respiratory Exam***)
- Infants and young children should have the respiratory exam done while sitting on a parent's lap – if they become agitated by the examiner's presence, they may need to be observed from a distance to better assess their respiratory status at rest

Inspection
- Anteroposterior (AP) diameter
  - In neonates/infants, the chest is rounder than in older children
  - Increased AP diameter is seen in cystic fibrosis, chronic asthma or chronic diffuse small airway obstruction
- Chest wall deformities
  - Pectus excavatum may be an isolated finding or may be associated with a chronic cardiorespiratory problem
  - Other chest wall deformities may be congenital or due to surgery
- Spinal configuration
  - Kyphoscoliosis can affect shape of thoracic cage and pulmonary function
- Signs of respiratory distress
  - Retractions in suprasternal and lower sternal region suggest extrathoracic (upper airway) obstruction
  - Retractions in subcostal or intercostal regions with increased AP diameter suggests air trapping
  - Nasal flaring is nonspecific, but is an important distress sign
- Respiration phases, depth and rhythm
  - Infants display more abdominal breathing, with a shift to chest excursion as they get older (thoracic breathing at ~6 years of age)

- Rhythm irregularities may signify abnormalities such as apnea
- Periodic breathing (up to 20 seconds of apnea) can be normal, especially in premature infants
- Finger clubbing: may indicate cystic fibrosis, respiratory, cardiac, and GI disorders
- Cyanosis: central cyanosis indicates cardiorespiratory disease

> **Clinical Pearl**
> Percussion is of little clinical benefit in young children and should be avoided, especially in low birth-weight or preterm infants, as it may cause injury or bruising.

> **Evidence-Based Medicine: Pneumonia in Infants**
> The respiratory rate should be determined by observing the chest of a quiet infant over two 30-second intervals, or over a full minute. When examining infants, auscultation is relatively unreliable.
>
> To rule out pneumonia, the best individual finding is the absence of tachypnea. Signs that can be helpful for ruling in pneumonia include abnormal auscultatory findings, chest indrawing and other signs suggesting increased work of breathing (e.g. nasal flaring). In developed countries, multiple findings are needed to increase the likelihood of pneumonia.
>
> If all clinical signs (i.e. respiratory rate, auscultation, and work of breathing) are negative, a CXR is less likely to be positive.
>
> Margolis P, Gadomski A. 1998. JAMA 279(4):308-313.

Palpation
- use 1 or two fingers (based on size) to assess tracheal position
- Chest expansion and tactile fremitus have little use in young children

Percussion
- Diaphragmatic excursion is usually only performed on older child
- Can be used to assess for consolidation/atelectasis

Auscultation
- The bell of an adult stethoscope, or a pediatric stethoscope diaphragm, should be used in young children
- The examiner should ask about and listen for respiratory sounds (see **Respiratory Exam** p. 341)
- The patient or the parent should be asked about congenital stridor
- As in the adult exam, always compare both sides

CARDIOVASCULAR

Inspection
- See **Cardiovascular Exam**
- General signs of health: nutritional status, responsiveness; failure to thrive is one presentation of heart failure
- Noncardiac findings that may indicate cardiac disease – i.e. poor feeding may be due to tachypnea, shortness of breath on exertion; fingernail clubbing may be associated with cardiogenic cyanosis
- Respiratory rate and pattern: effortless tachypnea is seen in acidosis (e.g. salicylate toxicity, diabetic ketoacidosis) and cardiac disease. Increase in respiratory effort is primarily seen in pulmonary disease

Table 9. Cardiac Causes of Central Cyanosis in Children

Onset	Potential Cardiac Cause
Directly after birth	Transposition of great arteries, pulmonary valve atresia, severe pulmonary valve stenosis, Ebstein's malformation (of tricuspid valve)
A few days after birth	See above, plus: Total anomalous pulmonary venous return, hypoplastic left heart syndrome, truncus arteriosus, signal ventricular variants
Within weeks, months or years after birth	See above, plus: Pulmonary vascular disease with atrial, ventricular, or great vessel shunting

Palpation
- Chest wall to assess volume change in heart and thrills
- Peripheral pulses help assess major branches of the aorta: palpate brachial artery pulse (antecubital fossa), temporal arteries in front of the ear and femoral pulses
- Normal pulse has sharp rise, is firm and well localized
- Point of maximal impulse is found in the 4th intercostal space before age 7, 5th space after age 7
- Patent Ductus Arteriosus is indicated by bounding pulses
- Coarctation of the aorta is indicated by absence of femoral pulse, or its diminution relative to the brachial pulse

Auscultation
- Note rate, rhythm, S1 and S2, murmurs (very difficult to distinguish for the novice)
- Listen to the back, neck and axillae as murmurs can radiate there
- Listen over both sides of the skull for an intracranial arteriovenous malformation
- Sinus arrhythmia is a normal finding in children, with heart rate increasing on inspiration and decreasing on expiration

Table 10. Benign Heart Murmurs in Children

Murmur (age of presentation)	Location	Timing	Intensity, Quality and Pitch
Closing ductus (neonate to 1 year)	Upper left sternal border	Transient	Soft
Peripheral pulmonary flow murmur (neonate to 1 yr)	Left of upper left sternal border, and in lung fields and axillae	Systole	Soft, slightly ejectile
Still's murmur (preschool to early school age)	Mid/lower left sternal border and over carotid arteries	Early and mid-systole	Grade I-II/VI Musical, vibratory, multiple overtones
Venous hum (preschool to early school age)	Under clavicle	Continuous	Soft, hollow, louder in diastole, can be eliminated by maneuvers that affect venous return, or by contralateral neck rotation

Adapted from: "Assessing Children: Infancy Through Adolescence". In Bickley LS, Szilagyi PG, Bates B. 2007. *Bates' Guide to Physical Examination and History Taking.* Philadelphia: Lippincott Williams and Wilkins.

Murmurs

- Up to 80% of children have heart murmurs, but only 0.35% have confirmed organic heart disease
- Soft precordial systolic murmur common in first few days after birth
  - May indicate patent ductus arteriosus if it persists and is heard over the back

---

Evidence-Based Medicine: Pneumonia in Infants

In a study of 30 office-based pediatricians, the average sensitivity was 82% and average specificity was 72% for differentiating innocent murmurs from pathological ones by auscultation, as compared to the gold standard of complete echocardiographic assessment.

Haney I et al. 1998. *Arch Dis Childhood* 81:409-412.

- *Innocent murmurs* (vibratory murmurs, venous hum, carotid bruits)
  - short duration systolic, low pitch, vibratory, and < grade 3
  - heard best with bell of stethoscope and may change with patient position
- *Organic (non-innocent) murmurs*
  - systolic or diastolic, coarse, > grade 3
  - < age 3: congenital heart disease
  - > age 3: acquired heart disease (e.g. rheumatic carditis)

Table 11. Murmurs Associated with Childhood Cardiac Defects

Defect	Location	Timing	Intensity	Pitch	Quality
Atrial septal defect (acyanotic)	Second left intercostals space	Wide, fixed split S2, peaks in mid-systole	Soft	Medium	Nonmusical
Ventricular septal defect (acyanotic)	Left sternal border, third and fourth interspaces	Between S1 and S2	Very loud	High	Blowing
Patent ductus arteriosus	Second left interspace; may radiate to left clavicle/sternum	Continuous; louder in late systole (just before S2); obscures S2; softer in diastole	Loud	Medium	Harsh
Tetralogy of Fallot (cyanotic)	Second and third left interspaces	Between S1 and S2	Not well transmitted		No distinct characteristics

Adapted from Engel J. 1989. *Pocket Guide to Pediatric Assessment*. St. Louis: Mosby.

Table 12. Congenital Heart Lesions

Congenital Heart Lesion	Manifestation	Examples
Obstructive	Pressure overload	AS, coarctation of the aorta, PS
Left-to-right shunts	Volume overload	ASD, VSD, PDA
Cyanotic heart lesions	Central cyanosis	Tetralogy of Fallot, transposition of the great arteries, triscuspid atresia

Legend: AS = aortic stenosis; PS = pulmonic stenosis; ASD = atrial septal defect; VSD = ventricular septal defect; PDA = patent ductus arteriosus

GASTROINTESTINAL

- It is important when inspecting the abdomen to relax the child
- Useful tips include flexing the child's knees, talking and playing with the child and putting your hand flat on the abdomen
- Make sure your hand is warm
- Distract older children by asking simple questions
- Common causes of gastrointestinal problems vary with age (e.g. in the neonate, one must consider congenital abnormalities like Hirschsprung disease or fistulas)

Inspection

- Protuberant abdomen
  - Expected in infants; feature disappears as early as 4 years of age
  - Distended abdomen may indicate obstruction
  - A large abdomen, with thin limbs and wasted buttocks, suggests severe malnutrition; seen in celiac disease or cystic fibrosis
  - Scaphoid abdomen together with respiratory distress may suggest congenital diaphragmatic hernia in a neonate
- Umbilicus
  - check for umbilical hernia
  - Neonate:
    + Check umbilical cord for 2 umbilical arteries and 1 umbilical vein
    + Examine cord for discharge or signs of infection
    + Presence of a single umbilical artery has a high correlation with a variety of congenital anomalies (e.g. sensorineural hearing loss)
- Abdominal Wall
  - *Omphalocele:* incomplete closure of anterior abdominal wall; herniated bowel, stomach, liver, spleen in peritoneum covered sac; associated with other abnormalities
  - *Gastroschisis:* defect in anterior abdominal wall just lateral to umbilicus; herniated intestine with no covering sac; no associated abnormalities
- Signs of jaundice, especially in neonates
  - Look for passage of meconium in newborns; ask if meconium passage was delayed in a neonate or infant with constipation
- Anus
  - Examine peri-anal skin for redness
  - Check for imperforation and prolapse
  - Asymmetry of buttocks and thigh folds suggests congenital hip dysplasia
  - Redness and rash may indicate inadequate cleaning, diaper rash, or irritation from diarrhea

Auscultation

- Listen for bowel sounds over each quadrant
- Bowel sounds normally present every 10-30 seconds, but must listen for several minutes before determining that sounds are absent
- Can use 'scratch test' to delineate liver size by listening for change in quality of sound when scratching over top and bottom edge of liver

Percussion

- Systematically percuss all areas of the abdomen
- Should be tympanic except over the liver, fecal masses, or full bladder

Palpation

- Observe child's face carefully for pain while lightly palpating for tenderness and deeply palpating for abnormal masses
- Localized tenderness with guarding and rebound is a sign of peritoneal irritation
- Liver edge, spleen tip and kidneys are often palpable in the normal infant
- Palpate for an umbilical or inguinal hernia

Clinical Pearl

While the digital rectal examination (DRE) is only performed if required for diagnosis or treatment, physicians should not forget its utility. DRE can help differentiate functional constipation from constipation due to organic causes. Functional fecal retention is the most common cause of childhood constipation.

- Liver size and position
  - Palpate liver's lower margin; if margin indefinite, use percussion
  - Normal liver margin is palpated no more than 1-2 cm below costal margin
- Pyloric stenosis: a mass described as an "olive" – should be palpable just to the right of the midline in the epigastric area (usually in the first few months of life)
- Rectal exam should be done only if abdominal or pelvic disease suspected
- Prostate gland is not palpable in the young male

Table 14. Differential Diagnosis of Abdominal Pain

Area of Pain	Differential Diagnosis
Right upper quadrant	Hepatitis, enlarged liver
Right lower quadrant or around the umbilicus	Appendicitis
Lower quadrants	Feces, gastroenteritis[†], pelvic infection, tumour
Left upper quadrant	Intussusception[‡], splenic enlargement

[†]Infants/children under the age of 5 experience gastroenteritis 1-2 times/year (episodes usually resolve in 3-7 days; causes: bacterial or viral; signs/symptoms: nausea, vomiting, fever, pain)
[‡]Intussusception: most common cause of bowel obstruction under age 5 (signs/symptoms: "currant jelly" stools and colicky pain)

GENITOURINARY AND REPRODUCTIVE SYSTEM

- In some newborns the genitalia may appear ambiguous as to gender indicating either a chromosomal or endocrine abnormality. This may result in problems of gender assignment and may be associated with life-threatening electrolyte imbalance

Male

Inspection
Infant
- Penis
  - Foreskin completely covers the glans penis and is not retractable until months to years after birth
  - Shaft of penis: ensure penis appears straight, and note any ventral surface abnormalities. Fixed downward bowing of the penis is a chordee, and may accompany a hypospadias
  - Look for fibrous ring around meatus of foreskin (phimosis)
  - A small amount of white, cheesy material under the foreskin around the glans (smegma) is normal
- Scrotum
  - Note rugae and presence or absence of testes in sac

Child
- In precocious puberty, the penis and testes are enlarged due to conditions of excess androgens, including pituitary and adrenal tumours
- As with adult men, swelling in the inguinal canal, especially after a Valsalva maneuver may indicate inguinal hernia

Palpation
Infant
- Palpate the testes in the scrotum and proceed downward to the external inguinal ring, and then to the scrotum
- If testis is palpated in the inguinal canal, gentle pressure can ease them down
- Testes should be ~10 mm width and 15 mm length
- Poorly developed scrotum indicates cryptorchidism (undescended testes)
- Differentiate any swelling found in the scrotum from the testes
  - Hydroceles and inguinal hernias are two common scrotal masses

Child
- An extremely active cremasteric reflex may cause testis to retract upwards and appear undescended
  - To minimize retraction, examine when child is relaxed, use warm hands, and palpate from the lower abdomen, along inguinal canal toward scrotum
- Cremasteric reflex test: scratch the medial aspect of the thigh, ipsilateral testis moves upward
- Common causes of painful testicle are infection, trauma, torsion of the testicle and torsion of the appendix testis

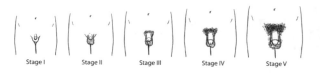

Figure 2. Male Tanner Stages

Diana Kryski 2010

Female

Inspection
- Examine child in supine position; in younger children, child can sit in parent's lap with parent holding knees outstretched
- Inspect labia majora, labia minora, size of clitoris, presence of rashes, bruises or other lesions
- To examine more internal structures, separate the labia majora at midpoint to inspect urethral orifice and labia minora
  - *infant:* use the thumbs of each hand
  - *older children:* grasp labia between thumb and index finger of each hand
  - note condition of labia minora, urethra, hymen and proximal vagina

Child
- Labia majora and minora flatten out after infancy
- Check for any rashes, bruises or external lesions
- Examine labia minora, urethra, hymen, and proximal vagina by inspection only
- Hymen becomes thin, translucent and vascular, often with easily identifiable edges
- Pubic hair before age 7 indicates precocious puberty
- Labial adhesions (fusion of the labia minora) posteriorly may be noted in prepubertal girls

MUSCULOSKELETAL
- Inspection, palpation, and range of motion with the greatest number of findings involving the spine and lower extremities
- Become familiar with normal MSK changes during development to recognize abnormalities and conditions that spontaneously regress
- Range of motion is greatest in the infant and then decreases with age

Newborn
- Full-term newborns exhibit 20-30° hip and knee relative flexion 'contractures' that will disappear by 4-6 months

Infant
- Feet
  - Club foot: plantar flexion of foot, heel inversion, medial forefoot deviation
  - Toeing-in:
    - 6-18 months: commonly caused by internal tibial torsion
      - Rotate knees so patella faces forward, feet should face inwards (usually disappears at age 2)
    - 3-12 years: commonly caused by internal femoral torsion
      - Rotate knees so patella faces forward, feet should now face forward
  - Flat feet are normal in children under 2-3 years of age

PEDIATRIC

- Knee Alignment
  - Mild bow-legged (genu varum) pattern is normal until age 2
  - Mild knock-knee (genu valgum) pattern is normal from 2 to 8 years of age
- Hips
  - Barlow's and Ortolani's tests are useful in the first 6 weeks of life; after this time the radiological exam provides a more accurate diagnosis
  - Check for an unstable or potentially dislocatable hip using Barlow's test
    - Place infant supine; stabilize pelvis by placing thumb on symphysis and fingers on sacrum; with other hand over knee, flex and slightly adduct hip while lifting femur and applying pressure to trochanter
    - In the presence of a dislocatable hip, the femoral head can be felt to slide or dislocate across the posterior lip of the acetabulum
  - Check hips for congenital dislocation using Ortolani's test
    - Congenital hip dislocation is often seen in breech babies
    - Place infant supine; with your thumbs on the inside of both thighs and fingertips resting over the thigh muscles, flex both hips and knees; abduct each knee until lateral aspects of the knees touch the table
    - If hip is dislocated, an audible and palpable "clunk" will be produced as the femoral head re-enters the acetabulum
- Spine
  - Look for vertebral deformities and pigmented spots, hairy patches, or overlying skin in lumbosacral region (spina bifida)

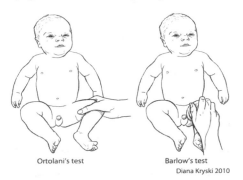

Ortolani's test   Barlow's test
                         Diana Kryski 2010

Figure 3. Ortolani's and Barlow's Tests for Hip Dislocation

Child
- As child gets older, MSK exam is generally the same as an adult exam (see *Musculoskeletal Exam*)
- Hips: check for hip pain or instability using Trendelenburg Test
- Spine
  - Look for vertebral deformities and pigmented spots, hairy patches, or overlying skin in lumbosacral region (spina bifida)
  - Check for scoliosis – ask child to lean forward and mark spinous processes with a pen; look for a curve in the dots when child stands up
  - Also look for asymmetry in the hips, rib cage, and scapulae
- Common Injuries
  - Ankle sprains are one of most common childhood MSK injuries
    - Signs and symptoms: pain, bruising, swelling
    - Ottawa ankle rules to determine presence of fracture do not apply for children

NEUROLOGICAL

- Findings are greatly affected by internal factors: alertness, timing from last feeding, sleeping, and external factors: fear and anxiety, presence of parents
- Neurologic and developmental exams are often combined, since neurologic abnormalities can present in young children as developmental abnormalities

Neonate

- Please see table of neonatal primitive reflexes under **Common Clinical Scenarios and Disorders**

Infant

Mental status
- Observe activities during child's alert periods

Motor exam
- Watch position at rest and as the infant moves spontaneously
- Test resistance to passive movement noting any spasticity or flaccidity, increased or decreased tone

Deep tendon reflexes
- Variable in newborns since corticospinal pathways are not yet developed, so little diagnostic significance unless response is extreme or different from previous
- Can substitute index or middle finger for reflex hammer
- Triceps, brachioradialis and abdominal reflexes are hard to elicit before 6 months
- Anal reflex is present at birth and should be elicited if spinal cord lesion is suspected
- Ankle reflex elicited by grasping infant's malleolus with one hand and abruptly dorsiflexing child's foot; up to 10 plantar flexion beats are normal in newborn (clonus)
- Normal downgoing plantar response is seen in 90% of infants, but a normal infant can manifest an upgoing plantar (Babinski) response until 2 years of age
- Progressive increase in deep tendon reflexes in first year coupled with increased tone may indicate CNS disease such as cerebral palsy

Sensory function
- Pain sensation: touch or flick infant's palm or sole with your finger and observe for withdrawal, arousal and change in facial expression

Child

Motor Exam
- Observe child's gait while walking and running, noting any asymmetry, tripping, or clumsiness
- Heel-to-toe walking, hopping, jumping (if developmentally appropriate)
- Use toy to test for coordination, strength of upper extremities
- If concerned about strength, test by having child lie of the floor and then stand up
- In certain forms of muscular dystrophy, children rise by rolling over prone and pushing off the floor with the arms while legs stay extended, then achieve upright position using arms to walk up legs (Gower's sign)

Deep tendon reflexes
- As assessed for adults (see **Neurological Exam** p. 190)

Sensory exam
- Test with cotton ball with child's eyes closed; do not use pinprick with young child

Cerebellar exam
- Finger-to-nose test with rapid alternating movements – make this a game

Table 15. Cranial Nerves Assessment in Infants

Cranial Nerve	Strategy
I Olfactory	Difficult to test
II Visual acuity	Have baby look at your face; observe facial response and tracking
II, III Response to light	Darken room and use light to test for optic blink reflex Use otoscope to assess papillary response
III, IV, VI Extraocular movements	Observe tracking as baby regards your face moving side to side
V Motor	Test rooting reflex and suckling reflex
VII Facial	Observe baby crying and smiling, noting symmetry of face and forehead
VIII Acoustic	Test acoustic blink reflex and observe tracking in response to sound
IX, X Swallow, Gag	Observe coordination during swallowing; test gag reflex
XI Spinal accessory	Observe for symmetry in shoulders
XII Hypoglossal	Observe coordination of swallowing, sucking and tongue thrusting Occlude nostrils and observe reflex opening of mouth with tip of tongue to midline

Table 16. Cranial Nerves Assessment Strategies with Young Children

Cranial Nerve	Strategy
I Olfactory	Testable in older children
II Visual acuity	>3 years, use Snellen chart Test visual field as for an adult
III, IV, VI Extraocular movements	Have child track a light or a toy
V Trigeminal	Play a game with a soft cotton ball to test sensation Have child clench teeth and chew food
VII Facial	Have child imitate you as you make faces, observing for symmetry and facial movements
VIII Acoustic	>4 years, perform auditory tests and whisper test
IX, X Swallow, Gag	Tell child to "stick your tongue out" and "say ah", observing movement of uvular and soft palate Test gag reflex
XI Spinal accessory	Have child push your hand away with his/her head Have child shrug shoulders against your resistance
XII Hypoglossal	Ask child to "stick out your tongue all the way"

DERMATOLOGICAL

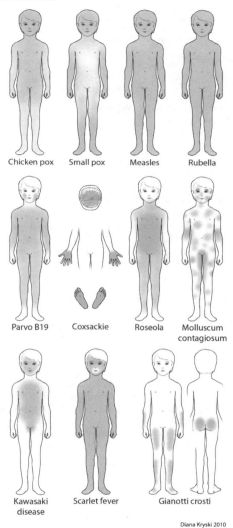

Chicken pox   Small pox   Measles   Rubella

Parvo B19   Coxsackie   Roseola   Molluscum contagiosum

Kawasaki disease   Scarlet fever   Gianotti crosti

Diana Kryski 2010

Figure 4. Distribution of Common Rashes

- Done almost entirely on history and inspection, with a good source of light
- Inspection should begin with a general observation of skin, hair and nail colour, pigmentation and texture
- Skin temperature should be assessed as well
- If lesions are present, describe their distribution, configuration, thickness primary/secondary changes present, and colour
- Be certain to distinguish physiological lesions and those from child abuse
- Dermatological findings vary with age

Evidence-Based Medicine: Assessing Anemia Using Pallor
A study of 2,540 children in Ethiopia indicated that the presence of any pallor clinically correlated with moderate anemia (hemoglobin <8 g/dL). This was detectable with a sensitivity of 95% and a specificity of 64-68% when the palm and nail bed were used.

Muhe L et al. 2000. *Trop Med Int Health* 5(11):805-810.

Young child

- Impetigo
  - pustule progresses to honey-coloured crust
  - most common on face
  - caused by group A β-hemolytic *Streptococcus*, *S. aureus* or both

APPROACH TO THE ADOLESCENT

APPROACH TO THE ADOLESCENT HISTORY AND PHYSICAL EXAM

- Adolescence is a time of tremendous physical and psychosocial change
- History and Physical should focus on the following:
  - *Puberty* – signs of normal vs. abnormal maturation
  - *Screening* – for safety and risk-taking behaviours

History

- With the adolescent's permission, at least part of the history should be obtained without parent in the room
- *Identifying Data* – name, age, school grade, siblings, cohabitants in home
- *Chief Complaint* – note that a teenager's initial CC may not represent his/her actual reason for seeking medical attention
- *History of Present Illness* – see **Focused History**
- *Past Medical History* – previous illnesses, surgeries, medications, allergies (medications and environmental), immunization history
- *Psychosocial History* – "HE²ADS³" (Home, Education, Eating, Activities, Drugs, Sexuality/Sex, Suicide/Mood, Safety) assessment, stressors, relationship with family
- *Family History* – recurrent illnesses, early deaths, genetic diseases, cancer, psychiatric conditions, suicide, alcohol/substance abuse
- *Review of Systems* – including menstrual patterns, urinary symptoms,

Physical Exam

- Knowledge of adult exam is assumed for adolescent exam
- As per adult exam except
  - *Growth and Development* – height, mass, body mass index (BMI) – should be plotted on curve to monitor development
  - *Head & Neck* – thyroid examination, screen for visual acuity and hearing
  - *Genitourinary*
    - ◆ *Male* – external genitalia (Tanner staging), secondary sexual characteristics (body hair, pubic hair)
    - ◆ *Female* – external genitalia (Tanner staging), if indicated speculum (vagina and cervix) and bimanual examination
  - *Dermatological* – skin (acne, petechiae, pallor, pigmentation), hair (amount, distribution, hirsutism), breasts (development in females, gynecomastia in males)

COMMON CHIEF COMPLAINTS

Disorders marked with (✓) are discussed in **Common Clinical Scenarios**

Growth and Development:
- Premature/delayed puberty
- ✓ Obesity

Respiratory:
- Cough
- ✓ Asthma

Neurological:
- Concussion
- Headache

Abdominal:
- Abdominal Pain

Dermatological:
- ✓ Acne

Genitourinary:
- ✓ Abnormal menstruation
- Urinary symptoms
- Contraception
- Teenage pregnancy
- ✓ Sexually transmitted infections

Musculoskeletal:
- ✓ Limping
- Sports injuries

Psychiatric:
- ✓ Depression/suicide
- Substance abuse
- ✓ Eating disorders

FOCUSED HISTORY

- The history should be obtained directly from the teenager, with parents absent
  - Broach delicate subjects without parent present during physical exam
- To promote disclosure about delicate subjects
  - Maintain environment of confidentiality so that teenager trusts you
  - Approach subjects directly, but be non-judgmental
  - Inform adolescent that you will have to discose to other people if they are suicidal or homocidal
- Always leave time for discussion of risk-taking behaviours such as drug usage, alcohol, drinking and driving, and legal difficulties

Chief Complaint (CC)

- A teenager's initial CC may not represent his/her actual reason for seeking medical attention

History of Present Illness (HPI)

- Often the HPI must be taken in context of adolescent's psychosocial history

Psychosocial History (HE²ADS³ Approach)

- **H**ome
  - Living arrangements, relationship with parents and siblings, other occupants
  - Attempts at running away, family issues, recent changes at home
- **E**ducation
  - Name of school, current grade, academic performance, school attendance, behaviour at school
- **E**ating
  - Diet: typical foods, types and frequency of skipped meals, vomiting, nutritional supplements, vitamin use, calcium/vitamin D intake
  - Body image: recent weight gain or loss, dieting, use of weight loss drugs
  - Compensatory behaviours: including vomiting, laxatives, exercise, diuretics, stimulants

- Eating Disorder Screen – **SCOFF**
  - Do you make yourself **S**ick because you feel uncomfortably full?
  - Do you worry that you have lost **C**ontrol over how much you eat?
  - In 3 months have you lost **O**ver 15 lbs?
  - Do you think you are **F**at when others think you are thin?
  - Does **F**ood dominate your life?
- **A**ctivities
  - After school or work; exercise, sports, hobbies, parties/clubs
  - Part-time work, income for activities
- **D**rugs
  - Do you have any friends who drink, smoke or use drugs?
  - Have you ever tried smoking or drinking alcohol? What did you think? What about other drugs?
  - Have you ever gotten in trouble because of using these substances?
- **S**ex/Sexuality
  - Current/past sexual activity, sexual identity, history of pregnancy
  - Sexually transmitted infections (STIs)
  - Contraception – what method(s)? is it used every time and used properly?
- **S**uicide/Mood
  - Screen for depression MSIGECAPS (See *Psychiatric Exam* p. 325)
  - Suicide assessment: past attempts, protective factors, current plan/means
- **S**afety
  - From physical and sexual abuse at home, school, in relationships
  - Recent injuries – motor vehicle accidents, sports injuries, concussions

---

Evidence-Based Medicine: Eating Disorders

A 2000 study indicated the 4 most sensitive questions to screen for an eating disorder:

"How many diets have you been on in the past year?"

"Do you feel you should be dieting?"

"Do you feel dissatisfied with your body size?"

"Does your weight affect the way you feel about yourself?"

Anstine D, Grinenko D. 2000. *J Adolesc Health* 26(5):338-342.

Past Medical History (PMHx)

- Current and Previous Illnesses
- Surgeries and Hospitalizations
  - Most recent hospitalization, length of stay
- Medications
  - Prescription, over the counter, supplements
- Allergies
  - Medications, food, environmental: reaction experienced, action taken
  - Previous anaphylactic reactions
  - Family history of atopy (genetic predisposition to asthma, atopic dermatitis, and environmental allergies)
- Immunization history
  - Adverse reactions: local, systemic, or allergic
  - Which and when?

Family History

- Family history of disease: early MI, headaches, diabetes, cancer, recurrent illnesses, atopy, asthma, genetic disorders (e.g. familial hypercholesterolemia)
- Psychiatric family history: suicide, alcohol/substance abuse, psychiatric disorders (ex. schizophrenia), mood disorders

Review of Systems

Similar to review of systems for infant/neonate, with the following highlights:

- *General:* health, diet, activity level, weight, fatigue, sleep, school performance
- *H & N:* infections: number, febrile/afebrile, sore throat, swallowing difficulties, swollen glands, cough, pressure/pain over sinuses
- *Resp:* respiratory difficulties (triggers: exercise/cold weather/seasonal allergens)
- *CVS:* syncope, ability to keep up with peers, chest pain
- *GI:* bowel movements: frequency, consistency, blood, mucous, pain associated with meals, diarrhea/loose stools
- *GU:*
  - Males and females:
    - Urinary symptoms (frequency, urgency, dysuria), UTIs
    - Sexual activity, sexually transmitted infections (genital lesions, discharge)
  - Males:
    - Testicular masses, testicular pain
  - Females:
    - *Menstrual history* – age at menarche, regularity, dysmenorrhea, menorrhagia, previous or current pregnancy, secondary amenorrhea
    - *Breast history* – lumps, mastalgia (breast pain), nipple discharge, breast development and enlargement
- *MSK:* recent injuries
- *Dermatological:* rash, pruritis, pigmented lesions, sun damage

FOCUSED PHYSICAL

- Often the genitourinary examination is left until the end, as teenagers can be embarrassed or sensitive about this area
  - There should always be a chaperone for the GU and breast exams
- Onset of puberty is variable; however, in general – onset is 8-13 in females, 9-14 in males
- Usual Sequence of pubertal sexual maturation:
  - *Females:* thelarche (breast budding) → adrenarche (pubic hair) → growth spurt → menarche (onset of menstruation)
  - *Males:* testes enlargement → penile enlargement → adrenarche + axillary hair → growth spurt

General Survey

- General Survey should consist of (a) General Inspection, (b) Growth Measurements
  1. *General Inspection* – does this adolescent look "sick?"
     - Respiratory distress, level of alertness, general affect, nutritional status

2. *Growth Measurements* – measure height, mass, calculate body-mass index (BMI)
   - Plot on growth chart and note trend and percentiles of growth
   - *Height* – growth spurt occurs during puberty, which accounts for 20-25% of final adult height; onset and duration of growth spurt is highly variable
     - Females: onset 9½-14½ years
     - Males: onset 10½-16 years
     - Growth spurt lasts about 2 years longer in males (into 3rd decade)
   - *Mass* – pubertal weight gain accounts for 50% of final adult body weight
     - Percentage body fat increases in females and decreases in males
   - *Body-Mass Index* = mass (kg) / height^2 (m^2)

Vital Signs
- As per adult
  - Ensure teenager is comfortable and not anxious before measuring vitals
  - Hypertension in *children* is often due to a secondary cause (see **Table 17**), whereas adolescent hypertension is usually essential hypertension

Table 17. Causes of Hypertension in Children and Adolescents

Causes
Vascular (coarctation of aorta, renal artery steosis/embolism)
Infectious (Hemolytic Uremic Syndrome, pyelonephritis)
Toxic (lead, mercury)
Autoimmune (arteritis, systemic lupus erythematosus)
Metabolic/Endocrine (cushing syndrome, thyrotoxicosis, diabetic nephropathy, pheochromocytma, congenital adrenal hyperplasia)
Iatrogenic (steroid therapy, sympathomimetic drugs, anxiety/stress)
Neurologic (poliomyelitis, encephalitis, increased ICP, spinal cord injury)
Renal (glomerulonephritis, Wilms' tumour, Polycystic Kidney Disease)
Essential Hypertension

Adapted from Kliegman R, Nelson WE. 2006. *Nelson Essentials of Pediatrics*. Philadelphia, PA: Elsevier Saunders. pp.764.

Head & Neck
1. Cranial Nerves – see the ***Neurological Exam*** p. 181
2. Oral Cavity and Pharynx – see the ***Head & Neck Exam*** p. 116
   - Of particular note in adolescents:
   - Teeth – check for poor dental hygene, enamel erosion from vomiting or tooth grinding (bruxism)
   - Tonsils
     - *Infectious mononucleosis* – can appear greyish
     - *Streptococcal infection (strep throat)* – erythema, edema
     - *Peritonsillar abscess* – asymmetric enlargement of tonsils (with lateral displacement of uvula towards unaffected tonsil)
     - *Viral pharyngitis* – diffuse redness across tonsils and pharynx (without tonsillar exudate)
3. Nose and Paranasal Sinuses – see the ***Head & Neck Exam*** p. 114

4. Thyroid – see the *Head & Neck Exam* p. 123
  - In adolescence, Hashimoto's thyroiditis > asymptomatic goiter > Grave's disease
  - *Hypothyroidism* – mostly caused by Hashimoto's thyroiditis in adolescence
    - Growth and pubertal delay, menstrual dysfunction
    - Abnormally high weight gain, cold and dry skin
  - *Hyperthyroidism* – almost always caused by Grave's disease in adolescence
    - Emotional lability and sleep disturbance, change in school performance
    - Skin changes – eczema, erythema, excoriations, or smooth skin
5. Neck – see the *Head & Neck Exam* p. 120
  - Lymph Nodes
    - Palpate the occipital, post auricular, pre auricular, anterior cervical, submandibular, submental, and supraclavicular nodes
    - Infection (vast majority) – red, <2 cm, mobile, anterior (often strep) vs. posterior (mono) location
    - Malignancy (rare) – hard, fixed, >2 cm, with constitutional symptoms
  - Neck stiffness – suggestive of *meningitis*

Eyes – see the *Ophthalmological Exam*
  - Adolescents should have visual acuity screened q2-3 years
    - Use standard Snellen chart, with one eye covered

Clinical Pearl
Neck stiffness is suggestive of meningitis and can be discerned with the following two clinical signs (both while the patient is supine):
Brudzinski's sign: flexion of the neck causes involuntary flexion of the knee and hip
Kernig's sign: extension ofthe knee while the hip is flexed 90° is limited by knee extensor spasm and hamstring pain

---

Ears – see the *Head & Neck Exam* p. 108
  - Teenagers should have at least one hearing screen during adolescence
    - High incidence of childhood middle ear infections can compromise hearing
    - Screen with tuning forks between 500-2,000 Hz frequency

Breast/Chest Wall – see the *Breast Exam*

Breast
  - Thelarche (budding of breast at onset of puberty) occurs at roughly 11 years old; is one of earliest signs of puberty
    - Age of onset variable among different ethnicities; earlier in black teenagers
  - Inspection
    - Inspection of breasts – **4 S**'s
      - **S**ize, **S**hape, **S**ymmetry, **S**kin changes
      - Normal to have asymmetry because one breast may develop more rapidly
    - Inspection of nipples – **6 S**'s
      - **S**ize, **S**hape, **S**ymmetry, **S**kin changes, **S**pontaneous secretions, **S**upernumerary nipples

- Sexual Maturation – can assign Tanner Stage (see *Gynecological Exam* p. 99)
  - Stage 1: *preadolescent breast*, with elevated papilla
  - Stage 2: *breast bud stage*; small elevation of breast and papilla; areola diameter enlarges
  - Stage 3: further enlargement of breast and areola, but their contours are not separated
  - Stage 4: projection of areola and papilla to form secondary mound
  - Stage 5: *mature breast*; areola recess to general contour of breast
- In males – inspect for gynecomastia
  - Usually benign, self-limited; seen in up to 50-60% of adolescent boys
  - *Etiology:* idiopathic, 1° or 2° hypogonadism, hyperthyroidism, anti-androgen drugs, cancer chemotherapy
  - *Typical appearance:* 1-3 cm, round, freely mobile, often tender, firm mass beneath areola
  - Further investigation if: large, hard, fixed enlargement or mass/nodules
- Palpation: see *Breast Exam*; see **Table 18** for causes of palpable breast masses

Table 18. Causes of Breast Masses in Children and Adolescents

Causes	
Classic or Juvenile Fibroadenoma	Intraductal Papilloma
Fibrocystic Changes	Fat necrosis/lipoma
Breast Cyst	Abscess/Mastitis
Neoplasm (carcinoma <1%)	Adenomatous Hyperplasia

Adapted from Kliegman R, Nelson WE. 2006. *Nelson Essentials of Pediatrics*. Philadelphia, PA: Elsevier Saunders. p 347.

Chest Wall
- Inspect for development of chest hair (characteristic of increased androgens)
  - Amount of chest hair highly variable
  - If chest hair present in females, suspect excess androgen

Respiratory – see the *Respiratory Exam*
- In adolescents, should be particularly aware of the following:
  - Asthma: wheezing, variable coughing (can be dry or wet), worsening with certain triggers (exercise, cold weather, environmental allergens)
  - Bronchitis: cough that is loose and "rattling," bronchial breath sounds
  - Cystic fibrosis: chronic cough, persistent crackles and wheezing, and digital clubbing due to recurrent respiratory infections

Cardiovascular – see the *Cardiovascular Exam* and the *Peripheral Vascular Exam*
- Specific sign in adolescents:
  - Bradycardia, postural hypotension – associated with anorexia nervosa

Abdominal – see the *Abdominal Exam*

Inspection
- Central adiposity vs. malnourishment/cachexia
- Lanugo (baby-like) hair – associated with anorexia nervosa

Auscultation and Percussion
- Bowel sounds
- Percuss all 4 quadrants, liver, and spleen
  - Splenomegaly in infectious mononucleosis, or leukemia/lymphoma

Palpation
- Light and deep palpation (tenderness, masses, peritoneal signs)
- Liver and spleen
- Kidney
- Special tests: appendicitis (see *Abdominal Exam* p. 43)
  - Appendicitis is the most common indication for emergency abdominal surgery in childhood; its frequency peaks between ages 15-30 years

Musculoskeletal – see the *Musculoskeletal Exam*
- Common MSK injuries in adolescents:
  - Knee
    - *Patellofemoral dysfunction* – deep, aching anterior knee pain worsened by prolonged sitting, knee instability (common in female athletes)
    - *Anterior cruciate ligament (ACL) tear* – after "cutting" movement in sports
    - *O'Donoghue's Unhappy Triad/Skier's Knee* (ACL, medical collateral ligamental, medial/lateral meniscus) – after valgus knee injury
  - Ankle – most common acute injury in adolescent athletes
    - Inversion – 85% acute ankle injuries
    - Eversion – often more serious because higher risk of fracture or injury to tibio-fibular syndesmosis
- Uncommon, but not to be missed:
  - *Slipped capital femoral epiphysis (SCFE)* – displacement of proximal femoral epiphysis (usually posteromedially) due to disruption of growth plate
    - Most common in obese adolescent males
    - *Common presentation:* acute, severe pain with limp
    - *Key signs:* limited internal rotation of hip + obligate external rotation on hip flexion (Whitman's sign)

Neurological – see the *Neurological Exam*

Dermatologic
- Pubertal changes
  - Acne (comedonal, papular or pustular inflammatory, nodulocystic); seen in 85% of adolescents
  - Pigmentation of areolae, external genitalia
  - Development of pubic and axillary hair
- Other
  - *Tinea pedis (athlete's foot)* – fungal infection
    - Scaling, fissuring, erythema at soles of feet and toe webs
  - *Contact dermatitis*
    - Vesicular, erythematous, well-defined lesions
  - *Atopic dermatitis (eczema)*
    - Itchy, dry, slightly elevated papular lesions that form plaques
    - Face, neck, hands, and flexor surfaces of joints
  - *Psoriasis* – 25% of cases have onset in adolescent years
    - Erythematous, circumscribed plaques with silvery scaly appearance
  - *Pitting and ridging nail changes* – associated with anorexia nervosa

Genitourinary

Female

- Please see the ***Gynecological Exam*** for detailed description
- Important points with respect to the adolescent female:
- *Indications for pelvic examination (otherwise not necessary until 18 years)*
  - Abnormal vaginal discharge, pelvic pain, history of unprotected sexual intercourse, menstrual irregularities, suspicion of anatomic abnormalities, patient request

Inspection
- External genitalia
- Pubic hair – assign Tanner staging based on amount and quality
  - Stage 1: prepubertal
  - Stage 2: sparse hair at labia/base of penis
  - Stage 3: hair over pubis
  - Stage 4: coarse adult hair
  - Stage 5: hair extends to medial thigh
- Internal genitalia (speculum examination)
  - Cervix, vagina

Palpation
- External genitalia (labia, clitoris, vagina), internal genitalia (cervix, uterus), adnexa – as in adult
- Not to be missed:
  - Triad of tender adnexal mass, vaginal bleeding, and abdominal/pelvic pain = ectopic pregnancy until proven otherwise

Evidence-Based Medicine: HPV Vaccine
In a 2007 systematic review of 9 RCTs, prophylactic HPV vaccination was found to be highly efficacious in the prevention of HPV infection, high- and low-grade precancerous lesions and genital warts amongst women aged 15-25 years.

Rambout et al. 2007. *CMAJ* 177(5):469-479.

Male

- Please see the ***Urological Exam*** for detailed description

Inspection
- Assign Tanner Stages of pubertal maturation (see **Table 20**)
- Pubic hair – assign Tanner staging (see above)

Palpation
- Supraclavicular lymaphdenopathy (metastasis from genitourinary neoplasm)
- Penis, scrotum, inguinal hernias, inguinal lymph nodes
- DDx of painless scrotal mass in adolescent male: testicular cancer, hydrocele, spermatocele, varicocele, indirect inguinal hernia, abscess

Table 20. Tanner Stages – Male Genitalia

Stage	Description
1	Testes: volume <1.5 mL Phallus: childlike
2	Testes: volume 1.6 – 6 mL Phallus: no change Scrotum: reddened, thinner, larger
3	Testes: volume 6-12 mL Phallus: increased length Scrotum: greater enlargement
4	Testes: volume 12-20 mL Phallus: increased length, circumference Scrotum: further enlargement, darkening
5	Testes: volume >20 mL Phallus: adult Scrotum: adult

Adapted from Neinstein LS. 2008. *Adolescent Health Care: A Practical Guide.* Philadelphia: Wolters Kluwer/Lippincott Williams & Wilkins.

COMMON INVESTIGATIONS

- Pap smear
- Gonorrheal and chlamydial swabs
- Sexually transmitted infections (STI) testing
- Please see the *Gynecological Exam* and the *Essentials of Infectious Diseases*

COMMON CLINICAL SCENARIOS AND DISORDERS

Head & Neck

Oral Candidal Thrush
- Common up to 3-4 months; investigate for underlying condition if persistent/recurrent episodes
- *Signs:* cracking at mouth corners and whitish patches on buccal mucosa
  - Milk can be scraped off with a tongue depressor, while thrush cannot

Otitis Media ("Ear Ache")
- *Chief Complaint:* ear pain, fever, irritability, pulling at ears, persistent crying
- *Signs:* bulging, immobile, erythematous tympanic membrane, and painful ear
- *Investigations:* usually none, tympanometry and audiometry if severe/uncertain diagnosis or hearing loss >3 mos
- *Causes: S. pneumoniae, H. influenzae, Moraxella catarrhalis* most common

Pharyngitis/Tonsillitis
- *Chief complaints:* sore throat, fever, stridor, shortness of breath, hoarseness, dysphagia, neck mass/swollen neck
- *Signs:* see **Table 21**
- *Investigations:* throat swab, rapid strep test, mono-spot

Table 21. Common and Serious Causes of Pharyngitis/URTI

Illness	Clinical Characteristics
Viral Pharyngitis†	Gradual onset; low grade fever; rhiorrhea/cough; conjunctivitis; hoarseness
Group A Strep	McIsaac Criteria: fever; age 3-14, anterior cervical lymphadenopathy; no cough; tonsillar erythema/exudate
Mononucleosis (EBV)	Fever, severely exudative, erythematous, hypertrophic tonsils; posterior cervical adenopathy; hepatosplenomegaly
Vincent's Angina/ Trench Mouth	High fever; halitosis; adenopathy; bleeding, engorged, exudative tonsils with grey pseudomemrane
Quincy/Peritonsilar abscess	Asymmetric hypertrophied, erythematous, exudative, ulcerated tonsil(s); uvula deviated away from affected side
Oral HSV (primary infection)	Gradual onset; high fever; acute gingivostomatitis; ulcerating vesicles throughout anterior mouth including lips, with sparing of posterior pharynx, pain with oral fluids
Epiglotitis	Sudden onset; high fever; drooling; dysphagia; dysphonia (hot potato voice); significant respiratory distress; tripod sit; irritability/lethargy; thumb print sign on neck AP x-ray
Croup	Sudden onset; fever; barking cough, non-productive cough; worse at night; stridor; hoarse voice; steeple sign CXR
Bacterial tracheitis	Similar to croup, then rapid deterioration, high fever and lack of response to treatment for croup

†Most common cause (80% of pharyngitis)

Respiratory

Asthma
- *Chief complaints:*
  - Shortness of breath from: physical activity, environmental allergens (animal dander, dust, house dust mites, pollen), food (eggs, seafood, peanut butter), smoke, weather changes, exposure to cold, and stress
  - Dry, tight, occasionally wheezy cough especially at night
  - Eczema in atopic child, especially in flexural surfaces
- *Signs:* expiratory phase longer than inspiratory phase, with high-pitched wheezes throughout inspiration and most of expiration
- *Investigations:* pulmonary function tests, eosinophil count, sputum examination, chest x-ray, allergen identification

---

Evidence-Based Medicine: Asthma
Asthma is considered well-controlled if daytime symptoms are <4 d/week, nighttime symptoms are <1 night/week, there is normal physical activity, infrequent exacerbations, no absence from school and the need for a β2-agonist is <4 doses/week.

Becker et al. 2007. *CMAJ* 173(6 suppl.):S12-S14.

Cough
- *Chief complaints:* productive or non-productive, worse at night/day
- *Signs:* see **Table 22**
- *Investigations:* CXR, ± CBC and sputum culture, mantoux test if suspect TB

Table 22. Qualities of Cough Associated with Common Respiratory Illnesses

Illness	Character of Cough
Asthma	Dry, "tight", occasionally wheezy; wet asthma cough can mimic cystic fibrosis cough; spasmodic asthma cough can mimic pertussis (without whoop)
Bacterial tracheitis	Brassy cough that does not respond to standard croup therapies; inspiratory and/or expiratory stridor; rapid decompensation
Bronchiolitis	Initially dry; may become "loose and rattling"
Croup	Sounds like a seal's bark; sudden hoarse voice and inspiratory stridor at night
Cystic fibrosis	Productive or purulent
Pertussis	During coughing spasm, sudden crowing inspiration (whoop) in between coughs, often followed by vomiting
Pneumonia	Paroxysmal, dry, and staccato (short inspiration between coughs)
Psychogenic	Uncommon, cough sounds like a loud goose "honk"; never occurs during sleep
Pulmonary aspiration	Dry or loose; often associated with lower airway obstruction; can be similar to cough of asthma or bronchitis
Tracheomalacia	Loud, brassy or vibratory; can be associated with a coarse inspiratory and expiratory stridor/wheeze

Adapted from Goldbloom RB. 2003. *Pediatric Clinical Skills*. Philadelphia: Saunders 2003

Cardiovascular

Heart Failure
- *Chief complaints:* shortness of breath, exercise intolerance, pre-syncope or sycopal episodes
- *Signs:* peripheral edema, failure to thrive, cyanosis, clubbing, heart murmur
- *Investigations:* CXR, ECG, 4 limb BPs, consider echocardiogram,

Table 23. Timing of Heart Failure

Timing of heart failure	Significance
At birth	Rare (hemolysis, fetal-maternal transfusion, neonatal lupus)
First week of life	Obstructive lesion or persistent pulmonary hypertension (this can present later in Trisomy 21 cases, as their lungs are more compliant to start with)
4-6 weeks	Left-to-right shunting
After 3 months	Myocarditis, cardiomyopathy or paroxysmal tachycardia

Gastrointestinal

Jaundice
- Common in the first week of life
- Visible at serum bilirubin levels of 85-120 μmol/L
- Etiology: see **Table 24**
- Clinical characteristics
  - Yellowed skin, scleral icterus
  - Acute bilirubin encephalopathy: lethargic, slight hypotonia, poor sucking, high pitched cry → no feeding, increased tone, coma

Table 24. Differential Diagnosis of Jaundice in the Neonatal Period

Time of Appearance	Possible Etiology
<24hrs of birth	***ALWAYS PATHOLOGIC*** Hemolysis: Rh/ABO incompatibility Sepsis: GBS/TORCH infection
24-72hrs	Physiologic Breastfeeding/Dehydration *Hemolytic:* G6PD/PKU deficiency, thalassemia, spherocytosis *Non-hemolytic:* hematoma, polycythemia, hypothyroidism, sepsis
72-96hrs	Physiologic Breastfeeding Sepsis
>1wk	Breast milk jaundice Inborn errors of metabolism: galactosemia Neonatal hepatitis Idiopathic: TPN Biliary atresia

Maisels MJ. 2006. Neonatal Jaundice. *Pediatr Rev* 27:443-454.

- Investigations
  - CBC, Blood group and screen, peripheral blood smear, Coombs test, Direct and Indirect Bilirubin
  - Other: TSH, G6PD
  - If suspect sepsis: CBC + differential, blood C+S, urine C+S; consider CXR and LP if fever

Rectal Bleeding
- *Chief complaints:* bright red blood on toilet paper, blood in underwear, blood tinged water in toilet bowl, blood coating stool
- Caution: large amounts of blood associated with hemodynamic instability and melena suggest more ominous source of GI bleeding
- *Etiology:* see **Table 25**
- *Investigations:* DRE, FOBT, stool cultures, O and P, abdominal x-ray, endoscopy only if serious bleed/uncertain diagnosis after initial investigations

Clinical Pearl

Physician assessment of neonatal jaundice, based on clinical appearance, is not consistent or precise enough to use for prediction of elevated bilirubin levels. Thus clinical judgement, with respect to bilirubin measurement, should be used on risk factors for severe hyperbilirubinemia and recognition of the extreme rarity of illness caused by hyperbilirubinemia in otherwise healthy infants.

Moyer VA, Ahn C, Sneed S. 2000. *Arch Pediatr Adolesc Med* 154(4):391-394.

Table 25. Differential Diagnosis of Rectal Bleeding

Category	Differential Diagnosis
Obstructive	Intussusception Volvulus Hirshsprung's enterocolitis
Anatomical	Anal fissures[†] Polyps (hamartoma) Neoplasms (rare)
Inflammatory/ Allergic	IBD (>4 yrs) Henoch-Schönlein Purpura Milk protein allergy Celiac disease (gluten-sensitive enteropathy)
Vascular/ Hematologic	Rectal or colonic varices Vascular lesions Coagulopathy
Infectious	Bacterial: *Yersinia, Campylobacter, Shigella, E.Coli, Salmonella,* Perianal streptococcal cellulitis ("strep bum") Amebiasis
Other	Sexual abuse/rectal trauma Necrotizing enterocolitis

[†]Most common

Genitourinary

Enuresis/Incontinence
- May be nocturnal (nightime only), diurnal (day and night)
- Decreasing prevalence with age; 7% of 8 yr olds, 1% of 15 yr olds
- Classification:
  - *Primary* – child has never achieved dryness; associated with family history of delayed bladder control
  - *Secondary* – child had achieved dryness for at least 6 months before new onset of "accidents"
- *DDx:* psychosocial stressors, constipation, UTI, behaviour, diabetes, abuse, neurodevelopmental condition, cauda equina syndrome

Urinary Tract Infection (UTI)
- *Chief Compaint:* primarily age dependent, may present with fever, irritability and smelly/cloudy urine at any age
- Signs:
  - *Infant and young child (<2 years)*
    - Asymptomatic, or GI symptoms such as vomiting, poor feeding, diarrhea or abdominal pain
  - Child (>2 years)
    - *Cystitis:* dysuria, frequency, urgency, hematuria, urinary retention, suprapubic pain, pruritis, incontinence, enuresis, foul-smelling urine
    - *Pyelonephritis:* fever, chills, costovertebral pain and tenderness

- *Investigations:* urine culture, ultrasound, voiding cystourethrogram (VCUG)
- *Causes:* E. coli, *Klebsiella*, coagulase negative *Staphylococci* most common

Sexually-Transmitted Infections – See the **Essentials of Infectious Diseases** p. 454

MSK

Limp
- *Chief complaints:* painful or painless limp
- *Signs:* antalgic gait, swelling/erythema of hip or knee joint, leg length discrepancy, unusual/fixed positioning of leg at rest, fever
- *Investigations:* hip/pelvic x-ray A-P and frogleg, knee x-ray AP and lateral, CT scan of hip/knee as indicated
- *Differential Diagnosis* – painless vs. painful
  - *Painless Limp:* weakness secondary to hip dysplasia, cerebral palsy, leg-length discrepancy
  - *Painful Limp:* see **Table 26**

Table 26. Differential Diagnosis of Painful Limp

Differential Diagnosis	Peak Age (yr)	Features
Septic arthritis	All ages	Fever, antalgic gait, refusal to weight bear, severely limited internal roation and adduction of hip
Osteomyelitis	All ages	Point tenderness, local edema, erythema, restricted movement/pseudoparalysis, ± fever
Transient synovitis†	3-10	Antalgic gait, hip fixed in flexion/external rotation
Legg Calve Perthes	4-10	Mild, intermittent hip pain, referred to thigh/knee, limited internal rotation and abduction of hip
Osgood-Schlatter	11-18	Pain with activity, relieved by rest, insidious onset over months, tenderness over tibial tuberosity ± erythema
Slipped capital femoral epiphysis	8-17	Obese child, tenderness over hip joint capsule, restricted internal rotation and abduction; acute, painful limp
Malignancy		All: weight loss, constitutional symptoms
- Leukemia	2-10	Night pain, pallor, petechiae, infections, bruising
- Neuroblastoma	1-5	Abdominal Mass, night pain
- Osteosarcoma	5-20	Palpable mass, pathologic fracture
Juvenile Idiopathic Arthritis (JIA) (several types)	Varies	Persistent arthritis in children <16 years; classified by affected joints; may have constitutional symptoms, fever, extra-articular signs, nail and eye abnormalities

Table 26. Differential Diagnosis of Painful Limp (continued)

Differential Diagnosis	Peak Age (yr)	Features
Henoch-Schönlein Purpura	3-7	Following respiratory illness, purpuric rash over buttocks and legs, arthralgia, angioedema, abdo pain
Growing pains	3-10	Crampy night pain in calves and thighs, occasionally wakes child from sleep, bilateral; exam unremarkable

†Most common cause of hip pain/limp in children

Neurological

Table 27. Neonatal Primitive Reflexes

Reflex	How to Elicit	Reaction	Time Period
Galant	Stroke back approx 1 cm from midline with baby held prone	Trunk curves toward stroked side	Birth to 4-6 mos
Placing	Baby upright, touch top of foot to table edge	Child mimics walking onto table	Birth to 4-6 mos
Rooting	Stroke cheek	Head turns to same side	Birth to 4 mos
Palmar/Plantar grasp	Place finger into palm or sole of foot	Fingers and toes grasps together	Birth to 4-6 mos
Moro	Startle baby with loud noise or suddenly lower supine baby	Arms extend, abduct with hands open; then arms come together	Birth to 2 mos
Asymmetric Tonic Neck	Turn head to one side	Arm/leg on same side extend, flex on opposite side (fencing position)	Birth to 3-4 mos
Parachute reflex	Tilting the infant to side while in sitting position	Ipsilateral arm extension	6-8 mos

Febrile Seizures
- *Chief complaint*
  - Commonly in infants and young children 6 mos-5 yrs with febrile illness
  - Associated with fever but without evidence of 1) intracranial infection or 2) history of previous afebrile seizures
- Classic Features
  - <15 minutes, generalized seizure occurring once in 24-hour period
  - No focal neurological findings
  - Family history of febrile seizures
- *Investigations*
  - None unless
    - *Atypical seizure* – CT scan, EEG, LP
    - *Fever of unknown origin* – work up for possible sources of infection

Dermatological

Rashes

The following rashes will be described in the following Tables
- Infectious childhood diseases with cutaneous manifestations
- Non-infectious childhood skin disorders
- Differential diagnosis of diaper dermatitis

Table 28. Features of Infectious Childhood Diseases with Cutaneous Manifestations

Disease	Infectious Childhood Diseases Accompanying Lesions
Chicken pox (Varicella)	Pruritic rash progresses from macule-papule-vesicle-crust; begins on trunk and spreads to face, extremities
Measles	Erythematous maculopapular rash appears 5d after prodromal URTI, may be preceeded by white "Koplik" spots on buccal mucosa
Rubella	Fever, suboccipital lymphadenopathy, maculopapular rash, red spots on soft palate
Parvovirus B19	Erythematous maculopapular rash on trunk, with "slapped cheek" appearance to face
Roseola	Preceded by fever, pharyngitis, and posterior cervical lympadenopathy; pink, non-pruritic maculopapular rash erupts 1-2d after fever resolves.
Gianotti Crosti	Papular acrodermatitis rash on cheeks and extremities, trunk-sparing; viral prodrome
Coxsackie	Vesicular rash on hands and feet, accompanied by ulcers in mouth. Highly contagious.
Scarlet Fever	Strawberry tongue, circumoral pallor, generalized sandpaper rash, prominent in skin folds, ends with desquamation.
Molluscum Contagiosum	Small pearly nontender papules with central umbilication; primarily affects axillae, groin, neck
Tinea Corporis	Pruritic, annular papule/ plaque that expands outward; raised area of erythema and scale surrounds central clearing
Scabies	Pruritic rash, usually linear burrows and excoriation, particularly between finger webs, flexoral surfaces of wrists, armpits, and genital region

Table 29. Distribution and Characteristics Non-infectious Childhood Skin Disorders

Disorder	Childhood Disorders Accompanying Lesions
Eczema *(Atopic Dermatitis)*	*Acute:* erythema, vesicles, exudate and crusts *Chronic:* pruritic, dry, scaly and thickened rash *Infantile:* on cheeks, forehead, scalp and extensor surfaces *Childhood:* on wrists, ankles and flexor surfaces
Urticaria	Wheals may be small or large, discrete or confluent, sparse or profuse; wheals tend to come in crops, and fade in a few hours
Contact Dermatitis	Pruritic red swelling; may be well demarcated from normal skin; papules and bullae may be present

Table 30. Differential Diagnosis of Diaper Dermatitis

Disease	Primary Lesion	Secondary Lesion	Flexural Involvement	Other sites
Contact irritant dermatitis	Shiny, red macules/patches	Ulcerations, superficial erosions	Absent	None
Seborrheic dermatitis	Yellow, greasy papules/ plaques on an erythematous base	Scales	Present	Scalp, axilla, trunk
Candidal dermatitis	Bright red patches with peripheral scale, 'satellite lesions'	None	Present	Oral thrush
Psoriasis	Sharply well demarcated ares of papules/ plaques with thin scale	None	Present	Trunk, extremities, nails, scalp
Bullous impetigo	Bullae on an erythematous base	Superficial erosions, crusts	Present	Axillae or other areas

GENETIC DISORDERS

Table 31. Common Genetic Disorders – Autosomal

Condition	Cause	Signs
Down syndrome (Trisomy 21) 1/650-1,000 live births	Chromosomal abnormality, extra chr. 21 Associated with ↑ maternal age	Hypotonia and microcephaly Epicanthal folds Upward slanting palpebral fissures Stenotic Eustachian tubes Single palmar creases Congenital heart and abdominal defects Mild to moderate mental retardation Frequent respiratory infections
Edwards syndrome (Trisomy 18) 1/5,000 births <5% infants survive past 1 year	Chromosomal abnormality, extra chr. 18 Associated with ↑ maternal age	Growth retardation Simple, low-set ears Prominent occiput Micrognathia Overlapping fingers Rocker bottom feet Congenital heart, genital and CNS defects Hypertonia

Table 32. Common Genetic Disorders – Sex Chromosomal

Condition	Cause	Signs
Klinefelter syndrome (1/1,000 live male births; XXY in 80% of cases)	Aneuploidy of sex chromosomes Associated with ↑ maternal age	Long arms and legs, slim build Small testes 1-2 cm Gynecomastia Delays in language and emotional development Cognitive deficits variable; average IQ ~90 Often not diagnosed until adolescence
Turner syndrome (1/2,000-5,000 live female births)	Aneuploidy of sex chromosomes, usually XO	Short stature Streak gonads Webbed neck Lymphedema Coarctation of aorta Hypoplastic nails Learning disabilities

PSYCHIATRIC AND BEHAVIOURAL ISSUES

Anxiety Disorders (AD) (see *Psychiatric Exam* p. 326)
- Suggested that ~10% of children and adolescents experience some form of AD
- Note that transient development of age appropriate fears are common in childhood; therefore must evaluate degree of life disruption
- Watch for frequent repeat occurrences of anxiety related behaviours

Attention Deficit/Hyperactivity Disorder (ADHD)

- Common neurodevelopmental disorder (3-5% school-aged children)
- Triad of *inattentiveness, impulsivity and hyperactivity* such that behaviour interferes with functional ability (social and academic)
- Hyperactivity can be associated with this disorder; not always present
- Signs: distractible, tendency to fidget, tendency to interrupt, low attention span

Autism Spectrum Disorders

- Prevalence of Autistic Disorder is 20/10,000; prevalence of all Pervasive Developmental Disorders is 60-70/10,000
- M > F; early onset (15-30 months)
- Spectrum of developmental disorders characterized by impairment in:
  - *Social interaction:* non-verbal behaviour, peer relationships, and social/emotional reciprocity, sharing of enjoyment/interests
  - *Communication:* delayed spoken language, difficulty conversing, repetitive use of language, lack of imaginative/make-believe play
  - *Stereotyped behaviours:* preoccupation with narrow interests or parts of objects, inflexible adherence to routines, motor mannerisms
- Checklist for Autism in Toddlers (CHAT Screening Tool) is available and has a good specificity; PPV=83%, but a low sensitivity of 18%

Depression

- 1-3% of children, 4-8% adolescents, females:males = 2:1
- Persistent depressed or irritable mood present for most of nearly every day, or anhedonia (markedly diminished interest/pleasure activities)
- *Symptoms and Signs:*
  - Changes in sleeping patterns and appetite, inability to concentrate, feelings of worthlessness, fatigue, suicidal ideations and behaviours
  - Atypical presentations in adolescents include anger, oppositional behaviours
  - Highly associated with other psychiatric issues – anxiety, somatic complaints, relationship problems, academic concerns, drug usage
- Take suicide threats seriously; 80% of suicidal teens seek help beforehand

Sleep Disorders

- 20-30% of children experience sleep disturbances at some point in their first 4 years; 10-12% experience by school-age
- Common parasomnias: night terrors, sleepwalking and sleep-talking; considered developmentally normal; treatment is reassurance

Eating Disorders (Anorexia Nervosa and Bulimia Nervosa)

- *Prevalence:* 0.5% anorexia, 2-4% bulimia; female:male ratio = 9:1, highest in adolescent females of developed nations
- *Risk Factors:* family history, low self-esteem, immaturity, poor family dynamics
- Expresses fears of obesity associated with alteration in perception of body image, and preoccupation with becoming or staying thin
- Disordered eating (especially AN) can be found as part of the *"Female Athletic Triad"* – disordered eating, osteoporosis, and amenorrhea
- See comparison in **Table 33**

Table 33. Anorexia Nervosa and Bulimia Nervosa

	Anorexia Nervosa	Bulimia Nervosa
Key feature	Refusal to maintain body weight at or above 85% expected	Recurrent binge eating with inappropriate compensatory behaviours (self-induced vomiting, laxatives, diuretics)
Amenorrhea	Yes	No
Epidemiology	0.5% adolescent females 0.05% adolescent males Peak incidence 15-19 yrs	1-5% adolescent females Peak incidence early 20s
Subtypes	1. Restricting (no compensatory behaviours) 2. Binge-eating/purging	1. Purging (vomiting, laxatives, diuretics) 2. Non-purging (compensatory behaviours: fasting, excessive exercise)
Physical signs	Emaciation, muscle wasting, lanugo, hypothermia, starvation edema, bradycardia, arrhythmias, carotenemia (from excess carrot ingestion)	Muscle weakness, tooth decay, parotid gland enlargement, Russell's sign (knuckle calluses from self-induced vomiting), bloodshot eyes
Body weight	BMI <18	Normal or higher than average

Aggressive Behaviours
- *Oppositional Defiant Disorder*
  - Negativistic, hostile, and defiant behaviour
  - Features: losing temper, arguing with parents, refusal to comply with rules, blames others for mistakes, angry/resentful
  - Must cause clinically significant impairment in social, academic, or occupational functioning
  - May progress to Conduct Disorder; usually onset before age 8
- *Conduct Disorder*
  - Repetitive, persistent pattern of behaviour in which basic rights of others and age-appropriate social norms/rules are violated
  - Features:
    - Aggression: bullying, initiating fights, cruelty to animals or people
    - Property destruction: setting fires, destroying others' property
    - Deceitfulness or theft: lying to obtain goods, breaking and entering
    - Serious violation of rules: staying out, running away from home, truancy

CHILD ABUSE
- *Definition:* violence, mistreatment, or neglect of a child while in the care of a parent, sibling, relative, caregiver, or guardian

Physician's Role
- *Mandatory Reporting Requirement:* physicians are responsible to report any "reasonable grounds to suspect" child abuse; not reporting to Children's Aid Society is an offence (in Ontario)
- Physician's duty to report overrides provisions of confidentiality

History
- Listen and believe reports with non-judgmental and caring attitude
- Any statements made by a child about abuse should be recorded as direct quotes
- Questions about what, who, when, how often, threats, bribes must be open-ended
- Observe behaviours of child and caretaker
  - Are caretaker responses appropriate and consistent?
  - Does the child have exaggerated aggressiveness or passivity, or suggest sexualized overtones?

Physical Exam
- Always do a complete physical exam (pictorializing on a diagram whenever possible), but especially noting the following:
  - *General:* height, weight, head circumference percentile
  - *H&N:* retina, eardrums, and oral cavity for signs of occult trauma
  - *GU:* genitalia, rectum
  - *MSK:* bone and joint tenderness, fractures (new or healed), ROM
  - *Derm:* bruises, bites, bruises, cuts, scars, puncture wounds; unusual number, shape and location warrant further investigation
- Red flags: lack of reasonable explanation, changing/vague history, history inconsistent with injury, or inappropriate level of concern by caretaker

---

Clinical Pearl
Rib fractures in children are highly predictive of non-accidental injury

---

Common Disorders Related to Abuse
- Malnutrition; developmental delay
- Emotional difficulty: anxiety, depression, self-harm, suicide attempts, PTSD
- Head injury – leading cause of death from child abuse
- Physical and mental health problems as adults and high risk lifestyle choices

Table 34. Indicators of Child Abuse

Types of Abuse	Signs and Symptoms	
Neglect: Failing to provide basic needs	*Behavioural indicators:* Frequent absence from school Poor hygiene Delinquent acts, alcohol/drug abuse	*Physical indicators:* Pale, listless, unkempt Poor hygiene Failure to thrive without identifiable organic disease Indiscriminately seeks affection
Physical abuse: Deliberately using force against child	*Behavioural indicators:* Cringe/flinch if touched unexpectedly Infants may have a vacant stare Extremely aggressive or withdrawn Extremely compliant and/or eager to please Delay in seeking medical attention Fear, anxiety, depression, low self-esteem, social withdrawal, poor school performance, self-harm	*Physical indicators:* Posterior rib fractures Distinct marks: cigarette burns, loop marks, belt buckles Untreated fractures Presence of several injuries over a period of time and/or in various stages of healing
Sexual abuse: Includes fondling, sexual touching, intercourse, rape, sodomy, exhibitionism or child pornography	*Behavioural indicators:* Age inappropriate play with toys, self or others displaying explicit sexual acts Age inappropriate sexually explicit drawing/description Bizarre, sophisticated or unusual sexual knowledge Prostitution and seductive behaviours	*Physical indicators:* Unusual or excessive itching in genital or anal area Torn, stained or bloody underwear Pregnancy; bruising, swelling or infection in genital or anal area, venereal disease, STDs
Shaken Baby Syndrome: Forceful shaking of infant or young child	*Behavioural indicators:* *Acute:* spectrum from vomiting, irritability to loss of consciousness or death *Long-term:* Developmental Disability, speech/learning disability	*Physical indicators:* Minimal to no evidence of external trauma Severe closed head injury, diffuse brain injury and swelling, subdural/subarachnoid and retinal hemorrhages Fractures, especially posterior ribs Paralysis, hearing loss, seizure, death

PEDIATRIC

GROWTH AND DEVELOPMENT

Obesity

- 26.5% of the American adolescent population is obese (age 12-19 years)
- Overweight (BMI 25.0-29.9), obese class I (BMI 30.0-34.9), obese class II (BMI 35.0-39.9)
- *Risk Factors:* absence of family meals, excessive consumption, excessive television viewing, sedentary lifestyle
- Assessment should include:
  - *Measurements* – height, weight, calculation of BMI
  - *History* – diet (meals and snacks, portion sizes, frequency of meals outside of home, family meals), activity (sedentary activities, vigorous activities)
  - *Physical examination* – BP, adipose distribution (central vs. generalized), markers of comorbidities (hepatomegaly, hirsutism, etc.)

REFERENCES

Canadian Immunization Guide. Ottawa: Health Canada, Population and Public Health Branch.

Anstine D, Grinenko D. 2000. Rapid screening for disordered eating in college-aged females in the primary care setting. *J Adolesc Health* 26(5):338-342.

Becker A, Berube D, Chad Z, Dolovich M, Ducharme F, et al. 2005. Canadian Pediatric Asthma Consensus guidelines, 2003 (updated to December 2004): introduction. *CMAJ* 173(6 Suppl):S12-14.

Bickley VA, Szilagyi PG, Bates B. 2007. *Bates' Guide to Physical Examination and History Taking*. Philadelphia: Lippincott Williams & Wilkins.

Engel J. 2002. *Pocket Guide to Pediatric Assessment*. St. Louis: Mosby.

Feldman W. 2000. *Evidence-Based Pediatrics*. Hamilton, ON; St. Louis: B.C. Decker.

Goldbloom RB. 2003. *Pediatric Clinical Skills*. Philadelphia: Saunders.

Haney I, Ipp M, Feldman W, McCrindle BW. 1999. Accuracy of clinical assessment of heart murmurs by office based (general practice) paediatricians. *Arch Dis Child* 81(5):409-412.

Hay W, Levin M, Deterding R, Sondheimer J. 2009. *Current Diagnosis and Treatment Pediatrics*. New York: McGraw-Hill Professional.

Kliegman R, Nelson WE. 2006. *Nelson Essentials of Pediatrics*. Philadelphia, PA.: Elsevier Saunders.

Lalani A, Schneeweiss S, Hospital for Sick Children. 2008. *Handbook of Pediatric Emergency Medicine*. Sudbury, Mass.: Jones and Bartlett Publishers.

Maisels MJ. 2006. Neonatal jaundice. *Pediatr Rev* 27(12):443-454.

Margolis P, Gadomski A. 1998. The rational clinical examination. Does this infant have pneumonia? *JAMA* 279(4):308-313.

Moyer VA, Ahn C, Sneed S. 2000. Accuracy of clinical judgment in neonatal jaundice. *Arch Pediatr Adolesc Med* 154(4):391-394.

Muhe L, Oljira B, Degefu H, Jaffar S, Weber MW. 2000. Evaluation of clinical pallor in the identification and treatment of children with moderate and severe anaemia. *Trop Med Int Health* 5(11):805-810.

Neinstein LS. 2008. *Adolescent Health Care: a Practical Guide*. Philadelphia: Wolters Kluwer/Lippincott Williams & Wilkins.

Rambout L, Hopkins L, Hutton B, Fergusson D. 2007. Prophylactic vaccination against human papillomavirus infection and disease in women: a systematic review of randomized controlled trials. *CMAJ* 177(5):469-479.

Rothman R, Owens T, Simel DL. 2003. Does this child have acute otitis media? *JAMA* 290(12):1633-1640.

Schafermeyer R. 1993. Pediatric trauma. *Emerg Med Clin North Am* 11(1):187-205.

The Peripheral Vascular Exam

Editors:
Hana Farhang Khoee, Sylvia Papp &
Ilana Saltzman

Faculty Reviewers:
Alan Barolet, MD, PhD, FRCP(C)
George Oreopoulos, MD, FRCS(C)

TABLE OF CONTENTS

Approach to Peripheral Vascular History and Physical Exam 299
Common Chief Complaints 299
Common Disorders 300
Focused History 300
Focused Physical 302
Common Investigations 306
Common Clinical Scenarios 307

APPROACH TO PERIPHERAL VASCULAR HISTORY AND PHYSICAL EXAM

In addition to general history taking, important aspects of the peripheral vascular history include:

- Risk factors for atherosclerosis
- Description of pain
- Skin changes – including colour, temperature, swelling, ulceration, gangrene
- History of thromboembolic diseases

Overview of the Physical Exam

- Inspection
  - Arterial (colour, temperature of skin)
  - Venous (erythema, pigmentation, inflammation, edema)
- Palpation
  - Presence and quality of pulses
  - Arterial: carotid, radial, brachial, abdominal aorta, femoral, popliteal, posterior tibial and dorsalis pedis
  - Venous: quality of edema – pitting vs. non-pitting
- Auscultation
  - Presence and quality of bruits – carotid, abdominal aorta, renal, and femoral
- Special Maneuvers
  - Arterial: Allen Test, Straight Leg Raise, and Rubor on Dependency
  - Venous: saphenous vein incompetence and Brodie-Trendelenburg Maneuver

COMMON CHIEF COMPLAINTS

- Chest, abdominal, or back pain (in the setting of acute aortic emergency)
- Pain in calf (especially on exercise)
- Skin ulceration
- Swelling
- Changes in skin temperature and colour

COMMON DISORDERS

Disorders marked with (✓) are discussed in **Common Clinical Scenarios**

Arterial
✓ Acute occlusion (embolus/thrombus)
✓ Chronic occlusion (claudication, limb threatening ischemia
✓ Abdominal aortic aneurysm (AAA)
✓ Cerebrovascular disease (carotid stenosis)

✓ **Vasculitides**

Venous
✓ Deep vein thrombosis
✓ Deep venous insufficiency
✓ Varicose veins
✓ Superficial thrombophlebitis

Lymphatic (see *Lymphatic System and Lymph Node Exam*)
Lymphangitis
Lymphedema

FOCUSED HISTORY

History of:
- Atherosclerotic risk factors
  - Smoking
  - Hypertension
  - Diabetes mellitus
  - Family history
  - Lifestyle (exercise, diet)
  - Elevated cholesterol
- Myocardial Infarction (MI) or Coronary Artery Disease (CAD)
  - Signs and symptoms of MI or CAD (see *Cardiovascular Exam* p. 67)
  - PVD often considered a "CAD equivalent"
  - Course of disease, hospitalization, medical and surgical treatment
- Congestive heart failure
  - Peripheral edema, pulmonary congestion, exercise intolerance
- Cerebrovascular Occlusive Disease
  - Signs and symptoms of stroke (see *Neurological Exam* p. 197) including: unilateral or bilateral weakness/paralysis of limbs, sensory deficits, speech difficulties, diplopia or amaurosis fugax, and facial droop
  - Neurological symptoms – e.g. dizziness, pre-syncope and syncope
  - Hemispheric symptoms
- Precipitants of venous thrombosis
  - Recent prolonged immobilization (DVT)
  - Post-operatively (esp. orthopedic, thoracic, GI, GU)
    - Trauma (esp. fractures of femur, pelvis, spine, tibia)
    - Post-MI, CHF
    - Long travel
  - Hormone-related: pregnancy, oral contraceptive pill use, hormone replacement therapy, SERMs
  - Inheritable hypercoaguability states:
    - APLA syndrome, Factor V Leiden, Prothrombin G20210A, etc.
  - Underlying malignancy or blood dyscrasias
- Risk factors for thromboembolic event
  - Atrial Fibrillation, post-MI <3 months, valvular disease, prosthetic valves, endocarditis, cardiomyopathy
- Vasculitis
  - Skin changes, mucosal ulcerations
  - Joint pain
  - Changes in vision and/or eye pain

Symptoms of Ischemia

6P's

- **P**olar (cold): this comes first
- **P**ain: absent in 20% of cases due to prompt onset of anesthesia and paralysis
- **P**allor: replaced by mottled (network-like appearance) cyanosis within a few hours
- **P**aresthesia: light touch lost first (small fibers) followed by other sensory modalities (larger fibers)
- **P**aralysis/**P**ower loss: further progression of ischemia, heralds severity
- **P**ulselessness
- Do NOT expect all of the 6 P's to be present and do NOT rely on pulses
- Of the 6 P's, the most important are parasthesia and paralysis, as they suggest critical ischemia

Pain

- **OPQRSTUVW** with emphasis on:
    - Onset (acute, associated with parasthesia)
    - Location (temple, muscles, abdomen)
    - Pain in lower extremities during exercise (e.g. pain in calves, thighs, hips, buttocks)
    - Dependent upon exertion (amount of walking, rate of walking, degree of incline)
    - Reproducible pain with similar exertion (consistent pattern)

Critical Ischemia

- Acute
    - 6 P's
    - Neuromotor dysfunction
- Chronic
    - Night pain
    - Rest pain (pain at all times and not relieved by dependency)
    - Tissue loss (ulceration/gangrene)

Skin

- Changes in colour, temperature, appearance
- Ulceration
    - Classification (traumatic, ischemic, neoplastic, venous, mixed, malignant)
    - Time and rate of development
    - If resulting from minor trauma (e.g. toes, heel), may indicate chronic ischemia
- Gangrene: wet (infectious) vs. dry (non-infectious)

FOCUSED PHYSICAL EXAM

General
- Ensure the patient is adequately exposed with draping in between the legs
- Remember to compare sides

Inspection
- **Specific locations**
  - Upper extremities (from the finger tips to the shoulder)
  - Lower extremities (from the groin and buttocks to the toes)
  - Inspect for:
    - Masses, scars, lesions
    - Symmetry – muscle bulk (atrophy/hypertrophy)
    - Size – swelling, thickening
    - Skin – colour, shiny, hair loss, erythema/discolouration, gangrene
    - Ulcers – arterial: between toes and heel; venous: medial malleolus
    - Nails – note colour and texture
- **Arterial Insufficiency**
  - Cyanosis: central (frenulum and buccal mucosa) and peripheral (fingernails)
  - Skin: cool, pale extremities, increased pigmentation, swelling, heaviness and aching in legs (usually medial lower third of legs)
  - Ulcers: ischemic ulceration due to trauma of the toes and heel, develops rapidly, painful and has discretely visible edges
- **Venous stasis**
  - Skin: warm, thickening and erythema over the ankle and lower leg (dependent areas), thickened (woody) fibrosis/lipodermatosclerosis
  - Ulcers: stasis ulceration of ankle or above medial malleolus, develops slowly, painless, diffuse with no distinct borders
  - Veins: engorgement, varicosities
    - Prominent veins in edematous limb may be venous obstruction
  - Chronic venous insufficiency: warm, erythematous, thickened skin, increased pigmentation, ± brown ulcers around ankles
  - Superficial phlebitis: warm, painful, erythema secondary to inflammation around vein
  - Acute DVT: pain secondary to inflammation in absence superficial changes, swelling of distal part of extremity
- **Vasculitis**
  - Skin:
    - Livedo reticularis rash (bluish-red discolouration, network pattern)
    - Malar or discoid rash on face in SLE
    - Raynaud's phenomenon: episodes of sharply demarcated pallor and/or cyanosis, then erythema of the digits
    - Purpura
  - Mucosa: Oral or nasal ulcers (SLE, Wegener's, Behçet's)
  - Joints: Look for "active" swollen joints
  - Eyes: Episcleritis, scleritis, anterior uveitis (iritis)
  - Venous and arterial thrombosis/ulcers, ulcers, gangrene as above

Palpation and Auscultation
- **Arterial**
  - Assess skin temperature (feel with back of hand – warm vs. cool)
  - Look for capillary refill by compressing nailbeds and assessing the duration for return of circulation – normal = 2-3 seconds

- **Pulses**
  - Rate: tachycardia >100 bpm, bradycardia <60 bpm
  - Rhythm: regular, regularly irregular (consistent pattern), irregularly irregular
  - Amplitude:
    - 0 = Absent
    - 1 = Diminished
    - 2 = Normal
    - 3 = Increased
    - 4 = Aneurysmal (often exaggerated, widened pulse)
  - Always compare both sides for presence and symmetry
  - Rate and rhythm generally described for radial pulse only
- Examine the following pulses (see **Figure 1**):
  - **Carotid**
    - Auscultate for bruits (absent, mild/soft, harsh/loud)
    - If no bruits, palpate one carotid artery at a time
  - **Brachial**
    - May use thumb to palpate
  - **Radial**
    - Use the pads/tips of three fingers
    - Significant delay of the radial pulse after the brachial pulse may suggest aortic stenosis
  - **Abdominal Aorta**
    - Palpate deeply for pulsations (lay patient flat, ensure abdomen is relaxed)
    - Auscultate for abdominal bruits
    - Midline pulsatile abdominal mass may be an AAA
    - Midline abdominal bruit suggests atherosclerotic disease of the aorta or renal vessels
  - **Renal Arteries**
    - Auscultate for bruits at positions 5 cm above the umbilicus and 3-5 cm to either side of the midline or from the back
  - **Femoral**
    - Palpate at mid point of the inguinal ligament
    - Auscultate for bruits
    - Compare timing of femoral pulse with radial pulse to rule out radio-femoral delay
    - Significant delay of the femoral pulse after the radial pulse suggests coarctation of the upstream aorta (most commonly thoracic, however abdominal coarctation is also possible)
  - **Popliteal**
    - Flex the knee approximately 10-20°
    - Using two hands, place thumbs on the tibial tuberosity and palpate deeply in the popliteal fossa with 3 to 4 fingers from each hand (allow knee to relax/fall into 2 hands)
    - A decreased or absent pulse indicates partial or complete arterial occlusion proximally; all pulses distal to occlusion are typically affected
    - Prominent pulse may predict popliteal aneurysm
  - **Posterior Tibial**
    - Palpate behind and slightly below the medial malleolus
    - Chronic arterial occlusion of the legs causes intermittent claudication, postural colour changes and skin alterations
  - **Dorsalis Pedis** (absent in 15% of normal population)
    - Palpate on dorsum of the foot, lateral to extensor tendon the big toe

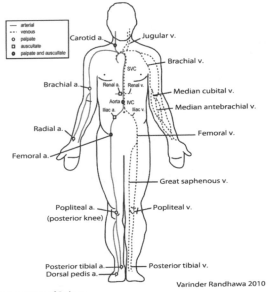

Figure 1. Location of Pulses

- Characteristic pulse patterns
  - **Hyperkinetic pulse**
    - Strong, bounding pulse
    - Increased stroke volume in heart block
    - Hyperdynamic circulation and increase stoke volume in fever, anemia, exercise, anxiety
    - Reduced peripheral resistance in patent ductus arteriosus, AV fistula
  - **Pulsus tardus**
    - Small, slowly rising pulse that is delayed with respect to heart sounds
    - Seen in aortic stenosis
  - **Pulsus parvus (hypokinetic)**
    - Small, weak pulse due to diminished LV stroke volume
    - Seen in hypovolemia, LV failure, MI, restrictive pericardial disease, shock, arrhythmia

Table 1. Description of Characteristic Wave Forms

Waveform	Description	Associated with/Etiology
Pulsus parvus et tardus (Anacrotic)	Small, slow rising pulse with drop or notch in ascending portion	Aortic stenosis
Collapsing	Quick rise, quick fall	Increased CO
Water-hammer	Sudden rapid pulse with full expansion followed by sudden collapse	Aortic regurgitation or arterial obstruction
Bisferiens	Double-peaked pulse with mid-systolic dip	Aortic regurgitation, ± aortic stenosis, hypertrophic cardiomyopathy
Alternans	Alternating amplitude of pulses	CHF, more easily detected in conjunction with BP measurement

Venous

Edema
- Check for pitting (venous) or non-pitting (lymphatic) edema
  - Press firmly with thumb over bony prominences for >5 sec
    - Over the dorsum of each foot
    - Behind each medial malleolus
    - Over the shins
    - If non-ambulatory, check for sacral edema
  - Pitting: depression caused by the pressure from your thumb
  - Pitting suggests orthostasis, chronic venous sufficiency or CHF
  - Firm, non-pitting edema (lymphedema) suggests lymphatic obstruction (see **Lymphatic System and Lymph Node Exam** p. 138)
  - Note height of leg edema and if swelling is unilateral or bilateral
  - Unilateral edema may suggest DVT
- When following patients with chronic edema (venous or lymphatic), it may be useful to document calf circumference at serial visits
  - A difference between the two sides suggests edema
  - >1 cm at the ankles and 2 cm at the calf
  - Muscular atrophy can also cause differences in leg circumference
- Note unusually prominent veins
- Chronic venous insufficiency can lead to dependent edema ('heaviness in the legs')
- With DVT, extent of edema may suggest location of occlusion:
  - A calf DVT if the lower leg or ankle is swollen
  - An iliofemoral DVT when the entire leg is swollen

SPECIAL TESTS

Arterial: Arterial Insufficiency

Allen Test
- Purpose: test for good collateral flow through the ulnar artery before proceeding with puncture of the radial artery for arterial blood gases
- Method
  - Using your thumbs, occlude the patient's radial and ulnar arteries at the wrist
  - At the same time, ask the patient to clench and open their fist several times (with patient's arm raised)
  - Ask patient to open their hand with the palm up – palm should be blanched
  - Then release pressure on the ulnar artery only, watch palm for "blushing"
- Normal Result: Colour returns to the hand in 5-10 seconds
- **Abnormal Result**: If colour does not return within 10 seconds, DO NOT perform arterial puncture at this site, as this may indicate incomplete palmar arch or insufficient collateral flow

Straight Leg Raise (Pallor on Elevation)
- Raise the leg 45-60° for 30 sec., or until pallor of the feet develops
- Normal Result: mild pallor on elevation
- **Abnormal Result**: Marked pallor on elevation may suggest arterial insufficiency

Rubor on Dependency
- After performing the Straight Leg Raise, ask the patient to sit up and dangle both legs over the side of the bed

- Normal Result: Return of colour within 10 seconds, filling of the superficial veins of the foot within 15 seconds
- **Abnormal Result**: Persistant pallor of the feet for >10 seconds followed by rubor (marked redness) on dependency (after 1-2 minutes) may be seen in patients with critical ischemia. The marked redness is due to arterial dilation following the tissue hypoxia induced by elevation of a leg with arterial insufficiency

Venous: Incompetent Saphenous Vein

Test for Incompetent Saphenous Vein
- Instruct patient to stand (dilated varicose vein will become obvious – note the location and distribution)
- Compress the vein proximally with one hand and place other hand 15-20 cm distally on the vein
- Briskly decompress/compress the distal site
- Normal Result: the hand on the proximal site should feel no impulse
- **Abnormal Result**: Any impulse transmitted to the proximal site indicates incompetent saphenous valves between the two sites

Brodie-Trendelenburg Maneuver
- Ask the patient to lie supine and raise his/her legs 90° for 15 seconds to empty the veins
- Place a tourniquet around the patient's upper thigh after the veins have drained (do not occlude arterial pulse)
- Instruct the patient to stand
- Watch for venous filling with the tourniquet still on for 60 seconds
- Normal Result: Superficial saphenous system should fill slowly from below the tourniquet within 35 seconds
- **Abnormal Results**: Early filling indicates incompetence of the deep and perforator veins. If refill is slower than normal, remove the tourniquet and observe the superficial venous system. Filling of veins from above (retrograde flow) suggests superficial venous incompetence
- Tourniquet can be used above and below knee to differentiate between long and short saphenous incompetence

COMMON INVESTIGATIONS

Angiography
- Inject a radio-opaque contrast agent into the blood vessel and image using x-ray based techniques
- Detects narrowing of vessels and vessel anatomy
- CTA and MRA can also be used as alternatives

Ankle Brachial Index
- ABI = ankle systolic pressure/brachial systolic pressure
- Measures the reduction in arterial blood pressure of the legs
- A Doppler U/S probe is placed over the artery (ankle and antecubital fossa). Distal to this, the sphygmomanometer is inflated until the pulse ceases. The cuff is then deflated until the Doppler probe detect the peripheral pulse again, allowing for the detection of systolic pressure
- ABI = 1.0-1.3 is normal
- ABI <0.5 warrants detailed investigation

Bloodwork

- Hypercoagulability workup:
  - PTT, PT/INR, factor assay
  - Deficiency of antithrombin III, protein C or S
  - Lupus anticoagulant, anti-cardiolipin antibody
  - C-ANCA, P-ANCA
  - D-dimers: useful to rule out DVT if negative and low clinical suspicion

Doppler Ultrasounography

- Detects the direction, velocity, and turbulence of blood flow by converting sound waves into images

COMMON CLINICAL SCENARIOS

ARTERIAL

Acute Arterial Occlusion/Insufficiency

- Patient has 6 hours before irreversible muscle injury (in the setting of complete ischemia)

Etiology

- Important to differentiate embolism from thrombosis because the treatment for the two varies dramatically
- **Embolus**
  - Cardiac source: (80-90%)
    - Palpitations, atrial fibrillation
    - MI (<3 mo. ago) – anterior MI most common
    - Rheumatic heart disease (rheumatic fever)
    - Known murmurs, abnormal or prosthetic valves
    - Mitral stenosis
    - Cardiomyopathy
    - Endocarditis
    - Atrial myxoma
  - Arterial source
    - Atheroembolism from plaques
    - Aneurysms
  - Paradoxical embolism
    - History of venous embolus passing through intracardiac shunt
  - Other with a history of
    - Medications (e.g. oral contraceptives increase DVT risk)
    - Previous emboli
    - Neurologic/TIAs (hemiplegias, sensory/visual deficits)
    - Abdominal pain
    - Peripheral pain, paresthesias in extremities
- **Arterial thrombosis**
  - Usually occurs in: a previously atherosclerotic artery, congenital anomaly, infection, hematologic disorders and low flow rates (e.g. CHF)
  - Occurs secondary to endothelial damage, stasis and hypercoagulability, however is frequently associated with a critical arterial stenosis
  - Check for a history of
    - Atherosclerosis risk factors
    - Claudication
    - Blood disorders (hypercoagulable states)
    - Recent bed rest

- ◆ Congestive heart failure
- ◆ Pregnancy
- ◆ Medications (i.e. oral contraceptive)
- **Trauma**
  - Check for a history of: trauma, arterial catheterization, intra-arterial drug injection

Symptoms/Signs
- **6 Ps** (refer to **Focused History** section)
- Depends on the etiology
- Presentation of embolus
  - Sudden onset of pain
  - Splenic, intestinal, renal artery emboli can cause acute abdominal or flank pain
  - Pulmonary emboli from the venous system can cause shortness of breath and pleuritic chest pain
  - Paresthesia can be caused by peripheral artery emboli
  - No past history of claudication
  - Pulses often present on contralateral limb
  - Emboli usually lodge at bifurcation of arteries
- Presentation of thrombosis
  - Onset over a few days or can be acute
  - Past history of claudication
  - Atrophic changes obvious
  - No contralateral pulses usually noted (this is evidence of chronic peripheral arterial diseases with bilateral disease)

Physical Exam
- Examine arterial pulses
- Assess colour and temperature of extremities (e.g. unilateral cool limb)

Investigations
- Doppler ultrasonography

Chronic Arterial Occlusion/Insufficiency

Etiology
- **Atherosclerosis** – most common
- **Arterial spasm**
- **Arteritis**
- **Buerger's disease** (thromboangiitis obliterans)
  - Rare disease characterized by a combination of acute inflammation and thrombosis (clotting) of the arteries and veins in the hands and feet
  - Typically in young male heavy smokers
- **Raynaud's Phenomenon**
  - Disease characterized by a combination of acute inflammation and thrombosis (clotting) of the arteries and veins in the hands and feet
  - Vasospasm of arterioles supplying toes and fingers producing sequential: pallor (white), cyanosis (blue), rubor (red)
  - Often induced by stress and cold
  - Often associated with connective tissue diseases, immune related diseases, ergotamine drugs

Symptoms/Signs
- Intermittent claudication
  - Pain in muscles of lower extremity during exercise (e.g. calves, thighs, hips, buttocks)
  - Dependent on amount of walking (time or distance), rate of walking, degree of incline
  - Discomfort arises when muscle exceeds its metabolic requirement because of arterial stenosis or occlusion
  - Relieved by rest (promptly)
  - Reproducible with specific exertion and not other maneuver (e.g. palpation)
  - Distinguish from neurospinal compression and osteoarthritis of knee or hip
- Neurogenic claudication
  - Discomfort with locomotion
  - Pain usually proximal/thigh, can be in a nerve distribution
  - Relieved by rest (prolonged) and flexion of spine
  - Climb hill – pain decreases, flex spine
- Osteoarthritic claudication:
  - Discomfort with locomotion
  - Pain usually localized to affected joints
  - Pain is often insidious and gradually progresses over years, with flare-ups and remissions relieved by rest (prolonged)
- Leriche's syndrome: if male patient complains of buttock or thigh pain while walking, inquire about impotence (intermittent claudication and impotence are features caused by chronic aortoiliac obstruction)
- Critical ischemia

Physical Exam
- Decreased or absent pulses
  - Look for abnormal femoral pulse in aortoiliac disease
- Significant bruits may be heard if 50% occlusion – if severe stenosis, no bruits
- Necrosis and atrophy
- Pallor on elevation/rubor on dependency

Investigations
- Ankle brachial index (ABI) <0.9
- Allen Test
- Straight Leg Raise and Refill Test
- Doppler ultrasonography

Abdominal Aortic Aneurysm (AAA)
- Definition – localized dilatation of an artery that is 2X normal diameter
- Clinically significant aneurysms are ≥5 cm in diameter or greater
- True Aneurysm – wall is made up of all 3 layers of the artery
- False Aneurysm – wall is made up of fibrous tissue or graft (e.g. organized hematoma)
- Location – 90% begin below the renal arteries
- Relevant history:
  - Previous diagnosis of AAA
  - Smoker or previous smoking (in 95%)
  - Atherosclerosis risk factors (esp. hypertension – see p. 300)
  - Family history of AAA
  - Cardiovascular disease
  - High risk groups

- >65 years old
- Male (4x more prevalent in males than females, women tend to present older and have worse outcomes, e.g. higher risk of rupture, higher rupture-related mortality, higher mortality after elective repair)
- Hypertension, PVD, CVD, CAD, COPD
- Positive family history of AAA

Etiology
- Degenerative (may manifest with secondary atherosclerosis)
- Hypertension and smoking can contribute to degeneration
- Genetic (e.g. Ehlers-Danlos and Marfan's syndrome)
- Trauma
- Mycotic, infection (syphilis)

Signs/Symptoms
- Asymptomatic (75%), often found on U/S or abdominal exam
- Ruptured
  - Classic triad: abdominal pain, pulsatile mass, hypotension
  - Pain typically radiates to back or flank
  - Other symptoms include syncope and shock (pale skin, hypotension, shallow, fast respirations, decreased level of consciousness)
  - Surgical emergency – rush to OR
  - Classic presentation is most often misdiagnosed as renal colic
    - e.g. severe abdominal pain radiating to the back or flank
    - 90% of abdominal aneurysms are infrarenal
    - Misdiagnosis can be avoided by having a high index of suspicion in patients with relevant history

Physical Exam – see **Evidence-Based Medicine** p. 311
- Classic triad
- Typical symptoms in triad may not be complete
  - Pulsatile mass may be hard to feel if person is obese or aneurysm is well tamponaded
  - Hypotension may be absent in person who is normally hypertensive
  - If in doubt, get imaging (plain non contrast CT), but if strongly suspect a ruptured AAA then get patient to OR immediately

Investigations
- CT scan
  - Done to assess extent of aneurysms
  - Usually abdomen and pelvis, however include chest if thorax involved
  - Also identifies anatomic abnormalities: retro aortic renal vein, left sided vena cava, dilatation of ureters, enhancing rim of aorta seen with inflammatory aneurysm
- Angiography
  - Done when considering operation or angioplasty or considering endo-vascular aneurysm repair (not used for diagnosis)
  - Risk of false aneurysm, hematoma or atheroembolism is 1-2%

Evidence-Based Medicine: Abdominal Aortic Aneurysm (AAA)
The only physical exam maneuver of demonstrated value for diagnosis of an AAA is abdominal palpation to detect a widened aorta.

Width of aorta by palpation	Sensitivity (%)	LR +	LR-
≥3.0 cm (all)	39	12.0	0.72
3.0 cm – 3.9 cm	29		
≥4.0 cm		15.6	0.51
4.0 cm – 4.9 cm	50		
≥5.0 cm	76		

Reference standard – abdominal ultrasound
• Positive findings on abdominal palpation greatly increase likelihood of large AAA
• Abdominal palpation is useful in detecting AAA large enough to require surgery, but cannot be relied on to exclude the diagnosis
• Sensitivity is diminished by abdominal obesity and by routine abdominal exam not specifically targeted at measuring aortic width

Lederle FA, Simel DL. 1999. *JAMA* 281: 77-82.

The long-term follow-up in the United Kingdom Small Aneurysm Trial (diameter 4.0 to 5.5 cm) indicated that, "there was no long-term survival benefit of early elective open repair of small abdominal aortic aneurysms. Even after successful aneurysm repair, the mortality among these patients was higher than in the general population."

Powell JT et al. 2007. Br J Surg 94:702-708.

Physical Sign	Sensitivity (%)	Specificity (%)
Definite pulsatile mass	28	97
Definite or suggestive pulsatile mass	50	91
Abdominal bruit	11	95
Femoral bruit	17	87
Femoral pulse deficit	22	91

Adapted from Swartz MH. 2006. *Textbook of Physical Diagnosis: History and Examination.*

Carotid Artery Disease

Etiology
- Atherosclerosis
- Dissection

Signs/Symptoms
- Transient Ischemic Attack (TIA) – lateralizing neurologic deficit (motor or sensory) lasting less than 24 hrs (usually 1 hr) and that completely reverses (CT normal)
- Amaurosis Fugax – transient blindness (total or sectorial) ipsilateral to side of pathology
- Stroke – similar to a TIA but lasting more than 24 hrs
- Check for a history of atherosclerotic risk factors, previous TIA, previous embolus/arrhythmias

Physical Exam
- Bruit
  - Carotid, but examine for bruits elsewhere as stenosis of any vessel provides evidence for the initiation of the atherosclerotic process
- Heart murmur
- Neurologic exam
- Fundoscopy
  - look for "Hollenhorst plaques": emboli that are visible as small bright flecks lodged in arterial bifurcations in the retina

Investigation
- Doppler ultrasonography
  - Duplex examination can diagnose the degree of stenosis
  - Symptomatic stenoses >70% benefit from carotid endarterectomy
  - 70% in asymptomatic stenosis also benefit from surgery
- PVD exam
  - Assess for atherosclerotic disease

Evidence-Based Medicine: Carotid Artery Stenosis
In the Northern Manhattan Study, the sensitivity and specificity of auscultation for the detection of clinically significant carotid stenosis was 56% and 98%, respectively. "The low false-negative rate suggests that auscultation is not sufficient to exclude carotid stenosis. An ultrasonography may be considered in high-risk asymptomatic patients, irrespective of findings on auscultation."

Ratchford EV et al. 2009. *Neurol Res* 21(7):748-752.

VENOUS

Deep Vein Thrombosis (Acute)

Etiology
- Virchow's Triad: Stasis, Hypercoagulability, Endothelial damage
  - Stasis causes:
    - Post-operative bed rest
    - Long airplane trip
    - Trauma and subsequent immobilization
    - Immobilization in acute MI, CHF, stroke and post-op surgical patients
    - Right heart failure, obstruction, shock
  - Hypercoagulability causes:
    - Estrogen use (e.g. oral contraceptive, HRT)
    - Pregnancy
    - Neoplasms (adenocarcinomas secreting mucins)
    - Tissue trauma (activation of coagulation)
    - Nephrotic syndrome
    - Hyperviscosity (polycythemia)
  - Endothelial damage causes:
    - Venulitis
    - Trauma

Signs/Symptoms
- A painful ache in the leg along with swelling after a long period of immobility
- Distinguishing between deep vein thrombosis and superficial vein thrombosis is critical because deep thrombi are far more prone to embolization than superficial
- Unilateral swelling
- Sudden swelling of thigh, ankle or hand, relieved by elevation or recumbence
- Erythema, warmth
- Tenderness over the involved vein may be present
- Pulmonary emboli (as a result of DVT)
  - Symptoms of PE are present in 10% of DVT patients
  - Shortness of breath, tachycardia, tachypnea

- Anxiety
- Generalized malaise
- Fever
- Venous distention
- Erythema
- Fever
- Tachycardia
- Warmth

Physical Exam
- Examine the patient both upright and supine, as venous distension is exacerbated in the upright position
- Look for clinical manifestations of swelling and pain
- Check for temperature differences along the extremities

Investigations
- Doppler ultrasonography
- Plethysmography (less commonly used compared to ultrasound)
- Venography (rarely used)
- Hypercoagulability work-up

Evidence-Based Medicine: Deep Vein Thrombosis
Signs and symptoms that are commonly associated with deep vein thrombosis (DVT), such as leg pain, swelling, pitting edema, warmth, dilated superficial veins, and erythema are neither sensitive nor specific in isolation.

Anand SS et al. 1998. *JAMA* 279:1094-1099.

Superficial Thrombophlebitis

Etiology
- 20% associated with occult DVT
- DVTs may be caused by intravenous indwelling catheters

Signs/Symptoms
- Tenderness, induration, redness along course of vein
- Generally no swelling of the limb
- Low-grade fever

Physical Exam
- Inspect the area for redness and swelling (may not always be present)
  - Differential is cellulitis: diffuse infection and inflammation of the der-mis and subcutaneous tissues
- Palpate the affected vein and determine if it is hard and cord like
- Tests are usually not needed
- DVT can occur concomitantly with superficial thrombophlebitis in up to 30% of cases, thus need to rule out DVT

Investigations
- Ultrasound
- Magnetic resonance venography
- Invasive contrast venography

Chronic Deep Vein Insufficiency (Post Phlebitis Syndrome)

Etiology
- Development of venous insufficiency after deep vein thrombosis leading to lower extremity discomfort and pain, edema, skin hyperpigmentation

Signs/Symptoms
- Leg swells as the day progresses, but swelling goes away overnight
- Pain – relieved on recumbency or elevation
- Pruritis
- Brawny induration
- Hyperpigmentation
- Brownish darkening – due to hemosiderin from extravasation of RBCs
- Ulceration (stasis dermatitis)
  - Ulcers are non-healing, typically around the medial malleolus
  - Venous ulcers are not as painful as ischemic arterial ulcers where pain is made worse with elevation
  - Arterial ulcers are often deep, extending through the fascia, whereas venous ulcers are shallow
  - Venous ulcers are weeping (wet) and not well demarcated (opposite is true for arterial ulcers)

Physical Exam
- Inspection for 6 common signs:
  - Edema
  - Hyperpigmentation
  - Induration
  - Venous ectasia
  - Blanching hyperemia
  - Pain with calf compression
- Venous Clinical Severity Score: use the following signs and symptoms and give them each a rating of 0 to 3
  - 0=absent, 1=mild, 2=moderate, 3=severe
  - Symptoms: pain, varicose veins, venous edema, skin pigmentation, inflammation, induration, ulcer number and ulcer diameter, compression therapy
  - Scores of 5 to 14 on two visits separated by ≥6 months indicate mild to moderate disease, and scores of ≥5 indicate severe disease

Investigations
- Doppler bidirectional flow studies with colour to exclude DVT
- Assess venous flow, its direction and presence of occluded veins
- Identification of incompetent veins and incompetent perforating veins

Varicose Veins

- Definition: distended tortuous superficial veins with incompetent valves in the lower extremities
- Occurs in equal frequency in males and females

Etiology
- Thrombophlebitis
- Congenital
- Situation of increased pressure (pregnancy, prolonged standing, ascites, tricuspid regurgitation)

Signs/Symptoms
- Dull aching, burning, or cramping in leg
- Worsening discomfort with standing, warm temperature or menses
- Edema which resolves overnight and can be relieved by elastic stockings and leg elevation

Physical Examination – (Refer also to **Special Tests** p. 305)
- Test for Incompetent Saphenous Vein
- Brodie-Trendelenburg Maneuver

Investigations
- Duplex ultrasonography

Treatment
- **Non-surgical**:
  - Elastic/compression stockings
  - Leg elevation
  - Sclerotherapy: injection of sclerosant drug into vein to cause vein shrinkage
- **Surgical**:
  - Stripping: removal of all or part of saphenous vein trunk
  - Phlebectomy: removal of affected superficial veins through skin
  - Vein ligation with a surgical suture

Vasculitis

Etiology
- Inflammation of any blood vessel, including arteries, arterioles, capillaries, venules and veins
- Clinical presentation is diverse depending on the type of blood vessel involved and their location
- Can involve any organ system, but some may present with symptoms of peripheral vascular disease

Disease-specific Findings
- Behcet's Disease
  - Multi-system leukoclastic vasculitis
  - Ocular involvement
  - Recurrent oral and vaginal ulcers
  - Venous thrombosis
  - Skin & joint inflammation
- Buerger's Disease
  - Inflammation 2° to clotting of small and medium-sized vessels
  - Most common in Asian males
  - Association with cigarette smoking
  - May lead to distal claudication and gangrene
- Giant Cell (Temporal) Arteritis
  - Inflammation of aorta and its branches
  - New headache, jaw claudication
  - Scalp tenderness, may have pulseless or "ropy"/thickened temporal artery
  - F>M, age >50, elevated ESR
  - May present with sudden, painless loss of vision ± diplopia
  - Aortic arch syndrome: involvement of subclavian and brachial arteries
    - Pulseless disease, aortic aneurysm ± rupture

- Polyarteritis Nodosa
  - Necrotizing vasculitis of small to medium-sized vessels
  - May lead to thrombosis, aneurysm or dilatation at any lesion site
  - Associated with Hepatitis B surface antigen positivity
  - Livedo reticularis of the skin
  - Diastolic BP >90 mmHg
  - Renal failure
  - Neuropathy
- Takayasu's Arteritis
  - "Pulseless" disease
  - Chronic inflammation of aorta and its branches
  - Usually in young Asian females
  - Constitutional symptoms
- Raynaud's Phenomenon
  - Pain and tingling in the digits due to vasospasm
  - Episodes of sharply demarcated pallor and/or cyanosis followed by erythema
  - Normal pulses present
  - Triggered by cold or emotional stress
  - May be primary or secondary, associated with SLE, scleroderma, RA, cryoglobulinemia
- Anti-Phospholipid Antibody Syndrome
  - Multi-system vasculopathy often associated with SLE
  - Recurrent thromboembolic events (arterial and venous)
  - Recurrent spontaneous abortions
  - Skin changes: livedo reticularis, purpura, leg ulcers, gangrene

Investigations
- Biopsy of affected organ, skin or suspected blood vessel
- Angiography
- CT scan
- Autoimmune workup: ESR, CRP, ANCA, RF, C3 and C4, ANA, ferritin, anticardiolipin and lupus anticoagulant antibodies
- Urinalysis (active sediment, proteinuria), BUN, creatinine
- Consider synovial fluid analysis if joint involvement
- Fundoscopy ± slit lamp examination

Treatment
- Often dependent on condition
- Mainstay of treatment is immunosuppressive agents, most often with corticosteroids and/or cyclophosamide
- If involves thromboembolism, may require anticoagulation with warfarin or heparin
- NSAIDs for pain control with joints, eye and/or skin involvement

Lymphatics
- See *Lymphatic System and Lymph Node Exam*

REFERENCES

Anand SS, Wells PS, Hunt D, Brill-Edwards P, Cook D, Ginsberg JS. 1998. Does this patient have deep vein thrombosis? *JAMA* 279(14):1094-1099.

Bickley LS, Szilagyi PG, Bates B. 2007. *Bates' Guide to Physical Examination and History Taking.* Philadelphia: Lippincott Williams & Wilkins.

Ratchford EV, Jin Z, Di Tullio MR, Salameh MJ, Homma S, Gan R, Boden-Albala B, Sacco RL, Rundek T. 2009. Carotid bruit for detection of hemodynamically significant carotid stenosis: the Northern Manhattan Study. *Neurol Res* 31(7):748-752.

Ricci MA, Emmerich J, Callas PW, Rosendaal FR, Stanley AC, Naud S, Vossen C, Bovill EG. 2003. Evaluating chronic venous disease with a new venous severity scoring system. *J Vasc Surg* 38(5):909-915.

Swartz MH. 2006. *Textbook of Physical Diagnosis: History and Examination.* Philadelphia: Saunders Elsevier.

The Psychiatric Exam

Editors:
Amy Ng & Julia Zhu

Faculty Reviewers:
Paul Kurdyak, MD, PhD, FRCP(C)
Jodi Lofchy, MD, FRCP(C)

PSYCHIATRIC

TABLE OF CONTENTS

Approach to Psychiatric History 317
Common Chief Complaints 317
Common Disorders 318
Focused History 318
Mental Status Examination 320
Folstein Mini-Mental Status Exam 322
Suicide Risk Assessment 323
Multiaxial Assessment 324
Common Investigations 324
Common Clinical Scenarios 324
Mental Health Act Forms 333
Pharmacology 334

APPROACH TO THE PSYCHIATRIC HISTORY

- The psychiatric history has a similar organization to the traditional medical history but places more emphasis on the psychosocial aspects of the patient's background, family and upbringing (see **Past Personal History**)
- The Mental Status Examination is the psychiatric equivalent of the physical exam and provides information about the patient's current mental status
- If the patient seems disoriented or cognitively impaired, the Folstein Mini-Mental Status Exam (MMSE) should be used to screen for cognitive problems – **Table 1**
- All elderly patients should undergo a cognitive screen
- A corroborative source for history (e.g. parent, child, spouse, friend) is almost always helpful
- The patient's previous psychiatric history needs to be collected and a suicide screen should be done on every patient
- The following aspects are particularly important in the psychiatric interview:
  - The privacy and confidentiality of the patient
  - Your safety: conduct the interview in a safe place with other staff and security available if needed

COMMON CHIEF COMPLAINTS

- Fears and concerns (delusions)
- Hearing voices (auditory hallucinations)
- Mood changes (depression, mania)
- Thoughts of suicide (suicidal ideation)
- Anxiety
- Confusion
- Medication side effects
- Agitation

COMMON DISORDERS

Disorders marked with (✓) are discussed in **Common Clinical Scenarios**

Mood Disorders
✓ Mood episodes
✓ Major depressive disorder
✓ Postpartum depression
✓ Dysthymia
✓ Bipolar disorders

Psychotic Disorders
✓ Schizophrenia
▪ Brief psychotic episode
▪ Schizoaffective disorder
▪ Delusional disorder
▪ Schizophreniform disorder
  (secondary to substance abuse)

Anxiety Disorders
✓ Panic attacks/disorder
✓ Agoraphobia
▪ Specific phobia
✓ Social phobia
✓ Obsessive compulsive disorder
✓ Post-traumatic stress disorder
✓ Generalized anxiety disorder

Substance abuse disorders
▪ Substance abuse
▪ Substance dependence
✓ Substance intoxication
✓ Substance withdrawal

Eating Disorders
✓ Anorexia nervosa
✓ Bulimia nervosa

Cognitive Disorders
✓ Delirium
✓ Dementia

Adjustment Disorders

Personality Disorders
✓ Cluster A
✓ Cluster B
✓ Cluster C

FOCUSED PSYCHIATRIC HISTORY

Identifying Data
▪ Age and date of birth (DOB) are an easy way of doing an initial cognitive screen
▪ Include age, employment (or most recent job) and relationship status, living arrangements, dependents, source of income, country of origin

Reason for Referral
▪ Who is referring this patient?
▪ What is the reason for referral? There may be a specific question to ask that can help you avoid taking a full psychiatric history

Chief Complaint
▪ Open-ended questions may help to elicit a thought disorder if present, so allow some time initially for an uninterrupted response
▪ Document patient's words verbatim

History of Present Illness
▪ Onset, frequency, progression of symptoms (see **Common Clinical Scenarios** for specific criteria)
▪ Screening questions for psychiatric disorders:
▪ "I want to ask you about some experiences that people sometimes have when they feel this way"
  ▪ Psychosis: hallucination, delusion
    ◆ "Have you noticed that you hear the voices of people speaking to you or about you when you are alone?"
    ◆ "Have you seen things and wondered if they were really there?"

- "Have you felt afraid that people you don't know might be taking special notice of you or even wanting to hurt you in any way?"
  - Mood: depression, mania
    - "Have you had little interest or pleasure in doing things?"
    - "Have you been feeling down, depressed, or hopeless?" "How is it different from usual feelings of sadness for you?"
    - "Have you been feeling euphoric or more irritable than usual?"
    - "Have these feelings been associated with a change in your sleep, energy, speed of your thinking?"
  - Organic: alcohol, drugs, illness
    - "Have you been using drugs/alcohol to help cope with your problems?"
  - Anxiety: panic, agoraphobia, obsessions, compulsions
    - "Do you ever feel anxious or on edge?"
    - "Do you find yourself worrying about a lot of different things?"
    - "Do you have worries or fears that you know are not rational but are unable to suppress?"
  - Eating disorders
    - "Do you feel fat?"
    - "Do you find yourself preoccupied with your weight? With food?"
  - Cognitive: memory, concentration, dementia
    - "Have you had trouble concentrating or remembering things lately?"
- Somatic Symptoms:
  - Anorexia, weight loss/gain, insomnia/hypersomnia, lethargy, agitation, decreased sexual energy or interest
  - Neurological symptoms (e.g. seizures, recent head injury)
  - Somatic problems with no known physical basis (psychosomatic)
- Possible precipitating factors (e.g. stressful life event, substance abuse)
- Effects on functioning (i.e. work, social, family, daily activities)
- Current medications and adherence – see **Pharmacology**
- Suicidal and/or homicidal ideation – see **Suicide Risk Assessment**
- Functional inquiry of symptoms associated with possible co-morbid conditions (e.g. anxiety and depression)

Past Psychiatric/Medical History

- Past psychiatric, psychosomatic, medical, or neurological history
  - Age of first symptoms and first contact with psychiatry
  - Hospitalizations: number, diagnosis, treatment, outcome, date of last discharge
  - Outpatient contacts: type, medications
- Suicide attempts: lethality, medical attention, date of last attempt
- Legal history: violence, charges
- Medications: adherence, response, top dose, duration, side effects
- Substance use
  - Alcohol (type of alcohol and weekly consumption)
  - Recreational drugs, smoking, caffeine
  - Over-the-counter medications, alternative medicines
- If alcohol abuse is suspected, the **CAGE** questionnaire should be used as a screening tool:
  - **C** = "Have you ever felt the need to **Cut** down on your drinking?"
  - **A** = "Have people **Annoyed** you by criticizing your drinking?"
  - **G** = "Have you ever felt **Guilty** about your drinking?"
  - **E** = "Have you ever taken a morning 'Eye Opener'?"
    - 4 affirmative responses are highly predictive of alcoholism, while 2 or 3 create a high level of suspicion

PSYCHIATRIC

- ◆ 2/4 affirmative answers for men or 1/4 for women prompts further exploration
- ◆ If all answers are negative, alcoholism can generally be excluded

Family History of Psychiatric Illness
- Determine if any of the patient's biological relatives have:
  - Major psychiatric illness (symptoms, diagnosis, duration, treatment, response, hospitalization)
  - Contact with a mental health professional
  - Attempted or completed suicide
  - Substance abuse
  - Legal history

Past Personal History
- Adjust detail for age of patient
- A summary of the patient's life from infancy to present, paying particular attention to relationships with family and major life events (e.g. illness, divorce, deaths, etc.)
- Prenatal and perinatal – maternal substance use, pregnancy/delivery complications
- Early childhood (to age 3) – developmental milestones, temperament, attachment figures, separations, earliest memories
- Middle/late childhood (ages 3-11) – school performances, socialization
- Puberty and adolescence – early relationships, friends, psychosexual development, experimentation with drugs and alcohol
- Adulthood – education, occupational history, marital and relationship history, sexual history, religions, social activity and current social support system

MENTAL STATUS EXAMINATION (MSE)
Note: The MSE should reflect the patient's condition in the "here and now." Much of the evaluation can be gleaned from your observations during the interview.

Objective
- Appearance and behaviour
- Speech
- Affect
- Thought process
- Cognition
- Insight/Judgement

Subjective
- Mood
- Thought content
- Perception
- Cognition
- Insight
- Judgement

General Appearance and Behaviour
- Appearance – apparent vs. chronological age, dress, grooming, posture, facial expression, apparent physical health
- Behaviour and psychomotor activity – psychomotor agitation/retardation, gestures, mannerisms, rigidity/posturing, gait
- Specific movements:
  - Repetitive gestures (e.g. tics)
  - Agitated behaviour (e.g. hair pulling, hand wringing)
  - Tardive dyskinesia (involuntary movement of the tongue, mouth, or extremities) in people taking antipsychotics
- Attitude toward examiner – cooperation, accessibility, hostility, eye contact

Speech
- Rate (pressured, rapid, slowed, mutism), rhythm/fluency, spontaneity
- Pitch, volume, clarity
- Specific abnormalities (e.g. stuttering, speech impediments, aphasia)

Mood and Affect
- Mood – subjective emotional state; in patient's own words
  - Find out how the patient feels here and now
- Affect – objective; patient's mood as observed by you
  - Describe quality (euthymic, depressed, elevated, anxious), range (full, restricted, flat), intensity, stability/lability, appropriateness (to thought content)

Thought Process and Content
- *Thought process* – the way that a patient comes to a conclusion
  - Coherence, logic
  - Rate and flow of ideas (paucity/overabundance of ideas, slow/rapid):
    - Blocking – sudden cessation of flow of thought and speech
    - Perseveration – inability to switch ideas, echolalia (parrot-like repetition of phrases and words)
  - Presence/absence of goal-directed thinking:
    - Circumstantiality – indirect and delayed in reaching the goal, but eventually answers the question
    - Tangentiality – digresses from initial topic, never returns to original point
    - Loosening of associations – shifting between topics illogically (seen in schizophrenia and mania)
    - Flight of ideas– continuous, rapid jumping from one topic to another with superficial connections between topics (common in mania)
    - Word salad – jumble of words/phrases with no coherent meaning
    - Clang associations– speech based on sound such as rhyming/punning
- *Thought content* – ideas/themes that the patient communicates
  - Obsessions – recurrent and persistent thoughts, intrusive impulses or images that are recognized as irrational and that the patient cannot suppress
  - Preoccupations, phobias, somatic concerns
  - Overvalued ideas, ideas of reference – unusual, sustained beliefs but not fixed like a delusion
  - Delusions (see **Psychotic Disorders**)
  - Suicidal/homicidal ideation (see **Suicide Risk Assessment**)

Perception
- *Hallucinations* – sensory perception in absence of external stimuli; can be auditory, visual, olfactory, gustatory, or tactile; note the circumstances (e.g. precipitating factor) and content of the hallucination
- *Illusions* – misperception of a real external stimulus
- *Depersonalization* – feeling detached from his/her body or that parts of his/her body are detached (seen in anxiety and dissociative disorders)
- *Derealization* – feeling detached from environment or that surroundings are unreal

Cognition

- Can use Folstein Mini-Mental Status Exam for an assessment of cognition
- Consciousness (hyperalert, alert, drowsy, confused, stuporous, unconscious)
- Orientation (to time, person, place)
- Attention and concentration
- Memory
  - Immediate – ask patient to repeat a series of numbers forwards, then backwards (on average, 7 forward and 5 backwards is normal)
  - Recent – "What is my name?" "What did you have for breakfast/lunch/dinner?"
  - Remote – names and dates from patient's past (ask verifiable data)
- Knowledge
  - Test patient's lifelong knowledge base – "Who is the prime minister of Canada?"
- Abstraction
  - Take into consideration patient's education, IQ, and native language
  - Proverb interpretation – "How would you explain the meaning of the grass is always greener on the other side?"
  - Similarities test – "What do a baseball and an orange have in common?"

Insight and Judgement

- *Insight* – determine the patient's degree of awareness and understanding of the nature of his/her illness and the need for help
- *Judgement* – determine the patient's ability to understand the likely outcomes of his/her behaviour and to act accordingly

FOLSTEIN MINI-MENTAL STATUS EXAM (MMSE)

- Brief summary of the mental status examination is used to quickly screen for but not diagnose dementia (see **Cognitive Disorders**)
- Some patients may become agitated by the nature of the questions. Use introductory comments such as: "How would you describe your memory? I have a few questions that will help me see how your memory and concentration are functioning" (avoid using the word 'test')
- Note that MMSE scores may be low in patients with sensory impairment, dysphasia, depression, poor English or low education level

Table 1. Folstein Mini-Mental Status Exam

	Points	Question/ Direction
Orientation	5	What is the year, season, month, day and date?
	5	Where are we (country, province, city, hospital, and floor)?
Registration	3	Name 3 objects (e.g. apple, penny, table). Number of items patient is able to recall on first attempt.
		Number of trials to learn all 3 items should be noted (remind patients that they must recall these items in a few minutes)
Attention and Concentration	5	Serial sevens (100, 93, 86, 79, 72) OR Spell 'WORLD' backwards. OR Name months of the year backwards from December

Table 1. Folstein Mini-Mental Status Exam (continued)

	Points	Question/ Direction
Recall	3	Ask patient to recall the three objects mentioned above.
Language	2	Point to and ask patient to name pencil and watch.
	1	Ask patient to repeat "No ifs, ands, or buts".
	3	Ask patient to follow a 3-stage command: "Take this piece of paper in your right hand, fold it in half, and return it to me".
	1	Ask patient to read a phrase you wrote on a piece of paper and obey the command (e.g. close your eyes); make sure the patient can see the words on the paper (e.g. is wearing his/her glasses).
	1	Ask patient to write a sentence (store it with the patient's file for subsequent comparative purposes).
	1	Ask patient to copy a design that you sketched – draw intersecting pentagons

- Note if the patient is alert or drowsy.
- Optional clock drawing test: ask patient to draw a clock with the instruction: "set the time to 10 past 11"
- If score is less than 24/30, suspect cognitive impairment (sensitivity = 0.69, specificity = 0.99; Tangalos *et al.* 1996). Interpretation of the score should be correlated with history from informants to determine need for further cognitive assessment
  - Normal range (24-30)
  - Mild cognitive impairment (20-23)
  - Moderate cognitive impairment (10-19)
  - Severe cognitive impairment (0-9)

SUICIDE RISK ASSESSMENT

> **Clinical Pearl**
> Discussing suicidal thoughts and plans does not put ideas into a patient's head; it is important to screen every patient for suicidal tendencies. It is appropriate to ask directly i.e. ask if he/she feels so low that he/ has been thinking of killing him/herself.

- **Suicidal ideation**:
  - Pervasiveness of suicidal thoughts (fleeting/sustained)
  - Extent and details of any suicide plans including lethality and availability of method, likelihood of rescue

- Motive (e.g. want help, want to make someone feel guilty)
- Passive ideation
  - "Have you ever felt so low that you thought life was not worth living?"
- Active ideation
  - "Have you ever thought of how you might end your life/kill yourself?"
- Current stressors that might precipitate the suicide
- Past attempted suicides
- Family history of suicide
- Risk factors for suicide – **SAD PERSONS** scale:
  - **S**ex – male
  - **A**ge >60 years old
  - **D**epression
  - **P**revious attempts
  - **E**thanol abuse
  - **R**ational thinking loss (delusions/hallucinations/hopelessness)
  - **S**uicide in family
  - **O**rganized plan
  - **N**o spouse/no support systems
  - **S**erious illness, intractable pain

MULTIAXIAL ASSESSMENT

Use this diagnostic approach provided by the DSM-IV to organize your assessment of a psychiatric patient based on the psychiatric history and MSE

Axis I – differential diagnosis of primary psychiatric disorder
Axis II – personality disorders, mental retardation
Axis III – relevant general medical conditions
Axis IV – psychosocial and environmental stressors
Axis V – global assessment of functioning (GAF 0-100) incorporating effects of Axes I to IV (refer to the DSM-IV for detailed scale)

COMMON INVESTIGATIONS

1. Laboratory Tests: TSH, vitamin B12, folate, ferritin, CBC, electrolytes, calcium profile, blood glucose, blood culture, serum and urine toxicology screen, BUN, creatinine, liver enzymes and liver function tests, serum medication level
2. Imaging: CT head (e.g. first episode psychosis), MRI head
3. Weight and BMI
4. ECG
5. Psychiatric Assessments: Folstein Mini-Mental Status Exam (MMSE), Montreal Cognitive Assessment (MoCA), clock drawing test

COMMON CLINICAL SCENARIOS

Note: Please see specific criteria for diagnosis in the DSM-IV

I. MOOD DISORDERS

Mood Episodes

Major Depressive Episode (MDE)
- Patient has experienced 5 or more of the following for at least 2 weeks; at least 1 is either 1) depressed mood or 2) loss of interest or pleasure (anhedonia):

- **M**ood – depressed
- **S**leep – increased/decreased (ask about early morning awakenings)
- **I**nterest or pleasure – decreased (anhedonia)
- **G**uilt or worthlessness
- **E**nergy – decreased
- **C**oncentration – decreased
- **A**ppetite or weight – decreased/increased
- **P**sychomotor agitation or retardation
- **S**uicidal ideation (see **Suicide Risk Assessment**)
- Symptoms cause significant distress or impairment in social, occupational, or other important areas of functioning
- Rule out conditions that can cause this symptomatology:
  - Mixed episodes (see below)
  - General medical conditions (e.g. hypothyroidism) or medications/substances
  - Bereavement due to loss of a loved one (should not persist past 2 months)

Manic Episode
- A period of abnormally elevated, expansive, or irritable mood for at least 1 week
- Requires at least 3 of the following symptoms (4 if mood is only irritable):
  - **G**randiosity (inflated self-esteem)
  - **S**leep, decreased need
  - **T**alkative, more so than usual or feel pressured to keep talking
  - **P**leasurable activities excessive with potentially painful consequences (e.g. spending, sex, substance abuse)
  - **A**ctivity, increase in goal-directed activity or psychomotor agitation
  - **I**deas, flight of (racing thoughts)
  - **D**istractible by irrelevant environmental stimuli
- Symptoms are severe enough to cause marked impairment in social or occupational functioning; or to necessitate hospitalization to prevent harm to self or others; or psychotic features are present
- Ruled out mixed episodes, general medical conditions (e.g. hyperthyroidism), or effects of medications/substances (e.g. antidepressant)

Mixed Episode
- Fulfill criteria for both a manic episode and a MDE in one week

Hypomanic Episode
- Abnormally elevated, expansive, or irritable mood lasts ≥4 days
- Other symptoms identical to those of a manic episode
- No marked social or occupational functional impairment, no need for hospitalization, and no psychotic features

Depressive Disorders

Major Depressive Disorder
- Single Episode: at least one MDE, or recurrent, 2 or more MDEs with ≥2 months between episodes)
- Never had a manic, hypomanic, or mixed episode
- Not better accounted for by schizoaffective disorder and not superimposed on a psychotic disorder
- Features: psychotic, atypical (increased sleep, weight gain, leaden paralysis (heavy feelings in arms/legs), interpersonal rejection sensitivity), chronic (≥2 years), postpartum, seasonal, catatonic, melancholic
- Lifetime prevalence ~ 17%, F:M = 2:1, average age of onset is 32 years

Depression, Postpartum Onset
- MDE starting within first 4 weeks postpartum, may present with psychosis
- Typically lasts 2-6 months, residual symptoms up to 1 year
- Must ask about suicidal and infanticidal ideation
- Occurs in 10% of mothers
- Distinguish from postpartum "blues": transient period of mild depression with onset 2-4 days postpartum, usually lasting 48 hours up to 10 days; 50-80% of mothers, where no medication is required

Dysthymic Disorder
- Depressed mood for most of the day, for more days than not for ≥2 years (in children and adolescents, mood can be irritable, lasting ≥1 year), causing significant distress or impairment in social or occupational functioning
- Patient has 2 or more of the following for ≥2 years:
  - Anorexia or hyperphagia
  - Insomnia or hypersomnia
  - Low energy or fatigue
  - Low self-esteem
  - Poor concentration or difficulty making decisions
  - Feelings of hopelessness
- Asymptomatic for no longer than 2 months at a time
- No MDE present in first 2 years, never a manic, hypomanic or mixed episode or met criteria for cyclothymia
- Does not only occur during psychosis
- Not due to substance use or a general medical condition

Bipolar Disorders
- Lifetime prevalence 2%; peak age of onset is 20-25 years

Bipolar I Disorder
- At least one manic or mixed episode
- Commonly with at least 1 MDE but not required

Bipolar II Disorder
- At least 1 MDE and at least 1 hypomanic episode
- No past manic or mixed episodes

Cyclothymia
- Ongoing hypomanic and depressive symptoms ≥2 years, never asymptomatic >2 months, causing significant distress or impairment in social or occupational functioning
- No MDE, manic, or mixed episodes; no psychosis
- Not due to substance use or a general medical condition

II. ANXIETY DISORDERS

Panic Attack
- A period of intense fear or discomfort, in which ≥4 of the following symptoms occur abruptly and peak within 10 minutes

- Mnemonic: **STUDENTS FEAR the 3 C's**
  - **S**weating
  - **T**rembling or shaking
  - **U**nsteadiness or dizziness
  - **D**erealization or **D**epersonalization
  - **E**xcessive heart rate, palpitations
  - **N**ausea or abdominal distress
  - **T**ingling and numbness (paresthesia)
  - **S**hortness of breath or **S**mothering sensation
  - **Fear** of loss of control, going crazy, or dying
  - **C**hest pain or discomfort
  - **C**hoking sensation
  - **C**hills or hot flushes

Panic Disorder
- Recurrent, unexpected panic attacks and ≥1 month of:
  - Worries about having additional attacks (anticipatory anxiety) or
  - Worries about what the attacks might mean or
  - Demonstrates a significant change in behaviour related to the attacks
- Not better accounted for by another mental disorder, substance use or a general medical condition
- Diagnosed with or without agoraphobia

Agoraphobia
- Anxiety about being in situations from which escape might be difficult or embarrassing, or in which help is unavailable during a panic attack
- Fears may include being alone outside the home, being in a crowd, standing in line, traveling
- Such situations are avoided, endured with anxiety about developing panic-like symptoms or a panic attack, or require the presence of a companion
- Not better accounted for by another mental disorder

Social Phobia
- Fear of social or performance situations in which one might be exposed to the scrutiny of others and be embarrassed
- Exposure to these situations causes marked anxiety or a panic attack
- Recognize that the fear is unreasonable or excessive
- Anxiety and fear causing significant impairment in daily functioning
- Generalized if fear applies to most social situations

Obsessive-Compulsive Disorder
- Obsessions and/or compulsions which are time-consuming (>1 hour/day) and adversely affect social or occupational functioning
- Lifetime prevalence of 2.5% in general population; peak onset < age 15 or in 20s
- Obsession:
  - Recurrent or persistent thought, impulse or image that is intrusive, inappropriate, or excessive (not a real-life worry)
  - Inability to suppress the thought
  - Anxiety-provoking thoughts perceived as irrational or not in keeping with the person's belief system (ego-dystonic)
- Compulsion:
  - Repetitive behaviour (e.g. hand washing, counting) often adopted to reduce the stress of an obsession
  - Behaviour is distressing and recognized as irrational

Post-Traumatic Stress Disorder
- Patient experienced, witnessed, or heard about a traumatic event which caused intense fear, and now has recurrent and distressing thoughts, nightmares, hallucinations, flashbacks, etc.
- Incidence up to 80% in people following a traumatic incident
- Avoidance of anything that will stimulate memories of the trauma
- Symptoms of increased arousal (e.g. difficulty falling or staying asleep, irritability, difficulty concentrating, hypervigilance)
- Decreased range of affect, feeling detached from others

Generalized Anxiety Disorder
- Excessive anxiety about a number of real-life concerns, occurring for a majority of days within a 6 month period, and causing social or occupational distress
- Lifetime prevalence is 5%
- Difficulty controlling the anxiety, but realize it is excessive
- Associated with restlessness, difficulty concentrating, and irritability

III. PSYCHOTIC DISORDERS

Psychosis
- Loss of contact with reality, often characterized by delusions, hallucinations, and disorganized behaviour
- In assessing psychotic disorders, be sure to ask about:
  - Delusions and hallucinations (see below)
  - Mood changes (onset and duration relative to psychosis)
  - Details of psychosis
    - Precipitating events (e.g. drug use, medication changes)
    - Duration of the active psychotic symptom phase
    - Changes in level of functioning (e.g. work, school, social)
- Differential Diagnosis of Psychosis:
  - **G**eneral medical condition (tumour, head trauma, dementia, delirium)
  - **A**ffective disorders (depression with psychotic features, bipolar disorder)
  - **S**ubstance induced (intoxication/withdrawal)
  - **P**sychotic disorders (schizophrenia, schizoaffective disorder, delusional disorder and brief psychotic disorder)
  - **P**ersonality disorders (schizotypal, schizoid)

Psychotic Symptoms
- *Hallucination*
  - Sensory perception in the absence of external stimuli
  - Types: auditory, visual, tactile, olfactory, gustatory – "Did you ever hear/see/feel/smell/taste things that other people couldn't?"
- *Delusion*
  - Fixed, false belief that continues despite proof to the contrary and is not understandable on the basis of the person's cultural or religious background
  - Common delusions and screening questions:
    - Grandiosity – "Did you ever feel that you were especially important in some way, or that you had special powers or abilities?"
    - Persecution (paranoid) – "Have you felt afraid that people may be trying to hurt you or are out to 'get you'?"
    - Reference – "Did it ever seem that people were talking about you?" "When watching TV or listening to the radio, did you feel that there are special messages intended specifically for you?"

- Thought broadcasting – "Did you ever feel as if your thoughts were being broadcast out loud so that other people could hear what you were thinking?"
- Thought insertion/withdrawal – "Did you ever feel that certain thoughts were put into or taken out of your head?"
- Mind reading – "Did you ever feel that people are able to read your mind and know what you're thinking?"
- Delusion of control – "Did you ever feel like you are being controlled against your will by someone or some power from outside yourself?"
- Delusion of guilt – "Did you ever blame yourself for bad things in the world?" "Did you ever feel like you have done something terrible and deserved to be punished?"
- Somatic delusion – "Do you fear that something is terribly wrong with your body?"

Schizophrenia

- Lifetime prevalence of 1%; onset often in adolescence and early 20s (onset in men earlier than in women (men 20-25; women 25-30)
- Chronic disorder characterized by psychotic symptoms that significantly impair functioning and involve disturbances in emotions, thoughts, and behaviours
- Active phase symptoms: 2 or more of the following (each present for a significant portion of time in a 1 month period):
  - Delusions
  - Hallucinations
  - Disorganized speech (e.g. incoherence, loosening of associations, word salad)
  - Disorganized or catatonic behaviour
  - Negative symptoms (e.g. flattening of affect, avolition – inability to initiate and persist in goal-directed activities, alogia – inability to speak)
- Social or occupational dysfunction (e.g. work, interpersonal relations, self-care)
- Signs of disturbance persist for at least 6 months, including at least 1 month of active phase symptoms (may include prodromal or residual phases)
- Rule out schizoaffective and mood disorders, general medical conditions, substances/medications
- Subtypes:
  - **Paranoid** – preoccupation with 1 or more delusions or auditory hallucinations
  - **Catatonic** – at least 2 of: motor immobility (catalepsy or stupor), excessive motor activity, extreme negativism or mutism, peculiar voluntary movement, echolalia or echopraxia (repetition of movements, gestures)
  - **Disorganized** – disorganized speech and behaviour, flat/inappropriate affect
  - **Undifferentiated** – meet criteria but does not fall into 3 previous subtypes
  - **Residual** – absence of prominent delusions, hallucinations, disorganized speech or behaviour; but evidence of persisting disturbance (negative symptoms or attenuated positive symptoms present)

Table 2. Differentiating Psychotic Disorders

Disorder	Psychotic Symptoms	Duration	Mood Symptoms
Schizophrenia	Active phase symptoms	>6 months	None
Schizophreniform disorder	Active phase symptoms	1 – 6 months	None
Schizoaffective disorder	≥2 weeks delusions / hallucinations	>1 month	Present
Delusional disorder	Non-bizarre delusions, hallucinations	>1 month	If present, 2°
Brief psychotic disorder	≥1 positive symptom(s)	<1 month	None
2° to substance intoxication/ withdrawal	Active phase symptoms	During intox. or ≤1 month after withdrawal	Variable
2° to mood disorder	Delusions/ hallucinations (mood congruent)	Unspecified	1°

IV. SUBSTANCE USE DISORDERS

Substance Abuse
- A maladaptive pattern of substance use leading to significant impairment or distress in at least one of four areas over a 12 month period: (1) occupation, (2) physical hazard, (3) legal, and (4) interpersonal
- Has never met the criteria for substance dependence

Substance Dependence
- A maladaptive pattern of substance use during a 12 month period focusing on:
    - Substance use behaviour (great deal of time spent in activities necessary to obtain substance, persistent desire or unsuccessful efforts to control or cut down substance use, using larger amounts or for longer period than intended)
    - Impairment caused by the substance (giving up social/occupational/ recreational activities, continued use despite knowledge of persistent physical or psychological problems)
    - Development of tolerance or withdrawal symptoms

V. EATING DISORDERS

Anorexia Nervosa
- Prevalence: 1-2% of women (F:M = 9:1); peak ages of onset at 14 and 18 years
- All 4 of the following criteria are present:
    - Refusal to maintain minimal body weight for age and height (i.e. body weight <85% of expected)
    - Intense fear of becoming obese even though underweight
    - Body image distortion
    - Amenorrhea (absence of at least 3 consecutive menstrual cycles)

Bulimia Nervosa

- Prevalence: 1-3% of young adult females; 0.2% of young males
- All 3 of the following criteria are present:
  - Recurrent episodes of binge eating (eating a large amount of food in a short period of time and feeling a lack of control over eating behaviour)
  - Inappropriate compensatory behaviours to prevent weight gain such as self-induced vomiting, use of laxatives or diuretics, strict dieting, vigorous exercise
  - Binge eating and inappropriate compensatory behaviours both occur at least twice a week for 3 months

VI. COGNITIVE DISORDERS

- Folstein MMSE (**Table 1**) and clock-drawing can be used to measure changes in cognition

Dementia

- Memory impairment and 1 or more of:
  - Aphasia – language disturbance
  - Apraxia – inability to carry out motor activities despite intact motor function
  - Agnosia – inability to identify objects despite intact sensory function
  - Disturbance in executive functioning – planning, organizing, sequencing, abstracting
- Gradual onset (vascular dementia following stroke may begin abruptly) and continuing cognitive decline
- Predominant in the elderly; 1% at 65 years and doubling every 5 years thereafter (8%, 65 and over; 25%, 80 and over)
- Common types of dementia include:
  - Alzheimer's Disease
  - Vascular Dementia
  - Lewy Body Dementia
  - Fronto-temporal Dementia (Pick's disease)
  - Sub-cortical (e.g. Parkinson's)

Delirium

- Characterized by transient changes in cognition and levels of consciousness
- Disturbance is caused by direct physiological consequences of a general medical condition or a medication/substance and develops over a short period of time

Table 3. Differentiating Between Dementia and Delirium

	Delirium	Dementia
Onset	Acute (hours to days)	Insidious
Duration	Days to weeks	Months to years
Natural history	Fluctuating, reversible	Progressive, usually irreversible
Consciousness	Reduced	Normal
Attention	Impaired	Variable
Medical status	Acute illness, drug toxicity	Variable

VII. PERSONALITY DISORDERS (PD)

- Enduring pattern of inner experience and behaviour that deviates markedly from expectations of the individual's culture
- Usually established by adolescence or early adulthood
- Affects ≥2 of: cognition, affect, interpersonal functioning, impulse control
- Inflexible and pervasive across a range of situations
- Individuals who present with an Axis I disorder may have a co-morbid Axis II personality disorder, so it is important to assess for a PD as it has many complications with respect to treatment outcomes

Table 4. Classification of Personality Disorders

Cluster	Personality Disorder	Main Features
A "Mad"	Paranoid	Pervasive distrust and suspiciousness of others such that their motives are interpreted as malevolent
	Schizoid	Detachment from social relationships and a restricted range of expression of emotions in interpersonal settings
	Schizotypal	Interpersonal deficits marked by acute discomfort with close relationships as well as by cognitive/perceptual distortions and odd, eccentric behaviour
B "Bad"	Borderline	Instability of interpersonal relationships, self-image, and marked impulsivity; recurrent suicidal behaviour, gestures or threats may be present; self-harm
	Antisocial	Criminal, aggressive, irresponsible behaviour; symptoms of conduct disorder before age 15
	Narcissistic	Grandiosity, need for admiration, lack of empathy
	Histrionic	Excessive emotionality and attention seeking; uncomfortable unless centre of attention
C "Sad"	Avoidant	Social inhibition, feelings of inadequacy, and hypersensitivity to negative evaluation
	Dependent	Excessive need to be taken care of that leads to submissive and clinging behaviour and fears of separation
	Obsessive-Compulsive	Preoccupation with orderliness, perfectionism and mental and interpersonal control, at the expense of flexibility and efficiency

VIII. MENTAL HEALTH ISSUES IN CHILDREN

- See *Pediatric Exam* p. 292

MENTAL HEALTH ACT FORMS

* Below are examples of the Ontario Mental Health Act Forms

Basic Criteria for Certification:
1. serious bodily harm to the person
2. serious bodily harm to another person or
3. imminent and serious physical harm of the person

Table 5. Mental Health Act Forms

Form	Form Name/Function	Purpose
FORM 1 (FORM 42 to patient)	Application by Physician for Psychiatric Assessment	Duration: 72 hours from admission Reason: meets criteria for certification and for psychiatric assessment Issued: by examining physician within 7 days
FORM 2	Order for Examination under Section 16	Duration: 7 days Reason: hospitalization and psychiatric assessment Issued: by Justice of the Peace
FORM 3 (FORM 30 to patient)	Certificate of Involuntary Admission	Duration: first Form 3 lasts 2 weeks from date signed Reason: meets criteria for certification Issued: by attending physician
FORM 5	Change to Informal or Voluntary Status	Reason: when physician feels that patient does not need involuntary admission, but does not necessarily mean that patient is ready for discharge
FORM 33	Notice to Patient that Patient is Incompetent	Reason: patient is not mentally capable to consent to collection, use or disclosure of personal health information; patient is not mentally capable to manage his/her property; patient is not mentally capable to consent to treatment of mental disorder

PHARMACOLOGY

Table 6. Commonly Used Psychiatric Pharmacological Agents by Class

Subcategory	Examples
Antidepressants	Tricyclic Antidepressants (TCAs): amitriptyline, imipramine, clomipramine, doxepin, nortriptyline, trimipramine, desipramine
	Selective Serotonin Reuptake Inhibitors (SSRIs): fluoxetine, paroxetine, citalopram, escitalopram, sertraline, fluvoxamine
	Serotonin-Norepinephrine Reuptake Inhibitors (SNRIs): venlafaxine, duloxetine
	Monoamine Oxidase Inhibitors (MAOIs): phenelzine, tranylcypromine
	Other: bupropion, mirtazapine, tryptophan
Antipsychotics	Typical: haloperidol, chlorpromazine, perphenazine, flupenthixol
	Atypical: olanzapine, risperidone, quetiapine, clozapine, ziprasidone
Anti-Anxiety Agents	SSRIs, TCAs, MAOIs
	Benzodiazepines: alprazolam, lorazepam, clonazepam
	β-blockers: propranolol, atenolol, oxprenolol, pindolol
	Other: venlafaxine, buspirone, hydroxyzine, pregabalin
Mood Stabilizers	Lithium
	Anti-convulsants: valproic acid, carbamazepine, lamotrigene
Opiate Agonist	Methadone
	Buprenorphine

Notes:
1. Cognitive behavioural therapy is an effective first line treatment for mild to moderate depression and anxiety disorders.
2. Electroconvulsive therapy is indicated and effective for severe and medically refractory depression.

REFERENCES

American Psychiatric Association, Task Force on DSM-IV. 2000. *Diagnostic and Statistical Manual of Mental Disorders: DSM-IV-TR*. Washington: American Psychiatric Association.

Andreasen NC, Black DW. 2006. *Introductory Textbook of Psychiatry*. Washington: American Psychiatric Pub.

First MB, Spitzer RL, Gibbon M, Williams JBW. 1997. *User's Guide for the Structured Clinical Interview for DSM-IV Axis I Disorders: SCID-1 Clinician Version*. Arlington: American Psychiatric Publishing.

Goldman HH. 2000. *Review of General Psychiatry*. New York: Lange Medical Books/McGraw-Hill, Medical Pub. Division.

Tangalos EG, Smith GE, Ivnik RJ, Petersen RC, Kokmen E, Kurland LT, Offord KP, Parisi JE. 1996. The Mini-Mental State Examination in general medical practice: clinical utility and acceptance. *Mayo Clin Proc* 71(9):829-837.

Zimmerman M. 1994. *Interview Guide for Evaluating DSM-IV Psychiatric Disorders and the Mental Status Examination*. East Greenwich: Psych Products Press.

The Respiratory Exam

Editors:
Michael Hill & Moises Maria

Faculty Reviewers:
Sheldon Mintz MD, FRCP(C), MEd

TABLE OF CONTENTS

Essential Anatomy   335
Approach to the Respiratory History and Physical Exam   335
Common Chief Complaints   336
Common Disorders   336
Focused History   337
Focused Physical Exam   339
Common Investigations   343
Common Clinical Scenarios   345

RESPIRATORY

ESSENTIAL ANATOMY

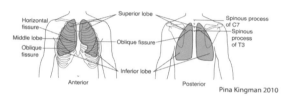

Figure 1. Locations of Lobes and Landmarks

Landmarks

- *Apex* – 2-4 cm above medial third of clavicle
- *Oblique fissure* (both lungs) – line from T3 spinous process, through 5th rib in the mid-axillary line, ending at the 6th rib in the mid-clavicular line
  - Right oblique fissure – separates the lower lobe from the upper and middle lobes
  - Left oblique fissure – separates the upper and lower lobes
- *Horizontal fissure* (right lung) – separates the upper and middle lobes; extends from the 5th rib in the mid-axillary line right to the 4th rib at the sternal border
- *Inferior margins* of the lungs extend from T10 posteriorly, through the 8th rib in the mid-axillary line to the 6th rib in the mid-clavicular line
- *Carina* – located at the level of the angle of Louis (T4)
- *Right hemi-diaphragm* – at the level of the 5th rib anteriorly and T9 posteriorly at end of respiration. Higher than left due to liver

APPROACH TO THE RESPIRATORY HISTORY AND PHYSICAL EXAM

In addition to general history taking, important aspects of the respiratory history include:

- Cough ± sputum production
- Wheezing/stridor
- Dyspnea
- Hemoptysis

- Pleuritic chest pain
- Cyanosis, edema
- Past history of respiratory infections
- Family history of atopy
- Smoking
- Previous CXR or pulmonary function test results
- Animal exposure, allergies
- Environmental/occupational exposures
- Travel history/birthplace (tuberculosis)

Overview of the Physical Exam
- Inspection
  - Rate and pattern of respiration
  - Signs of respiratory effort and distress
  - Cyanosis (central, peripheral)
  - Chest configuration (kyphosis, scoliosis, barrel chest)
  - Clubbing
  - Pursed-lip breathing
  - Presence of equipment (e.g. oximeter, supplementary oxygen)
- Palpation
  - General tenderness and deformities
  - Position of trachea
  - Chest expansion
  - Tactile fremitus
- Percussion
  - General percussion (resonance, dullness)
  - Diaphragmatic excursion
- Auscultation
  - Type of breath sounds (vesicular, bronchovesicular, bronchial, tracheal)
  - Symmetry of breath sounds
  - Presence of adventitious sounds (crackles, wheezes, stridor, pleural rub)

COMMON CHIEF COMPLAINTS
- Cough
- Phlegm production (sputum)
- Wheezing
- Shortness of breath (dyspnea)
- Coughing up blood (hemoptysis)
- Chest pain
- Chest radiographic abnormalities

COMMON DISORDERS
Disorders marked with (✓) are discussed in **Common Clinical Scenarios**
✓ Asthma
✓ COPD (chronic bronchitis, emphysema)
✓ Pneumonia
✓ Pulmonary embolism
- Interstitial lung disease
- Obstructive sleep apnea
- Pneumothorax
- Atelectesis
- Bronchogenic carcinoma
- Acute respiratory distress syndrome

FOCUSED HISTORY

Cough

- Onset/duration: acute/chronic, time of day, frequency, quality, progression, ± sputum (see **Table 1**)
- Aggravating/alleviating factors: body position, season, different environments
- Associated symptoms: fever, chills, night sweats, weight loss, post-nasal drip, runny nose, hoarseness, wheezing
- Risk factors: smoking, sick contacts, travel history, pets, occupational history

Table 1. Cough Descriptors and Etiology

Cough Descriptors	Etiology
Dry, hacking	Viral pneumonia, interstitial lung disease, tumour, laryngitis, allergies, anxiety
Chronic, productive	Bronchiectasis, chronic bronchitis, abscess, pneumonia, TB
Wheezing	Bronchospasm, asthma, allergies, congestive heart failure
Barking	Epiglottal disease (e.g. croup)
Stridor	Tracheal obstruction
Morning	Smoking
Nocturnal	Post-nasal drip, congestive heart failure, asthma
Upon eating/drinking	Neuromuscular disease of the upper esophagus

Adapted from Swartz M. 2006. *Textbook of Physical Diagnosis.*

Sputum

- Onset/duration, frequency, progression, quantity, colour, consistency, odour, hemoptysis
- Mucoid (uninfected) sputum is odourless, transparent and whitish-grey
- Purulent (infected) sputum is yellow, green
- Foul-smelling sputum is suggestive of a lung abscess

Wheezing/Stridor

- A high-pitched sound caused by a partially obstructed airway
  - Wheezing – due to intrathoracic obstruction, usually on expiration
  - Stridor – due to extrathoracic tracheal obstruction, on inspiration
- Causes: bronchospasm (e.g. asthma), mucosal edema, loss of elastic support, tortuosity of airways
- Onset, frequency, progression, duration of episodes
- Aggravating/precipitating factors: food, odours, emotions, animals, allergens (dust, pollen)
- Alleviating factors, associated symptoms
- Risk factors: history of nasal polyps, cardiac disease (e.g. congestive heart failure), smoking

Dyspnea
- Onset: gradual vs. sudden, provoking/palliating factors, duration, body position (see **Table 2**)
- Dyspnea on exertion:
  - Quantify with exercise tolerance (e.g. number of blocks walked or flights of stairs climbed before onset)
  - Compare before and after onset
- Progression of symptoms – compare present to 6 months prior
- Paroxysmal nocturnal dyspnea (PND) – sudden onset of dyspnea that awakens an individual from sleep. Patient classically describes need to get up and run to a window for air
- Associated symptoms:
  - Fever, chills, night sweats
  - Cough, hemoptysis, sputum
  - Fatigue, chest pain, palpitations, peripheral edema
- Risk factors: sick contacts, industrial exposure (asbestos, sandblasting), travel history

Table 2. Positional Dyspnea

Type	Etiology
Orthopnea (dyspnea when lying horizontally)	Congestive heart failure Mitral valve disease Severe asthma (rare) COPD (rare) Neurological diseases (rare)
Trepopnea (dyspnea when lying on one side)	Congestive heart failure
Platypnea (dyspnea when seated)	Status post-pneumonectomy Neurological diseases Cirrhosis (intrapulmonary shunts) Hypovolemia

Adapted from Swartz M. 2006. *Textbook of Physical Diagnosis.*

Hemoptysis
- Onset, number of episodes, quantity, quality (clots or blood-tinged sputum)
- Precipitating factors: cough, nausea, vomiting
- Associated symptoms
  - Fevers, chills, night sweats, weight loss
  - Pleuritic chest pain, leg pain, leg edema
  - Persistent cough, dyspnea, palpitations, arrhythmias
- Risk factors: recent surgery (DVT/pulmonary embolism), smoking, anti-coagulants, clotting disorders, oral contraceptives, TB exposure
- Be sure to distinguish hemoptysis from hematemesis
  - Hemoptysis: associated with coughing and dyspnea; red, frothy, mixed with sputum
  - Hematemesis: associated with nausea and vomiting; red/brown, not frothy, may be mixed with food

Pleuritic Chest Pain
- Localized "knife-like" pain associated with inspiration or coughing
- Suggests involvement of parietal pleura
  - Primary diseases of the pleura: mesothelioma and pleuritis
  - Pulmonary diseases that can extend to the pleura: pneumonia and pulmonary thromboembolism

Exposure History
- Domestic exposures – pets, hobbies, pollution
- Occupational exposures – see **Table 3**
- Recent travel and immigration history

Table 3. Occupational Exposures

Exposure	Associated Disease
Grain dust, wood dust, tobacco, pollens, many others	Occupational asthma
Asbestos	Pleural mesothelioma
Coal	Pneumoconiosis
Sandblasting and quarries	Silicosis
Industrial dusts	Chronic bronchitis

FOCUSED PHYSICAL EXAM

Inspection
- **Signs of respiratory distress**
  - General difficulty breathing (nasal flaring, stridor or wheezing, pursed-lip breathing on expiration)
  - Use of accessory muscles (trapezius, sternocleidomastoids, retraction of intercostal muscles)
  - Orthopnea – dyspnea that occurs when lying down and improves upon sitting up
  - Tripoding – sitting upright and leaning forward on outstretched arms
  - Paradoxical breathing – inward movement of abdomen on inspiration
  - Use of O_2 therapy/respiratory equipment (e.g. nasal prongs, mask, transtracheal O_2, endotracheal/tracheostomy tube with ventilator, oximeter)
- **Cyanosis (central or peripheral)**
  - Signs of peripheral cyanosis including coolness and bluish colour of extremities (fingers, toes, nose, ears)
  - Signs of central cyanosis including bluish mucous membranes (lips, frenulum, buccal mucosa)
  - Central cyanosis occurs when oxygen saturation falls below 85%
- **Clubbing**
  - Loss of Lovibond's angle between the nail bed and the axial plane of the DIP
  - Look for Schamroth sign: loss of diamond-shaped window when dorsal surfaces of terminal phalanges on opposite fingers are opposed
  - Sponginess of nail bed
- **Chest configuration (AP and lateral)**
  - Masses, scars, lesions, lacerations
  - Normal – AP diameter < lateral diameter
  - Barrel chest – AP diameter equal to lateral diameter
  - Pectus excavatum (funnel chest) – a depression of the sternum; associated with mitral valve disease
  - Pectus carinatum (pigeon breast) – an anterior protrusion of the sternum
  - Kyphosis – abnormal AP curvature of spine
  - Scoliosis – abnormal lateral curvature and torsion of spine

- **Respiratory rate (RR) and pattern** (assessed immediately after measuring pulse so patient is unaware of it being done)
  - Normal adults: RR = 12-16 breaths/minute
  - Apnea – a period without breathing
  - Bradypnea – abnormally slow rate of respiration (RR <12)
  - Cheyne-Stokes breathing – periods of deep breathing alternating with periods of apnea
  - Hyperpnea (Kussmaul's breathing) – increased depth and rate of breathing
  - Tachypnea – abnormally fast rate of respiration (RR >16)

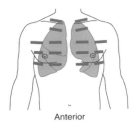
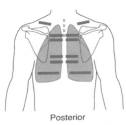

Anterior

Posterior

Pina Kingman 2010

Figure 2. Sites of Lung Percussion

Palpation
- **Chest wall tenderness**
  - Gently palpate all areas of chest for tenderness and deformities; check for MSK pain (beware of rib fractures)
- **Tactile fremitus**
  - Place ulnar side of the hand against chest wall and ask patient to say "ninety-nine" or "boy-o-boy"
  - The hand must be moved from side-to-side (to compare) and from the top downwards (see **Figure 2**)
  - Each lung field should be palpated both posteriorly and anteriorly (including the supraclavicular fossae, mid-axillary line and anterior intercostal spaces beginning at the clavicle)
- **Evaluation of position of trachea**
  - Palpate the trachea in the suprasternal notch to determine if it is midline
  - Trachea is deviated to ipsilateral side in atelectasis, fibrosis, lung collapse
  - Trachea is deviated to contralateral side in pleural effusion, hemothorax, tension pneumothorax
  - Nonpulmonary causes: lateral tracheal deviation can be caused by neck mass or retrosternal goiter
- **Evaluation of mobility of trachea**
  - A tracheal tug may be used to assess if the trachea is fixed in the mediastinum
  - With the patient's slightly flexed, support the back of the patient's head and position the middle fingers of the opposite hand into the cricothyroid space
  - Push the larynx upward
  - Normally, the trachea and larynx will move up 1-2 cm. Slowly lower the larynx before removing fingers
  - A fixed trachea may be due to mediastinal fixation (neoplasm or TB)

- **Chest expansion**
  - Place hands flat on back with thumbs parallel to the midline at the level of the 10th rib and fingers gripping the flanks
  - Ask patient to exhale completely and then inhale deeply – look for symmetry in outward movement of hands
  - Asymmetrical with pleural effusion, lobar pneumonia, pulmonary fibrosis, bronchial obstruction, pleuritic pain with splinting, pneumothorax

Table 4. Interpretation of Tactile Fremitus

Transmission	Pathologies
Increased	Consolidation (e.g. pneumonia)
Decreased – unilateral	Atelectasis, bronchial obstruction, pleural effusion, pneumothorax, pleural thickening
Decreased – bilateral	Chest wall thickening (muscle, fat), COPD, bilateral pleural effusion

Adapted from Swartz M. 2006. *Textbook of Physical Diagnosis.*

Percussion
- Percussion is performed in the same areas as tactile fremitus (see **Figure 3**)
- Normally, chest is resonant everywhere except in the left 3rd to 5th intercostal spaces anteriorly (cardiac dullness). Loss of dullness suggests hyperinflation (e.g. emphysema), see **Table 5**

Table 5. Interpretation of Percussion Notes

Percussion Note	Pathologies
Flat	Large pleural effusion
Dull	Lobar pneumonia, pleural effusion, hemothorax, empyema, atelectasis, tumour
Resonant	Simple chronic bronchitis
Hyperresonant	Emphysema, pneumothorax, asthma
Tympanic	Large pneumothorax

Adapted from Bickley LS et al. 2007. *Bates' Guide to Physical Examination.*

- **Diaphragmatic excursion**
  - Locate level of diaphragm during quiet respiration by percussing in an inferior direction for a change from tympanic to dull. The level of the diaphragm may be stated in reference to the vertebral level by counting down the vertebrae starting with the vertebral prominence (C7)
  - Ask the patient to breathe in deeply and hold breath. Locate new level of diaphragm (moved inferiorly)
  - Ask the patient to exhale as much as possible and hold and re-evaluate level of diaphragm (moved superiorly)
  - Normal diaphragmatic excursion is 4-5 cm
  - It may be necessary to percuss on both sides to compare excursion (check for hemiparalysis)

Auscultation
- Listen to breath sounds with diaphragm of stethoscope in the same areas as was done for tactile fremitus (**Figure 2**) after instructing patient to breathe deeply through an open mouth

RESPIRATORY

- When listening for breath sounds, note: intensity, pitch and ratio of duration of inspiration to expiration (see **Table 6**)
- Silent gap between inspiratory and expiratory sounds suggests bronchial breath sounds
- Compare breath sounds on both sides
- Over peripheral lung fields:
  - Bronchial breath sounds usually indicate consolidation
  - Bronchovesicular breath sounds may indicate bronchospasm or interstitial fibrosis

Table 6. Normal Auscultatory Sounds

Characteristic	Tracheal	Bronchial	Bronchovesicular	Vesicular
Description	Harsh	Air rushing through tube	Rustling but tubular	Gentle rustling
Intensity	Very loud	Loud	Moderate	Soft
Pitch	Very high	High	Moderate	Low
Inspiration: Expiration	1:1	1:3	1:1	3:1
Normal location	Extrathoracic trachea	Manubrium	Mainstem bronchi	Peripheral lung fields

Adapted from Swartz M. 2006. *Textbook of Physical Diagnosis.*

- **Adventitious sounds**
  - Listen for any sounds that are superimposed upon the usual breath sounds (see **Table 7**)

Table 7. Adventitious Sounds

Sound	Description	Mechanism	Causes
Crackles/ rales	Short, discontinuous, nonmusical sounds heard mostly during inspiration Fine: high-pitched Coarse: low-pitched	Excess airway secretions	Bronchitis, respiratory infections, pulmonary edema, atelectasis, fibrosis, CHF
Wheezes	Continuous, musical, high-pitched sounds; usually heard on expiration	Rapid airflow through obstructed airway	Asthma, pulmonary edema, bronchitis, CHF, secretions, tumour, foreign body
Rhonchi	Low-pitched, deep sound; may disappear following cough	Transient obstruction of larger airway by mucus	Bronchitis
Stridor	Inspiratory musical sounds best heard over trachea during inspiration	Upper airway extrathoracic obstruction	Partial obstruction of larynx or trachea
Pleural rub	Grating or creaking sounds best heard at end of inspiration and beginning of expiration	Inflammation of the pleura	Pneumonia, pulmonary infarction

Adapted from Swartz M. 2006. *Textbook of Physical Diagnosis* and Bickley, L. 2007. *Bates' Guide to Physical Examination.*

- **Consolidation**
  - Higher-pitched sounds are better transmitted through consolidated lung than air-filled lung
  - **Egophony**: when patient utters "E-E-E", sounds like "A-A-A" when over area of consolidation
  - **Whispered pectoriloquy**: whispered words (e.g. "one-two-three") by patient are auscultated more clearly over area of consolidation

COMMON INVESTIGATIONS

Pulse Oximetry
- LED device on finger, toe or earlobe measures oxygen saturation of hemoglobin
- Does not measure the oxygen tension; interpret O_2 stauration with the oxyhemoglobin dissociation curve in mind
- Reads incorrectly high (100%) during carbon monoxide poisoning

Arterial Blood Gasses
- Arterial oxygen tension (P_aO_2), carbon dioxide tension (P_aCO_2) and pH are measured; bicarbonate concentration is calculated using Henderson-Hasselbalch equation
- Useful for assessing acid/base disturbances (see *Essentials of Fluids, Electrolytes and Acid/Base Disturbances*)
  - Respiratory acidosis: hypoventilation causing increased P_aCO_2, bicarbonate increases to compensate
  - Respiratory alkalosis: hyperventilation causing decreased P_aCO_2, bicarbonate decreases to compensate
- Alveolar air equation used to determine theoretical alveolar oxygen tension (P_AO_2)
- $P_AO_2 = PO_{2\,(inspired)} - (P_aCO_2/0.8) = 150 - (P_aCO_2/0.8)$
- The alveolar-arterial oxygen gradient (A-a D_{O2}) is the difference between the calculated P_AO_2 and the measured P_aO_2
  - Normally not greater than 15 mmHg in healthy patients
  - Elevated A-a D_{O2} occurs with ventilation-perfusion mismatch or shunting
  - A-a D_{O2} increases with normal aging

Ventilation Perfusion Scanning
- Radioactive gas is respired; radiolabelled albumin is injected intravenously and deposits in the pulmonary capillaries
- Radiation from both sources is measured simultaneously to visualize the distribution of both ventilation and perfusion

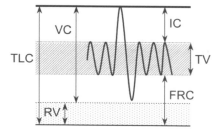

Figure 3. Lung Volumes
TLC = total lung capacity; VC = vital capacity; IC = inspiratory capacity; TV = tidal volume;
FRC = functional residual capacity; RV = residual volume

Pulmonary Function Tests

- Patient exhales into a spirometer from TLC down to RV with maximum effort; the maximum expiratory flow-volume envelope is plotted (see **Figure 5**)
  - FEV_1 = forced expired volume in first second
  - FVC = forced vital capacity
  - V50 = forced expired flow at 50% of vital capacity
  - V25 = forced expired flow at 25% of vital capacity
  - Response to bronchodilator and/or methacholine can be used to test for asthma
- A plethysmograph measures TLC, FRC and RV; panting against a closed shutter allows total airway resistance (Raw) to be measured
- Carbon monoxide is used to measure diffusion capacity (D_{CO})

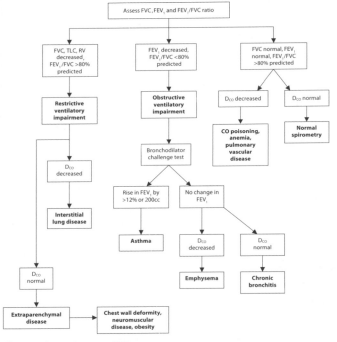

Figure 4. How to Interpret PFTs

Chest X-Ray

- See *Essentials of Medical Imaging* p. 478

Table 8. Characteristic Results of Pulmonary Function Tests in Obstructive and Restrictive Lung Disease

		Obstructive	Restrictive
Lung volumes	VC	Decreased or N	Decreased
	FRC	Increased	Decreased
	RV	Increased	Decreased
	TLC	Increased or N	Decreased
Flow rates	FEV_1	Decreased	Decreased or N
	FEV_1/FVC	Decreased	Increased or N
	V50	Decreased	Increased, decreased or N
	V25	Decreased	Increased, decreased or N
Diffusion capacity	D_{CO}	Increased, decreased or N	Decreased or N
Airway resistance	Raw	Increased	N

N = normal

COMMON CLINICAL SCENARIOS

Obstructive Lung Disease
- Characteristic "scooped-out" expiratory flow-volume curve (see **Figure 5**)
- Asthma
- COPD (emphysema, chronic bronchitis)
- Bronchiectasis (immotile cilia syndrome, hypogammaglobulinemia)
- Cystic fibrosis

Evidence-Based Medicine: Obstructive Airway Disease (OAD)
4 elements of history and physical exam are significantly associated with the diagnosis of OAD:

Finding	Likelihood Ratio
Smoking for more than 40 pack-years	8.3
Self-reported history of chronic OAD	7.3
Maximum laryngeal height of ≤4 cm	2.8
Age at least 45 years	1.3

Patients with all 4 findings had LR+ of 220. Those with none had LR– of 0.13.

Straus SE et al. 2000. *JAMA* 283:1853-57.

Restrictive Lung Disease
- Generally decreased lung volumes (see **Figure 5**)
- Interstitial lung disease (IPF, pneumoconiosis, hypersensitivity pneumonitis, iatrogenic)
- Neuromuscular disease (polio, myaesthenia gravis)
- Chest wall disease (kyphoscoliosis)
- Space-occupying lesions (tumours, cysts)
- Pleural disease (effusions, pneumothorax)
- Extrathoracic conditions (obesity, ascites, pregnancy)

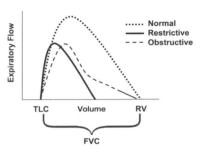

Figure 5. Flow-Volume Curves for Normal, Obstructed and Restricted Lungs

Asthma
- Chronic inflammatory disorder of the airways
- Association with: atopy/allergy, ASA sensitivity, sinusitis, nasal polyps
- Signs and symptoms:
    - Dyspnea
    - Chest tightness
    - Wheezing
    - Sputum production (white, scant)
    - Cough (especially nocturnal)
    - Respiratory distress (nasal flare, use of accessory muscles, intercostal indrawing, pulsus paradoxus [drop in SBP >5 to 10 mmHg during inspiration when compared to SBP in expiration], inability to speak)
    - Life-threatening episodes include silent chest, fatigue, cyanosis, diminished respiratory effort and/or decreased level of consciousness
- Investigations
    - Arterial blood gases (ABGs)
        - P_aO_2 during attack
        - P_aCO_2 decreased in mild asthma due to hyperventilation
        - Normal or increased P_aCO_2 in severe attack (ominous sign)
    - PFTs (may not be possible during severe attacks)
    - Indices of expiratory flow rate reduced
    - Decreased FEV_1, FEV_1/FVC, FVC, V50, V25
    - Increased FRC, RV, TLC
    - Flow-volume curve – typical obstructive pattern
- Management:
    - Life-threatening episodes:
        - Supportive therapy: sit upright, O_2 by mask, cardiac monitor, oximetry, IV fluids
        - Continuous β2-agonists and anticholinergics (nebulizer or meter-dose inhaler)
        - Methylprednisolone IV in ER
        - Intubation with decreased LOC, exhaustion, cyanosis, acidemia, silent chest
    - Short-term management:
        - Bronchodilators (selective β2-agonists, anticholinergics, theophylline)
        - Inhaled corticosteroids should be initiated early to prevent lung changes/scarring

- Long-term management:
  - Inhaled corticosteroids and long-acting β2-agonists (LABAs) or leukotriene receptor antagonists (LTRAs) as add-on therapy
  - Environmental control
  - Asthma education

Chronic Obstructive Pulmonary Disease (COPD)

- Characterized by progressive, partially reversible airway obstruction and lung hyperinflation and increasing frequency and severity of exacerbations
- Includes chronic bronchitis ("blue bloaters") and emphysema ("pink puffers")

Chronic Bronchitis

- Signs and symptoms:
  - Clinical diagnosis of chronic cough and sputum production on most days for at least 3 consecutive months over 2 successive years
  - Mild dyspnea with onset noted after cough
  - Sputum often purulent
  - Crackles
  - Wheezes
  - Hemoptysis
  - Often cyanotic due to ventilation-perfusion (V/Q) abnormalities ("blue")
  - Peripheral edema from RV failure (cor pulmonale) may be present ("bloater")
  - Hypoxemia causes secondary polycythemia and pulmonary vasoconstriction with pulmonary hypertension and eventual cor pulmonale
  - Obesity is often part of the clinical picture
- Investigations:
  - CXR (normal or increased bronchovascular markings, enlarged heart with cor pulmonale)
  - ABGs (hypoxemia with V/Q mismatch, hypercapnia with abnormal central respiratory drive and increased work of breathing)
  - PFTs
- Decreased FEV_1, FVC, FEV_1/FVC, V50, V25

Emphysema

- Signs and symptoms:
  - Exertional dyspnea with minimal cough
  - Tachypnea
  - Hyperinflation/barrel chest
  - Use of accessory muscles
  - Pursed-lip breathing
  - Hyperresonant on percussion (absent cardiac dullness)
  - Decreased diaphragmatic excursion
  - Decreased breath sounds
  - Pneumothorax due to bulla formation
- Investigations:
  - CXR (hyperinflation, flat hemidiaphragm, increased AP diameter, increased restrosternal airspace, bullae, reduced peripheral vascular markings, small heart)
  - ABGs (P_aO_2 and P_aCO_2 are normal or mildly decreased)
  - PFTs
    - Decreased FEV_1, FVC, FEV_1/FVC, $FEF_{25-75\%}$, V50 and V25, DC_{CO}
    - Increased TLC, FRC, RV

Management of COPD (emphysema and chronic bronchitis)
- Nonpharmacological:
  - Smoking cessation
  - Chest physiotherapy
  - Eliminate allergens/irritants
  - Exercise/multidisciplinary pulmonary rehabilitation
  - Nutrition
- Pharmacological:
  - Aggressive treatment of respiratory infections
  - Influenza vaccine and Pneumovax to prevent pneumonia
  - Short-acting bronchodilators (anticholinergics and/or β2-agonists)
  - Long-acting bronchodilators (e.g. tiotropium, salmeterol or formoterol) with short-acting β2-agonists as needed and inhaled corticosteroids for patients with moderate to severe COPD
  - Oral theophylline in some patients
- Others:
  - Home oxygen
  - Lung transplant
  - Lung volume reduction surgery

RESPIRATORY

Pneumonia
- Infection of the pulmonary parenchyma
- Separated into 3 classes: community-acquired (CAP), hospital-acquired (HAP) and ventilator-associated (VAP)

Table 9. Common Organisms in Community-Acquired and Hospital-Acquired Pneumonias

Site of Pathogen Acquistion	Organism	Typical or Atypical
Community	*S. pneumoniae*	Typical
	M. pneumoniae	Typical
	C. pneumoniae	Atypical
	H. influenza	Atypical
	Respiratory viruses: influenzas A and B, adenoviruses, coronavirus (responsible for severe acute respiratory syndrome, SARS)	Atypical
Hospital	*S. pneumoniae*	Typical
	S. aureus (commonly MRSA)	Typical
	C. pneumoniae	Atypical
	Legionella species	Atypical
	H. influenza	Atypical
	Gram-negative bacilli	Typical

- Predisposing factors:
  - Asthma, COPD
  - Smoking
  - Nursing home residents, often with a history of dementia
  - Age >70
  - Alcoholism
  - Travel

- Exposure to animals
- Hospitalization
- Past medical history: cardiac disease, lung cancer, renal failure
- Immunocompromised patients
- Signs and symptoms:
  - Sudden onset productive cough
  - Pleuritic chest pain
  - Fever
  - Chills, rigors
  - Dyspnea, tachypnea
  - Nausea, diarrhea
  - Cough may be more insidious and dry in atypical infections
  - Headache and myalgias may be present in atypical infections
  - Signs of consolidation (dullness to percussion, increased tactile and vocal fremitus, crackles, bronchial breath sounds, egophony, whispered pectoriloquy)
- Investigations:
  - Typical pneumonia:
    - ABGs
    - Blood culture
    - CXR (infiltrate ± cavitations)
    - Routine labs (CBC, electrolytes, others if indicated)
    - Sputum culture and Gram stain
  - Atypical pneumonia:
    - Nasopharyngeal culture
    - Pleural fluid culture
    - Bronchoalveolar lavage
    - Bronchoscopy
    - Serology
- Management:
  - Determine need for hospitalization
  - Empiric antibiotic therapy
  - For out-patients without COPD or macro-aspiration → macrolide (erythromycin, azithromycin or clarithromycin) or doxycycline
  - For out-patients with macro-aspiration → macrolide plus amoxicillin/clavunate or anaerobic fluoroquinolone (e.g. moxifloxacin)
  - For out-patients with COPD and recent treatment → respiratory fluoroquinolone
  - For hospitalized patients → respiratory fluoroquinolone (e.g. levofloxacin)

Evidence-Based Medicine: Community-Acquired Pneumonia
Individual signs and symptoms cannot reliably rule in or rule out the diagnosis of pneumonia. The absence of tachypnea, tachycardia and fever (i.e. RR <30, HR <100, temp <37.8ºC) among ambulatory patients with respiratory illness reduces the predicted probability of pneumonia to less than 1%. No combination of history and physical examination findings confirms the diagnosis of pneumonia. A chest radiograph should be obtained where diagnostic certainty is required.

Metlay JP et al. 1997. *JAMA* 278:1440-1445.

Pulmonary Embolism (PE)

- Signs and symptoms depend on the size of the embolus and the patient's underlying cardiovascular status but may include:
  - Dyspnea
  - Tachypnea
  - Chest pain
  - Hemoptysis
  - Syncope
  - Pleuritic chest pain
  - Stabbing pain on inspiration
  - Tachypnea is the only physical exam finding found reliably in more than 50% of patients with PE
  - Predisposition to venous thrombosis increase risk of PE (see *Peripheral Vascular Exam* p. 312)
  - Many substances other than thrombus can embolize to the pulmonary circulation including:
    - Air
    - Amniotic fluid (during active labour)
    - Fat (as a complication of long-bone fractures)
    - Foreign bodies (talc in IV drug users)
    - Parasite eggs (schistosomiasis)
    - Septic emboli (infectious endocarditis)
    - Tumour cells (renal cell carcinoma)
- Investigations:
  - Arterial blood gas
    - Arterial hypoxemia and elevated alveolar-arterial oxygen gradient
    - Acute respiratory alkalosis due to hyperventilation
    - These changes along with a normal CXR in a patient with no pre-existing lung disease are highly suspicious for PE
  - CXR helpful only in excluding other lung diseases and interpreting the V/Q scan
  - V/Q Scan:
    - Two or more lung segments with perfusion defects and normal ventilation are highly suggestive of PE
    - Defects in perfusion are interpreted in conjunction with ventilation and assigned either a high, low, or indeterminate probability that PE is the cause of the abnormality
  - Helical CT arteriography involves IV injection of radiocontrast dye. It is sensitive for detection of PE in the proximal pulmonary arteries, but not as much for the segmental and sub-segmental arteries
  - Venous thrombosis studies (see *Peripheral Vascular Exam* p. 312)
  - Pulmonary angiography is the gold standard for diagnosis of PE. An intraluminal filling defect in more than one projection is diagnostic of PE
- Management:
  - Anticoagulation: regimen of heparin followed by oral warfarin reduces risk of recurrent DVT and death from PE. Duration of anticoagulation will depend on potentially reversible risk factors including the patient's age, the likelihood of potential consequences of hemorrhage and the patient's preferences
  - Thrombolyic therapy: streptokinase, urokinase or TPA; shown to accelerate resolution of PE if administered within the first 24 hours
  - Should be used in patients at high risk of death and for whom the faster resolution may be life-saving
  - Inferior vena cava filter: recommended for patients in whom anticoagulation is contraindicated or who have experienced repeated PEs in spite of anticoagulation

REFERENCES

Andreoli TE, Cecil RL. 2004. Cecil Essentials of Medicine. Philadelphia: Saunders.

Bickley LS, Szilagyi PG, Bates B. 2007. *Bates' Guide to Physical Examination and History Taking*. Philadelphia: Lippincott Williams & Wilkins.

Lemiere C, Bai T, Balter M, Bayliff C, Becker A, Boulet LP, Bowie D, Cartier A, Cave A, Chapman K, Cowie R, Coyle S, Cockcroft D, Ducharme FM, Ernst P, Finlayson S, FitzGerald JM, Hargreave FE, Hogg D, Kaplan A, Kim H, Kelm C, O'Byrne P, Sears M, Markham AW. 2004. Adult Asthma Consensus Guidelines update 2003. *Can Respir J* 11 Suppl A9A-18A.

Mandell LA, Marrie TJ, Grossman RF, Chow AW, Hyland RH. 2000. Canadian guidelines for the initial management of community-acquired pneumonia: an evidence-based update by the Canadian Infectious Diseases Society and the Canadian Thoracic Society. The Canadian Community-Acquired Pneumonia Working Group. *Clin Infect Dis* 31(2):383-421.

McPhee SJ, Papadakis M. 2010. *Current Medical Diagnosis and Treatment 2010*. New York: Lange Medical Books/McGraw-Hill, Medical Pub. Division.

Metlay JP, Kapoor WN, Fine MJ. 1997. Does this patient have community-acquired pneumonia? Diagnosing pneumonia by history and physical examination. *JAMA* 278(17):1440-1445.

O'Donnell DE, Aaron S, Bourbeau J, Hernandez P, Marciniuk D, Balter M, Ford G, Gervais A, Goldstein R, Hodder R, Maltais F, Road J. 2003. Canadian Thoracic Society recommendations for management of chronic obstructive pulmonary disease--2003. *Can Respir J* 10 Suppl A11A-65A.

Sin DD, Man J, Sharpe H, Gan WQ, Man SF. 2004. Pharmacological management to reduce exacerbations in adults with asthma: a systematic review and meta-analysis. *JAMA* 292(3):367-376.

Swartz MH. 2006. *Textbook of Physical Diagnosis: History and Examination*. Philadelphia: Saunders Elsevier.

The Urological Exam

Editors:
Lindsay MacKenzie &
Yonah Krakowsky

Faculty Reviewers:
Sender Herschorn, MDCM, FRCS(C)
Michael A.S. Jewett, MD, FRCS(C), FACS

TABLE OF CONTENTS

THE MALE UROLOGICAL EXAM
Essential Male Anatomy   353
Approach to the Male Urological History and Physical Exam   354
Common Chief Complaints in a Male   354
Common Disorders in a Male   354
Focused Male History   355
Focused Male Physical Exam   357
Common Investigations   360
Common Clinical Scenarios in a Male   361

THE FEMALE UROLOGICAL EXAM
Essential Female Anatomy   363
Approach to the Female Urological History and Physical Exam   363
Common Chief Complaints in a Female   364
Common Disorders in a Female   365
Focused Female History   367
Focused Female Physical Exam   368
Common Investigations   368
Common Clinical Scenarios in a Female   368

THE MALE UROLOGICAL EXAM

ESSENTIAL ANATOMY

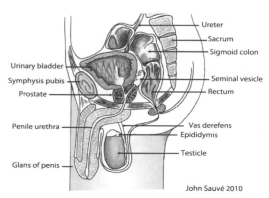

Ureter
Sacrum
Sigmoid colon
Urinary bladder
Symphysis pubis
Prostate
Seminal vesicle
Rectum
Penile urethra
Vas derefens
Epididymis
Glans of penis
Testicle

John Sauvé 2010

Figure 1. Anatomy of the Male Genitourinary Tract and Organs

APPROACH TO THE MALE UROLOGICAL HISTORY AND PHYSICAL EXAM

- Ensure proper draping throughout the exam
- Explain each procedure to the patient
- The genital exam can be performed with the patient standing or supine, however when checking for hernias or varicoceles the patient should be standing
- Wear gloves throughout the exam

Overview of the Physical Exam
- Inspection
  - Supraclavicular lymph nodes
  - Abdomen
  - Inguinal region
  - Penis and foreskin
  - Scrotum
- Palpation/Percussion
  - Kidneys
  - Bladder
  - Penis
  - Scrotum and contents
  - Inguinal region
  - Lymph nodes
- Digital Rectal Exam (DRE)

COMMON CHIEF COMPLAINTS IN A MALE

- Pain (costovertebral angle, suprapubic, genitals)
- Blood in urine (hematuria)
- Pain while urinating (dysuria)
- Hesitancy, intermittency, post-void dribbling
- Urine frequency
- Urinary urgency
- Incontinence
- Impotence (erectile dysfunction)
- Urethral discharge
- Blood in semen (hematospermia)
- Testicular mass
- Fever, chills, nausea
- Bathroom trips at night (nocturia)

COMMON DISORDERS IN A MALE

Disorders marked with (✓) are discussed in **Common Clinical Scenarios**
Renal
✓ Renal Colic
- Renal Mass (benign or malignant)
- Pyelonephritis
- Stones

Bladder
- Carcinoma

Prostate
✓ Benign Prostatic Hyperplasia (BPH)
✓ Prostate Cancer
- Prostatitis

Penis
- Erectile dysfunction
- Infertility
- Phimosis (inability to retract foreskin over glans)
- Paraphimosis (inability to reduce foreskin – an emergency)
- Peyronie's disease (induration of corpus cavernosa due to fibrosis)
- Priapism (persistent, painful erection)

Testicles
- Testicular tumours
- Spermatocele (pea-sized, nontender mass filled with spermatozoa at top of testicle)
- Epididymitis/orchitis
- ✓ Hernias
- Hydrocele (abnormal collection of clear fluid around testis in the tunica vaginalis)
- ✓ Testicular Torsion
- ✓ Varicocele (enlargement of spermatic cord due to dilation of pampiniform plexus)

FOCUSED MALE HISTORY

Genitourinary Pain
- Location (see **Table 1**), onset, duration, quality, radiation, severity, alleviation/aggravation

Table 1. Genitourinary Pain

Type of Pain	Location	Cause
Renal capsule	Ipsilateral costovertebral angle (CVA) May radiate to upper abdomen/ umbilicus	Distension of renal capsule (inflammation or obstruction)
Ureteral	Mid-ureter – referred to lower quadrant of abdomen and scrotum Lower ureter – referred to suprapubic area and penis	Obstruction of ureter leading to distension and spastic peristalsis
Vesical	Suprapubic region	Overdistension of bladder due to urinary retention or inflammation, cystitis, carcinoma
Prostatic	Perineum Referred to lower back, inguinal region or testes	Inflammation
Penile	Glans and shaft of penis	Flaccid: cystitis/urethritis, paraphimosis Erect: Peyronie's disease, priapism
Testicular	Testicles and/or scrotum	Epididymitis Torsion Mass

Lower Urinary Tract Symptoms (LUTS)

Storage Symptoms
- Frequency – increased urination ± increased urine output (polyuria)
- Nocturia – nocturnal frequency
- Urgency – strong, sudden impulse to void
- Dysuria – painful urination; start and/or during (urethral origin) vs. end (bladder origin)

Voiding Symptoms
- Straining – use of abdominal musculature to urinate
- Hesitancy – delay in initiation of urination
- Intermittency – involuntary starting/stopping of urinary stream
- Post-void dribbling – continued release of drops of urine post-void
- Decreased force of urination
- Incomplete emptying (sensation that urine retained)

Hematuria

Incontinence
- Involuntary leakage of urine

Urethral Discharge
- Continuous vs. intermittent
- Bloody (uretheral carcinoma) vs. purulent (infection)
- Gonococcal pus: thick, profuse and yellow to grey (see *Essentials of Infectious Diseases*, p. 456)
- Ask about multiple partners, STIs and UTIs

Scrotal Swelling
- Painful vs. painless

Table 2. Differential Diagnosis for Scrotal Swelling

Painful	Painless
Epididymitis	Hydrocele
Orchitis	Spermatocele
Testicular Torsion	Varicocele
Tumour (hemorrhagic)	Tumour (non-hemorrhagic)
Hematocele	Unstrangulated inguinal hernia
Strangulated inguinal hernia	Scrotal Hematoma
Epididymal cyst	

Erectile Dysfunction (Impotence)
- Inability to achieve and/or maintain an erection adequate for intercourse
- Onset, grade, duration, alleviation/aggravation
- Psychogenic vs. organic
- Differentiate from other male sexual disorders (loss of libido, failure to ejaculate, anorgasmia, premature ejaculation)

Systemic Symptoms
- Fever, chills, weight loss, nausea, vomiting

Past Medical History
- Particularly relevant: TB, diabetes mellitus, MS, renal disease

Family History
- Prostate cancer, renal tumours, stones

Travel History
- Egypt or Africa (schistosomiasis)
- Dehydration may lead to renal stones

Other
- Previous medical illnesses with urologic sequelae
- Medications (anti-coagulants, ASA, etc.)
- Previous surgical procedures
- Smoking (bladder cancer and erectile dysfunction), alcohol (testicular atrophy)

FOCUSED MALE PHYSICAL EXAM
- Throughout the examination, explain each step so that patient knows what to expect

Inspection
- **Supraclavicular lymphadenopathy** (genitourinary neoplasm)
- **Abdomen**
  - Masses, scars, suprapubic distension (see *Abdominal Exam* p. 34)
- **Inguinal region**
  - Bulges, swelling (lymphadenopathy)
- **Penis**
  - Ask patient to retract foreskin, if problematic = phimosis
  - Ask patient to reduce foreskin after retraction, if problematic = para-phimosis
  - Inspect meatus: if on underside = hypospadias, if topside = epispadias
- **Scrotum**
  - Size
  - Swelling, lumps
  - Poorly developed scrotum on one/both sides suggests cryptorchidism
  - Skin
    - Rashes, epidermoid cysts (lift scrotum to inspect posterior surface)
  - Veins
    - Varicocele upon standing or straining (usually on left side)

Palpation/Percussion
- **Kidneys** (see *Abdominal Exam* p. 37)
- **Bladder**
  - Normal adult bladder cannot be palpated/percussed (lies below pubic symphysis) unless filled with at least 150 mL of urine
  - Palpation: deeply palpate the midline of the suprapubic abdomen
  - Percussion: percuss immediately above the symphysis pubis and move cephalad until there is a change in pitch from dull to resonant
- **Penis**
  - Urethral meatus
    - Open by gently pressing on the glans with thumb and index finger
    - Urethal discharge – gonococcal (profuse, thick, and yellow) vs. non-gonococcal (scant and watery) pus

- Shaft
  + Palpate shaft of penis from glans to base with index fingers
  + Assess tenderness/abnormalities
  + Note any unusual curvature or fibrosis of penis (Peyronie's Disease)
- **Scrotum and contents**
  - Testes
    + Palpate each testicle separately using both hands (left hand holding superior/inferior poles, right hand palpates and squeezes the anterior/posterior surfaces)
    + Note size, shape, and consistency (normal testicle = firm, rubbery consistency with smooth surface)
    + Abnormally small testicles suggest hypogonadism
    + Hard area or nodularity is malignant until proven otherwise
  - Epididymis
    + Palpable ridge on supero-posterior surface of each testicle
    + Palpate for tenderness, nodularity or masses
    + Epididymitis: epididymis is very tender or painful and indistinguishable from testis on palpation (*E. coli, C. trachomatis, N. gonorrhoeae*)
  - Spermatic cord
    + Palpate both cords simultaneously with thumbs and index fingers
    + Note size, tenderness, or beading
    + Cords should be firm from epididymis to superficial inguinal ring
    + Varicocele confirmed by pulsation when patient is asked to cough
  - Transilluminate scrotal masses to differentiate between solid or cystic
    + Darken room, apply light source to side of scrotal enlargement
    + Cystic masses (hydrocele, spermatocele) transilluminate
    + Solid masses (tumour, varicocele, hernia) do not transmit light
  - Inguinal area (hernias)
    + Patient should be standing
    + Invaginate scrotal skin with finger and palpate external inguinal ring
    + Place fingertips of other hand over the abdomen in the area of internal inguinal ring
    + Ask patient to strain (Valsalva)
    + Hernia is felt as a bulge that descends against index finger in external inguinal ring
    + Indicative of hernias if: masses return to the abdomen upon lying down, have bowel sounds on auscultation and/or do not transmit light when transilluminated
- **Femoral hernias**
  - May be palpated on the anterior thigh in the femoral canal
- **Lymph nodes** (see *Lymphatic System and Lymph Node Exam*)
  - Palpable inguinal and subinguinal lymph nodes may suggest:
    + Inflammatory lesions of the penis and scrotum
    + Metastases from malignant tumours of penis, glans or scrotal skin
  - Left supraclavicular nodes may suggest:
    + Tumours of the testes and prostate
  - Iliac nodes may suggest:
    + Metastases from tumours of bladder and prostate

Table 3. Types of Hernias

	Inguinal indirect	Inguinal direct	Femoral
Frequency	Most	Less	Least
Age and Sex	All ages, M>F, Congenital	Usually men > 40 Adult Onset	Women > Men
Point of Origin	Above inguinal ligament	Above inguinal ligament	Below inguinal ligament
Course	Through internal inguinal ring	Through external inguinal ring	
	Often into scrotum	Rarely into scrotum Bulges anteriorly (deep to superficial) against finger during straining	Never into scrotum Inguinal canal is empty

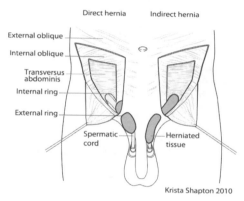

Krista Shapton 2010

Figure 2. Direct and Indirect Hernias

Digital Rectal Examination (DRE)
- If urinalysis is required, collect specimen before examination
- **Position**
  - Explain why and how examination is done, allow time for patient to prepare, relax, and be draped appropriately
  - Patient should either be supine, in left lateral decubitus, or standing bent over the examination table
  - Put on glove and lubricate the index finger thoroughly
- **Inspection (anus)**
  - Inflammation, excoriation
  - Anal carcinoma or melanoma
  - Hemorrhoids – ask patient to bear down while examining
- **Palpation** (see **Figure 3**)
  - Relax sphincter with pressure from palmar surface of gloved finger
  - Gently and slowly insert index finger into anus by rotating finger
  - Estimate sphincter tone
    - Flaccid or spastic sphincter suggests similar changes in urinary sphincter and may be suggestive of neurogenic disease

- Assess for the presence of any rectal masses
- Palpation of the prostate:
  - Do not massage prostate in patients with acute prostatitis
  - Assess size, consistency, sensitivity and shape (see **Table 4**)
- Withdraw index finger gently and slowly
- Note colour of stool on glove and test for occult blood
- Wipe the anal area of lubricant with a tissue and provide patient tissues to clean himself

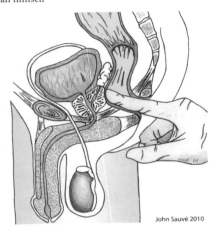

John Sauvé 2010

Figure 3. Digital Rectal Examination and Palpation of the Prostate

Table 4. Features of the Prostate on DRE

Feature	Normal	Pathologic
Size	Approx. 4 cm length and width (chestnut size)	Enlarged: benign prostatic hyperplasia, advanced prostatic carcinoma
Consistency	Rubbery	Firm/nodular in malignancy
Mobility	Variable	Fixed
Sensitivity	No pain (even on palpation)	Painful in prostatitis

COMMON INVESTIGATIONS

Urinalysis
- Should be performed in all urologic patients (see *Appendix 3* p. 547)
- A complete urinalysis includes both chemical and microscopic analyses

Gram Stain & Culture
- Including susceptibility testing if urethritis is suspected

Cytology
- Urine screened for cancer in:
  - High-risk individuals (e.g. environmental exposures)
  - Presence of painless hematuria
  - Evaluation for recurrence after bladder tumour resection

Cystoscopy

- Visualization of the bladder via insertion of fiberoptic instrument (rigid or flexible) through the urethra.
- Aids in diagnosis of bladder tumours and calculi, management of urethral stricture or accessing bladder for visualization of ureters (with x-ray) and stent placement
- Contraindicated in patients with an active UTI

Screening for Prostate Cancer

- Males 50 to 75 with life-expectancy of >10 years should be informed of the risks/benefits of PSA testing. Men over 75 should not be tested. Men at a higher risk for prostate cancer:
  - African-North American descent
  - 1st generation relative with prostate cancer
  - High fat diet
  - Prostatic nodule found on DRE
  - Abnormal-feeling prostate
  - Discrete change either in texture, fullness or symmetry
- PSA has limited specificity because elevations also occur in men with benign disease (i.e. prostatic hyperplasia, prostatitis)
- PSA levels vary according to age and degree of hyperplasia but cancer produces excess levels
- Consider tests such as PSA Velocity or Percent Free PSA (fPSA) to supplement investigation

> **Clinical Pearl**
> **PSA Measurements after Treatment of Prostate Cancer**
> PSA measurements become an integral part of follow-up visits post-treatment.
> The frequency and parameters of these measurements will depend on the modality of treatment and the physician's or hospital's protocol.

COMMON CLINICAL SCENARIOS IN A MALE

Renal Colic

- Symptoms/Signs
  - Intense, sudden onset, unilateral pain in flanks (or lower abdomen) radiating to groin/testis
  - Patient may writhe in pain unable to find relief in any position
  - Sweating, nausea and vomiting are common
  - Blood may be seen or detected in urine
- Physical Exam
  - Complete abdominal and urological exam (including DRE) → tenderness
  - Rule out aortic aneurysm by checking for pulsating mass
  - Rule out gallbladder by palpating right rib cage margin for tenderness
- Investigations
  - Urinalysis for blood
  - Non-contrast helical CT abdomen is diagnostic test of choice
  - Plain abdominal x-rays can track already detected stone

Hematuria

- Can be gross (visible in urine) or microscopic (>2-5 RBCs/HPF)
- Assess signs and symptoms:
  - Timing: initial stream, terminal stream, total stream
  - Pain (inflammation or obstruction from calculi/clots)

- Irritative urinary symptoms (suggests UTI)
- Voiding LUTS (fever, chills, nausea, vomiting)
- Other important aspects of hematuria history:
  - Recent sexual history (STIs)
  - Recent instumentation
  - Drugs: anti-coagulants, ASA, NSAIDs, phenytoin, chemotherapeutics
  - Others: trauma, sickle cell anemia, hemophilia, glomerulonephritis, malaria/schistosomiasis (travel history)
- Physical Exam
  - Complete abdominal and urological exam (including DRE) → tenderness, masses, distension and induration
- Investigations (see **Figure 4**)
  - Urinalysis
  - Urine cytology
  - Cystoscopy
  - Imaging (ultrasound, spiral CT, and/or IVP)

> **Clinical Pearl**
> Hematuria of any degree should never be ignored and, in adults, should be regarded as a symptom of urologic malignancy until proven otherwise.

Benign Prostatic Hyperplasia (BPH)
- Clinically appears in 25% men in their 50s, 33% men in their 60s, and 50% men in their 70s
- Symptoms/Signs
  - Storage/voiding LUTS
- Physical Exam
  - DRE – note size, and consistency (average prostate ~20 g)
  - Note: BPH is not a risk factor for prostate cancer
  - With BPH, prostate should be smooth, firm, elastic and enlarged
  - Induration found with DRE indicates further investigation for cancer
- Investigations
  - Urinalysis (to exclude infection/hematuria)
  - Creatinine
  - PSA (to exclude prostate cancer)
  - Transrectal ultrasound (TRUS) to assess size

Prostate Cancer
- Symptoms/Signs
  - Most are asymptomatic
  - Storage and voiding LUTS may suggest locally advanced or metastatic disease
  - Bone pain may be suggestive of metastases
  - Paresthesias, weakness of lower extremities and urinary or fecal incontinence may be observed in advanced disease with cord compression
- Physical Exam
  - Induration found with DRE indicates further investigation to rule out cancer (i.e. PSA screen/TRUS/biopsy)
- Investigations
  - PSA screen
  - Percent free PSA (fPSA)
  - PSA velocity
  - TRUS (if appropriate)
  - Biopsy (if appropriate)

Varicocele

- Symptoms/Signs
  - Most are asymptomatic
  - May present as infertile patient
  - May report scrotal heaviness
- Physical Exam
  - Careful inspection, may appear as "bag of worms" in scrotum
- Investigations
  - If unclear then high-resolution Doppler ultrasonography
  - Semen analysis to determine if surgery needed

Hernias

- Symptoms/Signs
  - Lump or swelling in groin or scrotum
  - Sudden pain in scrotum
  - Pain in scrotum while standing or moving
  - Heavy feeling in groin
- Physical Exam
  - Best performed seated with patient standing
  - Observe inguinal canal for bulge, size increased with cough
  - Invaginate scrotum with finger, ask patient to cough and feel for impulse
  - Investigations are often not necessary to make diagnosis

Testicular Torsion

- Symptoms/Signs
  - Sudden onset of severe testicular pain followed by inguinal and/or scrotal swelling
  - Testicle retracted upwards
  - $^1/_3$ have GI upset
  - May be preceded by trauma
- Physical Exam
  - Swollen, tender, high-riding, transverse testis
  - Lifting the testicle will increase pain (in epididymitis it will relieve pain)
  - Support diagnosis with the absence of the cremasteric reflex
- Investigations
  - If physical exam suggests testicular torsion, refer patient to OR for immediate scrotal exploration

ESSENTIAL FEMALE ANATOMY

Please see the *Gynecological Exam* for a depiction of the external female genital anatomy.

APPROACH TO THE FEMALE UROLOGICAL HISTORY AND PHYSICAL EXAM

In addition to a general history and physical, the following are important urologic symptoms/signs in a female:

- Genitourinary pain
- Hematuria
- Storage or voiding lower urinary tract symptoms (LUTS)
- Incontinence
- Systemic symptoms
- Vaginal bleeding

The urinary history is an important component of the urological history in a female, and should include specific questioning regarding:

- Difficulties passing urine
- Frequency
- Nocturia
- Polyuria/volume of urine passed
- Dysuria/burning sensation
- Incontinence (especially with sudden coughing, laughing, sneezing)
- Urgency
- Associated symptoms (fever, chills, hematuria, pain in abdomen, back or flank)

Overview of the Female Physical Exam
- Explain procedures to patient
- Inspection
  - Supraclavicular lymphadenopathy
  - Abdomen
  - External genitalia
  - Internal genitalia (pelvic exam)
  - Inguinal region
- Palpation/percussion
  - Kidneys
  - Bladder
  - Vagina (pelvic exam)
  - Inguinal region
  - Lymph nodes
- Urinary Stress Test

COMMON CHIEF COMPLAINTS IN A FEMALE

- Pain (costovertebral angle, suprapubic, genitals)
- Pain (dysuria) or burning or pressure while urinating
- Blood in urine (hematuria)
- Urinary frequency
- Urinary urgency
- Bathroom trips at night (nocturia)
- Leaking urine (incontinence)
- Spotting (vaginal bleeding between menstrual periods or post-menopausally)
- Vaginal fullness

COMMON DISORDERS IN A FEMALE

Disorders marked with (✓) are discussed in **Common Clinical Scenarios**
✓ Asymptomatic Hematuria
- Bladder carcinoma
- Hernias
- Incontinence (stress, urge, overflow, functional, pharmacological)
✓ Pelvic Organ Prolapse (urethral prolapse, uterine prolapse, cystocele, rectocele)
- Renal colic
- Renal mass (benign or malignant)
- Stones
✓ Urinary tract infection (cystitis, pyelonephritis, urethritis)

FOCUSED FEMALE HISTORY

Genitourinary Pain

- Location, onset, quality, severity, radiation, duration, alleviation/aggravation
- Renal capsule pain (inflammation or obstruction of kidney) is felt in the costovertebral angle/flank and may radiate anteriorly towards the umbilicus. Pain is usually described as a constant, dull, aching
- Ureteral pain (sudden ureteral distension) can be felt in the costovertebral angle and can radiate around anteriorly into the lower abdominal quadrant and into the upper thigh/labium. Pain is usually described as severe and colicky
- Suprapubic pain or tenderness (inflammation of bladder) is only examinable if bladder is distended above pubic symphysis
- Always ask about associated urinary symptoms (see below for storage/voiding symptoms) fever, chills, nausea, vomiting or hematuria.
- Ask about risk factors for UTI including: female gender, recent antibiotic use, sexual intercourse/diaphragm/spermicide use, anatomic abnormality, catheterization, elderly

Hematuria

- Colour, duration, pattern, frequency
  - Initial stream hematuria – anterior urethral source
  - Terminal stream hematuria – bladder neck source
  - Hematuria throughout stream – bladder or upper urinary tract source
- Always ask about associated fever, dysuria, suprapubic, flank or perineal pain
- Ask about recent past history of stone passage, sore throat, catherterization, streptococcal skin infection, joint pain
- Medications commonly associated with hematuria: warfarin, coumadin, ASA, NSAIDs, phenytoin, chemotherapeutics
- Urine can appear red due to recent beet ingestion, levodopa, methyldopa, rifampin, food dyes
- Ensure you distinguish true hematuria from menstrual blood

Lower Urinary Tract Symptoms (LUTS)

Storage Symptoms
- Frequency – increased urinary output (polyuria ≥3 L 24 hrs) or decreased bladder capacity
- Nocturia – nocturnal frequency (awakening > once/night)
- Urgency – strong, sudden impulse to void
- Dysuria – painful urination

Voiding Symptoms
- Straining – use of abdominal musculature to urinate
- Hesitancy – delay in initiation of urination
- Intermittency – involuntary starting/stopping of urinary stream
- Post-void dribbling – release of drops of urine at the end of micturition
- Decreased force of urination
- Incomplete emptying

Incontinence

- Involuntary loss of urine
- Ask about "problems with urine leaking" or "difficulties getting to the toilet on time"

Table 5. Classification of Incontinence

Type of Incontinence	Definition	Possible Causes
Stress	Urine loss with increased intra-abdominal pressure (e.g. coughing, laughing, sneezing) and not associated with the urge to urinate	Post-partum, post-menopausal or surgical loss of anterior vaginal support of bladder and proximal urethra
Urge	Urine loss due to uninhibited bladder contractions – preceded by urge to urinate	Cystitis Neurogenic bladder (following stroke, dementia, cord lesion above sacral level) Deconditioned voiding reflexes (frequent voluntary voiding at low bladder volume)
Overflow	Urine loss due to chronically distended bladder – even after effort to void	Bladder outlet obstruction, weak detrusor muscle, impaired sensation (e.g. with diabetic neuropathy)
Functional	Urine loss due to functional inability to reach toilet in time	Impaired health, environmental conditions
Pharmacological	Urine loss secondary to medication	Sedatives, tranquilizers, anticholinergics, sympathetic blockers, potent diuretics

*More than one type of incontinence can be present in a given patient

Systemic Symptoms

- Fever, chills, weight loss, nausea, vomiting

Other

- Previous medical illnesses with urologic sequelae
- Medications
- Previous surgical procedures
- Smoking, alcohol and drug use
- Family history of urologic disease
- Spotting or non-menstrual vaginal bleeding (either between cycles or post-menopause)

FOCUSED FEMALE PHYSICAL EXAM

- A full explanation of what to expect throughout the exam is important for patient comfort, especially during the pelvic exam
- Proper draping is essential – only expose what is necessary for the exam

Inspection

- **Supraclavicular lymphadenopathy (genitourinary neoplasm)**
- **Abdomen**
  - Masses, scars, suprapubic distension (see *Abdominal Exam* p. 34)

- **Vagina**
  - Vulvar/vaginal atrophy (assess estrogenization)
  - Urethral Orifice
    - Examine for caruncle = small, red, benign tumour in urethral opening (posterior portion)
    - Examine for urethral prolapse = swollen red ring of urethral mucosa protruding from urethral opening
- **Inguinal region**
  - Bulges of inguinal or femoral hernia

Palpation/Percussion
- **Kidneys**
  - Place one hand under the patient's back and apply upwards pressure near the 12th rib. Attempt to 'catch' the kidney between your hands by placing the opposite hand firmly and deeply in the upper quadrant of the abdomen
  - Note that the normal kidney is difficult to palpate unless the patient is very thin
  - Fist percussion over costovertebral angle to examine for tenderness
- **Bladder**
  - The normal adult bladder cannot be palpated/percussed unless filled with at least 150 mL of urine (and above the symphysis pubis)
    - Palpation: deeply palpate the midline of the suprapubic abdomen
    - Percussion: percuss immediately above the symphysis pubis and move cephalad until there is a change in pitch from dull to resonant
    - Bimanual palpation: abdomen and vagina; assess bladder mobility, masses
- **Vagina**
  - All women presenting with urinary complaints should have a pelvic exam
  - Examine for cystocele = bulge in anterior vaginal wall
  - Examine for rectocele = bulge in posterior vaginal wall
  - Assess anterior wall mobility by having patient Valsalva (increase intra-abdominal pressure) in the lithotomy position with a Graves speculum retracting posterior vaginal wall
  - Assess pelvic floor musculature and bulk with digital vaginal examination in the fornices
- **Hernias**
  - Occurences in females are less common than in males. When occurring: indirect inguinal > femoral > direct inguinal hernia
  - Examination for inguinal hernias: palpate within the labia majora and move finger upwards, ending just lateral to the pubic tubercle. If present will feel bulge against finger tip when patient valsalvas
  - Femoral hernia is felt as a bulge under the inguinal ligament in the femoral triangle
- **Lymph nodes**
  - See *Lymphatic System and Lymph Node Exam*
  - Inguinal and subinguinal lymph nodes may suggest:
    - Inflammatory lesions of the vulva
    - Metastases from malignant tumours of vagina or distal urethra
  - Iliac nodes may suggest:
    - Metastases from tumours of bladder

UROLOGICAL

Special Maneuvers
- **Urinary Stress Test**
  - Have patient sit upright on the examining table with a full bladder. Legs are spread and perineal area is relaxed. Ask the patient to cough vigorously. If urine is lost, beginning and ending with the cough, the test is confirmatory for stress incontinence

COMMON INVESTIGATIONS

Urinalysis
- Should be performed in all urologic patients (see *Appendix 3* p. 547)
- A complete urinalysis includes both chemical and microscopic analyses

Gram Stain & Culture
- Including susceptibility testing if UTI is suspected

Cytology
- Urine screened for cancer in:
  - High-risk individuals (e.g. environmental exposures)
  - Presence of painless hematuria
  - Evaluation for recurrence after bladder tumour resection

Cystoscopy
- Visualization of the bladder via insertion of fiberoptic instrument (rigid or flexible) into the urethra
- Aids in diagnosis of bladder tumours and calculi, management of urethral stricture or accessing bladder for visualization of ureters (with x-ray) and stent placement
- Contraindicated in patients with an active UTI

Ultrasound
- Often used to determine post-void residual volume, total bladder capacity and bladder proprioception in the setting of incontinence

COMMON CLINICAL SCENARIOS IN A FEMALE

Urinary Tract Infection (UTI)
- Definition: >100,000 bacteria/mL in midstream urine (MSU); can be less if patient is symptomatic
- May be pyelonephritis, cystitis, and/or urethritis
- Uncomplicated if infection in a healthy patient with structurally and functionally normal urinary tract
- Complicated if infection in advanced age, chronic renal disease, diabetes mellitus, immunodeficiency, pregnancy, recurrent instrumentation, urological abnormalities
- Most commonly due to ascending GI organisms (*E. coli*, Entercocci) but also commonly due to *Klebsiella* spp., *Proteus* spp., *Pseudomonas* spp., *S. saprophyticus, S. fecalis*
- **Symptoms/Signs**
  - Storage/voiding LUTS
  - Hematuria
  - Cloudy/malodorous urine
  - Pain/tenderness (costovertebral angle – pyelonephritis, suprapubic, back)

- Urethral discharge
- Recent sexual history
- History of instrumentation
- Previous UTIs
- Fever, chills, nausea, vomiting (suggests pyelonephritis)
- Potential sequelae: sepsis/shock
- **Physical Exam**
  - Vitals – temperature
  - Suprapubic/Costovertebral tenderness
  - Complete urological exam
- **Investigations**
  - Urinalysis
  - Midstream urine culture
  - Urine cytology*
  - Cystoscopy*
  - Imaging (ultrasound, spiral CT and/or IVP)*

* only if indicated by MSU culture, pattern of recurrence or associated fever

> **Evidence-Based Medicine: Acute Uncomplicated UTI in Women**
> Up to 33% of women will develop at least one urinary tract infection over the course of their lives.
> The diagnosis of acute uncomplicated UTI can be made by primarily by history; women with dysuria AND urgency or frequency will have a diagnosis of UTI 80% of the time and should be treated with empiric antibiotics. If a woman presents with vaginal symptoms in addition to urinary symptoms the likelihood of UTI is significantly decreased.
> Consider Culture and Sensitivity testing only in the setting of pyelonephrits symptoms, complicating factors, persistence of symptoms, or history of recurrent UTIs.
>
> *Urinary Tract Infection Guidelines.* 2005. University of Michigan Health System.

Hematuria

- Can be gross (visible in urine) or microscopic (>2-5 RBCs/HPF)
- **Signs and symptoms**
  - Pain (inflammation or obstruction from calculi/clots)
  - Storage urinary symptoms (suggests UTI)
  - Systemic symptoms (fever, chills, nausea, vomiting)
- Other important aspects of hematuria history:
  - Recent sexual history (STIs)
  - Recent instumentation
  - Drugs: anti-coagulants, ASA, NSAIDs, phenytoin, chemotherapeutics
  - Others: trauma, sickle cell anemia, hemophilia, glomerulonephritis, malaria/schistosomiasis (travel history)
- **Physical Exam**
  - Complete abdominal and urological exam (including DRE) → tenderness, masses, distension and induration
- **Investigations**
  - See **Figure 4**

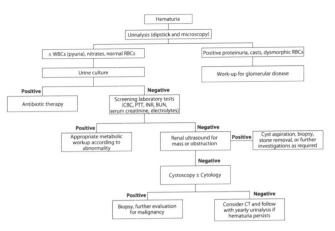

Figure 4. Investigations of Hematuria

Pelvic Organ Prolapse

- Descent or herniation of pelvic organs from their normal positions and attachment sites in the pelvis
  - Urethral Prolapse
  - Uterine Prolapse
  - Anterior Vaginal Wall Prolapse = Cystocele
  - Posterior Vaginal Wall Prolapse = Rectocele
- **Signs and Sympoms**
  - Often asymptomatic
  - Vaginal bleeding (from exposed/ulcerated mucous membrane)
  - Sensation of vaginal fullness/pressure
  - History of coital difficulties
  - History of voiding or defecation difficulty
  - Sacral back pain
  - Bulge protruding into vagina or through vaginal introitus
- Other important aspects of history with pelvic organ prolapse include:
  - Multiparous (higher risk for prolapse)
  - Other symptoms/signs of vaginal atrophy/hypoestrogenism
  - Increased intrabdominal pressure (obesity, COPD, etc.)
  - Connective tissue disease (e.g. Marfan disease)
- **Physical exam**: examine the patient in lithotomy as well as standing, both while relaxed and during maximal straining
  - Urethral prolapse – swollen, red, ring around urethral meatus
  - Cystocele if bulge in anterior vaginal wall
    - 1st Degree – protrusion to upper vagina
    - 2nd Degree – protrusion to the introitus
    - 3rd Degree – protrusion external to the introitus
  - Rectocele if bulge in posterior vaginal wall
  - Uterine prolapse (may be associated with cystocele and/or rectocele) – progressive retroversion of uterus and descent into vagina with lowering of cervix:
    - 1st Degree – cervix remains within vagina
    - 2nd Degree – cervix is at the introitus
    - 3rd Degree – cervix and vagina are outside the introitus

- **Investigations**
  - Assess for urinary retention – post-void residual volume (ultrasound)
  - Assess strength of pelvic floor musculature
  - If patient is asymptomatic and there is no urinary retention – may do nothing

REFERENCES

Bickley LS, Szilagyi PG, Bates B. 2007. *Bates' Guide to Physical Examination and History Taking.* Philadelphia: Lippincott Williams & Wilkins.

Campbell MF, Walsh PC, Retik AB. 2002. *Campbell's Urology.* Philadelphia: Saunders.

Fauci AS. 2008. *Harrison's Principles of Internal Medicine.* New York: McGraw-Hill.

Marcozzi D, Suner S. 2001. The nontraumatic, acute scrotum. *Emerg Med Clin North Am* 19(3):547-568.

Moul JW. 2003. Population screening for prostate cancer and emerging concepts for young men. *Clin Prostate Cancer* 2(2):87-97.

Tanagho EA, McAninch JW, Smith DR. 2008. *Smith's General Urology.* New York: McGraw-Hill Medical.

University of Michigan Health System. 2005. *Urinary Tract Infection.* Ann Arbor (MI): University of Michigan Health System.

UROLOGICAL

The Essentials of Clinical Pharmacology

Editors:
Alex Cheng & Janine Hutson

Faculty Reviewer:
Shinya Ito, MD, FRCP(C)

TABLE OF CONTENTS

Common Abbreviations for Orders	373
Essentials of Writing a Prescription	374
Modifying Factors of Drug Actions	375
Important Pharmacokinetic Formulae	376
Common Drug Interactions	377
Drug Safety in Pregnancy	379
Approach to the Toxic or Poisoned Patient	380
Common Recreational Drugs	381

The following chapter provides a brief overview of common topics in clinical pharmacology. Please refer to the Compendium of Pharmaceuticals and Specialties (CPS), USP DI or other pharmacology textbooks for more detailed information on the topics reviewed.

COMMON ABBREVIATIONS FOR ORDERS

Always consult the hospital formulary for approved abbreviations specific to each institution
Try to avoid abbreviations whenever possible

Table 1. Common Abbreviations for Orders

Abbreviation	Interpretation
ac	Before meals
amp	Ampoule
bid	Twice a day
cap	Capsule
CVL	Central venous line
D5W	Dextrose 5% in water
GT	Gastrostomy tube
hs	At bedtime
IM	Intramuscular
IT	Intrathecal
IV	Intravenous
mEq or meq	Milliequivalent
mitte	Dispense this number of tablets
mL	Millilitre
OTC	Over-the-counter
NG	Nasogastric

Table 1. Common Abbreviations for Orders (continued)

Abbreviation	Interpretation
Now	(For medications) give within 2 hours
NS	Normal saline
pc	After meals
po	By mouth
pr	Per rectum
prn	When required
q ( ) h	Every ( ) hour(s)
qam	Every morning
qid	Four times a day
SC, SQ	Subcutaneous
STAT	At once
supp or sup	Suppository
susp	Suspension
Tab	Tablet
tid	Three times a day
TPN	Total Parenteral Nutrition
v/v	Volume in volume
vag	Vaginal
w/v	Weight in volume
w/w	Weight in weight

Table 2. Error-prone Abbreviations to Avoid – To correct, write out the order in full

Full Order	Abbreviation	Misinterpretation
microgram	μg	mg
right eye	OD	AD (right ear) or qd
once daily	q1d or qd	q.i.d. (four times daily)
at every bedtime	qhs	qhr (every hour)
every other day	qod	q.d. (daily) or q.i.d. (four times daily)

ESSENTIALS OF WRITING A PRESCRIPTION

Essential Components of a Drug Prescription
- Hospital Name (for generic hospital prescriptions) or Prescriber Name and title i.e. MD
- Address and phone number of Hospital or Prescriber
- Date of the written prescription
- Patient information: name and address – important for verifying information
- May include age and weight of the patient, which can be helpful for dosing purposes

- Drug information: name, strength/dosage, and quantity
- Instructions for the patient e.g. take one pill by mouth daily
- Signature of Prescriber and if using a generic hospital prescription note, write down prescriber name as well
- Refill information – indicate how many refills you are prescribing

Other points to consider when writing a prescription drug order:
- Do not follow a decimal point with a zero (use 2 mg NOT 2.0 mg)
- Use zero before a decimal point when the dose is less than a whole unit (use 0.125 mg NOT .125 mg)
- Place adequate space between the drug name, dose, and unit of measure
- Use commas for dosing units at or above 1,000 or use words such as 100 'thousand' or 1 'million' to improve readability
- Use complete drug names; do not abbreviate drug names
- Avoid symbols such as @, and, +, °, and "u" for units (spell out "units")
- May include reason for prescribing drug to help avoid prescribing the wrong drug with a similar name
- Must be written in ink
- Ensure that the prescription can be read and is written eligibly
- If worried about a patient altering a prescription (e.g. for controlled substances), then the quantity of medication and any repeats should be written in words
- Should indicate in chart what prescription was written for patient

MODIFYING FACTORS OF DRUG ACTIONS

Individual factors may alter the effect of or how the body handles the drug. The following are common modifying factors, but a pharmacology text should be consulted for a complete list.

Table 3. Modifying Factors of Drug Actions

Modifying Factor		Effect
Age	Pediatrics	Changes in absorption, distribution, metabolism, and elimination occur with development
	Elderly	Changes in drug metabolism and elimination with geriatric diseases and change in distribution with changes in body composition
Alcohol		Chronic use can increase metabolism Acute use can inhibit metabolism
Concurrent Disease(s)		Renal disease, liver disease, cardiac failure, shock, and protein loss may alter pharmacokinetics
Concurrent Medications		May inhibit or induce metabolism or elimination
Food Intake		May alter absorption of medications taken by mouth
Genetics		Genetic variation in drug metabolizing enzymes and transporters may increase toxicity or decrease efficacy
Pregnancy		Increased plasma volume, decreased protein binding and changes in GFR may alter pharmacokinetics
Route of administration		Each differs in rates or amounts of absorption
Smoking		May induce drug metabolism

Table 4. Dosing Guidelines for Pediatric Population* (see *Pediatric Exam*)

Age	Weight (kg)	Surface Area (m²)	% of total adult dose
1 month	4	0.24	10
1 year	10	0.45	25
6 years	20	0.8	50
12 years	40	1.3	75
Adult	65	1.73	100

*Guidelines are an estimate – please check dosing guidelines specific to each drug when available

Table 5. Considerations for Drug Therapy in the Geriatric Population
(see *Geriatric Exam*)

General Considerations

Define the goal for drug therapy

Take a detailed drug history including over the counter and herbal products

Highly suspect drug reactions or drug interactions

Simplify the number of drugs taken and the number of times administered to increase compliance

Dosing Considerations

Concurrent diseases, such as renal failure, may increase the $t_{1/2}$

Changes in total body water and protein binding alter distribution

For drugs with a low TI, lower dose by $1/3$ and titrate to the desired effect

Wait at least 3 $t_{1/2}$ before increasing the dose

TI = therapeutic index = median toxic dose/median effective dose

IMPORTANT PHARMACOKINETIC FORMULAE

Clearance
$$Cl = \frac{\text{rate of drug elimination}}{\text{plasma drug concentration}}$$

Volume of distribution
$$V_d = \frac{\text{amount of drug in body}}{\text{plasma drug concentration}}$$

Elimination Half-life
$$t_{1/2} = \frac{(0.7)(V_d)}{Cl}$$

Ideal Body Weight (IBW)

for males $IBW = 50 \text{ kg} + [2.3 \text{ kg} \times (\text{no. of inches} > 5 \text{ ft})]$

for females $IBW = 45.5 \text{ kg} + [2.3 \text{ kg} \times (\text{no. of inches} > 5 \text{ ft})]$

(Doses of drugs such as acyclovir should be calculated with IBW to avoid toxicity)

Steady State Drug Concentration (Css)
$$C_{ss} = \frac{(F)(\text{Rate of drug administration})}{Cl}$$
Where F = bioavailability

PHARMACOLOGY

| Loading Dose (LD) | $LD = Cp \times V_d / F$ |
| | Where, Cp = target plasma drug concentration |

Maintenance Dose	$MD = Cp \times Cl \times \tau / F$
	Where τ = dosing interval
With renal impairment:	$MD = CrCl \text{ (patient)} / CrCl \text{ (normal)} \times$ Standard Dose of Drug
(when drug is renally excreted)	Where CrCl = Creatinine clearance

---

Clinical Pearl
With repeated dosing at the regular dosing interval, it takes 3 to 4 $t_{1/2}$ to reach 90% of the steady state concentration. To clear the body of 90% of the drug, it takes 3 to 4 $t_{1/2}$ from the last dose.

COMMON DRUG INTERACTIONS

Interacting agents can increase or decrease the actions of the following drugs (refer to CPS or other text for complete lists). Drug interactions may increase the risk for toxicity/overdose or may decrease the therapeutic response. Drug-drug interactions commonly result from changes in drug metabolism, drug transport, amount of absorption, and alterations in protein binding or additive pharmacological responses. Changes in drug metabolism can be predicted by consulting a table of known cytochrome P450 substrates. Therapeutic drug monitoring may be required (i.e. for carbamazepine).

Table 6. Common Drug Interactions

Affected Drug	Change in Drug Concentration/Action	Interacting Agent
Antidiabetic Agents	↑	MAO Inhibitors
Azole antifungals	↓	Antacids, barbiturates, didanosine, H2 blockers, PPIs, rifampin
Benzodiazepines	↑	Alcohol
Beta-blockers	↑	Cimetidine
	↓	Barbituates, Phenytoin, Rifampin
Calcium channel blockers	↑	Azole antifungals, cimetidine
	↓	Barbituates, phenytoin, rifampin
Carbamazepine	↑	Azole antifungals, cimetidine, clarithromycin, dilitazem, erythromycin, isoniazid, SSRIs, verapamil
Codeine	↓	Amiodarone, haloperidol, paroxetine

MAO-monoamine oxidase; SSRI – selective serotonin reuptake inhibitor

Table 6. Common Drug Interactions (continued)

Affected Drug	Change in Drug Concentration/Action	Interacting Agent
Cyclosporine	↑	Azole antifungals, clarithromycin, erythromycin, grapefruit juice, nefazodone, ritonavir
	↓	Barbituates, carbamazepine, phenytoin, rifampin, St. John's wort
Digoxin/digitoxin	↑	Amiodarone, cyclosporine, macrolide antibiotics, potassium depleting drugs, propafenone, quinidine, verapamil
Glyburide	↑	Fluconazole, fluoxetine, metronidazole, sulfamethoxazole/trimethoprim
HMG-CoA reductase inhibitors (Statins)	↑	Azole antifungals, clarithromycin, cyclosporine, erythromycin, grapefruit juice
Imidazoles (e.g. ketoconazole)	↑	Phenytoin
	↓	Antacids, Barbituates, PPIs, Rifampin
Lithium	↑	Diuretics, NSAIDs, sodium retention
	↓	Theophylline
Methotrexate	↑	Probenecid, salicylates
NSAIDs	↓	Bile acid sequestrants
Phenytoin	↑	Amiodarone, cimetidine, felbamate, fluconazole, miconazole, NSAIDS, proton pump inhibitors
Quinidine	↑	Acetazolamide, cimetidine
	↓	Barbituates, phenytoin, rifampin
Quinolones	↓	Antacids, iron, sucralfate
SSRIs	↑	MAO Inhibitors – contraindicated
Tetracycline	↓	Metal-containing products
TCAs	↑	SSRIs, MAO Inhibitors
	↓	Barbituates, Rifampin

MAO-monoamine oxidase; SSRI – selective serotonin reuptake inhibitor

PHARMACOLOGY

Table 6. Common Drug Interactions (continued)

Affected Drug	Change in Drug Concentration/ Action	Interacting Agent
Theophylline	↑	Cimetidine, clarithromycin, dilitazem, erythromycin, fluvoxamine, isoniazid, mexiletine, quinolones, tacrine, thiabendazole, troleandomycin, verapamil, zileuton
	↓	Barbituates, phenytoin, rifampin, smoking
Warfarin/dicumarol	↑	Acetominophen, amiodarone, ASA, cimetidine, clarithromycin, clopidogrel, erythromycin, fibrates, fluconazole, hyperthyroidism, metronidazole, trimethoprim-sulfamethoxazole, quinolones, hyperthyroidism
	↓	Barbiturates, carbamazepine, cholestyramine, rifampin

MAO-monoamine oxidase; SSRI – selective serotonin reuptake inhibitor

DRUG SAFETY IN PREGNANCY

Proper counselling should be given to pregnant women who use medications. When considering therapeutics in pregnancy, the risk of the medication together with the benefit of treatment must be weighed. Please consult a teratogen information service for more information i.e. Motherisk (CDN) or the Organization of Teratology Information Specialists (USA).

The following are selected medications that are teratogenic (but not all are absolutely contraindicated in pregnancy, please consult an information service). Pre-pregnancy planning is advised for patients using these medications.

- ACE Inhibitors
- Carbamazepine
- Isotretinoin/Retinoids
- Lithium
- Methotrexate
- Mycophenolate
- Misoprostol
- Phenytoin
- Thalidomide
- Valproic Acid
- Warfarin

The following are selected drugs that are considered safe at recommended doses in pregnancy.

- Acetaminophen
- Antihistamines
- Beta-lactams
- Doxylamine
- Flu vaccine
- Ranitidine

APPROACH TO THE TOXIC OR POISONED PATIENT

Drug toxicity can result from drug overdose, impaired drug metabolism, drug interactions, and idiosyncratic hypersensitivity. Altered mental status, seizures, or cardiovascular changes may lead to the suspicion of poisoning. Contact the local poison control center for consultation. The following includes an approach to taking the history of a poisoned patient after the ABCs and glucose level have been assessed.

- Take the history from family/friends, police officers, paramedics about what substance was taken. Often the history is unreliable and if possible, ask for any bottles, syringes, or household products that were found around the patient
- To aid in the differential of possible poisons, assess the following and determine any characteristic toxic syndrome (**Table 7**)
    - Assess vital signs including pulse, respiratory rate, blood pressure and temperature
    - Observe the eyes for miosis, mydriasis, nystagmus, or ptosis
    - Assess the colour, dryness and temperature of the skin
    - Auscultate for bowel sounds to determine ileus or increased sounds
    - Perform a neurological exam
- A broad toxicology screen can be ordered
- Decontamination procedures (including administration of activated charcoal and whole bowel irrigation) should be individualized according to age, properties of substances ingested, and the time that has elapsed since ingestion

Table 7. Common Toxic Syndromes and Treatment

Agents	Signs and Symptoms	Treatment
Acetaminophen	Gastrointestinal upset, liver injury	N-acetylcysteine (Mucomyst®) for liver injury
Amphetamines and other stimulants	Agitation, acute psychosis, hypertension, tachycardia, seizures, hyperthermia	Manage seizures with benzodiazepines
Anticholinergic agents	Blurred vision, dry skin and mucous membranes, confusion, hyperthermia, flushed	Benzodiazepines, general support, physostigmine
Antipsychotics	CNS depression, seizures, hypotension, arrhythmia, dystonia	Fluids, sodium bicarbonate
Aspirin (salicylate)	Hyperventilation, respiratory alkalosis, then metabolic acidosis, hyperthermia	IV sodium bicarbonate and fluids
Benzodiazepines	Amnestic effects, confusion, respiratory depression	General support – flumazenil under supervision
Beta-adrenergic blockers	Bradycardia, hypotension	Glucagon
Calcium channel blockers	Hypotension	Calcium, high dose insulin + glucose
Carbon monoxide (and other toxic gases)	Headache, confusion, nausea tachypnea	Oxygen

Table 7. Common Toxic Syndromes and Treatment (continued)

Agents	Signs and Symptoms	Treatment
Cholinesterase inhibitors (e.g. insecticides)	Abdominal cramps, diarrhea, sweating, muscle twitching, seizures	Pralidoxime and atropine
Digoxin (and related cardiac glycosides)	Vomiting, variety of cardiac rhythm disturbances	Digoxin antibodies (Digibind®), avoid calcium
Ethylene glycol and methanol	Metabolic acidosis, hyperventilation, visual disturbances	Ethanol or fomepizole
Iron salts	Vomiting, abdominal pain, bloody diarrhea	Deferoxamine (Desferal®)
Opioids	Respiratory depression, nausea, vomiting, constipation	Naloxone (Narcan®)
Tricyclic antidepressants (TCAs)	Seizures, hypotension, arrhythmia, tachycardia, hypotension	Sodium bicarbonate

COMMON RECREATIONAL DRUGS

It is not uncommon for patients to be using street drugs in addition to pre-scribed medications. Knowledge about the health effects produced by these drugs along with some of the various street terms is useful.

Table 8. Common Recreational Drugs and Effects on Health

Drug	Alternative Street Names	Short-term Health Effects
Amphetamine family i.e. amphetamines, methamphetamines, dextroamphetamine	Amphetamine family - Speed, bennies, glass, crystal, crank, uppers, pep pills	CNS stimulant drug; increased alertness, energy, restlessness, increased breathing, blood pressure, respiratory rate
	Methamphetamine – speed, crystal meth, meth, chalk, ice, crystal, jib	
Benzodiazepines	benzos, tranks, downers	CNS depressant; often used in conjunction with opioids or stimulants (to decrease their effect); produces calming and relaxing effect

Table 8. Common Recreational Drugs and Effects on Health (continued)

Drug	Alternative Street Names	Short-term Health Effects
Cannabis – includes marijuana, hashish, and hash oil	Marijuna – grass, weed, pot, dope, ganja Hashish – hash Hash Oil – weed oil, honey oil	Hallucinogen; perceptual distortions, drowsiness, spontaneous laughter, relaxation or anxiety, increased appetite and heart rate; decreased blood pressure and balance
Cocaine	Blow, C, coke, flake, rock, snow, marching powder, nose candy	CNS stimulant drug; increased alertness, awareness of senses, and energy; decreased sleep and hunger; increased heart rate, temperature, blood pressure, restlessness, anxiety
Crack	Freebase, rooster, tornado	Smoking form of cocaine; same as above
Ecstasy/ Methylenedioxymethamphetamine (MDMA)	E, XTC, Adam, the love drug	Effects of both a stimulant and a hallucinogen; stimulant effects include increase blood pressure, heart rate, sense of euphoria; hallucinogen effects include hallucinations, distortion of perception
Gamma hydroxybutyrate (GHB)	Goop, G, liquid ecstasy, liquid x	CNS depressant; at low doses, can allow user to feel euphoric, less inhibited, and more sociable; at higher doses, dizziness, memory loss, decreased consciousness, breathing, heart rate; loss of coordination
Gravol® (dimenhydrinate)		Antinausea medication available OTC, can cause euphoria and hallucinations
Jimson Weed	Jamestown weed, angel's trumpet, devil's trumpet, devil's snare, devil's seed, mad hatter, zombie cucumber	Plant that contains atropine and scopolamine, may lead to confusion, euphoria, hallucinations, delirium, and an anticholinergic toxidrome

Table 8. Common Recreational Drugs and Effects on Health (continued)

Drug	Alternative Street Names	Short-term Health Effects
Ketamine	K, special K, ket, vitamin K, cat tranquilizers	Anesthetic drug and hallucinogen; produces intense hallucinations and sense that mind is detached from body (dissociation); also loss of coordination, confusion, memory loss, increased sleepiness
Heroin	Big H, china white, mexican brown, smack, junk, dope	Opioid type of drug; sedative effect; sense of euphoria; detachment from physical and emotional pain; slowed breathing, constipation
Lysergic acid diethylamide (LSD)	Acid, blotter, microdot, windowpane	Hallucinogen; variable effects from person to person; can experience sense of joy, confusion, anxiety; vivid visual effects and altered sense of hearing, smelling, taste
Mescaline	Cactus, cactus heads, cactus buttons, buttons, mesc, mese	Hallucinogen; component of ecstasy producing hallucinogenic effects
Oxycodone	Hillbilly heroin, killers, OC, oxy, oxycotton, oxy80	Opioid, sedative effect; causes a sense of well-being or euphoria
Phencyclidine (PCP)	Angel dust, dust, crystal joint, tic tac, zoom, boat	Hallucinogen; unpredictable and variable effects including hallucinations, anxiety, panic, increased heart rate, blood pressure, drowsiness, lack of coordination
Psilocybin	Mushrooms, shrooms, magic mushrooms, musk, magic	Hallucinogen; unpredictable and variable effects including hallucinations, calming effect, anxiety, panic, increased heart rate, blood pressure, drowsiness, lack of coordination
Rohypnol	Roofies, roachies, rope, rophies, ruffies	CNS depressant (part of the benzodiazepine family); can lead to calming effect, drowsiness and loss of consciousness at higher doses
Steroids	Juice, pumpers, weight trainers, roids	Increased muscle bulk, energy, irritability, anxiety, aggression; reduced fertility

PHARMACOLOGY

REFERENCES

Katzung B, Masters S, Trevor A. 2009. *Basic and Clinical Pharmacology*. New York: Lange Medical Books/McGraw-Hill, Medical Pub. Division.

Fauci AS. 2008. *Harrison's Principles of Internal Medicine*. New York: McGraw-Hill.

Goldfrank LR, Flomenbaum N. 2006. *Goldfrank's Toxicologic Emergencies*. New York: McGraw-Hill Medical Pub. Division.

PHARMACOLOGY

The Essentials of Dermatology

Editors:
Lea Luketic &
Weronika Harris-Thompson

Faculty Reviewers:
Vince Bartucci, MD, FRCP(C)
Miriam Weinstein, MD, FRCP(C)
Siobhan Ryan, MD, FRCP(C)

TABLE OF CONTENTS

Essential Anatomy   385
Approach to the Dermatological History and Physical Exam   385
Common Chief Complaints   386
Common Disorders   386
Focused History   386
Focused Physical   386
Common Clinical Scenarios   391

ESSENTIAL ANATOMY

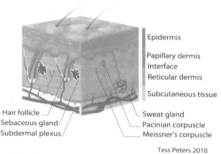

Epidermis
Papillary dermis
Interface
Reticular dermis
Subcutaneous tissue

Hair follicle
Sebaceous gland
Subdermal plexus

Sweat gland
Pacinian corpuscle
Meissner's corpuscle

Tess Peters 2010

Figure 1. Layers of the Skin

APPROACH TO THE DERMATOLOGICAL HISTORY AND PHYSICAL EXAM

In addition to general history taking in regards to the chief compliant, important aspects of the history include:

- Systemic symptoms (e.g. fever, arthralgias, weight loss, malaise)
- History of skin disease
- History of chronic disease (e.g. rheumatologic, thyroid, diabetes, collagen vascular)
- Exposure history (e.g. toxins, commercial skin and hair products, chemicals, sun/tanning beds, medications)
- Allergies (medication and environmental) and resulting symptoms
- Family history (skin diseases, allergies or atopic diseases such as hay fever and asthma, skin cancer)

Overview of the physical exam:

- Confirm location and distribution of lesions
- Describe the characteristics of the lesion (see **Tables 1-3**, **Figures 2 and 3**)
- Examine remainder of the skin, including important secondary sites (e.g. nails, mouth, genital/anal regions, peripheral lymph nodes)
- Palpate lesions to assess texture and tenderness

DERMATOLOGY

COMMON CHIEF COMPLAINTS

- Itch
- Rash
- Acne
- "Strange mole"
- Ulcer

COMMON DISORDERS

Disorders marked with (✓) are discussed in **Common Clinical Scenarios**

- ✓ Acne vulgaris/Common acne
- ✓ Rosacea
- ✓ Dermatitis
- ✓ Psoriasis
- ✓ Fungal infections
- ✓ Cysts
- ✓ Scars
- ✓ Nevi
- ✓ Malignant skin tumours
- Lumps and bumps
- Alopecia
- Others

FOCUSED HISTORY

In contrast to most areas of medicine, it can be helpful to do a physical exam before taking a detailed history; this allows for interpretation of the lesion without predetermined ideas, and for a more objective interpretation of the history.

History of Presenting Illness

- Changes in moles/birthmarks (e.g. colour, size, shape, scaling, bleeding, pain)
- Itch, change in sweating or dryness of the skin
- Non-healing lesions that may be red, scaly or crusted
- Systemic symptoms (e.g. fever, arthralgias, weight loss, malaise)
- Family history of atopy, autoimmunity, skin cancer, psoriasis

Skin Lesions

- Initial appearance of new lesion/growth (e.g. flat, raised, blistered)
- Change in lesion over time; new areas of involvement
- Associated symptoms (e.g. pruritus, pain, numbness)
- Aggravating factors (e.g. sunlight, temperature)
- Alleviating factors (e.g. herbal treatments, medications)

Changes in Hair or Nails

- Recent illnesses or stressors
- Exposures (e.g. toxins, commercial hair or nail products, chemicals)
- Hair loss: symmetric/asymmetric, focal/diffuse, rash/no rash
- Associated symptoms (e.g. pruritus, fever)

Past Medical History

- Skin cancer (non-melanocytic, melanocytic)
- Chronic disease (e.g. diabetes, rheumatologic, thyroid, collagen vascular)
- Allergies and resulting symptoms

Exposure History

- Occupation and hobbies (e.g. chemical, sun, travel, animals/pets)
- Medications (e.g. tetracycline – photosensitizing, sulfonamides – Stevens-Johnson syndrome)
- Recent contact with an individual with similar skin lesions

DERMATOLOGY

FOCUSED PHYSICAL

The focused physical exam includes (1) a general examination of the skin, (2) inspection of skin lesions, (3) palpation of lesion and (4) examination of secondary sites such as the nails and hair. Ensure appropriate lighting for this exam.

> **Clinical Pearl**
> Some skin eruptions are so characteristic they do not require an initial history; seeing the lesion first can allow for more objective interpretation of the complaint.

General Skin Inspection

- Colour: erythema, cyanosis, jaundice, pigmentary abnormalities, skin type
- Excessive moisture: fever, emotions, neoplastic diseases, hyperthyroidism
- Dryness: normal aging, myxedema, nephritis

Inspection of Skin Lesions

- The ability to correctly characterize the lesion is half the battle in dermatology. When describing lesions, avoid the word "rash" and use this mnemonic:

    S ize/Surface area
    C olour (refer to **Table 1** for common colours seen in dermatology)
    A rrangement (refer to **Table 2** and **Figure 2** for arrangements seen in dermatology)
    L esion morphology (refer to **Table 3**)
    D istribution
    A lways check hair, nails, mucous membranes and intertriginous areas

Table 1. Colours in Dermatology

Colour	Examples
Black	Melanin, exogenous pigments (e.g. tattoos, ink), exogenous chemicals (e.g. silver nitrate, gold salts)
Blue-grey	Deep blood (angioma), deep melanin (blue nevus), drugs (e.g. phenothiazines)
Dark brown	Melanin near surface (melanocytic nevi)
Green	Exogenous pigment (e.g. copper salts)
Pink-red	Psoriasis
Purple	Vascular lesions (angioma)
Red-brown	Hemosiderin (pigmented purpuric dermatoses)
Scarlet-red	Lesions with a strong arterial supply (spider nevi)
Violet	Lichen planus
White-ivory	Lichen sclerosus
Yellow-green	Jaundice
Yellow-orange	Carotenemia (ingested carotene, myxedema)
Yellow-white, yellow-pink	Xanthomatous disorders

DERMATOLOGY

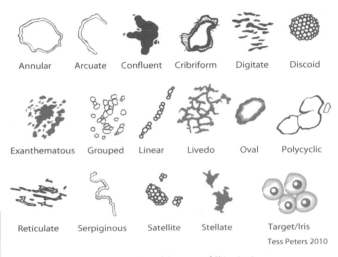

Annular   Arcuate   Confluent   Cribriform   Digitate   Discoid

Exanthematous   Grouped   Linear   Livedo   Oval   Polycyclic

Reticulate   Serpiginous   Satellite   Stellate   Target/Iris

Tess Peters 2010

Figure 2. Common Arrangement and Patterns of Skins Lesions

Table 2. Arrangements and Patterns

Shape/Pattern	Description	Examples
Annular	Ring/empty circle shape	Granuloma annulare (non-scaling), tinea (scaling)
Arcuate	Curved with the appearance of an arc/part of a circle	SLE, urticaria
Confluent	Merging lesions	Psoriasis plaques, scaly macules of pityriasis versicolour (yeast)
Cribiform	Strand-like patterning of scar tissue	Pyoderma gangrenosum heals with this pattern
Dermatomal	Lesions confined to particular nerve or dermatome distribution	Shingles (herpes zoster)
Digitate	Elongated ovals, long and thin/finger-shaped	Digitate dermatosis
Discoid/ nummular	Filled circle/ "coin-shaped"	Discoid eczema, psoriasis
Exanthematous	Macular-papular (or morbilliform) eruption	Infections, drug eruptions
Grouped	Discrete lesions in localized areas	Insect bites, herpes simplex

DERMATOLOGY

Table 2. Arrangement and Patterns (continued)

Shape/Pattern	Description	Examples
Linear	Linear patterns	Striae, scabetic burrows, insect bites, excoriations
Livedo	Reticulate eruption that follows vascular supply to the skin	Cutis marmorata, erythema ab igne, vasculitis
Oval	Oval shape commonly found on trunk (aligned with long axis)	Pityriasis rosea
Polycyclic	Interlocking/coalesced, unfilled circles	Psoriasis, tinea
Reticulate	Lace-like appearance of an eruption of individual lesions	Wickham's striae in lichen planus
Serpiginous	Wavy, angulated, "snake-like"	Track left by larva migrans
Satellite	Initial large lesions with adjacent spreading lesions	Local malignant spread, Candidal diaper dermatitis
Scattered and disseminated	Lesions on various parts of skin without any other specific patterns	Varicella, disseminated metastases, cutaneous lymphoma, benign nevi
Stellate (rare)	Star-shaped	Meningococcemia
Target/iris	Arrangement of concentric rings in a bull's eye pattern	Erythema multiforme

Table 3. Primary Lesion Morphology

Lesion Profile	General Size	
	<1 cm diameter	**>1 cm diameter**
Flat, smooth	Macule (e.g. freckle)	Patch (e.g. vitiligo)
Raised, superficial	Papule (e.g. wart)	Plaque (e.g. psoriasis)
If edematous	Wheal (e.g. urticaria)	
Raised, fluid-filled	Vesicle (e.g. HSV)	Bulla (e.g. bullous pemphigoid)
If purulent	Pustule	
Palpable deep (dermal)	Nodule (e.g. dermatofibroma)	Tumour (e.g. lipoma)
If semi-solid or fluid-filled	Cyst	

Secondary Skin Lesion Morphology

Scaling: increase in keratin, dead cells on surface of skin (e.g. dermatitis, psoriasis)

Crust: dried fluid (pus, blood, serum) originating from lesion (e.g. impetigo)

Lichenification: thickening of skin with accentuated skin markings (e.g. chronic atopic dermatitis, lichen simplex chronicus)

Other Morphology

Purpura: bleeding into dermis
- Petechiae (small red or brown spots)
- Ecchymoses (bruises)

Telangiectasia: dilated superficial blood vessels; blanchable

Excoriation: a scratch mark

Erosion: disruption of skin involving epidermis alone; heals without scarring

Ulcer: disruption of skin into the dermis or beyond; heals with scarring
- Can form dark-coloured crust, called eschar

Palpation

- Wear gloves when palpating a lesion
- Assess for texture, consistency, fluid, adjacent edema, tenderness, blanching
- Texture:
  - Superficial (largely epidermal) or deep (more likely in dermis)
  - Soft (e.g. lipoma) or doughy (e.g. hypothyroidism) versus hard (e.g. scleroderma, calcification), firm (e.g. lichen planus, sarcoid, amyloid) or indurated (e.g. pretibial myxedema)
  - Dry (e.g. hypothyroidism) versus wet
  - Velvety – acanthosis nigricans, Ehlers-Danlos syndrome
  - Leathery and bark-like (lichenification) – epidermal hypertrophy from prolonged rubbing/scratching, pruritic cutaneous disorder (e.g. lichen simplex chronicus, neurodermatitis)

Hair

- Texture should be examined (e.g. coarse – hypothyroidism, fine – hyperthyroidism)
- Alopecia (loss of hair): anemia, thyroid disease, androgenetic alopecia, heavy metal poisoning, hypopituitarism, pellagra (niacin deficiency), discoid lupus/lichen planopilaris (each of these exhibit scarring)
- Hirsutism (abnormally exuberant hair growth, especially male pattern of hair distribution in women): Cushing's disease, polycystic ovarian disease, neoplasm of the adrenals and gonads

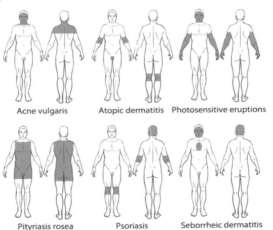

Acne vulgaris   Atopic dermatitis   Photosensitive eruptions

Pityriasis rosea   Psoriasis   Seborrheic dermatitis

Tess Peters 2010

Figure 3. Distribution Patterns of Skin Lesions

Nails
- Shape, size, colour and brittleness should be noted
- Hemorrhages under the nail (e.g. splinter hemorrhages in bacterial endocarditis)
- Grooves in the nail (e.g. trauma, Beau's lines)
- Increased white area under the nail bed (e.g. renal disease, liver disease)

COMMON CLINICAL SCENARIOS
- The type, prevalence, and incidence of many skin diseases varies with age, gender, race, geographic location, culture, and socio-economic status
- Appropriate management includes psychosocial interventions as skin diseases can have a major impact on the quality of life of the patient

Acne Vulgaris
- A common disease of the pilosebaceous unit
- Epidemiology: teens to adulthood (85% of individuals), more severe in males
- Presentation:
  - **Type I:** comedonal, sparse, with no scarring
  - **Type II:** comedonal and pustular (with possible scarring)
  - **Type III:** comedonal, pustular, and papular (with possible scarring)
  - **Type IV:** nodulocystic, risk of severe scarring
- Distribution: face, chest, back
- Lesion:
  - Non-inflammatory: hallmark comedones (blocked follicles)
    - Closed comedones = whiteheads
    - Open comedones = blackheads (black due to melanin, not dirt)
  - Inflammatory: papules/pustules with a core of purulent material and suppurative or hemorrhagic nodules

> **Clinical Pearl**
> Emotional stress and mechanical pressure can exacerbate acne; contrary to popular belief, chocolate and fatty foods do not.

Rosacea
- Epidemiology: found in all skin types, but most common in those with fair skin; females > males; usual age of onset is greater than 30 years
- Exacerbating factors: hot food/drink, spices, alcohol (especially red wine), sun exposure
- Lesion:
  - Vascular component: erythema, flushing, blushing, and telangiectasia (visible dilatation of dermal venules)
  - Eruptive component: papules and pustules
- Distribution: eruptions on the forehead, cheeks, nose, chin
- Associated symptoms: mild conjunctivitis with soreness, grittiness and lacrimation; chronic, deep inflammation of the nose leading to irreversible hypertrophy in men, known as rhinophyma
- Clinical diagnosis: bacterial culture to rule out folliculitis, KOH test to rule out tinea, biopsy to rule out SLE if not responsive to standard therapy

Dermatitis/Eczema
- Non-infectious inflammation of the skin accompanied by edema and blistering

Contact Dermatitis

- Generic term for acute or chronic inflammatory reaction to substances which contact the skin (endogenous and exogenous agents)
- *Irritant contact dermatitis:* caused by exposure to chemical irritant; given enough exposure, all individuals react to irritants
- *Allergic contact dermatitis:* caused by antigen with type IV (cell mediated/delayed-type) hypersensitivity reaction (e.g. reaction to poison ivy)
- Common allergens: nickel, chromate, cobalt, rubber additives in gloves and shoes, preservatives in water-based cosmetics, fragrances, dyes
- Lesion: vesicles, edema, erythema, extreme pruritus; bullae may be present
- Distribution (for both irritant and allergic contact dermatitis):
  - Appearance at a specific site suggests contact with certain objects
  - Hands, forearms and face
  - Usually first confined to the area of exposure
  - Distributed in linear streaks if caused by plants
  - May be patchy and asymmetric if caused by topical products
  - May spread beyond the area of contact in chronic exposure

Atopic Dermatitis/Eczema

- A skin disorder defined by the presence of 4 of the following major diagnostic criteria:
  - Pruritus
  - Young age of onset
  - Typical morphology and distribution
  - Chronic and relapsing course
  - Personal or family history of atopy – asthma, allergic rhinoconjunctivitis
- Aggravated by contact irritants, allergens, perspiration, excessive heat, stress
- Lesion:
  - Papular lesions with erythema, scale, and severe pruritus
  - Acute lesions may be oozing and vesicular
  - Subacute lesions: scaly and crusted
  - Chronic lesions: dull red and lichenified
- Distribution (varies with age):
  - *Infantile* (2 months-2 years) – often exudative lesions: cheeks, perioral area, scalp, around ears, extensor surfaces of feet and elbows; spares the diaper area if present on the body
  - *Childhood* (2-12 years) – flexural involvement: antecubital and popliteal fossae, neck, wrists and ankles
  - *Adult* – flexural involvement, hands, face

Psoriasis

- Chronic, non-infectious, inflammatory condition with increased epidermal cell proliferation (epidermal turnover reduced from 28 to 4 days)
- Recurrent exacerbations and remissions; may be associated with arthritis
- Epidemiology: equal sex incidence; onset at any age, peaks in 20s and 30s
- Etiology: recognized familial genetic component (family history important)
- Lesion:
  - Well-demarcated, disc-shaped, erythematous (red or salmon-pink) plaques topped with silvery scales; redness is constant
  - May bleed when scales detached (Auspitz's sign)
  - Symmetrical distribution
  - Classical presentation involves elbows, knees, sacrum and scalp hair margins

- ◆ Extensor > flexor surfaces
- ◆ Palms and soles may be spared
- ◆ Scalp: scaling is very dense and may be very thick
- ◆ Nails (matrix or nail bed involvement): thimble pitting, onycholysis (separation of nail plate from nail-bed), discolouration (oily or salmon-pink)
- ◆ Nail changes support diagnosis if skin changes are questionable or absent
- Precipitating factors:
  - *Koebner phenomenon:* trauma to epidermis and dermis (e.g. scratching)
  - Infection: Streptococcal pharyngitis (for guttate psoriasis)
  - Drugs: β-blockers, lithium, antimalarials
  - Stress, dry winter weather, possibly alcohol and smoking
- Associated conditions: psoriatic arthritis, increased cardiovascular risk, diabetes, obesity, depression, IBD

Guttate Psoriasis (youths and adolescents)
- Acute symmetrical appearance of small, bright red, well-demarcated, "drop-like" lesions on trunk and limbs
- Streptococcal pharyngitis may stimulate first episode: confirm presence of streptococci; may be widespread
- May develop rapidly; may disappear spontaneously in 2-3 months
- *Differential diagnosis:* secondary syphilis (no malaise, lymphadenopathy, or may see lesions on palms and soles), pityriasis rosea (light pink, scaling only around the edge of plaques)

Flexural Psoriasis (elderly)
- Located in the axillae, sub-mammary flexures, other intertriginous areas
- Scales may only be present on the edge

Pustular Psoriasis
In contrast to regular psoriasis, pustules, not papules are predominant in two subtypes:
- Localized pustular psoriasis (*pustulosis palmaris et plantaris*)
  - Palmoplantar pustules – chronic, relapsing eruption on palms and soles
  - Pustule can be white, yellow, orange, or brown; do not rupture - turn brown and scaly as they reach the surface
- Generalized pustular psoriasis (Von Zumbusch)
  - Life threatening, rare, and serious – requires immediate hospitalization
  - Small, sterile, yellow pustules on bright red, burning, erythematous background
  - Rapid spread
  - Accompanied by acute fever, malaise, leukocytosis, "toxic" appearance

> **Clinical Pearl**
> In psoriasis, pustules on the palms and soles vary in colour; this can help distinguish localized psoriasis from both tinea and eczema (which have a uniform colour).

Fungal Infections
Cutaneous Fungal "Ringworm" Infections
- Due to dermatophytes (*Trichophyton, Microsporum, Epidermophyton*)

Table 4. Different Forms of Cutaneous Fungal Infections

Infection	Lesion Description	Lesion Location
Tinea capitis	Annular patches of alopecia with surface scaling	Invasion of stratum corneum and hair shaft on scalp
Tinea corporis	Annular lesions in a classic ringworm pattern begin as flat scaly spots; develop a raised advancing border extending in all directions with central clearing; lesions can coalesce	Trunk and limbs, face (*Tinea faceii*), beard (*Tinea barbae*)
Tinea cruris (Jock itch)	Often bilateral beginning in the crural fold; half-moon red plaque with a well-defined scaling border advancing onto thigh	Groin: moist environment with excessive sweating/itching
Tinea pedis (Athlete's foot)	Classic ring-worm pattern: scaly advancing border, may present with an acute vesicular eruption	Plantar surface/dorsum of foot, soles of feet, interdigital: toe webs between 4th and 5th digits

Tinea Versicolor

Common infection caused by the yeast *Malassezia spp.* (commensal flora)

- Epidemiology: adolescents and young adults, often first noticed after sun exposure
- Characteristics: pruritic but usually asymptomatic; may be infectious
- Risk factors: adrenalectomy, Cushing's disease, pregnancy, malnutrition, burns, corticosteroid therapy, immunosupression, oral contraceptives
- Lesion:
  - Multiple, small, circular macules with superficial, subtle scale
  - Hypopigmented or hyperpigmented, minimally scaly papules
- Distribution: upper trunk, upper arms, neck, and abdomen
- Clinical Diagnosis: scale scrapings for culture; Wood's light: irregular, pale, yellow-to-white fluorescence which in some cases fades with improvement

Cysts

- Cysts can contain air, fluid or semi-solid material; if pus is present then considered an abscess
- Most cysts in body are benign, however a few have potential to become malignant (e.g. dermoid cysts)

DERMATOLOGY

Table 5. Differentiating Cysts

Cyst	Description	Signs and symptoms
Epidermal	Keratin-containing cyst lined by squamous epithelium; most common cutaneous cyst; youth to middle age	Present on parts of body with little hair; round, flesh-coloured and slow growing, firm and mobile nodule; punctum often visible
Pilar	Keratin-containing cysts that form in hair follicles; 2nd most common cutaneous cyst; F > M	Present most often on scalp; smooth, hard and mobile, can be tender; do not have central punctum
Dermoid	Cystic lesion often filled with skin and/or skin appendages and other mature tissue	Most common location is at the lateral third of eyebrow or midline under nose (along embryonal cleft closure lines); grow slowly and non-tender
Ganglion	Cyst filled with clear, gelatinous fluid that originated from joint or tendon sheath; F > M; usually found in older patients	Around joints and tendons; solitary, rubbery and translucent

Scars

- Scars are a natural part of the healing process. Two types of scars can result from the overproduction of collagen (hypertrophic and keloid scars)
- Epidemiology: keloid scars are more common in people with darker skin types and may have a familial tendency
- Can be caused by surgery, trauma or body piercing

Table 6. Hypertrophic vs. Keloid Scars

Scar	Description	Distinguishing Features
Hypertrophic	Erythematous, pruritic, raised lesion	Does not grow beyond the boundaries of the original wound
Keloid	Dense, thick nodules, can be single or multiple	Grows beyond the boundaries of the original wound

Nevi

- Epidemiology: nevi (which are often referred to as moles) are very common (each person on average has 10-40 nevi)
- Lesion:
  - Colour: pink, tan, brown or flesh coloured; may darken with sun exposure
  - Shape: flat or raised
  - Can change over time
- Distribution: over entire body
- Classification:
  - *Junctional Nevi:* usually flat with dark brown colour; appear in childhood and adolescence; nevus cells are found at the dermal-epidermal junction
  - *Compound Nevi:* slightly raised with less intense colour than junctional nevi; the nevus cells are migrating into the dermis

DERMATOLOGY

- *Dermal Nevi:* dome-like nevi with even less pigmentation; nevus cells are completely within the dermis
- *Dysplastic Nevi:* usually appear in adolescence and have more "dysplastic features" (larger with irregular and indistinct borders and non-uniform colour); large numbers are a risk factor for melanoma

Common Skin Malignancies
Basal Cell Carcinoma (BCC)
- Most common primary skin malignancy (>75%)
- Increased prevalence in elderly, M > F
- Clinical variants: sclerosing, noduloulcerative, superficial, and pigmented BCC
- Characterized by local destruction and slow growth
- Risk factors: chronic sun exposure, ionizing radiation
- Rarely metastatic but local tissue destruction can be debilitating
- Distribution: face (80%), scalp, ears, neck; less often on sun-exposed areas of the trunk and extremities; rarely on the dorsum of the hand

Squamous Cell Carcinoma (SCC)
- Second most common primary skin malignancy
- Primarily in elderly, M > F
- Clinical variants: keratoacanthoma (benign), SCC in situ (Bowen's disease), SCC
- Risk factors – chronic sun exposure, immunosuppression, HPV
- More rapid enlargement and more likely to metastasize than BCC
- Clinically looks like crusted nodule with erythematous base

Malignant Melanoma (MM)
- Potentially curable, thus early diagnosis is important
- All pigmented lesions should be examined periodically: 30% of melanomas develop from a pre-existing nevus, 70% develop *de novo*
- Early signs: changes in the colour, shape, or size of a nevus (mole)
- Early symptom: pruritus
- Later symptoms: tenderness, bleeding, ulceration
- Associated symptoms: regional lymphadenopathy; sentinel node biopsy is an important factor in determining prognosis
- Lesion: variable in appearance; no one colour/change is diagnostic

Superficial Spreading Melanoma (>50%)
- Most common form
- Affects mainly Caucasians
- Trunk and extremities distribution; spreads laterally
- Lesions >6 mm, flat, asymmetric with varying colouration – ulcerate and bleed withgrowth

Nodular Melanoma (30%)
- Extremities; extends vertically – rapidly fatal
- Lesions are elevated, brown to black, appear rapidly and develop papules
- May be accompanied by local hemorrhage

Lentigo Maligna Melanoma (15%)
- Affects older Caucasian patients with a history of chronic sun exposure
- Distribution: face, neck, dorsal arms
- Lesions: flat and irregular in shape, brown in colour but mottled; nodules and ulceration may indicate local invasion

Evidence-Based Medicine: Melanoma
The gold standard for diagnosing melanoma is the histopathological evaluation of the excised lesion. When referring patients to dermatologists, GPs will use one of two checklists:

Checklist	ABCD(E)	Revised 7-point
Criteria	**A**symmetry **B**order irregularity **C**olour variation **D**iameter >6 mm **(E)**levation Elevation is often excluded because many benign nevi are elevated and elevation may not be apparent with early melanoma	*Major (2 points each)* Change in size Irregular in shape Irregular colour *Minor (1 point each)* Inflammation Crusting or bleeding Sensory change Diameter >7 mm
Refer	When 1 of the above is present	Score of ≥3 points
Sensitivity	92-100%	79-100%
Specificity	98%	30-37%

Whited JD, Grichnik JM. 1998. *JAMA* 279:696-701.

Acral Lentiginous Melanoma (5%)
▪ Occurs mainly on the extremities of darker skinned individuals

Clinical Pearl
Not all black-blue pigmentation is due to melanoma (e.g. benign blue nevus).

Premalignant Skin Tumours
▪ May transform into malignancies (in parentheses) and should be carefully monitored
▪ Precursors include nevus sebaceous (BCC), actinic keratosis (SCC), dysplastic nevi, giant/congenital hairy nevi (>20 cm in diameter) (MM), lentigo maligna (MM)

Table 8. Dermatological Manifestations of Systemic Diseases

Systemic Disease	Skin Manifestations
Addison's disease	Generalized hyperpigmentation
Breast carcinoma	Paget's Disease: persistent unilateral dermatitic-looking lesion(s) on the breast
Cushing's syndrome	Moon facies, purple striae, acne, hyperpigmentation, hirsutism, atrophic skin with telangiectasias
HIV	Kaposi's sarcoma, seborrheic dermatitis, psoriasis
Hyperthyroidism	Moist warm skin, seborrheic dermatitis, acne, hirsutism, nail atrophy, onycholysis
Hypothyroidism	Cool dry scaly thickened skin, toxic alopecia, coarse hair, brittle nails
Liver disease	Spider nevi, palmar erythema, alopecia
Rheumatic fever	Nodules over bony prominences, erythema marginatum
Systemic Lupus Erythematosus (SLE)	Malar erythema, discoid rash, patchy/diffuse alopecia, photosensitivity
Thyroid carcinoma	Sipple's syndrome: multiple mucosal neuromas
Inflammatory Bowel Disease (IBD)	Pyoderma gangrenosum, erythyma nodosum

REFERENCES

Ashton R, Leppard B. 2005. *Differential Diagnosis in Dermatology.* Abingdon: Radcliffe.

Cole JM, Gray-Miceli D. 2002. The necessary elements of a dermatologic history and physical evaluation. *Dermatol Nurs* 14(6):377-383.

Dugani S, Lam D (eds.) 2009. *The Toronto Notes 2009: Comprehensive Medical Reference.* Toronto: Toronto Notes for Medical Students, Inc.

Gawkrodger DJ. 2008. *Dermatology: An Illustrated Colour Text.* Edinburgh: Churchill Livingstone Elsevier.

Habif TP. 2005. *Skin Disease: Diagnosis and Treatment.* Philadelphia: Elsevier Mosby.

Kittler H, Pehamberger H, Wolff K, Binder M. 2002. Diagnostic accuracy of dermoscopy. *Lancet Oncol* 3(3):159-165.

Leggett P, Gilliland AE, Cupples ME, McGlade K, Corbett R, et al. 2004. A randomized controlled trial using instant photography to diagnose and manage dermatology referrals. *Fam Pract* 21(1):54-56.

Whited JD, Grichnik JM. 1998. The rational clinical examination. Does this patient have a mole or a melanoma? *JAMA* 279(9):696-701.

DERMATOLOGY

The Essentials of Emergency Medicine

Editors:
Ishtiaq Ahmed &
Caroline Chan

Faculty Reviewers:
Norman Chu, MD CCFP(EM)
Paul Hawkins, MD, MCFP(EM)
David J. MacKinnon, MD, CCFP(EM)

TABLE OF CONTENTS

Rapid Primary Survey (RPS) of Trauma	399
Secondary Survey	401
Common Clinical Scenarios	402
Anaphylaxis/Anaphylactoid	402
Hypothermia	403
Hyperthermia	404
Burns	405
Wound Care	406
Abdominal Pain	407
Chest Pain	409
Headache	412

RAPID PRIMARY SURVEY (RPS) OF TRAUMA

In order of priority, **ABCDE**:

Airway

- Assume cervical spine injury for trauma patient and use collar for immobilization
- Assess airway (ability to speak, respiratory distress, lethargy, cyanosis)
- Management:

Basic Airway

- To open airway: head-tilt or if C-spine injury suspected, use jaw thrust
- To remove foreign material, sweep and suction
- Maintain airway: nasopharyngeal airway, oropharyngeal airway

Definitive Airway

- Indications for intubation:
  - Respiratory insufficiency (apnea)
  - Airway obstruction/trauma
  - Inability to protect airway (altered mental status)
  - Potential airway compromise (profound shock)
- Endotracheal intubation
- If intubation not successful:
  - Bag-valve-mask, laryngeal mask airway (LMA), Combitube, bougie
  - Consider advanced airway intervention such as Glide Scope bronchoscope
- If intubation and ventilation not possible:
  - Cricothyroidotomy or jet ventilation

Breathing
- Look: respiratory rate, decreased LOC, anxiety, cyanosis, nasal flaring, pursed-lip breathing, tracheal tug, intercostal indrawing
- Listen: equal breath sounds (including signs of obstruction like stridor, gurgling)
- Feel: air flow, tactile fremitus, tracheal shift, chest tenderness, flail segments, sucking chest wound, subcutaneous emphysema

Circulation
- Shock = insufficient perfusion of organs and tissue with oxygenated blood
- Treat cause of shock and replace fluids based on % blood volume lost
  - See *Fluids, Electrolytes and Acid/Base Disturbances* for details on fluid replacement

Table 1. Classes of Shock

Class	I	II	III	IV
Respiratory rate	20	30	35	>45
Pulse	<100	100-120	>120	>140
Blood pressure	Normal	Normal	↓	↓
Capillary refill	Normal	↓	↓	↓
% blood volume	<15%	15-30%	30-40%	>40%
Fluid replacement	Crystalloid	Crystalloid	Crystalloid and blood	Crystalloid and blood

Disability
- Assess level of consciousness using Glasgow Coma Scale (GCS)

Table 2. Glasgow Coma Scale

Eye Opening		Verbal Response		Motor Response	
Spontaneous	4	Oriented	5	Obeys commands	6
To verbal command	3	Confused	4	Localizes to pain	5
To pain	2	Inappropriate words	3	Withdraws from pain	4
None	1	Incomprehensible sounds	2	Flexion (decorticate)	3
		No verbal response	1	Extension (decerebrate)	2
				No response	1

- GCS score = eye + verbal + motor
  - Mild disability (13-15)
  - Moderate disability (9-12)
  - Severe disability (≤8)
- **AVPU** scale:
  - **A** lert
  - **V** erbal stimulus response
  - **P** ainful stimulus response
  - **U** nresponsive

Exposure/Environment
- Expose entire body and assess for injuries
- Avoid hypothermia with warm blankets, warm IV blood/fluids

EMERGENCY

SECONDARY SURVEY

A more detailed head-to-toe exam to identify significant injuries and concerns.

SAMPLE History
- **S** igns and symptoms
- **A** llergies
- **M** edications
- **P** ast medical history
- **L** ast meal
- **E** vents surrounding episode

Focused Physical Exam

Neurological
- Evaluate GCS
- Cranial nerve exams
- Evaluate for spinal cord injury: sensory level and motor exam

Head and Neck/Ophthalmological
- Pupillary reactivity and reflex
  - Reactive pupils (symmetrical) + decreased LOC: metabolic/structural cause
  - Nonreactive pupils (or asymmetrical) + decreased LOC: structural cause
- Extraocular movements
- Fundoscopy
- Assess tympanic membrane for CSF leakage/hemotympanum
- Evaluate for facial trauma
- Signs of basal skull fracture: hemotympanum, CSF rhinorrhea, CSF otorrhea, Battle's sign (retroauricular hematoma), raccoon eyes (periorbital ecchymosis)
- Evaluate for neck pain

Chest
- Inspection: contusions, flail segments, symmetrical chest expansion
- Palpation: subcutaneous emphysema
- Auscultation: all lung fields

Abdomen/Pelvis
- Assess for intraperitoneal bleeding, acute abdomen
- DRE, bimanual exam

MSK
- Palpate cervical, thoracic and lumbar spines for fractures
- Palpate pelvic girdle, pubic symphysis for instability indicating fracture
- Extremity exam for fracture and neurovascular status

Investigations
- X-rays: C-, T-, and L-spine, chest, pelvis
- Focused abdominal sonography in trauma (FAST)
- CT scans (head, chest, abdomen, pelvis)

COMMON CLINICAL SCENARIOS

Anaphylaxis/Anaphylactoid Reaction

Immune response mediated by massive release of histamine, leukotrienes, prostaglandins and tryptase resulting in severe systemic reaction occurring within minutes.

History
- Age
- Exposure to anaphylactic agent and time of exposure
- Symptoms from exposure
- Past history of allergic/systemic reactions, previous ICU admissions
- Common agents causing anaphylaxis:
  - IgE-mediated: medications (usually antibiotics), food (peanuts, tree nuts, shellfish, wheat, milk, eggs, soybeans, nitrates/nitrites), latex, hormones, animal/human proteins, exercise, venom, allergen vaccines, enzymes, polysaccharides, colourants
  - Non-IgE-mediated: IVIg, opioids, physical factors (temperature, exercise), radiocontrast media, ACE inhibitor administered with dialysis, quaternary ammonium muscle relaxants, ethylene oxide gas on dialysis tubing, transfusion reaction to cellular elements, psychogenic, idiopathic

Clinical Features
- Key presenting features:
  - Bronchospasm (wheezing)
  - Upper airway obstruction or laryngeal edema (urticaria or angioedema)
  - Vasodilation (e.g. hypotension)
- General: marked anxiety, tremor, weakness, cold sensation
- CNS: weakness, syncope, dizziness, seizures
- Eyes: lacrimation, ocular pruritis
- Respiratory: tachypnea, accessory muscle use, cyanosis, respiratory arrest, laryngeal edema(lump in throat, hoarseness, stridor), bronchospasm (cough, wheezing, chest tightness, respiratory distress)
- CVS: tachycardia, hypotension, arrhythmia, chest pain, MI
- GI: nausea, vomiting, crampy abdominal pain, bloody diarrhea
- Skin: pruritic urticaria (occasionally), edema, erythema

Management
- ABCDE
- Identify and treat responsible agent as soon as anaphylaxis is suspected
- IV normal saline
- Epinephrine (depends on signs and symptoms):
  - Pre-hospital care: Epi-pen and oral antihistamine
  - Mild to moderate: minimal airway edema, mild bronchospasm, cutaneous reactions
    - IM epinephrine (adults: 0.3-0.5 mL of 1:1000, children: 0.01 mL/kg per dose to 0.4 mL/dose of 1:1000 epinephrine)
  - Critical: laryngeal edema, severe bronchospasm, shock
    - IV drip or ETT epinephrine if unable to obtain IV access (adults: 1 mL of 1:10,000, children: 0.01 mL/kg). Repeat every 5-10 min until symptoms resolve
- Diphenhydramine (adults: 50 mg IM or IV q4-6h; children: 2 mg/kg)
- Histamine blockers for moderate to severe reaction (ranitidine 50 mg or famotidine 20 mg IV)

- Glucocorticoids as adjunct to epinephrine (hydrocortisone sodium succinate 100-250 mg IV or prednisone 50 mg PO)
- If bronchospasm, β-agonist aerosol (salbultamol) via nebulizer

Hypothermia

Decline in core temperature below 35°C due to increased heat loss (convection, radiation, conduction, evaporation) or decreased heat production (metabolic, behavioural)
- Primary hypothermia from environmental exposure
- Secondary hypothermia from underlying medical condition which disrupts thermoregulatory mechanism (e.g. bacterial infection, thyroid disease, malnutrition, stroke, diabetes, spinal cord injury, use of medication or substance which affects brain or spinal cord (e.g. alcohol))

History
- Age (extremes of age most at risk)
- Duration of exposure
- Pre-disposing factors: drug or alcohol overdose, toxins, cold water immersion, trauma, outdoor sports, impaired thermoregulation due to central CNS conditions affecting hypothalamus, spinal cord injury or surgery, malnutrition, endocrine failure

Table 3. Clinical Features of Hypothermia

Type	°C	Clinical Features	Management
Mild	32-34.9	Lethargy, shivering, tachypnea, tachycardia, altered judgment, confusion, dysarthria, ataxia, shivering	Passive rewarming (since thermoregulatory mechanism is intact)
Moderate	28-31.9	Stupor, delirium, loss of ability to shiver, dilated pupils, arrhythmias, slowed reflexes, muscle rigidity	Active external rewarming
Severe	<28	Unresponsive, coma, hypotension, fixed pupils, ventricular fibrillation, apnea, areflexia, acidemia, cold skin	Active core rewarming

Investigations
- ECG: prolongation of conduction interval, atrial fibrillation, J or Osborne wave (positive deflection in RT segment)
- Bloodwork: hypoglycemia, hypomagnesemia, hypophosphatemia

Management
- ABCDE
- Secondary survey
- Monitor core temperature – rectal or esophageal temperature probes are most accurate
- Rewarming: passive, active external (forced air blankets/"bear hugger", heated blanket, heating lamp, warm baths), active core (warmed humidified oxygen, IV fluids, peritoneal dialysis, irrigation of cavities, cardiopulmonary bypass – most effective and rapid but not readily available)

Hyperthermia

Increased heat production (muscular activity, metabolism, drugs, severe infection) and/or decreased heat loss ($\downarrow$ sweating, $\downarrow$ CNS response, $\downarrow$ cardiovascular reserve, drugs) leading to:
- Dilation of peripheral venous system, $\uparrow$ blood flow to skin, stimulation of sweat glands
- Severe hyperthermia: dehydration with electrolyte abnormalities → dysfunction of thermoregulatory mechanism → multi-system organ failure

History
- Duration of exposure
- Peak ambient temperature
- Insidious onset of symptoms: fatigue, dizziness, irritability, weakness, headache, nausea, vomiting, myalgias, muscle cramps
- Susceptible individuals have circulatory insufficiency: extremes of age, obesity, dehydration, CHF, diuretics, laxatives
- Excessive heat load: fever, environment, lack of acclimatization, exertional
- Medications: sympathomimetics (e.g. cocaine, ecstasy), anticholinergics, antihistamines, LSD, MAO inhibitors, PCP, drug or alcohol withdrawal, β-blockers, sympatholytics

Focused Physical Exam (for heat exhaustion and heat stroke)
- General: fatigue, malaise, sweating (anhydrosis when severe), fever
- CNS: confusion/lethargy, weakness, headache, agitation, delirium, seizure, ataxia, coma
- H&N: fixed dilated pupils (heat stroke), subconjunctival hemorrhage
- CVS: tachycardia, hypotension, dehydration
- Respiratory: tachypnea, alkalosis, hemoptysis
- GI: nausea, vomiting, diarrhea ± bright red blood or melena
- GU: oliguria or anuria (acute renal failure), hematuria
- Skin: dry, warm, diaphoretic, piloerection

Table 4. Clinical Features of Heat Disorders

Heat Disorder	Clinical Features	Management
Heat edema	Vasodilation and venous stasis → swelling of feet and ankles	Elevation of limbs
Heat syncope	Peripheral pooling of intravascular volume → $\downarrow$ pre-load → orthostatic hypotension → syncope	Rest, cooling and rehydration
Heat cramps	Dehydration → salt depletion (Na/K shifts) → spasms of voluntary muscles of abdomen and extremities	Fluid and salt replacement
Heat exhaustion	Prolonged heat exposure → primary water loss or primary sodium loss → dehydration signs, NO central nervous system symptoms	Rehydration and cooling
Heat stroke	Extremely high body temperature (>40.5°C) → multi-organ dysfunction (e.g. rhabdomyolysis and hepatic damage) including CNS → altered mental status, confusion, bizarre behaviour, hallucinations, disorientation, coma	Rapid reduction in body temperature

Management
- ABCDE
- Cooling measures: convection (fan), evaporation (spray bottle), conduction (ice packs to groin and axillae, gastric lavage, iced peritoneal lavage), cooling blanket

Burns

History
- Age
- Exposure: duration, type (thermal, chemical, UV, electrical, inhalation), environment (e.g. enclosed space), materials involved (e.g. smoke, fire, carbon monoxide, cyanide poisoning, UV)
- Onset, course, location and quality of pain
- Associated symptoms: respiratory illness (persistent cough, wheeze, hoarseness from respiratory burns, soot-stained sputum, delayed ARDS)
- Co-morbid conditions for increased risk of secondary infections: immunodeficiency, diabetes mellitus, respiratory illness
- Associated injuries

Focused Physical Examination
- Degree of burn assessed by:
  - Burn size: rule of nines for percentage of affected body surface area in 2° and 3° burns (see **Figure 1**)
  - Burn site: serious injuries if hands/feet, face, eyes, ears, perineum affected

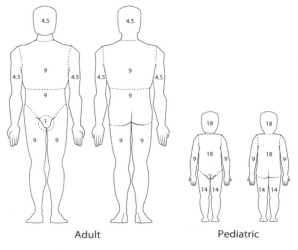

Adult   Pediatric

Caitlin O'Connell 2010

Figure 1. Rule of Nines

Table 5. Classification of Burns

Burn Depth	Layers Involved	Signs and Symptoms
First degree	Epidermis	Local erythema, pain
Second degree	Superficial partial thickness to deep partial thickness (dermis)	Blisters and bullae-covered skin that is erythematous, moist and swollen (intact sensation)
Third degree	All layers of skin	No sensation, charring if severe
Fourth degree	Fat, muscle, bone	

- H&N: corneal damage, singed nasal hair, facial charring
- Respiratory: hypoxic, respiratory obstruction (due to inhalational injury)
- CVS: cardiac irritability (electrical burns)
- CNS: neurologic dysfunction (due to electrical burns)
- GU: genital or perineal burns in children (suspect child abuse)
- MSK: reduced joint movement due to scarring over joints, mobility
- Skin: minimal surface wounds with extensive deep damage (electrical burns)

Management
- Airway: control early with ETT if signs of upper airway and laryngeal edema (severe burns to lower face and neck, inhalation of superheated air in confined space, carbonatious sputum), full thickness circumferential chest wall involvement
- Breathing: O_2 saturation
- Circulation: if hemodynamically unstable, initial fluid resuscitation with NS, then:
  - IV Ringer's lactate using Parkland formula:
    - Fluid for first 24 hours (mL) = Total body surface area burn (%) × Weight (kg) × 4; give ½ over first 8 hrs, ½ over next 16 hrs
- Disposition/drugs/draw bloods/drains: assess GCS, routine bloods and ABG/CO levels, CK if concern for tissue damage/rhabdomyolysis, sedatives/narcotics as needed, tetanus, Foley, NG
- Expose and secondary survey: dress wounds (irrigation with sterile saline ± dressing to prevent heat loss and infection), evaluate for other associated injuries (e.g. fractures)
- Imaging as needed

Wound Care
- Establishment of absolute hemostasis (prevent further blood loss and formation of hematoma) before wound care through indirect and direct methods
  - Indirect: elevation of injured part above level of heart, direct pressure over wound or tourniquets for complex injuries, epinephrine-containing solutions (contraindicated in wounds on penis, digits, tip of nose)
  - Direct: ligation, electrocautery, chemical cautery
- Types of injuries: lacerations, bites, puncture wounds, stretch injuries, compression or crush injuries

History
- Time of injury (increased risk of infection if sutured >6 hours after time of injury)
- Site of injury, contact with contaminants
- Mechanism of injury
- Tetanus immunization status

Focused Physical Examination
- ABCDE
- MSK: loss of function in injured part, involvement of underlying structures (e.g. nerves, major blood vessels, ligaments, bones), degree of contamination, foreign body

Management
- Assess neurovascular status before using anesthestic agents (lidocaine ± epinephrine) via local infiltration
- Cleansing: irrigation (normal saline), cleaning agent (e.g. iodine), mechanical scrubbing
- Debridement
- Wound closure (absorbable or nonabsorbable sutures, steri-strips, steel and metallic clips or staples, wound tapes, wound staples, tissue adhesives)

Abdominal Pain

Focused History
- OPQRSTUVW
- Anorexia, N/V
- Constipation, diarrhea
- Fever, rigors
- Pearls:
  - Abrupt, severe onset is suggestive of a vascular cause or viscus rupture
  - Gradual onset is more suggestive of inflammatory or infectious causes
  - Crampy, cyclic pain occurring in crescendo-decrescendo cycles may indicate small bowel obstruction
  - Consider referred pain (e.g. cholecystitis causing subscapular pain)
- See *Abdominal Exam*

Focused Physical Exam
- Establish stability of patient: evaluate appearance, responsiveness, ABCDE and vital signs
- Inspection: rigid/board-like abdomen, distension, ecchymosis, hepatic stigmata
- Auscultation
- Percussion
- Palpation
  - Cough tenderness, shake tenderness, CVA tenderness
- Special tests
  - Obturator, psoas and Murphy's signs
- DRE, pelvic exam (if indicated)

EMERGENCY

Table 6. Differential Diagnosis of Abdominal Pain

Type/Location	Differential	Type/Location	Differential
Diffuse pain	**Aortic dissection** **Ruptured AAA** **Ischemic bowel** **Perforated viscus** Gastroenteritis Bowel obstruction Peritonitis Appendicitis (early stage) Sickle cell crisis	**Localized pain**	Cystitis: suprapubic pain Pyelonephritis: flank pain
Right upper quadrant	Cholecystitis/biliary colic Hepatitis **MI** Lower lobe pneumonia	**Left upper quadrant**	Pancreatitis **Splenic injury** **MI** Lower lobe pneumonia
Right lower quadrant	Appendicitis (late stage) Meckel's/cecal/right-sided diverticulitis **Ectopic pregnancy** Ovarian cyst Ovarian torsion Pelvic inflammatory disease (PID) Tubo-ovarian abscess (TOA) Testicular torsion Renal colic	**Left lower quadrant**	Sigmoid diverticulitis **Ectopic pregnancy** Ovarian cyst Ovarian torsion PID TOA Testicular torsion Renal colic

Note: in bold are life-threatening conditions that always need to be ruled out

EMERGENCY

Table 7. Signs and Symptoms of Selected Causes of Abdominal Pain

Diagnosis	Signs and Symptoms
Appendicitis	Initially vague, colicky central abdominal pain progressing to localized RLQ pain over McBurney's point Anorexia, nausea/vomiting (N/V), fever (50% of patients), leukocytosis (50% of patients) Guarding, tenderness, psoas sign, obturator sign CT if diagnosis uncertain or U/S in females of reproductive age
Abdominal aortic aneurysm	Pulsatile abdominal mass If ruptured: shock, hypotension, mottled abdominal wall CT: aneurysm and free fluid seen U/S: aneurysm but not necessarily free fluid seen
Acute ischemic bowel	Tachycardia, hypotension, fever, lactic acidosis, bloody diarrhea, abdominal pain out of proportion with physical exam (hallmark) AXR upright and left lateral decubitis: free air, air-fluid level Contrast CT: thickened bowel wall loops (thumbprinting) Abdominal angiography: may show embolus or thrombus
Cholecystitis	RUQ pain, anorexia, N/V Positive Murphy's sign U/S: gallstones, gallbladder wall thickening (inflammation)
Ectopic pregnancy	Adnexal mass Transvaginal U/S: blood or mass in adnexa, ectopic cardiac activity or gestational sac β-hCG >1500 and no intrauterine pregnancy
Obstruction	Abdominal distension, N/V AXR: dilated bowel, air fluid levels
Splenic rupture	Hypotension, peritonitis CT: rupture seen, blood detected U/S: free fluid around spleen

Investigations
- CBC, differential, electrolytes
- Serum creatinine, BUN, lactate
- LFTs, amylase
- Urinalysis
- β-hCG in all women of reproductive age
- ECG (especially if >40 years old)
- AXR, CXR, CT, U/S as needed

Management
- NPO, NG tube, IV fluids
- Treat shock
- Analgesia: judicious use of IV narcotics has been shown to aid the diagnostic process by making the physical exam more reliable
- Antiemetics and NG suction if necessary
- Consider holding back antibiotics unless sepsis/infection is obvious or until diagnosis is established
- Immediate surgical consult if hemodynamically unstable, acute abdomen, pulsatile abdominal mass

Chest Pain

Focused History
- OPQRSTUVW
- N/V, diaphoresis
- Dyspnea, palpitations, syncope
- Cardiac or other risk factors
- Sense of doom
- Pearls:
    - Onset of post-emesis chest pain is suggestive of Boerhaave's syndrome
    - Consider drug use, especially cocaine and other sympathomimetics

Focused Physical Exam
- Establish stability of patient: evaluate appearance, responsiveness, ABCDE and vital signs
- Inspection: diaphoresis, pallor, anxiety, Levine's sign, JVP
    - Distinguish between central vs. peripheral cyanosis
- Palpation
    - Check pulses in all limbs – assess for any asymmetry
    - Capillary refill
- Auscultation
    - See ***Cardiovascular Exam*** p. 64 for details on heart sounds
    - Pleural rub may be heard in pulmonary embolism
    - Hamman's sign

Table 8. Differential Diagnosis of Chest Pain

Differential Diagnosis of Chest Pain	
CVS - **Aortic dissection** - **Cardiac tamponade** - **MI/Acute coronary syndrome** - Stable angina - Aortic stenosis, aortic insufficiency - **Mitral prolapse** - Pericarditis, myocarditis - Sickle cell crisis - Cocaine use **GI** - **Boerhaave's syndrome/Esopha-geal rupture** - Cholecystitis - Esophagitis - GERD - Gastritis - Peptic ulcer disease - Pancreatitis	**Respiratory** - Pleurisy - Pneumonia - Pneumothorax/**tension pneumothorax** - **Pulmonary embolism** **MSK** - Costochondritis - Intercostal muscle strain - Rib fractures - Thoracic outlet syndrome **Neurological & Psychogenic** - Spinal nerve root compression - Anxiety **Dermatological** - Herpes zoster

Note: in bold are life-threatening conditions that always need to be ruled out

EMERGENCY

Table 9. Signs and Symptoms of Selected Causes of Chest Pain

Diagnosis	Signs and Symptoms
MI/ACS	Pain can be retrosternal or radiating to arms, neck, epigastrum N/V, diaphoresis, restlessness Dyspnea, heart failure, shock CK-MB, elevated troponin ECG: can be diagnostic or normal
Aortic dissection	Retrosternal pain, often described as tearing, often presents atypically Absent pulses, limb ischemia, MI, stroke, hematuria Pulsatile abdominal mass CXR: widened mediastinum ECG: acute MI CT, angiography and echo are investigations of choice
Cardiac tamponade	Beck's triad: hypotension, increased JVP, muffled heart sounds Echo and U/S are diagnostic Pericardiocentisis can be used to confirm and treat diagnosis
Aortic stenosis	Triad of heart failure, angina, and syncope Crescendo-decrescendo, systolic ejection murmur ECG: left ventricular hypertrophy Echo is diagnostic
Mitral prolapse	Palpitations, dyspnea, dizziness Late systolic click, mitral regurgitation murmur Arrhythmia possible ECG: non-specific T-wave abnormalities Echo is diagnostic
Pulmonary embolism	Abrupt onset of pleuritic CP Dyspnea, tachypnea, hemoptysis (in some instances) Friction rub (rare) Hypoxemic, hypocapneic ECG: sinus tachycardia or non-specific ST-T changes most common; S1, Q3, T3 are the classic signs but uncommon CT pulmonary angiography V/Q scan if young female: areas of lung ventilated but not perfused
Pneumothorax	Dyspnea, tachycardia, collapsed lung If tension pneumothorax: shock, tracheal deviation CXR: absence of lung markings peripheral to visceral pleural line; if tension: mediastinal shift
Esophageal rupture	Retrosternal pain Subcutaneous emphysema, history of ++ vomiting, esophageal instrumentation CXR: pneumomediastinum, pleural effusion Esophagoscopy is diagnostic

Investigations
- CBC, lytes, serum glucose
- Serum creatinine, BUN
- Lipase, amylase
- Cardiac enzymes: CK-MB, troponins I and T
- Consider d-dimer to rule out PE
- ECG
- CXR

Management
- Supplemental oxygen by facemask, nasal prongs
- Establish IV access (saline lock)
- Continuous cardiac monitoring
- Evaluate for hypotension/shock
  - If hypovolemic: IV crystalloids, type and crossmatch 6-8 units PRBCs
- ECG
- Aspirin and nitroglycerin if not contraindicated for suspected ACS
- IV analgesia
- Correct arrhythmias if present
- Consider use of thrombolytics or catheterization in event of acute MI with ST elevation
- Percutaneous coronary intervention (PCI) is treatment of choice

Headache

Focused History
- OPQRSTUVW
  - Onset: acute onset or sudden change in pattern is serious
  - Quality: shooting pain in V1, V2 distribution indicative of trigeminal neuralgia; steady, band-like pain indicative of tension headaches
  - Timing: headaches secondary to raised ICP are often worst on awakening (prolonged supine position)
- N/V, myalgia, jaw claudication, scalp tenderness
- Photopobia, phonophobia, aura, vision changes
- Meningeal signs
- Hx of recent head trauma
- Pregnancy status
- Highest risk for traumatic bleed: alcoholics, elderly, patients on coumadin

Focused Physical Exam
- Establish stability of patient: evaluate appearance, LOC and responsiveness, vital signs (especially BP and temperature)
- Inspection: neurofibromas, café-au-lait spots, cutaneous hemangiomas, purpuric rash
- Neurological exam and fundoscopy: neurological deficits or papilledema are suggestive of intracranial lesion
- Meningeal signs
- Palpate for scalp tenderness, suggestive of temporal arteritis

Table 10. Differential Diagnosis of Headache

Differential Diagnosis of Headache (H/A)		
Acute onset H/A	**Subacute H/A**	**Chronic H/A**
Cerebrovascular accident	Intracranial mass/ Pseudotumour/Increased ICP	Cervical spine disease
Meningitis	Meningitis/CNS infection	Cluster headache
Subarachnoid hemorrhage	**Pre-eclampsia/ Hypertensive crisis**	Migraine
Migraine	Trigeminal neuralgia	Tension headache
Trauma	Polymyalgia rheumatica	Sinusitis
Venous sinus thrombosis	**Temporal arteritis**	Temporomandibular joint (TMJ) disease
	Toxin exposure (e.g. CO)	Iritis
	Migraine	Glaucoma
		Occipital neuralgia

Note: in bold are life-threatening conditions that always need to be ruled out

Table 11. Signs and Symptoms of Selected Causes of Headache

Diagnosis	Signs and Symptoms
Increased ICP	Worst on awakening and during coughing, sneezing Focal neurological deficits develop over time Papilledema CT or MRI are diagnostic
Meningitis	Fever, N/V, decreased LOC Meningismus, purpuric rash LP for CSF profile, Gram stain, C&S, PCR
Subarachnoid hemorrhage	Sudden onset headache, "worst headache ever" N/V, meningismus Focal neurological deficits, decreased LOC C: 90-95% sensitivity → 5-10% will be negative 12 h after event LP if CT negative but diagnosis still suspected: elevated opening pressure, xanthochromia, total RBCs in tubes 1 and 4
Temporal arteritis	>50 years old, scalp tenderness, jaw claudication Fever, malaise, myalgia, weight loss Visual loss/disturbance ESR: elevated (>50 mm/h), temporal artery biopsy is definitive

Investigations
- CBC, electrolytes, ESR
- If focal neurological symptoms: CT, MRI or angiography/MRA
    - For subarachnoid hemorrhage, CT = 90-95% sensitive (5-10% will be false negative 12 hours after onset of headache)
- If meningismus present: blood culture, LP
- If temporal arteritis suspected: temporal artery biopsy

Management
- Varies depending on diagnosis:
    - Intracranial mass/subarachnoid hemorrhage: urgent neurosurgery consult
    - Meningitis: do not delay IV antibiotics for LP
    - Temporal arteritis: high-dose steroids

EMERGENCY

REFERENCES

Barrow MW, Clark KA. 1998. Heat-related illnesses. *Am Fam Physician* 58(3):749-756, 759.
Biem J, Koehncke N, Classen D, Dosman J. 2003. Out of the cold: management of hypothermia and frostbite. *CMAJ* 168(3):305-311.
Stiell IG, Wells GA, Vandemheen K, Clement C, Lesiuk H, Laupacis A, McKnight RD, Verbeek R, Brison R, Cass D, Eisenhauer ME, Greenberg G, Worthington J. 2001. The Canadian CT Head Rule for patients with minor head injury. *Lancet* 357(9266):1391-1396.
Tintinalli JE, Kelen GD, Stapczynski JS (eds.) 2003. *Emergency Medicine: A Comprehensive Study Guide.* New York: McGraw-Hill Medical Pub. Division.

The Essentials of Endocrinology

Editors:
Alyse Goldberg &
Sarah Troster

Faculty Reviewers:
Bruce Perkins, MD, FRCP(C)
Rosario Briones, MD, FRCP(C)

TABLE OF CONTENTS

Disorders of Carbohydrate Metabolism 415
Pituitary Disorders 417
Adrenal Disorders 419
Thyroid Disorders 422
Polycystic Ovarian Syndrome (PCOS) 424

DISORDERS OF CARBOHYDRATE METABOLISM

- Disorders of dysregulation of glucose, leading to hyperglycemia and/or hypoglycemia

Hyperglycemia: Diabetes Mellitus

The Essentials
Classification:
1. *Idiopathic Type 1 DM*
2. *Idiopathic Type 2 DM*

Table 1. Idiopathic Diabetes Mellitus

Condition	Type 1 DM	Type 2 DM
Definition	Lack of insulin due to auto-immune destruction of β-cell mass	Two-step pathophysiology: 1) insulin resistance, 2) β-cell failure
Etiology	Multifactorial: genetic predisposition, auto-immune reactions, environment	Multifactorial: genetic predisposition; obesity is major environmental RF
Age of Onset	Usually <40 yrs	Tends to be >40 yrs (type 2 DM in youth becoming an epidemic)
Family History	Usually none	Often present
Treatment	Require exogenous insulin for survival	Require diet modification and exercise, oral hypoglycemic agents, and eventually insulin for many patients

2. *Secondary DM:* accounts for <10% of all DM; causes include monogenic forms (MODY genes, e.g. HNFα), endocrinopathies (Cushing's disease, acromegaly, tumours), drugs (commonly prednisone; also pentamidine, immunosuppressive therapy), infectious (congenital rubella, CMV), other
3. *Gestational DM:* mainly caused by increased hPL in the 3rd trimester (24-38 weeks of gestation) in susceptible individuals (with underlying insulin resistance, which resolves)

Common Chief Complaints
- *Type 1 DM:* sub-acute hyperglycemic symptoms (e.g. polyuria, polydipsia, nocturia, hyperphagia, weight loss, blurred vision, fatigue)
- *Type 2 DM:* same, but often identified on asymptomatic blood glucose screening

Diagnostic Criteria
- Fasting plasma glucose (PG) ≥7.0 mM or random PG >11.1 mM with symptoms (polyuria, polydipsia, unexplained weight loss) or seen on 2 occasions
  - *Note:* can also diagnose on 2h PG in a 75g OGTT ≥11.1 mM
- Screening for hyperglycemia should begin at age 40

Focused History
- Document details of diagnosis (age, time, presenting signs, symptoms), episodes, management, family and past medical history (DM, other autoimmune disorders)
- Ask questions related to *risk factors:* family history, ethnicity, obesity (specifically subcutaneous truncal fat), lifestyle (smoking, exercise, dietary patterns)
- Ask questions related to *blood sugar control:* diet, exercise, oral hyperglycemic agents, drugs, home blood glucose monitoring, symptoms, severity of acute complications (e.g. diabetic ketoacidosis; infections; hypoglycemia: adrenergic = hunger, shakes, sweats and/or neuroglycopenic = confusion, coma, seizures (see below); hyperglycemia: as above)
- Ask questions related to *microvascular complications* of DM:
  - Retinopathy: cataracts, last ophthalmologist visit
  - Nephropathy: urinary albumin excretion, hypertension
  - Neuropathy:
    - Autonomic: postural hypotension, gastroparesis, urinary retention, impotence
    - Peripheral: numbness, tingling or decreased sensation in hands and/or feet, foot ulcers
- Ask questions related to *macrovascular complications* of DM:
  - Risk factors include smoking, hypertension, dyslipidemia, family history of premature CAD (e.g. angina, MI, stroke, TIA, PVD – intermittent claudication, gangrene, infection)
- Other complicatons: immunosuppression – recommend pneumovax

Focused Physical Exam
- General: height, weight, waist circumference (central obesity), BMI, BP (supine and standing), pulse
- H&N: eyes (pupillary reactions, extraocular movements, lens opacities, fundoscopy), thyroid
- CVS: signs of CHF, peripheral pulses and bruits
- GI: hepatomegaly from fatty liver
- MSK: foot inspection, limited joint mobility, arthropathy, colour/temperature of limbs
- Neuro: screen for peripheral neuropathy using vibration tuning fork or monofilament
- Derm: inspection for cutaneous infections, problems with injection sites, signs of dyslipidemias (tendon xanthomas, xanthelasmas)

Important Laboratory Markers
- Blood: hemoglobin A1C, glucose, lipids, creatinine
- Urine: albumin/creatinine ratio

Hypoglycemia

The Essentials

Clinical Classification:

- **FASTING:** resulting from an imbalance of hepatic glucose production (too little) and peripheral glucose utilization (too much)
  - Iatrogenic: most common causes is *side effect of drugs for diabetes mellitus* (hypoglycemic unawareness is a consequence of previous hypoglycemia) as well as alcohol
  - *Factitious hypoglycemia* is a consequence of covert or overutilization of glucose (serum insulin will be elevated in the absence of C-peptide)
    - ◆ Insulinoma
    - ◆ Non-B cell tumour: overproduction of insulin-like growth factor II (IGF-II)
- **POST-PRANDIAL:** within 4 hours of food consumption; glucose levels fall more rapidly than insulin levels
  - Alimentary hypoglycemia post gastric surgery
  - Idiopathic

Focused History

Ask questions relating to common symptoms:

- *Neurogenic:* sweating, pallor, tachycardia, palpitations, tremor, anxiety, tingling and paresthesisas of mouth and fingers, hunger, nausea/vomiting
- *Neuroglycopenic:* weakness, headache, fainting, dizziness, blurred vision, mental dullness/confusion, abnormal behaviour, amnesia, seizures

Diagnostic Test

- 72 hour fast for levels of plasma glucose, insulin, C-peptide, proinsulin, plasma sulfonylurea, IGF-II

PITUITARY DISORDERS

The Essentials

- Disorders of the pituitary gland that cause problems related to endocrine functions or mass effect leading to overproduction or underproduction of pituitary hormones

Hyperfunction (e.g. prolactinoma)

- *Etiology:* usually resulting from benign adenomas that overproduce one or more hormones (anterior pituitary: ACTH, GH, PRL, TSH, FSH/LH; posterior pituitary: ADH, OXY)
- *Mass Effect:* any tumour can either overproduce or compress adjacent normal tissue to cause it to underproduce; other mass effect symptoms include pressure on the optic nerve CN II (leading to bitemporal hemianopsia), and cranial nerves of the cavernous sinus (e.g. CN III, IV, V, VI)
  - Classified as either *micro* (<1 cm) or *macro* (>1 cm)
- Prolactinomas:
  - Account for 30% of all pituitary adenomas
  - 5 × greater prevalence in women (50% are microadenomas; larger tumours commonest in men)
  - Age of onset: <40 yrs, rare in children

Clinical Pearl

Over-production of PRL can also be caused by bisection of the pituitary stalk, mass effect or administration of psychiatric drugs

---

ENDOCRINOLOGY

Focused History and Physical Exam

Etiology: increased hormone secretion is most commonly due to adenomas

Table 2. Symptoms and Signs of Pituitary Hormone Overproduction

Hormones	Focused History	Physical Exam
	Symptoms of Overproduction	Signs of Overproduction
Anterior Pituitary		
ACTH (see adrenal)	Symptoms of Cushing's disease: symptoms of DM, weight gain, ecchymoses	Central obesity, dorsal and supraclavicular fat pads, hypertension, high cholesterol
GH	Symptoms of acromegaly: "change in shoe/ring size", symptoms of hyperglycemia, dental complaints	Hypertension, high cholesterol, "acral" features: thickening of hands, fingers and heel pad, prominent eyebrows and jaw, misaligned teeth, macroglossia, visual field changes
PRL	Symptoms of galactorrhea, amenorrhea, hirsutism, infertility, impotence	Galactorrhea
TSH (see thyroid)	Leads to symptoms of hyperthyroidism, very uncommon	Signs of hyperthyroidism
FSH/LH	Adenomas don't usually overproduce enough of these hormones to cause changes in the pituitary gonadal axis	Usually no signs
Posterior Pituitary		
ADH	Clinical syndromes arise from underproduction (see hypofunction)	
Oxytocin	Not seen as a clinical syndrome	

Note: for any adenoma, bitemporal hemianopsia may be present

Hypofunction (e.g. hypopituitarism)

- *Etiology:* cell destruction can occur by the following mechnisms:
    - Compression of normal cells by pituitary adenomas
    - Pituitary infarction (e.g. Sheehan's syndrome)
    - Pituitary surgery or radiation
    - Other rare causes such as cell infiltration (e.g. saroidosis)
- For each individual pituitary hormone, there exists a factor that stimulates its release arising from the hypothalamus; e.g. for the *anterior pituitary* (*stimulator → hormone*): CRH → ACTH, GHRH → GH, TRH → PRL/TSH, GnRH → FSH/LH
- Hypothalamic lesions (tumours, aneurysms, genetic syndromes) can cause pituitary hormone deficiencies, which are referred to as "tertiary" deficiencies

Table 3. Symptoms and Signs of Pituitary Hormone Underproduction

Hormones	Focused History	Physical Exam
	Symptoms of Underproduction	Signs of Underproduction
Anterior Pituitary		
ACTH (see adrenal)	Symptoms of adrenal insufficiency	Signs of adrenal insufficiency
GH	Low energy, osteoporosis, dyslipidemia	Short stature (in children)
PRL	Inability to lactate	None
TSH (see thyroid)	Symptoms of hypothyroidism	Signs of hypothyroidism
FSH/LH	*Women:* amenorrhea, infertility *Men:* erectile dysfunction, loss of libido, decreased sex-dependent hair growth	Decreased secondary sexual characteristics (body hair growth, breast development)
Posterior Pituitary		
ADH	Symptoms of diabetes insipidus: polyuria, polydipsia	Confusion and coma from hypernatremia
Oxytocin	Not seen as a clinical syndrome	

ADRENAL DISORDERS

The Essentials
- Disorders of the adrenal gland that cause problems related to endocrine functions leading to overproduction or underproduction of adrenal hormones
- The adrenal gland makes 3 classes of steroid hormones:
  - *Glucocorticoids* (regulate blood sugar, metabolism, and immunity)
  - *Mineralocorticoids* (regulate Na^+ and K^+, blood volume, and BP)
  - *Androgens* (affect secondary sex characteristics: axillary/pubic hair, libido)

Hyperfunction (e.g. Cushing's syndrome or hypercortisolism)
- *Etiology:* can result from overproduction of ACTH (corticotrophin-dependent) by the pituitary or an ectopic tumour (e.g. bronchial, pancreatic) or cortisol (corticotrophin-independent) by adrenal tumours; or from exogenous/iatrogenic use of glucocorticoids

Causes of Cushing Syndrome:
- *Primary:* adrenal neoplasia (adenoma, carcinoma); adrenal micronodular dysplasia (sporadic, familial e.g. Carney's syndrome); adrenal macronodular hyperplasia
- *Secondary:* adrenal hyperplasia (from ACTH stimulation) – pituitary ACTH-producing adenoma; 2° to ACTH- or CRH-producing tumours – bronchogenic carcinoma, carcinoid of the thymus, pancreatic carcinoma, bronchial adenoma
- *Exogenous/Iatrogenic:* prolonged glucocorticoid use

ENDOCRINOLOGY

Common Chief Complaints

- Weight gain: usually central distribution (frequently patients are evaluated for Cushing's because of a combination of DM, HTN, dyslipidemia, and/or obesity)
- Bruising/striae
- Hirsutism/acne

Focused History

- Ask questions related to the *cause of adrenal disease:* pituitary tumour symptoms (headache, peripheral vision loss), drug use (glucocorticoid)
- Ask questions related to *consequences* and *complications:* in >60% of patients, weakness and fatigue, oligomennorrhea/amenorrhea, personality changes (depression or euphoria); other findings include symptoms of DM, osteoporosis and fractures, thinning of skin, ecchymoses, weight gain

Focused Physical Exam

- General: hypertension (BP >150/90), centripetal obesity (with increased abdominal fat, dorsocervical and supraclavicular fat pads)
- H&N: plethoric, "moon facies"
- CVS: often evidence of CAD (e.g. ankle edema)
- GI: purple abdominal striae
- MSK: proximal muscle weakness (inability to rise from squatting position)
- Derm: acne, oily skin, thin skin, hirsutism, ecchymosis

Hypofunction (e.g. Addison's Disease or adrenal insufficiency)

- *Etiology:* can be caused by underproduction of adrenal gland hormones, as a result of secondary failure due to inadequate ACTH formation or release, or destruction of the adrenal gland

Causes of Adrenal Insufficiency

- *Primary (adrenal gland hypofunction, high ACTH):* autoimmune adrenalitis (may be associated with type 1 or 2 autoimmune polyglandular syndrome); infectious (TB, systemic fungal infection, opportunistic infection, e.g. in HIV); tumour (metastatic carcinoma, especially of breast, lung, kidney,or bilateral lymphoma); other (hemorrhage, necrosis, thrombosis, congenital)
- *Secondary (pituitary hypofunction, low ACTH):* tumour (pituitary, craniopharyngioma); pituitary surgery or radiation, necrosis (e.g. Sheehan syndrome); hemorrhage; trauma; infection (e.g. Histiocytosis X); other (lymphocytic hypophysitis, sarcoidosis, empty sella syndrome)
- *Tertiary (low CRH secretion, low ACTH):* hypothalamic tumours; long-term glucocorticoid therapy

Common Chief Complaints

- Fatigue, weakness, loss of appetite, weight loss
- Other: hyperpigmentation, nausea/vomiting or abdominal pain (signs of adrenal crisis), hypotension, muscle and joint pain, salt craving

Focused History

- *Associated symptoms:* Fatigue that worsens on exertion and improves on rest, weakness; anorexia, weight loss; salt craving; nausea/vomiting, abdominal pain; amenorrhea; more severe cases present with postural lightheadedness, myalgias, arthralgias, intractable hiccups
- Ask questions related to *cause of adrenal disease:* pituitary tumour symptoms (headache, loss of peripheral vision, symptoms of low levels of other pituitary hormones)

- Ask questions related to *consequences* and *complications*: adrenal crisis (shock = hypotension with loss-of-consciousness; preceded by fever, nausea/vomiting, and abdominal pain, weakness and fatigue, and confusion) can occur in primary adrenal insufficiency often due to infection, trauma or other stress; symptoms of hypoglycemia are more common in secondary/tertiary adrenal insufficiency

> **Clinical Pearl**
> Pseudo-Cushing's is a false-positive test that arises from increased cortisol secretion seen with obesity, depression, alcohol and/or stress. This must be ruled out when evaluating a true Cushing syndrome

Focused Physical Exam
- H&N: assess pituitary findings (headache, visual symptoms, diabetes insipidus), articular calcification
- CVS: postural hypotension
- GI: tenderness on palpation
- MSK: proximal muscle weakness (inability to rise from squatting position)
- Derm: vitiligo, hyperpigmentation (primary adrenal insufficiency) especially in areas exposed to light (e.g. face, neck, backs of hands) and to chronic mild trauma (e.g. elbows, knees, spine, knuckles, waist, shoulders, buccal mucosa along dental occlusion and inner surface of lips)

Table 4. Pharmacological Therapy for Endocrinology Common Clinical Scenarios

Common Clinical Scenario	Pharmacological Therapy
Addison's Disease	Hydrocortisone, fludrocortisone
Diabetes Mellitus Type I	*Insulin:* rapid (aspart, lispro), short (insulin), intermediate (NPH, lente), long (ultralente, glargine)
Diabetes Mellitus Type 2	*Sulfonylureas:* glyburide, glyclazide, glimepiride, chlorpropamide *Biguanides:* metformin *Glucosidase inhibitor:* acarbose *Thiazolidinediones:* pioglitazone, rosiglitazone *Meglitinides:* nateglinide, repaglinide *Insulin* *Sitagliptin (DPP-4 inhibitor):* Januvia™
Hypercalcemia	Bisphosphonates, osteoclast RNA synthesis inhibitors (mithramycin), calcitonin, bone reabsorption inhibitor (gallium nitrate), precipitating agents (Potassium Phosphate), calcimimetic agent (cinacalcet)
Hyperkalemia	Electrolyte supplements (calcium chloride, calcium gluconate), insulin with dextrose, sodium bicarbonate, β-agonists, furosemide, potassium binding resins (sodium polystyrene sulfonate)
Hyperthyroidism	methimazole, propylthiouracil, sodium iodide I-131, β-blocker to alleviate symptoms
Hypothyroidism	levothyroxine (T_4, Synthroid®, Eltroxin®), liothyroxine (T_3, Cytomel®) can be used in conjunction with levothyroxine

THYROID DISORDERS

The Essentials

- Disorders of the thyroid gland that cause problems related to endocrine function or mass effect leading to overproduction or underproduction of thyroid hormones
- The thyroid gland makes two main forms of thyroid hormone: main circulating hormone T_4 and small amounts of the active hormone T_3
- T_4 enters cells and is converted to T_3; T_3 has nuclear receptors that have different effects depending on the organ; in general, T_3 increases metabolic rate, heart rate, and energy levels, and regulates bone health

Thyrotoxicosis

- *Excess production (hyperthyroidism)*
  - *Primary ($\downarrow TSH$, $\uparrow T_4/T_3$):* Graves' disease, toxic multi-nodular goiter, toxic adenoma, hyperemesis gravidarum, trophoblastic tumours, struma ovarii, drugs (e.g. amiodarone)
  - *Secondary ($\uparrow TSH$, $\uparrow T_4/T_3$):* TSH-secreting anterior pituitary adenoma; pituitary resistance to T_4/T_3
- *Excess hormone release (thyroiditis, $\downarrow TSH$, $\uparrow T_4/T_3$):* thyroid gland inflammation and release of stored hormone; can be sub-acute, post-partum, drug-induced, or radiation-induced
- *Exogenous thyroid hormone ($\downarrow TSH$, $\uparrow T_4/T_3$):* thyroid medications (excess dosage or surreptitious use); Hamburger thyrotoxicosis

Common Chief Complaints

- "Anxiety," weight loss with increased appetite, fatigue and weakness, frequent bowel movements, heat intolerance/sweating, palpitations, chest pain, shortness of breath, insomnia

Focused History

- Ask questions related to the *cause of thyroid disease:* personal or family history of autoimmune, thyroid or endocrine disorders (e.g. DM, Cushing's, gonadal dysfunction), past management (drugs, surgery, head/neck irradiation), medication use (e.g. amiodarone), pregnancy, goitrogen ingestion (e.g. seaweed, kelp, iodine)
- Ask questions related to *symptoms associated with enlarged thyroid:* enlarged thyroid/nodule, "mass effects": dysarthria, dysphagia, dyspnea, dysphonia (pressure on laryngeal nerve)
- Ask questions related to *symptoms associated with high thyroid hormone:* see **Table 5**; eye symptoms (e.g. Graves' exalpthalmous, eye grittiness, discomfort, excess tearing)
- Ask questions related to *symptoms of complications of high thyroid hormone:* e.g. thyrotoxicosis can cause decompensation in heart disease leading to chest pain and osteoporosis leading to bone fractures

Focused Physical Exam

Table 5. Physical Signs and Symptoms of Thyrotoxicosis

System	Symptoms of Thyrotoxicosis	Signs of Thyrotoxicosis
General	Weight loss with good appetite, heat intolerance	Fever, decreased LOC
H & N	Anxious, irritability, short attention span	Eyes: exophthalmos, lid lag
CVS	Palpitations	Tachycardia, wide pulse pressure, bounding pulse, aortic systolic murmur
GI	Increased bowel movements	Increased bowel sounds
GU	Women: amenorrhea	None
Neuro	Feel shaky	Fine tremor, proximal muscle weakness, hyperreflexia
Derm	Warm smooth skin, increased perspiration, hair thinning	Diaphoresis, pretibial myxedema (Graves')

Hypothyroidism
- *Primary (↑TSH, ↓T_4/T_3):*
  - Iatrogenic: post-thyroid surgery or radioactive iodine ablation (e.g. in treatment of thyroid cancer or Graves' disease)
  - Autoimmune: Hashimoto's thyroiditis, recurrent thyroiditis
  - Drug-induced: goitrogens (iodine), thionamides (propylthiouracil, methimazole), Li, amiodarone
  - Infiltrative disease: progressive systemic sclerosis, amyloid
  - Other: iodine deficiency, congenital
- *Secondary (↓TSH, ↓T_4/T_3):*
  - Insufficiency of pituitary TSH
  - Bexarotene treatment
  - Hypopituitarism: tumours, surgery, trauma, infiltrative disorders
- *Tertiary:* hypothalamic disease leading to TRH release

Common Chief Complaints
- Weight gain, fatigue, constipation, cold intolerance

Focused History
- Ask questions related to *cause of thyroid disease*, and to *symptoms associated with enlarged thyroid:* as above
- Ask questions related to *symptoms associated with low thyroid hormone:* see **Table 6**
  - Compensated hypothyroidism is a milder disease: weight gain with normal or decreased appetite, fatigue and weakness, dyspnea, paresthesia, goiter (associated with Hashimoto's)
- Ask questions related to *symptoms of complications of low thyroid hormone:*
  - Decompensated hypothyroidism (myxedema coma) is a severe disease where the body cannot adapt to the hypothyroidic changes causing organ failure and is usually precipitated by another illness (leading to coma, hypothermia, hypotension, bradycardia and respiratory failure)

ENDOCRINOLOGY

Table 6. Physical Signs and Symptoms of Hypothyroidism

System	Symptoms of Hypothyroidism	Signs of Hypothyroidism
General	Weight gain, cold intolerance, fatigue	Increased weight, hypothermia
H & N	"Mass effects"; periorbital edema, hearing impairment, enlarged tongue	Queen Anne's sign: loss of lateral third of eyebrow, signs of goiter
CVS	Dizziness	Hypotension, bradycardia
GI	Constipation	None
GU	Women: menstrual irregularities	Heavy menses
Neuro	Difficulty concentrating	Delirium, coma, proximal muscle weakness, Carpal tunnel syndrome
Derm	Dry skin, hair loss	Dry skin, brittle hair

POLYCYSTIC OVARIAN SYNDROME (PCOS)
The Essentials
- PCOS is a metabolic syndrome characterized by oligomenorrhea, hirsutism, obesity and polycystic appearing ovaries.
- *Prevalence:* 5-10% of reproductive age women, leading cause of infertility, may be underdiagnosed because condition is masked by oral contraceptive pills. Age of onset is often around menarche, adolescence or in young adults.
- *Etiology:* Causes are not well understood, both genetic and environmental influences.

Diagnostic Criteria
- 2003 ESHRE/ASRM criteria require 2 of the following 3:
  1. Oligomenorrhea and/or amenorrhea
  2. Clinical and/or biochemical signs of hyperandrogenism
  3. Polycystic ovaries on transvaginal ultrasound (ovary size >7.5-10mL and/or >12 follicles 2-9 mm)
- PCOS is a diagnosis of exclusion
- Rule out androgen excess disorders, such as congenital adrenal hyperplasia (21-hydroxylase deficiency)

Table 7. Conditions for exclusion for the diagnosis of PCOS

Differential Diagnosis	Clinical Features	Laboratory Features
Androgen secreting tumour	Virilization (clitoromegaly, extreme hirsutism)	↑ DHEAS and ↑ Testosterone (very high)
Amenorrhea: primary (or secondary)	May be related to other autoimmune disorders	↑ FSH, normal/↓ Estradiol
Acromegaly	See **Table 2**	↑ IGF-1

Table 7. Conditions for exclusion for the diagnosis of PCOS (continued)

Differential Diagnosis	Clinical Features	Laboratory Features
Androgen secreting tumour	Virilization (clitoromegaly, extreme hirsutism)	↑ DHEAS and ↑ Testosterone (very high)
Amenorrhea: primary (or secondary)	May be related to other autoimmune disorders	↑ FSH, normal/↓ Estradiol
Acromegaly	See **Table 2**	↑ IGF-1
Congenital adrenal hyperplasia	Family history of infertility and hirsutism	↑ 17-hydroxyprogesterone
Cushing's syndrome	Hypertension, striae	↑ 24hr urinary cortisol
Hyperprolactinemia	Galactorrhea	↑ prolactin
Thyroid dysfunction	Goiter, signs of hypothyroidism (see **Table 6**)	↑ TSH and ↓ T$_4$
Idiopathic hirsutism		
Exogenous androgen administration		

Risks: Substantial risks of Type 2 Diabetes, Hypertension, Dyslipidemia, Cardiovascular disease, Stroke, Endometrial hyperplasia/cancer, Weight gain, Miscarriage

Treatment
- Lifestyle modification: diet and exercise
- Menstrual control: oral contraceptive pill, cyclic progestins
- Hirsutism: OCP (Diane 35*), spironolactone, flutamide, finasteride, ketoconazole
- Insulin resistance: spironolactone, metformin
- Infertility: clomiphene, metformin, ovarian drilling, GnRH therapy, IVF

Focused History
- Ask questions related to *presenting symptoms:* menstrual history, hair growth on face, back, chest and abdomen
- Ask questions related to *associated symptoms:* irregular vaginal bleeding, recent weight gain, impaired glucose tolerance, infertility, dyslipidemia, sleep apnea
- Ask questions related to *family history* of infertility, insulin resistance, diabetes and androgen excess

Focused Physical Exam
- **HAIR-AN** Syndrome: **H**yper**a**ndrogenism, **I**nsulin **R**esistance, **A**canthosis **N**igricans
- General: height, weight, BMI, waist circumference (>88 cm)
- H&N: thyroid exam, androgenic alopecia (male pattern baldness),
- CVS: blood pressure
- GU: adenexal size and masses
- Derm: Acanthosis nigricans (hyperpigmented skin, usually in the posterior folds of the neck, axilla, groin, and umbilicus), hirsutism, acne

REFERENCES

Ehrmann DA. 2005. Polycystic ovary syndrome. *N Engl J Med* 352(12):1223-1236.

Fauci AS. 2008. *Harrison's Principles of Internal Medicine.* New York: McGraw-Hill.

Franks S. 2006. Controversy in clinical endocrinology: diagnosis of polycystic ovarian syndrome: in defense of the Rotterdam criteria. *J Clin Endocrinol Metab* 91(3):786-789.

Hegedus L. 2004. Clinical practice. The thyroid nodule. *N Engl J Med* 351(17):1764-1771.

Reid JR, Wheeler SF. 2005. Hyperthyroidism: diagnosis and treatment. *Am Fam Physician* 72(4):623-630.

Rotterdam ESHRE/ASRM-Sponsored PCOS consensus workshop group. 2004. Revised 2003 consensus on diagnostic criteria and long-term health risks related to polycystic ovary syndrome (PCOS). *Hum Reprod* 19(1):41-47.

Rotterdam ESHRE/ASRM-Sponsored PCOS Consensus Workshop Group. 2004. Revised 2003 consensus on diagnostic criteria and long-term health risks related to polycystic ovary syndrome. *Fertil Steril* 81(1):19-25.

The Essentials of Fluid, Electrolytes and Acid/Base Disturbances

Editors:
Michal Bohdanowicz &
Derek Chew

Faculty Reviewers:
Martin Schrieber, MD, FRCP(C), MEd

TABLE OF CONTENTS

Volume Status   427
Disorders of Sodium Concentration   428
Disorders of Potassium Concentration   430
Disorders of Calcium Concentration   432
Disorders of Phosphate Concentration   434
Disorders of Magnesium Concentration   435
Disorders of Acid-Base Balance   437
Intravenous Fluids   440

VOLUME STATUS

Clinical Features of Volume Overload

- *Symptoms*
  - Swelling of ankles, especially at the end of the day
  - Swelling all over the body, including hands (rings feel tight) and around the eyes
  - Shortness of breath on exertion, paroxysmal nocturnal dyspnea, orthopnea
  - Recent weight gain
- *Signs*
  - Peripheral edema (ankle edema in patients who are ambulatory; sacral edema in patients who are mainly in bed)
  - Evidence of ascites and/or pleural effusion
  - Bibasilar crackles on lung auscultation (i.e. indicating pulmonary edema)
  - Elevated JVP, positive abdominal-jugular reflux
  - Blood pressure may be elevated

Clinical Features of Volume Depletion

- *History*: Excessive fluid loss
  - GI: Vomiting, diarrhea
  - Renal: Diuretics, polyuria
  - Skin: Excessive sweating (fever, exercise, hyperthermia), burns
  - Hematologic: Blood loss
  - Neurologic: Altered mental status leading to reduced intake
- *Symptoms*
  - Recent weight loss
  - Excessive thirst
  - Postural dizziness
  - Fatigue
  - Weakness
  - Cramps

FLUIDS

- *Signs*
  - Dry mucous membranes
  - Dry axilla
  - Oliguria or anuria
  - Hemodynamic changes
    - Resting supine tachycardia and hypotension
    - Orthostatic tachycardia (rise in HR >30 from supine to standing)
    - Orthostatic hypotension (fall in SBP >20 on standing, any fall in DBP)
    - Low JVP
  - Soft fontanelles, reduced skin turgor, dry cry, dry diaper (in newborns)

Evidence-Based Medicine: Hypovolemia
The finding of dry axilla has a LR+ of 2.8 and a LR- of 0.6 while the finding of orthostatic tachycardia has a LR+ of 1.7 and a LR- of 0.8.

Simel DL. Hypovolemic, Adult. In Simel D, Rennie D (eds.) 2008. *The Rational Clinical Examination: Evidence-Based Clinical Diagnosis.* McGraw-Hill.

DISORDERS OF SODIUM CONCENTRATION

Clinical Pearl
Correcting chronic hyponatremia and hypernatremia too quickly can lead to neurological damage (demyelination and brain swelling, respectively).

Hyponatremia
- Serum sodium <135 mmol/L

Clinical Features
- Symptoms: (vary depending on severity and speed of onset)
  - Slow onset, mild hyponatremia:
    - Often asymptomatic (due to compensation)
    - Nausea, anorexia, malaise
  - Rapid onset, severe hyponatremia:
    - Headache, lethargy, decreased LOC
    - Seizures and death may occur

Classification and Causes
- Pseudohyponatremia
  - Normal plasma osmolality: hyperlipidemia, hyperproteinemia
  - Increased plasma osmolality: hyperglycemia, hypermannitolemia
- Hyposmolar hyponatremia
  - Primary sodium loss with secondary water gain:
    - Skin: Sweating, burns
    - GI: Vomiting, diarrhea
    - Renal: Diuretics, osmotic diuresis
  - Primary water gain
    - Syndrome of inappropriate ADH
      - Ectopic production by neoplasm
      - CNS pathology
      - Respiratory pathology
      - Drugs
    - Severe stress (pain, nausea, surgery)

FLUIDS

- Addison's disease
- Hypothyroidism
- Primary sodium gain with excessive secondary water gain:
  - Heart failure
  - Liver cirrhosis
  - Nephrotic syndrome

Investigations
- Assess volume status (heart rate, blood pressure, signs of edema or volume depletion)
- Measure serum sodium, osmolality
- Measure urine sodium, osmolality

Management
- Treat underlying cause
- Water restrict
- Monitor serum sodium and urine osmolality to ensure that chronic hyponatremia is not corrected too rapidly (serum sodium concentration should never increase more than 8 mmol/L/day except in acute, symptomatic hyponatremia)
- For acute, symptomatic hyponatremia, treat with intravenous 3% sodium chloride

Hypernatremia
- Serum sodium >145 mmol/L

Clinical Features
- Symptoms: (mild unless thirst mechanism is defective or water access is restricted)
- Weakness, lethargy, irritability, confusion
- Intracerebral hemorrhage, seizures, coma and death if severe

Classification and Causes
- Net water loss
  - Extra-renal Causes:
    - Skin and respiratory tract: evaporation without water intake (fever, exercise)
    - GI: diarrhea or vomiting without water intake
  - Renal Causes:
    - Loop diuretics (e.g. furosemide)
    - Diabetes insipidus
      - Central (hypothalamic disease)
      - Nephrogenic (due to renal resistance to ADH)
    - Osmotic diuresis (e.g. mannitol or hyperglycemia)
- Salt gain
  - Intake of salt (orally or IV) either without water or with water in lower proportion to normal Na concentration

Investigations
- Assess ECF volume status
- Serum electrolytes, creatinine, urea, glucose
- If hypovolemic
  - Check urine osmolality (U_{osm}) and sodium (U_{Na})
    - Renal loss: U_{osm} 300-600 and U_{Na} >20
    - Nonrenal loss: U_{osm} >600 and U_{Na} <20
- If euvolemic

- Check urine osmolality (U_{osm})
- U_{osm} <300 suggests diabetes insipidus

Management
- Hypovolemic Hypernatremia
  - If evidence of hemodynamic instability, correct with bolus of NS;
  - Calculate free water deficit and replace with water PO/NG or IV hypotonic infusates (max. 12 mM decrease of [Na] over 24 hours)
  - Free H_2O deficit = TBW x (serum [Na] -140) / 140
- Hypervolemic Hypernatremia: Loop diuretic (or dialysis if renal failure); replace deficit with D5W

DISORDERS OF POTASSIUM CONCENTRATION

Hypokalemia
- Serum potassium <3.5 mmol/L

Clinical Features
- *Symptoms*
  - Skeletal muscle: fatigue, myalgia, cramps, weakness
- *Signs*
  - Metabolic alkalosis
  - Heart: arrhythmia
  - ECG changes: flattened T waves, premature ventricular beats, prolonged QT interval, U waves

Classification and Causes
- Increased losses
  - GI: diarrhea, bowel obstruction, ileus
  - Skin: sweating
  - Renal:
    + Increased distal flow: non-potassium-sparing diuretics, osmotic diuresis
    + Increased potassium secretion: vomiting (with bicarbonaturia), increased mineralocorticoid activity, diabetic ketoacidosis, hypomagnesemia
- Redistribution into cells: insulin, metabolic alkalosis, exogenous catacholamines (e.g. salbutamol at very high doses), thyrotoxic periodic paralysis, vitamin B_{12} treatment of pernicious anemia
- Decreased potassium intake (contributory rather than causative)

Investigations
- Rule out shift into cells
- 24-hour K excretion (U_K)
  - U_K <20 mEq/day suggests extrarenal loss
  - U_K >40 mEq/day suggests renal loss
- Transtubular potassium gradient (TTKG) = $(U_K /P_K) / (U_{osm}/P_{osm})$
  - TTKG >4 suggests renal loss due to increased distal K+ secretion
- If renal loss, check BP and acid-base status
- Assess serum renin, aldosterone and [Mg]

Management
- ECG if potassium level <3.0
- Treat underlying cause (if fluid repletion needed, avoid dextrose-containing solutions since dextrose → ↑ insulin → intracellular potassium shift)
- Potassium repletion – difficult to quantitate precisely

FLUIDS

- 100-200 mEq of K raises serum [K] by ~1 mEq/L
- Mild-moderate hypokalemia:
  - KCl (40 mEq) PO BID
- Severe hypokalemia or patient incapable of oral therapy:
  - Maximum IV concentration 40 mEq/L in peripheral veins or 60 mEq/L in central lines

Hyperkalemia
- Serum potassium >5.0 mmol/L
- N.B. serum potassium >7.0 mmol/L is life-threatening

Clinical Features
- Symptoms: none if mild
  - Skeletal muscle: weakness, stiffness
- Signs:
  - Heart: arrhythmia (sinus bradycardia, heart block, asystole, juntional rhythms, etc.)
  - ECG changes (if severe): peaked T waves, widened QRS, small/absent P waves, prolonged PR interval, "sine wave", asystole

Classification and Causes
- Decreased renal excretion (always present)
  - Decreased tubular fluid flow in cortical collecting duct:
    - Renal failure leading to low GFR
    - Low extracellular fluid volume
  - Decreased aldosterone action:
    - ACE-inhibitors, aldosterone receptor blockers
    - Potassium-sparing diuretics (spironolactone, amiloride, triamterene)
    - Mineralocorticoid deficiency or insensitivity
- Redistribution out of cells: insulin deficiency, rapid cell breakdown (e.g. hemolysis, rhabdomyolysis, acute tumour lysis syndrome), hyperglycemia, metabolic acidosis with non-organic anions
- Increased intake

Specific Physical Findings Depending on Cause of Hyperkalemia
- If patient is hypovolemic, consider these possibilities:
  - Decreased renal function and decreased potassium secretion.
  - Decreased mineralocorticoid level
    - Adrenal insufficiency (especially Addison's disease – may also have bronzing of skin due to excess proopiomelanocortin secretion from anterior pituitary)
    - Mineralocorticoid resistance
    - Aldosterone blockers (spironolactone), blockage of Na channel in cortical collecting duct (amiloride, trimethoprim, triamterene)
- If patient is hypervolemic, consider these possibilities:
  - Due to enhanced chloride absorption in cortical collecting duct (and therefore reduced intraluminal negative charge to attract potassium secretion)
    - Gordon's syndrome (rare)
    - Calcineurin toxicity (i.e. cyclosporine, tacrolimus)
    - Hyporeninemic hypoaldosteronism of diabetes

Investigations
- Rule out factitious hyperkalemia (e.g. hemolysis during venipuncture)

- Check to make sure if receiving IVF that there is not KCl in fluid
- Rule out shift of K^+ out of cells
- Estimate GFR
  - If normal GFR, calculate TTKG (see **Hypokalemia**)
  - TTKG <7 in patient with hyperkalemia →hypoaldosteronism
  - TTKG >7 in patient with hyperkalemia → normal aldosterone function

Management
- Emergent Rx if symptoms, ECG changes, or serum [K] >6.5 mEq
- Tailor Rx to severity of increase in K and ECG changes

Table 1. Treatment of Hyperkalemia

Intervention	Onset	Dose	Mechanism
Calcium Gluconate	minutes	1-2 amps (10 mL of 10% solution) IV	Protect heart
Insulin	15-30 min	1 amp D50W IV then 10-20 units insulin R IV	Shift K^+ into cells
Bicarbonate	15-30 min	1-3 amps IV	Shift K^+ into cells
β2-agonists	30-90 min	Salbutamol: 10 mg inh.	Shift K^+ into cells
Diuretics	30 min	≥40 mg furosemde IV ± IV NS to prevent hypovolemia	Enhance K^+ removal via urine
Cation-exchange resins	1-2 hrs	Kayexalate PR w/ tap water or calcium resonium/ Kayexalate and sorbitol PO	Enhance K^+ removal via gut
Dialysis			Enhance K^+ removal

DISORDERS OF CALCIUM CONCENTRATION

Hypocalcemia
- Total serum Ca <2.2 mmol/L

Clinical Features
- *Symptoms*
  - Acute, mild hypocalcemia: paraesthesia, hyperreflexia;
  - Acute, severe hypocalcemia: tetany, confusion, seizures, laryngospasm, bronchospasm
  - Chronic hypocalcemia: parkinsonism, dementia, catarcts, abnormal dentition, dry skin
- *Signs*
  - Chovstek's sign
    - Facial spasm when facial nerve or branch is tapped
  - Trousseau's sign
    - Carpal spasm induced with arterial occlusion using a BP cuff (1-3 minutes above systolic on the forearm)
  - Papilledema
  - ECG: prolonged QT interval

Classification and Causes
- **Associated with low PTH levels (hypoparathyroidism)**
  - Genetic disorders
  - Surgical removal of parathyroid glands
  - Autoimmune hypoparathyroidism
  - Hypomagnesemia
- **Associated with elevated PTH levels (secondary hyperparathyroidism)**
  - Deficiency of vitamin D
  - Renal failure
  - Malabsorption syndromes
  - Drugs: phosphate, calcitonin, aminoglycosides
  - Shift out of circulation: sepsis, osteoblastic metastases, pancreatitis, post parathyroidectomy (called the "hungry bone syndrome")
  - Respiratory alkalosis (total calcium level is normal, but a greater fraction is bound to albumin, so ionized fraction falls)
  - Hyperphosphatemia
  - Tumour lysis syndrome
  - Hypoalbmuinemia (ionized calcium will be normal)

Investigations
- Measure serum ionized calcium, phosphorus, magnesium, creatinine, and PTH
- Serum phosphorus usually elevated except in hypocalcemia from vit. D deficiency
- Serum PTH usually elevated except in hypoparathyroidism and magnesium deficiency

Management
- Treat underlying cause
- Do not treat hypocalcemia if suspected to be transient response
- Mild/asymptomatic
  - Oral calcium 1000 – 2000 mg/day (of elemental calcium)
- Acute/symptomatic
  - Calcium gluconate: 1 g IV over 10 min ± slow infusion (10 g in 1000 mL D5W over 10 hours)
  - Check serum calcium q4-6h
  - If hypomagnesemia present, must be treated to correct hypocalcemia
- If PTH recovery not expected (e.g. hypoparathyroidism), treat with vitamin D and calcium long-term (use calcitriol for vitamin D replacement if patients have hypoparathyroidism or renal failure)

Hypercalcemia
- Total serum Ca >2.6 mmol/L

Clinical Features
- *Symptoms*
  - "Bones, stones, abdominal groans with mental overtones"
    - Skeleton "bones":
      - Bone pain
    - Renal "stones":
      - Renal colic, polyuria, polydipsia
    - "Abdominal groans":
      - Nausea, vomitting, anorexia, constipation, pancreatitis, peptic ulcer disease
    - "Mental overtones":
      - Cognitive changes, decreased LOC

- *Signs*
  - Hypotonia, hypertension
  - ECG: shortened QT interval

Classification and Causes
- Parathyroid hormone (PTH)
  - Primary hyperparathyroidism
  - Tertiary hyperparathyroidism of renal failure
- Malignancy
  - Humoral hypercalcemia of malignancy (paraneoplastic PTHrP)
  - Solid tumours causing local bone resorption
  - Hematologic malignancy (e.g. multiple myeloma)
- Vitamin D elevation, as in sarcoidosis, TB or exogenous
- Drugs: thiazides, lithium, calcium carbonate
- Familial hypocalciuric hypercalcemia, Addison's disease, hyperthyroidism

Investigations
- Measure serum free calcium, chloride, phosphate, bicarbonate, PTH and PTHrP
- Measure urine calcium

Management
- Treat underlying cause
- Normal saline to restore extracellular fluid volume
- Use furosemide if and only if extracellular fluid volume overload develops
- Bisphosphonates (e.g. pamidronate) for hypercalcemia of malignancy
- If emergency situation, can use calcitonin subcutaneously
- In chronic situation with hyperparathyroidism, can use cinacalcet

DISORDERS OF PHOSPHATE CONCENTRATION

Hypophosphatemia
- Serum phosphate <0.84 mmol/L

Clinical Features
- *Symptoms*
  - Generally absent
  - Proximal muscle weakness, paresthesia, seizures, delirium, coma
- *Signs*
  - Hemolytic anemia
  - Muscle weakness, ventilatory failure, rhabdomyolysis
  - Heart failure

Classification and Causes
- Decreased intestinal absorption
  - Poor intake
  - Aluminum or magnesium containing antacids
  - Fat malabsorption
  - Vitamin D deficit
- Excessive renal excretion of phosphate (tends to be chronic)
  - Hyperparathyroidism
  - Fanconi syndrome
- Rapid shift of phosphate from ECF to bone or soft tissue
  - Insulin (either exogenous [treatment of DKA] or endogenous [refeeding in patients with severe malnutrition])
  - Acute respiratory alkalosis
  - Hungry bone syndrome

FLUIDS

- Measure serum phosphate, PTH
- Measure urine phosphate

Management
- Treat underlying cause
- Chronic cases can be treated with oral phosphate supplementation
- Can treat acute or symptomatic hypophosphatemia with intravenous potassium-phosphate

Hyperphosphatemia
- Serum phosphate >1.8 mmol/L

Clinical Features
- Ectopic soft tissue calcification leading to hypocalcemia
- Clinical features of hypocalcemia (i.e. muscle cramping)

Classification and Causes
- Increased intake
  - Phosphate-containing laxatives
- Decreased output
  - Renal failure
  - Hypoparathyroidism
- Shift of phosphate out of cells
  - Massive cell death (rhabdomyolysis, tumour lysis, hemolysis)
  - Respiratory acidosis

Investigations
- Measure serum phosphate, PTH
- Measure urine phosphate

Management
- Treat underlying cause
- Oral phosphate binders in severe cases

DISORDERS OF MAGNESIUM CONCENTRATION

Hypomagnesemia
- Serum magnesemia <0.7 mmol/L

Clinical Features
- *Symptoms*
  - CNS: altered mental status, seizure
  - Neuromuscular: muscle cramps
- *Signs*
  - Neuromuscular: increased deep tendon reflexes, tetany
  - Cardiac: arrhythmias
  - Metabolic: refractory hypokalemia and hypocalcemia

Classification and Causes
- Decreased intake
  - Malabsorption/malnutrition

FLUIDS

- Increased losses
  - Renal
    - Diuretics (thiazide, furosemide)
    - Alcohol
    - Nephrotoxic drugs (amphotericin, cisplatinum, cyclosporine)
    - Rare inherited renal tubular disorders (Bartter's, Gitelman's)
  - Diarrhea

Investigations
- Measure 24-hour urine Mg excretion (>2 mEq/day indicates excessive renal loss)
- Normal serum Mg does not exclude total body Mg deficiency

Treatment
- Mild/Chronic: 250-500 mg elemental Mg PO qd-bid
- Severe symptomatic: 1-2 g magnesium sulphate IV over 15 minutes followed by infusion of 6 g in ≥1 L over 24 hours, repeated over 7 days to replete Mg stores

Hypermagnesemia
- Serum magnesium >1.2 mmol/L

Clinical Features
- *Symptoms*
  - Mild hypermagnesemia: nausea, vomiting, skin flushing, bradycardia
  - Moderate hypermagnesemia: weakness, somnolence
  - Severe hypermagnesemia: muscle paralysis, coma
- *Signs*
  - Mild hypermagnesemia: decreased deep tendon reflexes
  - Moderate hypermagnesemia: hyporeflexia, hypotension
  - Severe hypermagnesemia: refractory hypotension, bradycardia, respiratory failure, decreased LOC

Classification and Causes
- Increased intake
  - Iatrogenic (most commonly in setting of treatment of preeclampsia)
- Decreased Output
  - Renal failure (most common cause)

Investigations
- Measure Serum [Mg]
- Assess kidney function (creatinine, urea)

Treatment
- Asymptomatic: stop Mg-containing products
- Severe Symptomatic: 1-2 g calcium gluconate IV over 10 min (+ dialysis in severe renal failure)

FLUIDS

DISORDERS OF ACID-BASE BALANCE

Information required to evaluate the status of a patient with an acid-base disturbance:

- Arterial blood gasses (for ABG see **Respiratory Exam** p. 343)
- Plasma anion gap (see below)
- Clinical evaluation of respiration

Table 2. Normal ABG Values

Normal ABG Values	
pH	7.35 – 7.45
pCO_2	35 – 45 mmHg
pO_2	80 – 100 mmHg
HCO_3^-	22 – 28 mmol/L

Respiratory Acidosis

Pathophysiology: hypoventilation leads to accumulation of CO_2 from metabolism, which lowers the pH of body fluids

Common Causes

- COPD or any severe lung disease associated with excessive work of breathing can lead eventually to respiratory muscle fatigue and hypoventilation
- Drugs (narcotics, anesthetics) or other causes of decreased LOC, hypothyroidism
- Problem with respiratory muscles or chest wall (e.g. nerve problem such as Guillain-Barre syndrome; neuromuscular junction disorder such as myasthenia gravis; severe chest wall abnormality such as kyphoscoliosis)

Normal Compensation

- Increased levels of bicarbonate raises the pH and buffers against respiratory acidosis
- Acute: bicarbonate increases 1 mmol/L for every 10 mmHg increase in pCO_2
- Chronic (after 2-3 days): the kidney increases rate of production of new bicarbonate, resulting in a rise of 3 mmol/L for every 10 mmHg increase in pCO_2

Respiratory Alkalosis

Pathophysiology: hyperventilation lowers pCO_2 and thereby raises pH of body fluids

Common Causes

- Any lung disease tends to cause hyperventilation and therefore respiratory alkalosis (provided work of breathing not so great that patient develops respiratory muscle fatigue)
- Examples: pneumonia, pulmonary embolism, asthma, pulmonary fibrosis, pulmonary edema
- Sepsis
- Pregnancy
- Liver failure
- Acetylsalicylic acid

Normal Compensation

- Reduction in bicarbonate lowers the pH and buffers against respiratory alkalosis

FLUIDS

- Acute: bicarbonate decreases 2 mmol/L for every 10 mmHg decrease in pCO_2
- Chronic: the kidney reduces bicarbonate production, resulting in a drop of 5 mmol/L for every 10 mmHg decrease in pCO_2

Metabolic Acidosis

Pathophysiology: reduction in ECF bicarbonate concentration results in a lower pH. This can be caused directly by the addition of H^+ (which binds to bicarbonate to reduce the concentration), loss of bicarbonate from the body; or the failure of the kidneys to produce bicarbonate at the usual rate. Use plasma anion gap to help determine etiology

Plasma anion gap (PAG)
- $PAG = Na^+ - (HCO_3^- + Cl^-)$, normal value is 12 (range 10-14)
- Proportional to albumin concentration
- If the compound that caused the acidosis contributes an anion, this will be reflected in an increased PAG
- In a pure increased anion gap acidosis, the drop in bicarbonate closely matches the increase in PAG
- If the drop in bicarbonate is significantly greater than the increase in PAG, then there is both an increased anion gap type of metabolic acidosis and also a normal anion-gap type of acidosis
- If the drop in bicarbonate is significantly less than the increase in PAG, then there is both an increased anion gap type of metabolic acidosis and also a metabolic alkalosis

Common causes of increased-PAG metabolic acidosis: **KARMEL**
- **K**etoacidosis
- **A**cetylsalicylic acid
- **R**enal failure (severe)
- **M**ethanol ingestion
- **E**thylene glycol ingestion
- **L**actic acidosis

Common causes of non-anion gap metabolic acidosis
- Diarrhea
- Mild to moderate renal failure
- Renal tubular acidosis
- Mineralocorticoid deficiency

Normal Compensation
- Hyperventilation should decrease the pCO_2 (in mmHg) by the same amount as the decrease in bicarbonate (in mmol/L)
- Kussmaul's breathing: respiratory compensation (i.e. hyperventilation) for metabolic acidosis may be clinically detectable in terms of deep and perhaps rapid breathing

Metabolic Alkalosis

- Pathophysiology: an increase in ECF bicarbonate raises the pH. The source of the bicarbonate is either:
  - Exogenous
  - Made in stomach when patient vomits
  - Made in kidneys
- Under normal conditions, the kidneys excrete the extra bicarbonate and thus prevent metabolic alkalosis. During volume and/or potassium depletion, the kidneys retain the extra bicarbonate and thus cause metabolic alkalosis

Common Causes
- Diuretics
- Vomiting
- Excess mineralocorticoid activity

Normal Compensation
- Hypoventilation with a variable increase in pCO_2 (range is 3-8 mmHg for each 10 mmol/L rise in bicarbonate level)

Table 3. Algorithm for Evaluation of Acid-Base Status

pH	PaCO₂	Bicarbonate	Diagnosis	Normal Compensation*
Acidemic		↑	Respiratory acidosis	Acute: Bicarbonate rises 1 mmol/L for every 10 mmHg rise in paCO₂ (from cells)
	↑			Chronic: Bicarbonate rises 3 mmol/L for every 10 mmHg rise in paCO₂ (renal formation of new bicarbonate)
		↓	Concurrent respiratory and metabolic acidoses	N/A
	↓	↓	Metabolic acidosis	Hyperventilate to lower the paCO₂ 1 mmHg for every 1 mmol/L drop in bicarbonate
Alkalemic		↓	Respiratory alkalosis	Acute: Bicarbonate falls 1 mmol/L for every 10 mmHg drop in paCO₂ (into cells)
	↓			Chronic: Bicarbonate falls 3 mmol/L for every 10 mmHg drop in paCO₂ (renal excretion)
		↑	Concurrent respiratory and metabolic alkaloses	N/A
	↑	↑	Metabolic alkalosis	Hypoventilate to raise the paCO₂ (not more than 50 mmHg)

* Failure of normal compensation or overcompensation indicates the presence of a second acid-base disturbance. For example, a patient with a bicarbonate of 10 mmol/L (i.e. a drop of 15) with a paCO₂ of 35 (i.e. a drop of only 5) would represent a combined metabolic and respiratory acidosis – manifested by a failure to reach normal compensation for the metabolic acidosis. When comparing changes in pCO₂ and HCO₃⁻ levels, use middle values of normal ranges: for pCO₂, 40 mm Hg; for HCO₃⁻ level, 24 mmol/L.

FLUIDS

INTRAVENOUS FLUIDS

Table 4. Commonly Used IV solutions (Crystalloids)

Fluid	Components	Tonicity	Indications
D5W (5% dextrose in water)	50 g/L Dextrose	Hypotonic (100% free water)	Hypernatremia
0.9% NaCl (Normal Saline NS)	154 mmol/L Na 154 mmol/L Cl	Isotonic	Fluid resuscitation Fluid maintenance Large volumes can cause hyperchloremic nonanion gap metabolic acidosis
0.45% NaCl (½ NS)	77 mmol/L Na 77 mmol/L Cl	Hypotonic (50% free water)	
Ringer's lactate	130 mmol/L Na 109 mmol/L Cl 4 mmol/L K 3 mmol/L Ca 28 mmol/L Lactate	(nearly) Isotonic	Avoid in hyperkalemia Useful in large volume resuscitation (lactate metabolized by liver to bicarbonate)
2/3rds 1/3rds	33 g/L Dextrose 51 mmol/L Na 51 mmol/L Cl	Hypotonic (66% free water)	
3% NaCl	513 mmol/L Na 513 mmol/L Cl	Hypertonic	Cerebral edema due to hyponatremia

Fluid Balance:
- TBW = 60% total body weight = $^2/_3$ ICF + $^1/_3$ ECF (where ECF = $^3/_4$ interstitial + ¼ intravascular)

Maintenance Fluids
- To calculate maintenance fluids (4/2/1 Rule):
  - 4 mL/kg/hr for first 10 kg of patient's body weight
  - 2 mL/kg/hr for second 10 kg
  - 1 mL/kg/hr for the patient's remaining weight
- To calculate maintenance electrolytes:
  - Na: 3 mEq/kg/day
  - K: 1 mEg/kg/day

REFERENCES

Fauci AS. 2008. *Harrison's Principles of Internal Medicine.* New York: McGraw-Hill.
McPhee SJ, Papadakis M. 2010. *Current Medical Diagnosis and Treatment 2010.* New York: Lange Medical Books/McGraw-Hill, Medical Pub. Division.
Simel DL, Rennie D, Keitz SA, American Medical Association. 2009. *The Rational Clinical Examination: Evidence-Based Clinical Diagnosis.* New York: McGraw-Hill, Medical/JAMA & Archives Journals, American Medical Association.
Washington University School of Medicine, Cooper DH, Krainik AJ, Lubner SJ, Reno HEL. 2007. *The Washington Manual of Medical Therapeutics.* Philadelphia: Lippincott Williams & Wilkins.

FLUIDS

The Essentials of General Surgery

Editors:
Emilie Lam & Jo Jo Leung

Faculty Reviewer:
Robert Mustard, MD

TABLE OF CONTENTS
Pre-operative Management   441
Operative Management   442
Post-operative Management   445

PRE-OPERATIVE MANAGEMENT

Surgical Emergency: SAMPLE History
- **S** igns/Symptoms
- **A** llergies
- **M** edications
- **P** ast Medical History
- **L** ast Meal
- **E** vents preceding the emergency

Investigations

Table 1. Indications for Pre-operative Laboratory Investigations

Investigation	Indications
Hb	Procedure associated with significant blood loss
WBC	Infection symptoms, myeloproliferative disease, myelotoxic medications
Platelets	Bleeding disorder, myeloproliferative disease, myelotoxic medications
PTT and INR	Bleeding disorder, chronic liver disease, malnutrition, long-term antibiotic or anticoagulant use
Electrolytes	Renal insufficiency, CHF, diuretic, digoxin, ACE inhibitors
Creatinine and BUN	Age >50, diabetes, hypertension, cardiac disease, medications influencing renal function (ACE inhibitors, NSAIDS), major surgery
Glucose	Obesity, known diabetes or symptoms thereof
Albumin	Liver disease, serious chronic illness, recent major illness, malnutrition
Urinalysis	No indication
Chest X-ray	Age >50, known cardiopulmonary disease or symptoms thereof
ECG	Males >40, females >50, CAD, hypertension, diabetes

Smetana GW, Macpherson DS. 2003. *Med Clin North Am* 87:7-40.

Cardiac Evaluation

- History: SOB, angina, syncope, palpitations, DM, MI, CABG, angioplasty, prosthetic heart valve, rheumatic heart disease, PMH, etc.
- Physical exam: vitals, postural vitals, JVP
- Assess Goldman cardiac risk to determine cardiac risk in a noncardiac surgical setting (**Table 2**)
- See *Cardiovascular Exam*

Table 2. Goldman Cardiac Risk Factors

Factor	Points
Third heart sound or jugular venous distension	11
Myocardial infarction in the past 6 months	10
Rhythm other than sinus	7
>5 premature ventricular depolarizations per minute	7
Age >70 years old	5
Emergency procedure	4
Hemodynamically significant aortic stenosis	3
Aortic, intraabodominal or intrathoracic procedure	3
Poor general health: respiratory insufficiency, electrolyte abnormality, metabolic acidosis, renal failure, hepatic dysfunction	3

	Total Points	Complications	Cardiac Death
Class I	0-5	0.7%	0.2%
Class II	6-12	5.0%	2.0%
Class III	13-25	11.0%	2.0%
Class IV	≥26	22.0%	56.0%

Goldman L et al. 1997. N Engl J Med. 297:845-850.

Pulmonary Evaluation

- History: smoking history, sputum production, wheezing, exertional dyspnea, COPD, asthma, occupational exposure, obesity, functional status (rake the yard, walk up a flight of stairs)
- Physical exam: body habitus, wasting, respiratory distress, clubbing, cyanosis, AP chest diameter, prolonged expiratory phase, auscultation
- See *Respiratory Exam*

OPERATIVE MANAGEMENT

Operative Note

- Date and time of procedure
- Pre-operative diagnosis
- Post-operative diagnosis
- Procedures
- Names of surgeons and assistants
- Operative findings
- Complications
- Anesthesia (e.g. general)
- Estimated blood loss (EBL)
- Crystalloid replaced (type and volume)

- Blood products administered
- Tubes and drains (e.g. NG, Foley, JP)
- Urine output
- Specimens collected: cultures, blood, pathology
- Intra-operative x-rays
- Condition of patient on transfer to post-anesthesia care unit (PACU)
- Disposition

Sutures

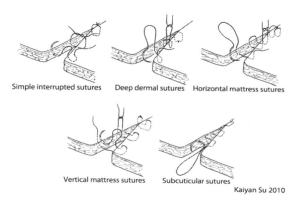

Simple interrupted sutures   Deep dermal sutures   Horizontal mattress sutures

Vertical mattress sutures   Subcuticular sutures

Kaiyan Su 2010

Figure 1. Common Stitch Types

Table 3. Timing of Suture Removal

Location	Time Frame (Days)
Face	5-7
▪ Eyelids	3-5
▪ Lip	5-7
Hands/Feet	10-14
Trunk	7-10
Breast	7-10

Souba WW et al. 2007. *ACS Surgery Principles and Practice.* WebMD Professional.

Table 4. Commonly Used Suture Materials

Absorbable	Non-Absorbable
Gut (plain, chromic)	Polypropylene (Prolene)
Polyglactic acid (Vicryl)	Nylon (Surgilon, Nurolon)
Polyglycolic acid (Dexon)	Silk
Polyglyconate (Maxon, Monocryl)	Other (e.g. staples, tape)
Polydiocanone (PDS)	

Taylor JA. 2004. *Blueprints Plastic Surgery: Outcomes and Beyond.* Lippincott Williams & Wilkins.

GENERAL SURGERY

*Admission/Post-operative Orders: **ADDAVID***

- **A dmit to ward/service** (under the care of Dr. _____)
- **D iagnosis**
- **D iet**
    - Pre-operative: NPO (nil per os = nothing by mouth)
    - Post-operative: NPO → sips/CF (clear fluids) → DAT (diet as tolerated)
    - TPN (total parenteral nutrition; requires interventional radiology consult to insert PICC line)
- **A ctivity**
    - AAT (activities as tolerated)
    - Bed rest/elevate head of bed
- **V ital signs**
    - VSR (vital signs routine, as per floor)
    - Vitals q4h (vitals every 4 hours)
    - Notify MD if: sBP <90 mmHg, HR >120 bpm, T >38.5°C or O_2 sat <92%
- **IV, investigations, nurses' orders**
    - IV
        - NS at 100 cc/h (+ 20meq/L KCl if hypokalemic)
        - If dehydrated, bolus with NS or Ringer's lactate
        - If patient drinking well post-operatively
            - IV TKVO WDW (IV to keep vein open when drinking well; means IV running at 5 cc/h)
            - IV to SL (saline lock)
            - D/C (discontinue) IV
    - Investigations (labs)
        - Routine b/w (blood work): CBC, lytes, BUN, creatinine
        - Assess for coagulopathy: PTT, INR, platelet count (in differential)
    - Imaging/tests (as indicated):
        - CXR, x-ray of extremity
        - ECG
    - Consults (as indicated)
        - Internal medicine
        - Anesthesia, Acute Pain Service
    - Nurses' orders
        - Nasogastric (NG) tube (to suction/straight drain); especially post-gastric surgery/upper GI obstruction; if excessive losses via NG, then replace losses 1:1 with NS + 20 meq/L KCl
        - Jackson-Pratt (JP) drains to bulb suction
        - Foley catheter to straight drain/urometer
        - Measure ins + outs
        - Maintain O_2 sat >92%
- **D rugs (6 As)**
    - Analgesics
        - Morphine 5-10 mg SC q3h prn for pain
        - Tylenol #3 1-2 tabs PO q4h prn for pain
        - Note: give laxatives with opioid pain medications (constipating)
    - Antiembolics
        - Heparin 5000 units SC q12h
    - Antecedents
        - Hold medications taken by patient prior to admission – e.g. anti-hypertensives, thyroid, hormone replacement, etc.
        - Note potential contribution of medications to coagulopathy and stop/reverse if possible pre-operatively:
            - Aspirin = antiplatelet → stop 1 week before surgery
            - Coumadin (warfarin)
            - NSAIDs
        - Post-operative: restart medications

- Antibiotics
  - Cefotetan (2nd gen. cephalosporin – 1 g IV q12h for bowel flora)
  - Cefazolin (Ancef®) (1st gen. cephalosporin – 1g IV q8h)
- Antiemetics
  - Dimenhydrinate (Gravol®) 25-50 mg IV/IM/PO q3-4h for nausea
- Anxiolytics
  - Benzodiazepines (e.g. diazepan, lorazepam)
- CAUTION: Do NOT order medications PO with concurrent NPO order

POST-OPERATIVE MANAGEMENT

*Progress Notes: **SOAP***
- **Date/Time, Service, POD#**
- **S ubjective**
  - Changes in symptoms, significant events, physical complaints in patient's own words, pain control
- **O bjective**
  - Vital signs
  - Intake and output (UO, NG, JP)
  - Physical exam: check incision site and dressing, neurovascular status
  - Lab results: CBC, electrolytes, imaging, etc.
- **A ssessment and P lan**
  - For each identified problem, devise an appropriate therapeutic regimen; note any plans for discharge or transfer

Sample Procedure Note
- **Procedure**: Diagnostic lumbar puncture
- **Indication**: Suspected meningitis
- **Consent**: Patient gave informed consent after indications, risks, alternative options were adequately explained
- **Complications**: None
- **Description**: Patient was placed in left lateral decubitus position with spine flexed and the L4-L5 interspace was identified. Under sterile conditions, the area was anesthetized with 1% lidocaine 5 cc, spinal needle was inserted in L4-L5 interspace without problems
- **Specimen**: 8 cc clear, nonturbid spinal fluid collected
- **Investigations**: Sent for protein, glucose, Gram stain, cell count, culture
- **Disposition**: Patient tolerated procedure well

Discharge Note
- Date and time
- Diagnoses
- Therapy during hospital stay
- Investigations: EKG, CXR, CT
- Discharge medications
- Follow-up arrangements

Discharge Summary
- Patient's name, medical record number
- Date of admission
- Date of discharge
- Admitting diagnosis
- Discharge diagnosis
- Name of attending or ward service

- Surgical procedures, diagnostic tests, invasive procedures
- History and physical exam on admission
- Course of illness while in hospital
- Discharge condition/arrangements (who will care for patient once out of hospital)
- Discharge medications (make note of medications added, discontinued or changed while in hospital)
- Discharge instructions and follow-up care: date of follow-up visit, diet, exercise, homecare
- Problem list: list all past and current problems

REFERENCES

Goldman L, Caldera DL, Nussbaum SR, Southwick FS, Krogstad D, Murray B, Burke DS, O'Malley TA, Goroll AH, Caplan CH, Nolan J, Carabello B, Slater EE. 1977. Multifactorial index of cardiac risk in noncardiac surgical procedures. *N Engl J Med* 297(16):845-850.

Lawrence PF, Bell RM, Dayton MT. 2006. *Essentials of General Surgery*. Philadelphia; Baltimore: Williams & Wilkins.

Smetana GW, Macpherson DS. 2003. The case against routine preoperative laboratory testing. *Med Clin North Am* 87(1):7-40.

Souba WW, Fink MP, Jurkovich GJ, Kaiser LP, Pearce WH, Pemberton JH, Soper NJ. 2007. *ACS Surgery: Principles and Practice*. Hamilton: BC Decker.

Taylor JA. 2005. *Blueprints Plastic Surgery*. Malden: Blackwell Pub.

The Essentials of Infectious Diseases

Editors:
Grace Lam &
Fiona Lovegrove

Faculty Reviewers:
W. Conrad Liles, MD, PhD, FACP, FIDSA, FRCP(C)
Susan M. Poutanen, MD, MPH, FRCP(C)

TABLE OF CONTENTS

Common Cold	447
Tuberculosis	448
HIV/AIDS	451
Sexually Transmitted Diseases (STIs)	454
Urinary Tract Infections	457
Infectious Diarrhea	457
Viral Hepatitis	460
Meningitis	463
Sepsis	465
Osteomyelitis	467
Skin, Muscle and Soft Tissue Infections	468
Travel-Related Illnesses	471
Special Populations	474

THE COMMON COLD

Definition
- Non-specific symptoms without localization to any one part of the URT, duration of approximately 1 week

Etiology
- Mostly viral – rhinovirus, influenza, parainfluenza, coronavirus, adenovirus and respiratory syncytial virus (RSV)

Focused History
- Signs and symptoms: very diverse, typically acute, mild, and self-limited
  - Rhinorrhea
  - Nasal congestion
  - Sore throat
  - Hoarseness (± reduced pitch or aphonia)
  - Sneezing
  - Dry cough
  - Mild malaise and fatigue
  - Conjunctivitis (suggests adenovirus or enterovirus)
  - Fever (uncommon in adults, more frequent in infants and children)

Focused Physical Exam
- ***Respiratory Exam*** p. 339
- ***Head and Neck Exam*** p. 107
- If specific localization of symptoms is observed – such as sinus, ears, pharynx, lower airway – then specific examination of those structures
  - Ear and mastoid: pneumatic otoscopy, focused neurological exam of CN VIII (see ***Neurological Exam*** p. 186)
  - Larynx: direct laryngoscopy

- Epiglottitis (a bacterial complication): may find respiratory distress, with inspiratory stridor and retraction of the chest wall

Investigations
- The common cold is generally self-resolving and with non-specific lab exams and thus rarely investigated
- Pharynx and oral cavity: key investigation is to distinguish Group A streptococcal pharyngitis from viral pharyngitis
  - Throat swab culture (takes 24-48h)
  - Rapid antigen detection testing for GABHS (less sensitive)
- Epiglottitis: Fiberoptic laryngoscopy in the OR for visualization and culture (direct examination in the exam room with tongue blade and laryngoscope NOT recommended)

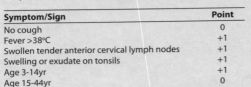

Evidence-Based Medicine: Sore Throat Score
Score of 0,1 –no need for antibiotics
Score of 2,3 – culture all; treat only if culture positive
Score of 4 – culture all; treat with penicillin if patient has high temperature or is clinically unwell early in disease course

Symptom/Sign	Point
No cough	0
Fever >38°C	+1
Swollen tender anterior cervical lymph nodes	+1
Swelling or exudate on tonsils	+1
Age 3-14yr	+1
Age 15-44yr	0
Age ≥45yr	-1

Adapted from McIsaac WJ et al. 1998. *CMAJ* 158(1);75-83.

Management
- Antibiotic therapy not indicated for uncomplicated common colds. Management of symptoms: decongestants, NSAIDs, dextromethorphan (for cough), lozenges, etc.
- Pharyngitis: see EBM for management criteria based on the quick diagnosis of presence of Group A beta-hemolytic streptococcal (GABHS) infection in adults

PNEUMONIA
- See *Respiratory Exam* p. 348

TUBERCULOSIS (TB)

Definitions
- Caused by the *Mycobacterium tuberculosis* complex, manifesting in the lungs with possible extra-pulmonary dissemination (see **Table 1**)
- Transmission via airborne droplets produced by coughing from individuals with active pulmonary TB

Pulmonary Tuberculosis

Focused History
- Risk Factors:
  - Endemic areas: Eastern Europe, Mediterranean, Russia, China, Southeast Asia, India, Pakistan, Africa, South America, and the Caribbean. Assume exposure regardless of whether the patient recognizes an exposure or not

- First Nations peoples
- Homeless, individuals with a history of prison or jail time, lack of social support, joblessness and poverty
- Substance abusers
- Family members with TB
- Actual exposure to known TB cases
- Non-specific symptoms (fever that persists more than 2 weeks, night sweats, weight loss, anorexia, chills, general malaise, weakness)
- Specific pulmonary symptoms
  - Cough – may be initially non-productive and subsequently purulent
  - Sputum ± hemoptysis
  - Pleuritic chest pain
  - Shortness of breath
  - Dyspnea or adult respiratory distress syndrome
  - Heaviness of chest

Focused Physical Exam
- General inspection (age, degree of nutrition, emotional and anxiety states, cyanosis)
- Fever
- Wasting
- Chest
  - Cough: frequency and character of cough
  - Dyspnea
  - Persistent rales in involved areas during inspiration, especially after coughing
  - Rhonchi due to partial bronchial obstruction
  - Whispered pectoriloquy may be helpful in finding small areas of local consolidation
  - Amphoric breath sounds in areas with large cavities
  - Percussion: fluid accumulation suggested by flat, wooden sounds
  - Grocco's sign: presence of para-vertebral area of dullness on the opposite side
- May have no detectable abnormalities

Extrapulmonary Tuberculosis

Table 1. Extrapulmonary Tuberculosis

Location	Physical Symptoms	History
Lymph Nodes	Accompanying HIV Infection	Painless swelling of lymph nodes, most commonly at cervical and supraclavicular sites
Upper Airways	Hoarseness, dysphagia, chronic productive cough	Ulcerations
Pleura	Asymptomatic, fever, pleuritic chest pain, and dyspnea	Pleural effusion, dullness to percussion, absence of breath sounds
Pericardial	Subacute or acute with fever, dull retrosternal pain	Friction rub, cardiac tamponade, effusion, constrictive pericarditis
Peritoneal	No specific physical findings	Abdominal/pelvic masses and/or ascites

Table 1. Extrapulmonary Tuberculosis (continued)

Location	Physical Symptoms	History
Genitourinary	Asymptomatic, urinary frequency, dysuria, hematuria, flank pain	Note: Females – infertility, pelvic pain, menstrual abnormalities Males – epididymitis, prostatitis, orchiditis
Musculoskeletal (spine)	Back pain, paraplegia, paraparesis	Kyphosis (gibbus deformity)
Sites outside spine	Monoarticular destructive arthritis	Monoarticular destructive arthritis
Miliary or disseminated	Accompanying HIV infection. Presenting symptoms: fever, night sweats, anorexia, weakness, weight loss Associated symptoms: cough, other respiratory symptoms and abdominal symptoms	Hepatomegaly, splenomegaly, lymphadenopathy, choroidal tubercles in retina
Central Nervous System	Headache, mental lethargy, altered sensorium, neck rigidity	Paresis of CN (especially ocular ones), hydrocephalus Note: hyponatremia typical

Investigations
- Diagnosis of latent TB infection
  - Tuberculin skin test (not used for acute TB infection)
    - False negatives common in immunocompromised patients
    - False positives with nontuberculous mycobacteria and by BCG vaccination
- Chest radiograph (usually showing upper-lobe infiltrates with cavities but in immunocompromised patients, atypical pattern of lower-lobe infiltration without cavities seen)
  - CT and MRI can be used for imaging of extrapulmonary TB
- AFB microscopy
  - Smear of sputum or tissue biopsy
  - 3 sputum specimens, taken early in the morning
- Mycobacterial culture or nucleic acid amplification
  - Isolation and identification of *M. tuberculosis*
- Interferon-gamma release assays (e.g. QuantiFERON-TB)
- Drug susceptibility testing
  - Upon isolation of the bacteria, drug susceptibility testing should be done to determine which antibiotics will be effective

Differential Diagnosis
- Non tuberculous conditions with similar symptoms:
  - Chronic pulmonary infections due to agents other than *M. tuberculosis*: chronic bronchitis (especially with emphysema), early bronchiectasis, pulmonary abscess, chronic empyema (interlobar), chronic or subclinical bronchopneumonia (e.g. with accompanying history of recent past influenza infection)
  - Focal infections: intranasal conditions, dental infections, diseased tonsils, middle ear disease and abdominal infections
  - Rarer conditions: malignancy, syphilis, mycotic infections, pneumonoconiosis (miners phthisis)

Basic Management Plan
- 6-month course of triple drug therapy:
  - Oral administration of first line agents: isoniazid, rifampin, pyrazinamide and ethambutol
  - Second line agents include: injectable aminoglycosides – streptomycin, kanamycin and amikacin; injectable polypeptide capreomucin; oral agents – gatifloxacin, levofloxacin, moxifloxacin, ethionamide, cycloserine and para-aminosalicylic acid.
- Regimen:
  - Initial phase of 2 month with the 4 first line drugs, followed by a continuation phase of 4 months with isoniazid and rifampin
  - Daily treatment throughout or intermittently (3x weekly throughout)
  - Referral to Public Health
  - Completion of treatment is defined by total doses taken and not duration of treatment.
  - Generally speaking, with each antibiotic's resistance (and especially in the immunocompromised population), the duration of treatment will have to increase
- Drug resistance and poor rates of adherence:
  - Multi-drug resistant (MDR) and extensive drug-resistant (XDR) strains of *M. tuberculosis* are on the rise due in part to poor rates of adherence. To combat this issue, direct observation of treatment (DOT), especially during the initial phase, has been implemented.
  - Concurrently with treatment, monthly sputum examination is conducted until AFB and cultures become negative
- Other treatment options:
  - Lobectomy or pneumonectomy may be a viable option for patients with localized disease

HIV DISEASE AND AIDS

Definition
- Infection with the Human Immunodeficiency Virus (subtypes 1 or 2) causing immunodeficiency through the progressive depletion of CD4+ lymphocyte populations
- Acquired Immunodeficiency Syndrome (AIDS) is characterized by CD4+ cell counts below 200/ml and opportunistic infections

Epidemiology
- Approximately 33 million people infected worldwide
- Risk factors
  - Unprotected sexual activity, injection drug use
  - High risk populations include: MSM, sex workers, marginalized populations (e.g. aboriginals), immigrants from endemic countries

Natural History of HIV Infection
- Acute HIV syndrome or acute seroconversion illness
  - 50-70% experience acute syndrome 3-6 wks after primary infection
  - Much like acute infectious mononucleosis
  - Unexplained fatigue, sore throat, myalgias, malaise, fevers, night sweats, diarrhea, rash, weight loss, aseptic meningitis, lymphadenopathy, neutropenia
  - Resolves spontaneously in 1-2 weeks

- Middle phase
  - Asymptomatic stage – clinical latency
  - May note persistent generalized lymphadenopathy, thrombocytopenia
  - Minor opportunistic infections (e.g. Herpes zoster (shingles), oral candidiasis, oral hairy leukoplakia, various skin disorders – i.e. seborrhea, eczema, warts, molluscum, chronic diarrhea)
  - Length of latent stage can vary greatly, median is 10 yrs for untreated patients
  - Progressive decline in CD4$^+$ cells, but viral load may remain relatively stable or slowly increase
- Final/Crisis phase
  - Persistent fever, fatigue, weight loss, diarrhea
  - AIDS defining illnesses: serious opportunistic infections (*Pneumocystis jiroveci* (previously known as *P. carinii*) pneumonia (PCP), TB – pulmonary or extrapulmonary, recurrent bacterial pneumonia, cryptococcal meningitis, central nervous system toxoplasmosis, cytomegalovirus retinitis), or neoplasms (Kaposi's sarcoma, lymphoma), clinical neurological disease-progressive multifocal leukoencephalopathy, HIV dementia

Focused History
Clinical presentation can vary widely depending on the stage of infection, underlying comorbid illness, and various aspects of patient history

History of Present Illness
- Pertinent medical assessments
  - Date and place of HIV testing and confirmation of test results
  - Any history of prior testing – i.e. for insurance, giving blood, pregnancy, other
  - CD4$^+$ count and viral load
  - TB skin test results
  - Syphilis test results
  - Date and results of last Pap smear
- Occurrence of opportunistic infections, malignancies or any other IVDU-associated conditions
  - STIs: hepatitis B and C, syphilis, genital warts, herpes simplex, gonorrhea, chlamydia, *Molluscum contagiosum*, crabs, lice
  - Other infections or malignancies (bacterial infections, fungal infections, parasitic infections, mycobacterial infections)
- Travel history, illness while away and use of preventative vaccines, etc.
- Medication history (certain clinical manifestations are due to side effects of medication and antiretrovirals)
  - Antiretroviral history (include response, CD4$^+$, viral load), adherence, toxicity, any resistance testing and results
  - Participation in clinical trials
  - Toxicity of ARV

Social History
- Sexual history – use of barrier protection
- Pregnancy – dates, mode of delivery, testing of offspring
- Significant relationships and support systems
- Disclosure
- Physical or emotional violence
- Work
- Housing

- Drug plan, % coverage and financial resources
- Depression, previous suicidal attempts or ideations
- Alcohol, tobacco, recreational drug use

Review of Systems

For history taking on HIV/AIDS patients, it is very important to do a thorough review of systems (see ***General History and Physical Exam***). It is also important to note symptoms of the opportunistic infections that often accompany AIDS

Focused Physical Exam
- General
  - Vitals (including temperature)
  - Weight changes (including fat redistribution)
- Head and Neck
  - Fundoscopy (e.g. HIV retinopathy (cotton wool spots), CMV retinitis)
  - Examine oral cavity
    + Candidiasis (thrush)
    + Kaposi's sarcoma (KS) lesions
    + Hairy leukoplakia on lateral tongue
    + Gingivitis
    + Bruises or bleeding form gums
    + Ulcer
  - Lymphadenopathy
- CVS
  - Signs of heart failure (edema, SOB)
  - Hypertension
- Respiratory
  - Focal chest findings associated with bacterial pneumonia
  - Chest findings may also be associated with TB
  - Absent chest findings associated with PCP (*P. carinii* pneumonia)
- Abdo
  - Liver (hepatitis B/C, drug toxicity) – stigmata of chronic liver disease, ascites, jaundice, hepatomegaly
  - Spleen – splenomegaly
  - Masses (lymphoma)
- GU
  - Ulcers or warts
  - Pelvic exam/PAP – cervical carcinoma
  - Rectal exam – anal/rectal carcinoma or KS
- Neurological
  - Mental status – depression, memory loss, dementia and psychosis
  - Sensory and motor exam
    + Focal neurological findings (e.g. weakness, photophobia) suggest CNS infection or tumour
    + Unsteady gait, poor balance, tremor
    + Loss of bladder or bowel control with myelopathy
    + Increased tone and deep tendon reflexes
    + Peripheral neuropathies
  - Meningeal irritation (see **Meningitis**)
- Musculoskeletal (MSK)
  - Arthritis in large joints – suggests HIV/AIDS-associated arthropathy
- Dermatological
  - Macular roseola-like rash (seen with acute seroconversion syndrome)
  - Dermatitis, folliculitis, seborrhea, eczema

INFECTIOUS DISEASES

- Herpes zoster
- Kaposi's Sarcoma

Investigations
- HIV antibody test
- CD4$^+$ T cell count
- HIV RNA level
- HIV Genotyping
- Routine bloodwork (CBC, electrolytes, Cr, LFTs, blood glucose, lipids)
- STI testing
- TB skin test
- Pap smear

Differential Diagnosis
- Idiopathic CD4$^+$ lymphocytopenia
- Sjögren's syndrome
- Sarcoidosis
- Lymphoma
- Congenital immunodeficiency syndromes affecting T cells (e.g. SCID)

Management
- Education and counseling
- Immunizations (pneumovax, hepatitis A/B, influenza)
- Combination anti-retroviral therapy (CART)
- Prophylaxis of opportunistic infection

SEXUALLY TRANSMITTED INFECTIONS (STIs)

Definition
Bacterial, viral or parasitic organisms transmitted by any mode of sexual activity (oral, vaginal, anal).

Epidemiology
- Most common infectious agents are *Chlamydia trachomatis* (chlamydia) and *Neisseria gonorrhoeae* (gonorrhea/gonococcus/GC), and HSV
- *C. trachomatis* and *N. gonorrhoeae* have similar clinical presentations but *C. trachomatis* infections are more common, more often asymptomatic, and clinically less severe than *N. gonorrhoeae* infections

Focused History
- Predisposing factors
  - Age (<25 years old)
  - History of previous STI
  - New sexual partner in past 3 months
  - Multiple partners
  - Not using barrier contraception
  - Oral contraceptive pill usage
  - Contact with infected person
- Signs and Symptoms
  - See **Table 2**
- Children
  - Infections typically acquired during childbirth include conjunctivitis, lower respiratory infection, pharyngitis, and anal canal infections
  - Suspect abuse if vaginal infection is found in pre-pubertal female prior to sexual activity

- Women and MSM
  - Rectal infections are possible: perianal discomfort, rectal discharge, mucopus coating on stools
  - Oral-genital contact can cause pharyngitis: usually asymptomatic, but can have sore throat, pain/discomfort on swallowing
- Both men and women can develop a reactive arthritis syndrome (Reiter's syndrome) following *C. trachomatis* infection: conjunctivitis, urethritis or cervicitis, arthritis, and mucocutaneous lesions

Focused Physical Exam
- General Inspection
  - Vitals (temperature)
  - Examine conjunctiva, inspect mouth and tonsils, look for skin lesions
- Abdominal
  - Adnexal masses
  - Tenderness and guarding in lower quadrants
  - Inspect rectum and stool for mucopus
- GU
  - In men: inspect and palpate penis (esp. meatus) and scrotum (esp. epididymis), inspect for secretions
  - Inspect for secretions
  - In women: inspection of Bartholin's gland for erythema and exudate, pelvic exam including inspection of cervix for redness, friability, discharge
- Musculoskeletal
  - Arthritis
  - Polyarthralgias (esp. wrists, knees, fingers, ankles)
  - Myalgias

Investigations
- See **Table 2**
- Direct microscopic examination of tissue scrapings
  - Gram stain of urethral discharge only useful for GC in men
  - Typically low sensitivity with large number of false interpretations
- Chlamydia cell culture of isolated organisms
  - Low and variable sensitivity (60%-80%), high cost, technically difficult
  - Only available in major medical settings
- Antigen and nucleic acid detection by immunologic and hybridization methods
  - Low and variable sensitivity (60%-80%)
  - High specificity (97%-99%)

Table 2. Signs/Symptoms and Diagnosis of Common STIs

Symptoms/Signs	Diagnosis	Epidemiology
Chlamydia (*Chlamydia trachomatis*)		
Asymptomatic (most)		
Muco-purulent cervical discharge; grossly red cervix, often with infected erosion Urethral syndrome (dysuria, frequency, urgency, pyuria with no bacteria) Pelvic pain; post-coital bleeding	Nucleic acid amplification Need tissue culture Cervical culture or monoclonal antibody	Most common STI Often associated with gonorrhea

Table 2. Signs/Symptoms and Diagnosis of Common STIs (continued)

Symptoms/Signs	Diagnosis	Epidemiology
Gonorrhea (*Neisseria gonorrhoeae*)		
Similar to chlamydia Offensive yellow-white recurrent discharge; tends to be thicker, more copious and painful than chlamydia	Nuclei acid amplification Gram stain Cervical, rectal and throat culture	Often associated with chlamydia
Trichomonas (*Trichomonas vaginalis*)		
Asymptomatic (up to 50%) Profuse thin, frothy grey/ yellow-green discharge, often foul-smelling Occasionally irritated, tender vulva; dysuria Petechiae on vagina and cervix (10%)	Saline wet mount	May not be transmitted sexually (e.g. whirlpools)
Condylomata Acuminata/Genital Warts (Human Papilloma Virus – HPV)		
Latent: no visible lesions, asymptomatic **Subclinical**: visible after acetic acid use **Clinical**: visible, wart-like hyperkeratotic, verrucous or flat, macular lesions; vulvar edema Lesions usually enlarge in pregnancy	Cytology (Pap) Colposcopic biopsy HPV DNA (nucleic acid probes – not routine)	>60 subtypes (>20 genital) Increased risk cervical and vulvar CA with HPV types 16, 18, 36, 45
Herpes Simplex (Herpes Simplex Virus – HSV)		
May be asymptomatic **Prodromal**: tingling, burning, pruritus Multiple painful shallow ulcerations with small vesicles – may coalesce **First infection**: inguinal lymphadenopathy, malaise, fever If affect urethral mucosa: dysuria, urinary retention **Recurrent**: decreased duration, frequency, severity	Viral culture Cytologic smear Electron microscope	Caused by HSV type II (genital) in 90% of cases; by type I (oral) in 10%

Table 2. Signs/Symptoms and Diagnosis of Common STIs (continued)

Symptoms/Signs	Diagnosis	Epidemiology
Syphilis (*Treponema pallidum*)		
1°: usually single painless vulval/vaginal/ cervical chancre, inguinal lymphadenopathy 3-4 weeks after infection **2°:** (2-6 months later): malaise, anorexia, headache, adenopathy; fever; generalized maculopapular rash; condylomata lata **3°:** CNS/asc. aorta progressively destroyed; may involve other organs **Congenital:** possible fetal anomalies/ stillbirth/neonatal death **Latent:** asymptomatic	Aspirate ulcer serum or node Serology (often negative for 1° syphilis)	Most cases: age 15-30

Basic Management
- Chlamydia: Azythromycin 1 g po once
- Gonorrhea: Cefixime, 400 mg po once
- Trichomonas: Metronidazole, 2 g po once
- Genital Warts: Cryotherapy, Aldara cream, Electrocautery
- Herpes: Anti-virals (acyclovir, valacyclovir, and famciclovir)
- Syphilis: Parenteral penicillin G (duration of therapy varies depending on the stage of disease and clinical manifestations)

URINARY TRACT INFECTIONS (UTIs)
- See *Urological Exam* p. 368

INFECTIOUS DIARRHEA

Definition
- Liquid or unformed stool passed at a higher frequency than usual
- >200 g/d
- 3 categories: acute (<2 wks), persistent (2-4 wks), chronic (>4 wks)

Etiology
- Infectious (90% of cases), see **Table 3**
- Non-infectious
  - Medication or toxin ingestion
  - Ischemic colitis
  - Diverticulitis
  - Partial bowel obstruction
  - Inflammatory Bowel Disease (IBD) – Crohn's Disease, Ulcerative Colitis
  - Irritable bowel syndrome

INFECTIOUS DISEASES

Table 3. Common Signs & Symptoms & Epidemiology of Infectious Diarrhea

	Signs and Symptoms	Epidemiology
Parasitic		
Giardia, Cryptosporidia, Cyclospora, Isospora	Persistent diarrhea (never blood) bloating; cramps; no fever May have malabsorption	Particularly important in HIV patients
Amoebiasis (E. histolytica)	Colitis with blood and mucus; absence of stool leukocytes	Rare, but serious
Bacterial (Inflammatory)		
Campylobacter, Salmonella, Shigella	Watery diarrhea progressing to bloody diarrhea Severe lower abdominal cramps; vomiting; fever	Increasing incidence of *Campylobacter* in travelers *Shigella* is more common in children and MSM
Listeria		Often foodborne, especially in ready-to-eat meats and soft cheeses
ETEC	Watery diarrhea; mild cramps; no fever	Traveller's diarrhea
EHEC (E. coli 0157:H7)	Bloody diarrhea May cause hemolytic uremic syndrome	Often foodborne, especially undercooked hamburgers
C. difficile	Diarrhea with mucus, sometimes blood Lower abdominal cramps Increased incidence and severity in Canadian and American hospitals	Associated with antibiotic use
Viral		
Hepatitis A		Often foodborne, especially raw seafood
Rotavirus, Norwalk-like virus (Norovirus)	Vomiting and diarrhea (blood is rare, only in severe cases)	Rotaviruses: children <2 yrs Norwalk-like viruses: Adults and children

ETEC = Enterotoxigenic *E. coli*; EHEC = Enterohemorrhagic *E. coli*

Focused History
- Predisposing factors, outlined in **Table 4**
- Features of diarrhea
  - Frequency, duration
  - Appearance of stool: blood, mucus
- Associated signs and symptoms
  - Fever
  - Abdominal pain
  - Tenesmus
  - Vomiting

Table 4. Predisposing Factors & Commonly Associated Causes of Infectious Diarrhea

Factor	Common Etiologic Agent
Traveller	
Sudden onset of abdominal cramps, anorexia, and watery diarrhea Onset usually 3d to 2wks after arrival in tropical country Self-limited illness, lasting 1 to 5 days Ingestion of contaminated food or water	Varies by area, but most commonly enterotoxigenic *E. coli* (ETEC) Also Noroviruses, *Shigella*, *Salmonella*, *Campylobacter* species *Giardia* (History of camping)
Location *Day-care centre*	
High attack rate High attack rate in family members	Rotavirus (age <2 y), also *Shigella*, *Campylobacter* species, and *Cryptosporidium parvum*
Hospital	
Intensive care units Wards (e.g. pediatric) - Inquire about antibiotic exposures	*C. difficile*-associated diarrhea; noroviruses (adults); rotavirus (children)
Toxin-mediated Bacterial Food Poisoning	
Non-inflammatory Common-source may exist Incubation period and food source may help pinpoint etiology/outbreak	*Staphylococcus aureus* (incubation period ~6h) *Bacillus cereus* (fried rice within last 6-24h) *Clostridium perfringens*

Focused Physical Examination
- Assess for of intravascular volume depletion
  - Postural lightheadedness and a reflex tachycardia >30 minute indicates moderate to severe intravascular volume depletion

Investigations
- Fecal WBC count
- Stool microbiology investigations
  - Gram stain
  - Culture
  - Polymerase chain reaction (PCR) (e.g. for noroviruses)
  - Electron microscopy (e.g. for noroviruses, rotaviruses)
- Imaging (if non-infectious etiology suspected):
  - Sigmoidoscopy
  - Colonoscopy
  - Abdominal CT scanning

Differential Diagnosis
- Pseudo-diarrhea (frequent passage of stool but total <200 g/d)
- Fecal incontinence
- Overflow diarrhea due to fecal impaction
- Post-infectious IBD
- *C. difficile* colonization
- Secondary lactose intolerance

Management
- Fluid and electrolyte replacement
- In mild cases, observe
- In non-febrile moderate cases without bloody stool or raised WBC, anti-diarrheal agents
- In febrile moderate to severe cases, treat empirically or with quinolone
- Note: antibiotic treatment of *E. coli* 0157:H7 is contraindicated due to an increased risk of progression to HUS and TTP

VIRAL HEPATITIS

Definition
- 5 classes: Hepatitis A-E (HAV, HBV, HCV, HDV and HEV)
- Can be classified into two categories: fecal-oral (HAV, HEV) vs parenteral
- Of the 5 classes, HBV and HCV can cause chronic disease
- All RNA viruses except for HBV
- Wide range of symptoms from mild to severe

Etiology
- HAV
  - Incubation period ~4wks
  - From raw seafood or food prepared by an individual with active HAV
  - Usually self limiting but occasional fulminant, life-threatening disease
- HBV
  - Incubation period: 8-12wks
  - Two peaks of exposure: infancy and adolescence
  - Exposure in infancy leads to chronic infection while adolescence exposure tends to lead to acute infections
  - Severe chronic and fulminant hepatitis can lead to cirrhosis and hepatocellular carcinoma
  - Extrahepatic sequelae include: polyathritis nodosa (vasculitis), cryoglobulinemia is a complication of HCV
- HDV
  - Incubation period ~8-12wks
  - Absolute co-infection or superinfection with HBV (i.e. never alone)
  - Cause of fulminant hepatic deterioration in individuals with active HBV
  - Duration of infection therefore depends on duration of HBV infection
- HCV
  - Incubation period ~7wks
  - At risk groups: injection drug users, tattoo recipients, prison inmates, HIV patients, health care workers
  - At least six different genotypes with different patterns of worldwide distribution
  - Due to diversity, patients exposed to HCV will not have immunity against subsequent HCV infections
  - Extrahepatic manifestation include immune-complex glomerulonephritis and cryoglubulinemia
  - Associated with cutaneous disorders such as porphyria cutanea tarda and lichen planus
- HEV
  - Incubation period ~5-6wks
  - Enteric virus predominantly in India, Asia, Africa and Central America
  - Animal reservoir in pigs among others

Focused History
- Associated signs and symptoms
  - Constitutional symptoms: nausea, vomiting, anorexia, fatigue, malaise, arthralgia, myalgia, headaches, photophobia, pharyngitis, cough, coryza
  - Fever: low grade (38°C-39°C) for HAV and HEV, high grade (39.5°C-40°C) for the rest
  - Dark urine and clay coloured stool
  - Jaundice
- Predisposing factors
  - Injection drug user
  - Use of immunosuppressive agents or history of immunosuppression (i.e. HIV+)
  - Prison inmate
  - Health care worker
- Exposure history
  - Dietary history
  - Travel history
  - Drug or medicine history
  - Alcohol usage

Focused Physical Examination
- Focused abdominal exam
  - Palpation of enlarged masses (see ***Abdominal Exam***)
- Surface examination for signs of liver disease

Investigations
- Most common investigation for patients suspected of viral hepatitis is a panel of serological tests: HBV surface antigen (HBsAg), HBV surface antibody (HBsAb), IgM anti-HAV, IgM anti-HBc and anti-HCV, plus viral load testing in patients with active HBV and HCV (see **Table 5** for diagnostic approach)
- HAV
  - Serology for anti-HAV IgM antibodies
  - Blood work: AST/ALT
- HBV
  - Immunoassay for HBsAg, keeping in mind that level of HBsAg does NOT correlate with the degree of liver damage
  - Serology for anti-HBV core protein antigen IgM antibodies (anti-HBc) in the beginning 8-12 weeks of infection and later, anti-HBsAg antibodies (anti-HBs)
    - In other words, immunoglobulin class gives indication of acute (IgM) vs chronic/past infection (IgG)
  - HBeAg
  - HBV DNA PCR
  - Blood work: AST/ALT, serum bilirubin, WBC, PT, glycemic index
- HDV
  - Anti-HDV IgM class antibodies in acute infection but may not be detectable until 30-40 days of infection
  - Detection of HDV RNA
- HCV
  - PCR or transcription mediated amplification (TMA) against viral RNA (detected days after exposure)
  - Blood work: AST/ALT
- HEV
  - HEV serology is available
  - Blood work: AST/ALT

Table 5. Simplified Approach to Diagnosis of Suspected Cases of Viral Hepatitis

HBsAg	IgM anti-HAV	IgM anti-HBc	Anti-HCV	Interpretation
-	+	-	-	Acute hepatitis A
+	-	+	-	Acute hepatitis B
+	-	-	-	Chronic hepatitis B
-	-	+	-	Acute hepatitis B (HBsAg below detection threshold)
-	-	-	+	Acute hepatitis C

*Adapted from Fauci AS et al. (eds.) *Harrison's Principles of Internal Medicine*, 17th edition.

Differential Diagnosis

Vascular
- Problems with venus return to heart: right atrial myxoma, constrictive pericarditis, Budd-Chiari syndrome venoocclusive disease
- Right ventricular failure with passive hepatic congestion
- Hypoperfusion syndromes (i.e. left ventricular failure or shock)

Infectious/Inflammatory/Autoimmune
- Infectious mononucleosis (caused by cytomegalovirus, herpes simplex and Coxsackie virus in particular)
- Toxoplasmosis
- Other causes of liver injury by: *Leptospira, Candida, Brucella, Mycobacteria,* and *Pneumocystis*
- Acute cholecystitis
- Ascending cholangitis
- Common duct stone
- Autoimmune hepatitis
- Primary sclerosing cholangitis
- Primary biliary cirrhosis

Neoplastic
- Pancreatic cancer
- Metastatic malignancy to the liver
- Hepatoma

Drug
- Medication/toxin poisoning

Congenital/Developmental/Inherited:
- α-1-antitrypsin deficiency
- Hemochromatosis
- Wilson's disease
- Aceruloplasminaemia
- Porphyria

Anatomic
- Complications of pregnancy: acute fatty liver of pregnancy, cholestasis of pregnancy, eclampsia, HELLP syndrome
- Primary parenchymal liver disease
- Non-alcoholic steatohepatitis (NASH)

Trauma

Environmental Exposure/Endocrine/Metabolic
- Alcoholic hepatitis
- Copper toxicity
- Iron overload
- Metabolic diseases of the liver such as Wilson's

Management
- HBV/HDV
  - No intervention needed unless disease is chronic/persistent (HBeAg+) (adefovir or lamivudine)
- HCV
  - 24wk course of long-acting pegylated interferon plus ribavirin
- In general, specific treatment not necessary
  - High calorie diet, possibly through IV in cases of persistent vomiting
  - If pruritus present, give bile salt-sequestering resin cholestyramine

MENINGITIS

Definition
Inflammation of the meninges which can be infectious or non-infectious in origin.

Epidemiology
- Viral and bacterial meningitis are most common (fungal/parasitic causes less common)
- Meningococcal and Pneumococcal infections are the most common causes of bacterial meningitis in adults
- Predisposing factors:
  - Infectious contacts
  - Travel to endemic regions
  - STIs (HSV, syphilis, HIV)
  - Exposure and infection with *Mycobacterium tuberculosis*
  - Parameningeal infections (e.g. otitis media, sinusitis)
  - Compromised immunity
  - Head trauma
  - Persistent CSF leaks
  - Anatomical defects (including dermal sinuses)
  - Previous neurosurgical procedures

Focused History
- Altered level of consciousness: irritability → confusion → drowsiness → stupor → coma
- Seizures
- Neonates: signs of sepsis (fever, respiratory distress, apnea, jaundice)
- Infants: fever, vomiting, irritability, convulsions, high-pitch cry, poor feeding, lethargy
- Older children and adults:
  - Fever
  - Headache
  - Neck stiffness
  - Photophobia

Focused Physical Exam
- Vitals (fever, bradycardia, irregular respiration)
- Neonates and infants: inspect anterior fontanelle for bulging or tightness
- Nuchal rigidity (stiff neck)
  - Brudzinski's Sign: abrupt neck flexion with patient in supine position – involuntary flexion of hips and knees is positive sign
  - Kernig's Sign: strong passive resistance to attempts to extend knee from flexed thigh position
- Assess lethargy, level of consciousness (MMSE, Glasgow Coma Scale)

- Cranial nerves: typically IV, VI, VII affected by raised ICP or basilar inflammation
- Petechial or purpuric rash (typically in extremities)

Evidence-Based Medicine: Adult Meningitis

History alone is not useful in establishing a diagnosis of meningitis. Physical exam is useful in ruling out meningitis, and in determining which patients should proceed to more definitive testing (lumbar puncture).

Physical Exam Finding	Sensitivity (%)	95% CI
Fever	85	78 to 91
Neck Stiffness	70	58 to 82
Altered Mental Status	67	52 to 82

The absence of all three signs of the classic triad of fever, neck stiffness, and altered mental status virtually eliminates a diagnosis of meningitis (sensitivity of >1 sign present = 99%)

Jolt accentuation of headache may aid in the decision to proceed to LP, while a negative result essentially excludes meningitis

Note: the applicability of these results is severely limited by the fact that most of the studies included in the analysis described were retrospective chart reviews, which lacked control populations. Only sensitivities could therefore be determined, and these are likely to overestimate the true sensitivities because the clinical examinations would have been performed with knowledge of the LP results.

Attia J et al. 1999. *JAMA* 282(2):175-181.

Investigations
- CBC and differential, electrolytes
- Blood cultures
- CT to exclude elevated ICP and mass lesion
- Lumbar puncture
- Opening pressure
  - Protein, glucose, cell count and differential, Gram stain

Differential Diagnosis
- Bacterial endocarditis
- Early tuberculous meningitis
- Amoebic meningoencephalitis
- Lyme disease
- Herpes encephalitis
- Cerebral toxoplasmosis
- Cerebral malaria
- Chemical or drug-induced meningitis
- Carcinomatous meningitis
- Sarcoid meningitis
- Parameningeal foci secondary to other lesions

Management Principles
- IV antibiotics should be initiated promptly after LP
- The chosen antimicrobial agent should be bactericidal and penetrate the CSF

- Examples of empiric antibiotic treatment of bacterial meningitis include:
  - Ceftriaxone 2g IV q12h
  - Vancomycin 1g IV q12h
- Adjuvant dexamethasone treatment in adults with acute pneumococcal meningitis lowers mortality/risk of unfavorable outcome

SEPSIS

Definitions

Sepsis
- Clinical evidence of infection as well as evidence of systemic inflammatory response to infection, with three or more of the following manifestations:
  - Oral temperature <36°C or >38°C
  - Heart rate >90 beats/min
  - Respiratory rate >20 breaths/min or $PaCO_2$ <32 mmHg or the use of mechanical ventilation
  - WBC >12 x 10^9/L or <4 x 10^9/L or >10% immature PMNs (bands)

Severe sepsis
- Sepsis associated with organ dysfunction due to hypoperfusion or hypotension, manifested by:
  - Oliguria
  - Lactic acidosis
  - Acute alteration in mental status

Septic shock
- Severe sepsis (as above) with refractory hypotension – systolic BP <90 mmHg or reduction of systolic BP >40 mmHg from patient's normal baseline level
- This clinical presentation persists despite fluid resuscitation of at least 500 mL saline solution

Epidemiology/Etiology
- Approximately ²/₃ of new cases are due to nosocomial infection
- See **Table 6** for common microorganisms that may generate the sepsis response

Table 6. Common Microorganisms that may Generate Sepsis Response

Microorganism	Common Examples
Gram-negative bacteria	Enterobacteriaceae, *Pseudomonas aeruginosa*
Gram-positive bacteria	*S. aureus, Enterococci, S. pneumoniae,* other *Streptococci*
Classic pathogens	*N. meningitidis, S. pneumoniae, H. influenzae, S. pyogenes*
Fungi	*Blastomyces dermatitidis* (in overwhelming TB), *Cryptococcus neoformans* (in HIV)

INFECTIOUS DISEASES

Focused History

In addition to general history taking, the following questions should be asked:

- Signs and symptoms
  - Related to the site of origin of infection (skin and soft-tissue, abdomen, genitourinary tract, lungs, central nervous system)
- Exposure history (diet, travel, infectious contacts)
- Predisposing factors
  - **Previous medical or surgical interventions**
    - e.g. chemotherapy, surgery, transplantation, etc.
  - **Use of immunosuppressive agents or history of immunosuppression**
    - e.g. HIV/AIDS, chemotherapy, splenectomy, organ transplant, corticosteroid therapy, immunomodulatory biologic therapy (anti-TNF therapy) hypogammaglobulinemia
  - **Previous infections and antimicrobial treatments** including medications and drug reactions (microbiological data from studies and investigations performed in the few weeks prior to presentation can be quite useful)
- Underlying chronic diseases affecting prognosis include:
  - Diabetes
  - Alcoholism and/or cirrhosis
  - Renal failure
  - Respiratory failure
  - Hematology malignancies and solid tumours
  - Invasive procedures or indwelling devices, vascular catheterization
  - Intravenous drug use
  - Structural abnormalities in urogenital tract

Focused Physical Exam

- Vitals (Temperature, RR, HR, BP)
- Respiratory
  - Cyanosis
  - Pulmonary infiltrates
- Cardiovascular
  - Signs of CHF
- Abdominal
  - Jaundice
  - Hepatosplenomegaly
- Skin
  - Lesions
  - Contusions
  - Purpuric rash
- Neurological
  - Altered mental status

Investigations

- Culture and sensitivity of microorganisms:
  - Local site
  - Blood samples (2 x 10 ml samples from different venipuncture sites)
  - Midstream urine
- CBC with differential, comprehensive metabolic panel
- Chest x-ray

Differential Diagnosis
- Infectious (with or without a source)
    - Bacterial (bacteremia, endocarditis)
    - Viral (e.g. viral hepatitis, dengue)
    - Parasitic (e.g. malaria)
- Non-infectious
    - Acute pancreatitis
    - Anaphylaxis
    - Drug intoxication/withdrawal
    - Heat stroke
    - Massive tissue injury (e.g. infarction, rhabdomyolysis)
    - Vasculitis

Management
- IV antibiotics (following sample collection)
- Source management (e.g. abscess drainage)
- Oxygen saturation and fluid management
- Respiratory support

OSTEOMYELITIS

Definition
An infection of bone, characterized by progressive inflammatory destruction of bone, bone necrosis, and new bone formation.

Epidemiology/Etiology
- Often community-acquired
- Commonly caused by staphlococci, streptococci, *Pseudomonas aeruginosa* and other GNR, anerobic bacteria and mycobacteria
- Microorganisms enter bone from a penetrating wound, or by spreading from a contiguous infectious focus or via hematogenous dissemination

Focused History
- HPI
    - Pain history (onset, duration, severity, localized skeletal pain, similar pain previously)
    - Trauma history
    - Constitutional symptoms
- Past medical history (pre-disposing factors)
    - Sickle cell anemia
    - Immunodeficiency
    - IV drug abuse
    - Prosthetic joints
    - Diabetes mellitus
    - Vascular insufficiency
    - Endocarditis

Focused Physical Exam
- Vitals (temperature, HR, RR, BP)
- Inspection:
    - Evidence of injury/trauma
    - Local source of infection (ingrown toenail, wound infection)
    - Cellulitis
- Peripheral vascular exam:
    - Hair/nail/skin changes, ulcerations, skin temperature
    - Capillary refill
    - Peripheral pulses, bruits
    - Pallor on elevation, rubor on dependency

INFECTIOUS DISEASES

- CBC, ESR, and C-reactive protein
- Blood cultures
- Bone biopsy – culture/sensitivity and histology
- X-ray, bone scan and other radiological examinations

Differential Diagnosis
- MSK
  - Traumatic or stress fractures
  - Altered biomechanics
- Vascular
  - Bone infarcts
- Inflammatory
  - Inflammatory arthritis
  - Psoriatic arthritis
  - Reiter's syndrome
  - Gout
- Neoplastic
  - Sarcoid
  - Lymphoma
  - Metastases

Management
- Medical
  - IV antibiotics, can step-down to PO in selected cases following IV therapy
- Surgical
  - Acute infection – debridement of dead tissue
  - Chronic infection – debridement of all devitalized bone and soft tissue and removal of foreign bodies

SKIN, MUSCLE AND SOFT TISSUE INFECTIONS

Definition
Tissue infection that involves the skin, subcutaneous fat, the fascia and/or muscle.

Epidemiology/Etiology
- Nosocomial vs. community-acquired
- Disruption of the epidermal layer by burns or bites, abrasions, foreign bodies, primary dermatologic disorders, surgery, or vascular/pressure ulcers allows penetration of bacteria to the deeper structures.
- Hair follicles are a route of infection either for normal flora (e.g. staphylococci) or for extrinsic bacteria (e.g. *Pseudomonas aeruginosa*).

Focused History
- HPI
  - Fever, chills, sweats
  - Pruritus
  - History of insect, tick, or animal/human bites
  - Travel history
  - Skin lesions
  - Erythema, warmth, edema
  - Pain, tenderness, myalgia

- Past Medical History
  - IV drug use
  - History of past disease (e.g. varicella zoster virus, herpes simplex virus)
  - Immune status
  - History of diabetes mellitus

Focused Physical Exam
- Lesion(s)
  - Type of lesion (see *Essentials of Dermatology* and **Table 7**)
  - Exudates, hemorrhage
  - Arrangement (e.g. linear, clustered, annular, arciform, dermatomal)
  - Distribution and location (e.g. exposed surfaces, extremities, along skin folds)
  - Colour (e.g. erythema in cellulitis)
  - Pain, tenderness; crepitus
  - Associated lymphangitis and regional lymph node involvement
  - Generalized lymph node enlargement
- Fever

Table 7. Common Skin Lesions and Conditions

Lesion	Associated Conditions
Vesicles	Smallpox, chickenpox (primary varicella zoster virus infection), shingles (herpes zoster virus), "cold sores" (herpes simplex virus), genital ulcers (herpes simplex virus), hand, foot and mouth disease (Coxsackie virus)
Bullae	Necrotising fasciitis (group A streptococci, mixed Gram-negative and anaerobic infections), staphylococcal scalded skin syndrome, gas gangrene (clostridial myonecrosis)
Crusted lesions	Impetigo (streptococcal, staphylococcal), ringworm (dermatophytes), histoplasmosis, blastomycosis, sporotrichosis, cutaneous leishmaniasis
Papules and nodules	Onchocerciasis nodule (Calabar swelling), lepromatous leprosy, secondary syphilis
Ulcers	Anthrax, leprosy, chancroid, primary syphilis (chancre). CA-MRSA
Necrotizing Fasciitis	Staphylococcal necrotizing fasciitis (CA-MRSA), streptococcal gangrene (*S. pyogenes*), Fournier's gangrene (mixed aerobic and anaerobic bacteria)
Myositis and Myonecrosis	Pyomyositis (*S. aureus*), streptococcal necrotizing myositis (*S. pyogenes*), nonclostridial (crepitant) myositis (mixed infection), synergistic nonclostridial anaerobic myonecrosis, (mixed infection), gas gangrene (*Clostridium* spp.)

Table 8. Common Soft Tissue Infections

Epidemiology/ Risk Factors	Body Location	Appearance of Lesions	Degree of Pain
Impetigo			
Common in children	Skin of face, often mouth and nose	Non-bullous honey-crust lesions, bullous – thin crust	Mild
Erysipelas			
Any age; may be spontaneous or post-traumatic; may complicate lymphedema	Face or extremities; involving the epidermis and dermis	Abrupt onset of fiery red swelling, well-defined indurated margins	Intense
Cellulitis			
As above	Epidermis, dermis, and subcutaneous fat	Swelling, erythema, warmth	Localized
Necrotising Fasciitis (Streptococcal gangrene or mixed infection involving gram-negative bacilli and anaerobes)			
Any age	Involves subcutaneous fascia	Swelling, edema, hemorrhagic bullae, cutaneous necrosis, patchy cutaneous anesthesia	Early course may be out of proportion to the extent of lesions

Investigations
- Aspiration or punch biopsy
- CT or MRI

Differential Diagnosis
- Infection localized to the skin or soft-tissues versus systemic viral and bacterial infections (e.g. measles, bacterial meningitis, infective endocarditis)
- Non-infectious
  - Drug reaction (e.g. Stevens-Johnson syndrome)
  - Inflammatory dermatologic conditions (e.g. psoriasis)
  - MSK
  - Vascular

Management
- Appropriate empirical antibiotic treatment (dependent on site, route of infection, exposure history)
- Early/aggressive surgical management if necrotizing fasciitis, myositis or gangrene is suspected:
  - Visualization of deep structures
  - Removal of necrotic tissue
  - Reduction of compartment pressure
  - Obtain samples for Gram staining and culture

TRAVEL-RELATED ILLNESSES

Definition
- Fever from the tropics is:
  - A medical emergency and assumed to be malaria until proven otherwise i.e. it is imperative to rule out malaria in any febrile traveler returning from the tropics or sub-tropics
  - However, travel-related illnesses are often not tropical ("flu", urinary tract infection, etc.)

Epidemiology
- The risk of acquiring tropical diseases is dependent on the travel environment, location and duration
- Disease distribution is complicated and varies with seasons (e.g. rainy seasons)
- For up-to-date information, it is best to visit a comprehensive website (e.g. CDC)

Focused History
- Pre-Travel Preparation
  - Immunizations (e.g. hepatitis, meningitis, rabies, typhoid, yellow fever, etc.)
  - Malaria chemoprophylaxis (drug dose, compliance, duration)
  - Medications
- Travel Itinerary
  - Countries visited, dates/duration
  - Accommodations (urban and/or rural, living conditions)
  - Purpose of travel
- Exposure History
  - Ingestion of:
    - Raw, undercooked or "exotic" foods
    - Contaminated mild or unpasteurized dairy products
    - Contaminated water
  - Fresh water exposure
  - Walking barefoot
  - Sexual contact with local residents or fellow travellers
  - Transfusions, injections, receiving tattoos or body piercings
  - Insect bites (time of day, urban or rural)
    - Mosquitoes
    - Ticks
    - Reduviid bugs
    - Mites and their larvae
    - Tsetse flies
    - Sand flies
    - Deerflies
  - Exposure to or bites from animals
  - Contact with ill persons
  - Accommodation (e.g. mud/thatched huts)
- Fever History
  - See **Table 10**
  - Onset
  - Duration: febrile symptoms may be self-limiting or prolonged
  - Peak temperature
  - Pattern

INFECTIOUS DISEASES

- Signs and Symptoms
  - See **Table 11**

Table 9. Incubation Periods for Selected Tropical Diseases

Incubation Period	Infection
Short (<10 d)	Enteric bacterial infections Plague Arboviral infections (yellow fever, dengue fever) Tularemia Marburg viral disease
Intermediate (10-21 d)	American trypanosomiasis Leptospirosis Malaria (except *P. malariae*) Rickettsial infections (Rocky Mountain spotted fever, scrub typhus, Q fever)
Long (>21 d)	Malaria (*P. malariae*) Schistosomiasis Tuberculosis Viral hepatitis B Visceral leishmaniasis Filariasis (*W. bancrofti*)

Table 10. Fever Pattern for Selected Tropical Diseases

Pattern	Infection
Continuous	Enteric (typhoid or paratyphoid) fever, Lassa fever
Remittent	Tuberculosis
Intermittent	Malaria, tuberculosis
Relapsing	Relapsing fever, dengue fever, *P. malariae*

Focused Physical Exam
- General
  - Hydration, level of consciousness, malnourishment
  - Inspect the skin and sclera for jaundice
- Head and Neck
  - Inspect the conjunctiva for infection
  - Assess for lymphadenopathy (see **Table 11**)
- Respiratory
  - Signs of pneumonia
- Gastrointestinal (GI)
  - Hepatomegaly
  - Splenomegaly
  - Diarrhea
- Musculoskeletal (MSK)
  - Myalgia, flu-like symptoms
- Dermatological
  - Rash, lesion, ulcer, nodule
  - Hemorrhage

Table 11. Basic Epidemiology and Symptoms of Major Tropical Diseases

Illness	Vector or Exposure	Distribution	Symptoms
African sleeping sickness (African Trypanosomiasis)	Tsetse Flies	Africa	Skin sore at the bite site, muscle and joint pain, swollen lymph nodes, fever
Chagas Disease (America Trypanosomiasis)	Night-biting reduviid bugs Mud, thatch or adobe houses	S. and Central America	Pain and swelling in the area of an infected bug bite followed by a flu-like illness
Dengue Fever	Mosquitoes	Tropical regions of Africa, S. and Central America, Caribbean, Asia and Oceania	Fever, bone and joint pain, headache, swollen glands, hepatomegaly fatigue, rash (e.g. hemorrhagic dengue fever)
Filariasis	Mosquitoes	Central and South America, Africa, Asia, India, Caribbean	Most asymptomatic or lymphedema of leg, scrotum, penis, arm, or breast
Leishmaniasis	Night-biting sandflies	Widespread	1) Cutaneous – slow healing skin sores 2) Visceral – fever, weight loss, hepatosplenomegaly, and anemia. Months to years after exposure
Malaria	Mosquitoes	Widespread	Fever, chills, headache, myalgia, malaise, hepatosplenomegaly, jaundice
Onchocerciasis (River Blindness)	Day biting black flies	Africa and S. America	Dermatitis, subcutaneous nodules, lymphadenitis, and ocular lesions (can progress to blindness). May occur months to years after exposure
Schistosomiasis (Bilharzias)	Wading, swimming or bathing in fresh water	Sub-Saharan Africa, southern China, the Philippines, and Brazil	Most acute infections asymptomatic. Acute syndrome: Katayama fever – fever, lack of appetite, weight loss, abdominal pain, hematuria, weakness, headaches, joint and muscle pain, diarrhea, nausea, and cough
Yellow Fever	Mosquito bites	Sub-Saharan Africa, Panama, Trinidad, South America	Sudden onset of fever, backache, headache, nausea, vomiting, slowed pulse, bleeding, jaundice

INFECTIOUS DISEASES

Diagnostic Investigations
- Blood films (thick and thin) × 3 (malaria) or rapid diagnostic test
- CBC, LFTs
- Blood, urine, stool cultures
- Serology (e.g. for dengue fever, schistosomiasis)
- Chest x-ray

SPECIAL POPULATIONS: IMMUNOCOMPROMISED AND PEDIATRIC

Immunocompromised Population

Table 12. Important Opportunistic Infections and Common Associated Symptoms in HIV-infected Individuals

Infections	Common Signs and Symptoms
Hepatitis C	Enlarged, tender liver, jaundice, splenomegaly, stigmata of liver disease
Pneumocystis jiroveci (previously *P. carinii*) pneumonia	Fever, progressive dyspnea, nonproductive cough, fatigue O/E: tachypnea, fever, inspiratory rales
Tuberculosis (pulmonary)	Fever, cough, sputum production, chest pain, night sweats, weight loss, and anorexia
Mycobacterium Avian Complex in HIV-infected individuals	Nonspecific symptoms: high fevers, night sweats, weight loss, anorexia, fatigue Hepatosplenomegaly
Cytomegalovirus	Retinitis: floaters, visual field defects, scotoma O/E: Creamy white retinal exudates with hemorrhage; lesions obscure visualization of underlying vessels and other retinal structures Colitis: fever, diarrhea, weight loss, colon ulceration (± bleeding) Esophagitis: Fever, odynophagia, and retrosternal pain
Candida	Thrush – white patches in oral cavity, scrape off with tongue depressor Esophagitis: fever, anorexia, dysphagia, retrosternal pain
Toxoplasmic encephalitis/Cryptococcal meningitis	Insidious onset Fever, headache, mental status changes Focal neurologic signs, seizures

Pediatric Populations

Table 13. Common Infections and Common Associated Symptoms in the Pediatric Population

Infections	Common Signs and Symptoms
Viral	
Rhinovirus, Enteroviruses (summer months)	Upper respiratory infections: low grade fever, runny nose, nasal congestion, sore throat, tearing, coughing, and sneezing More severe symptoms: otitis media, pneumonia, and sinusitis
Adenovirus	Upper respiratory infections: pneumonia, pharyngitis with tonsillitis and cervical adenopathy, conjunctivitis, rash, mild diarrheal diseases (short-lived, afebrile)
Influenza (winter months)	Fever, cough, pharyngitis, malaise and congestion, pneumonia, encephalitis
Parainfluenza	Fever, laryngitis, tracheobronchitis, croup, bronchiolitis
Respiratory syncytial virus (RSV) (late fall to early spring)	Low grade fever, diffuse wheezing, hyperinflation, crackles, tachypnea, apnea, bronchiolitis, pneumonia and cyanosis
Enteroviruses (summer-fall)	Acute febrile illness, headache, sore throat, rash, nonexudative pharyngitis, respiratory tract symptoms, aseptic meningitis
Bacterial	
Group A Streptococcus	Highly infectious, rapidly spreading skin rash, erythematous denuded areas with honey-coloured crusts
Group B Streptococcus	Pneumonia with respiratory failure, meningitis and sepsis
Pneumococcal Infections	Bacteremia with high grade fever, pneumonia, localized chest pain and rales, meningitis
Staphylococcal Infections	Skin diseases (i.e. furuncles, cellulitis, impetigo), osteomyelitis, septic arthritis, pneumonia, endocarditis, vomiting and diarrhea, sepsis and toxic shock syndrome
Meningococcal Infections	Fever, headache, vomiting, convulsions, shock, petechial or purpuric skin rash
Enterobacteriaceae infections	Diarrhea, hemorrhagic colitis and hemolytic-uremic syndrome, sepsis and meningitis, urinary tract infection
Salmonella, Shigella, Listeria, Campylobacter, Cholera	Nausea, vomiting (without nausea or fever with cholera), headache, meningismus, fever, diarrhea (pus and blood with *Shigella*, severe watery with cholera), abdominal pain, malaise
Mycobacterium tuberculosis	Fatigue, undernutrition, cough, with or without fever, meningitis, chronic cervical adenitis

INFECTIOUS DISEASES

Table 13. Common Infections and Common Associated Symptoms in the Pediatric Population (continued)

Infections	Common Signs and Symptoms
Parasitic and mycotic	
Toxoplasmosis	Lymphadenopathy, hepatosplenomegaly, rash, encephalitis, myocarditis, pneumonitis, chorioretinitis
Giardiasis	Chronic relapsing diarrhea, flatulence, bloating, poor weight gain
Enterobiasis (*Enterobius vermicularis*)	Anal pruritus
Cutaneous Larva Migrans (Canine and feline hookworm)	Erythematous, elevated, vesicular, serpiginous tracks (2-4 mm wide) usually confined to skin of feet, buttocks, or abdomen
Strongyloidiasis (*Strongyloides stercoralis*)	Abdominal pain, diarrhea, vomiting, pruritic rash at skin penetration, wheezing, cough and hemoptysis, abdominal pain, distention
Taeniasis (*Taenia saginata* from beef and *Taenia solium* from pork)	Mild abdominal pain, focal seizures, headaches, subcutaneous nodules, passage of fecal proglottids
Candida	Oral thrush, ulceration, vulvovaginitis, erythematous intertriginous rash, systemic infections, cotton-wool retinal lesions

REFERENCES

Attia J, Hatala R, Cook DJ, Wong JG. 1999. The rational clinical examination. Does this patient have acute meningitis? *JAMA* 282(2): 175-181.

Fauci AS. 2008. *Harrison's Principles of Internal Medicine*. New York: McGraw-Hill.

Heymann DL, American Public Health Association. 2008. *Control of Communicable Diseases Manual*. Washington, DC: American Public Health Association.

Mandell GL, Bennett JE, Dolin R. (ed.) 2009. *Mandell, Douglas and Bennett's Principles and Practice of Infectious Diseases*. New York: Churchill Livingstone/Elsevier.

McIsaac WJ, White D, Tannenbaum D, Low DE. 1998. A clinical score to reduce unnecessary antibiotic use in patients with sore throat. *CMAJ* 158(1): 75-83.

McPhee SJ, Papadakis M. 2010. *Current Medical Diagnosis and Treatment 2010*. New York: Lange Medical Books/McGraw-Hill, Medical Pub. Division.

Porter RS (ed.) 2006. *The Merck Manual of Diagnosis and Therapy*. Whitehouse Station: Merck Research Laboratories.

Stumacher RJ. 1987. *Clinical Infectious Diseases*. Philadelphia: Saunders.

The Essentials of Medical Imaging

Editors:
Alfonse Marchie, Lik Hang Lee &
Pearl Behl

Faculty Reviewers:
Nasir Jaffer, MD, FRCP(C)

TABLE OF CONTENTS

The Essentials	477
Approach to Chest Radiography	478
Approach to Abdominal Radiography	482
GI Contrast Studies	487
Approach to Musculoskeletal Radiography	488
Approach to Neuroimaging	490
Basics of Nuclear Medicine	494
Detailed Imaging Findings	496
Chest Imaging	504

THE ESSENTIALS

X-Ray (Radiography)

- Differences in density of body structures produce images of varying light or dark intensity
- Limited densities visible (metal, bone, fat, water, air)
- Soft tissues may not be well identified

Magnetic Resonance Imaging (MRI)

- Can generate images in all possible planes (axial, sagittal, coronal or oblique)
- No radiation
- Records data based on the magnetic properties of hydrogen nuclei
- Use of T1 vs. T2 relaxation times gives rise to MR signals that accentuate different tissues
- T1-weighted images: fat will give a high intensity signal (bright) whereas CSF and water will be low intensity (dark)
- T2-weighted images: fat is low intensity (dark), water is high intensity (bright)
- Excellent delineation of soft tissues

Computerized Tomography (CT) Scan

- Traditional images are limited to the axial or coronal plane, but newer scanners allow multiplanar imaging
- X-ray based technique – bones appear white and air appears black
- Delineates surrounding soft tissue better than a plain film
- CT scans are read as a cross section as if looking up from the feet in a supine position

Ultrasound (U/S)

- High frequency sound waves emitted from a transducer, penetrate tissues and are reflected back to generate an image
- No radiation

- Findings are described in terms of echogenicity:
  - Hyperechoic regions appear bright because tissue is reflective (e.g. gallstones)
  - Hypoechoic regions appear dark because sound waves pass freely through the tissue (e.g. water)
- Provides images in real time which is useful for mobile structures and can be used for U/S guided procedures (e.g. prostate biopsy)
- U/S cannot scan through gas – may be problematic with excess gas in the bowel
- U/S cannot penetrate bone

> **Clinical Pearl**
> Abnormal radiological findings only suggest certain types of disease. Findings must be used in combination with clinical history for an accurate diagnosis.

APPROACH TO CHEST RADIOGRAPHY

Types
- Posteroanterior (PA) and Left Lateral View
- Portable: Anteroposterior (AP) – done supine or upright
- Special views:
  - Lordotic: to assess the apex of lungs
  - Lateral decubitus: for effusions, pneumothorax

General Approach to Chest Radiography (ABCDs x2)

- Airway	- Aorta
- Breathing	- Bones
- Circulation	- Cardiac
- Diaphragm	- Deformity
- Soft Tissues	- Shoulder

> **Clinical Pearl**
> PA upright chest films are preferred because pleural disease (effusions, pneumothorax) and air fluid levels are harder to appreciate on AP supine films, which also magnify mediastinal structures.

PATHOLOGIES ASSESSED
- Pulmonary pathology (e.g. pneumothorax, consolidation)
- Disorders of the pleura, diaphragm and viscera
- Bony abnormalities (e.g. fractures, metastases)
- Cardiac enlargement
- Calcification (e.g. valves, coronary arteries, aorta, LV walls, costochondral junction)
- Mediastinal masses (see **Table 1**)

Table 1. Differential Diagnosis for a Mediastinal Mass

Mediastinal Compartment	Differential Diagnosis
Anterior mediastinal mass	Thyroid lesions, thymic lesions, parathyroid lesions, teratoma
Middle mediastinal mass	Bronchus carcinoma, bronchogenic cysts
Posterior mediastinal mass	Neurogenic tumours, esophageal lesions, hiatus hernia
All compartments	Lymphoma, hematoma, abscess, aortic aneurysm

Interpretation

Identifying Data

- Exam date, name, sex, age, history number, position (supine, decubitus, upright), view (e.g. AP, PA), markers (R and L)

> **Clinical Pearl**
> 4Ts of an Anterior Mediastinal Mass: Thyroid, Teratoma, Thymus, (terrible) Lymphoma.

Quality of Radiograph: RIP

Rotation

- To see if patient is turned more to one side or the other
- Medial ends of the clavicle should be equidistant from the spinous process
- Left and right ribcages, if not superimposed, should be within ~1-2 cm of each other on the lateral film (ideally <0.5 cm)

Inspiration

- Both the anterior segment of the 6th rib and the posterior segment of the 9th rib should be above the diaphragm (if inspiratory effort appropriate)

Penetration

- Vertebral bodies should be just visible through the cardiac shadow

ABCDs

Airway

- Follow trachea to carina and main bronchi

Aorta

- Frontal – follow contour from arch to descending aorta
- Lateral – follow path from arch to descending aorta

Mediastinum

- Mediastinal shift, abnormal widening and masses
- Trachea (midline or deviated)
- Heart borders
- Great vessels and mediastinal contours
- Determine location of abnormality with respect to mediastinal compartment
  - Anterior mediastinum – everything in front of and superior to the heart shadow on lateral film
    - e.g. thymus, thyroid and parathyroid, lymphatics and lymph nodes

- Middle mediastinum – between anterior and posterior compartments
    - e.g. heart, pericardium, aortic arch and great vessels, trachea, main bronchi
- Posterior mediastinum – everything behind the posterior side of the heart shadow and trachea on lateral film
    - e.g. esophagus, descending aorta, thoracic duct, and neurogenic structures (e.g. sympathetic chain)

Breathing (Lungs and Pleura)
- Lung fields: upper, middle and lower
    - Lung volumes, symmetry of markings (on frontal film)
    - Air space pathologies, interstitial pathologies, lobar collapse and nodules
    - Lung periphery for pneumothroax and effusions
    - Examples of lung findings:
        - Silhouette sign: loss of normally appearing interfaces implying opacification usually due to consolidation
        - Air bronchogram: bronchi become visualized because the lungs are opacified indicating air space disease, consolidation, etc.
        - Kerley B lines: thickened connective tissue planes that commonly occur in pulmonary edema
        - Net-like/reticular appearance: interstitial disease
        - "Batwing" or "butterfly" appearance: alveolar edema
- Pleura: costophrenic angles, entire perimeter of lung fields, position of fissures
    - Minor fissure from the right hilus to the 6th rib
    - Major fissure laterally from T4-5 to the diaphragm
    - Check for: blunting of costophrenic angles, focal or diffuse areas of pleural thickening, shifting of fissures, calcification, fluid collection

Bones
- Vertebrae, clavicles, ribs, sternum (best seen on lateral film)
- Check for vertebrae and disc spaces, lytic or sclerotic lesions, rib fractures, osteoporosis (osteopenia, compression fracture, wedged)
- Circulation (including hila)
- Central pulmonary arteries, veins, lymph nodes; main stem and lobar bronchi
    - Deviation – left hilum should be 1-2 cm above the right (deviation may be due to lobar collapse or lobectomy)
    - Hilar enlargement
        - Smooth enlargement suggests arteries
        - Lobulated enlargement suggests lymphadenopathy
        - Focal enlargement suggests a mass

Cardiac
- Assess width of heart borders via the cardiothoracic ratio
    - Maximum heart width in relation to chest should be less than half the greatest thoracic diameter
    - Right border = edge of right atrium, left border = edge of left ventricle
- Enlargement/distortion of cardiovascular shadow
    - Cardiomegaly, poor inspiration, supine position, obesity, pectus excavatum
    - Cardiomegaly suggests either myocardial hypertrophy, cardiac chamber dilatation or pericardial effusion
    - Cardiothoracic ratio may be <0.5 and still be enlarged due to multiple problems (i.e. cardiomegaly and emphysema)
    - On expiration, heart size appears larger and mediastinum appears wider

Diaphragm

- Assess: position and costophrenic angles
  - Right hemidiaphragm may be up to 2 cm higher than the left
  - Check for: free air, calcifications, high or low diaphragm
- Diaphragm findings:
  - Free air underneath diaphragm indicates pneumoperitoneum
  - Calcifications on diaphragm suggests asbestosis
  - Diaphragm will be deviated in conditions that greatly increase volume of peritoneal/thoracic structures or decrease volume leaving a void
  - Elevated diaphragm suggests abdominal distention, lung collapse, pneumonectomy, pregnancy, pleural effusion
  - Low diaphragm suggests asthma, emphysema, pleural effusion, tumour

Deformities

- Assess: spine for deformity, asymmetry of pedicles/spinous processes

Soft Tissues

- Assess: neck, supraclavicular area, axillae, breast tissue, muscles
- Check for: soft tissue masses, amount of soft tissue present

Shoulder

- Reminder to look at bones and periphery
- Continue in superior soft tissues/bones, up anterior chest wall, and down posterior ribs to the costophrenic angles

Detailed Chest Imaging Findings (see p. 504)

Table 2. Chest Pathology and Typical Radiographic Findings

Chest Pathology	Typical Findings	
Pulmonary nodules (XR, CT)	**Benign:** <3 cm, round, regular Smooth margin Calcified pattern; usually concentric and/or diffuse eccentric Doubles in <1 mo or >2 yrs	**Malignant:** 3 cm, irregular Fuzzy margin Usually not calcified; if calcified, pattern is eccentric Doubles in >1 mo or <2 yrs
Pneumothorax (XR)	Pleural air collects over the cupola of the lung apex and against the upper lateral chest wall Mediastinal shift if air is under tension	
Air space disease (XR)	Alveoli filled with fluid or exudate that displaces air Areas of alveolar filling can be small or large, single or multiple and appear white, radio-opaque and ill-defined (acinar shadows) Air-containing bronchi surrounded by dense, airless lung (air bronchogram) Silhouette sign DDx: fluid (pulmonary edema), pus (pneumonia), blood (hemorrhage), cells (lung CA/lymphoma), protein (alveolar proteinosis)	

Table 2. Chest Pathology and Typical Radiographic Findings (continued)

Chest Pathology	Typical Findings
Interstitial disease (XR, CT) (see p. 496)	Distributed through lung tissue that is well aerated Can produce thin, linear strands of densities (e.g. reticular pattern: net-like), Kerley B lines may be present Can also produce spherical densities (e.g. nodular pattern: multiple, discrete, nodular densities <5 mm diameter) Reticulonodular patterns are also seen Pleural Effusion: lateral decubitus > Lateral > PA in sensitivity DDx: pulmonary edema, miliary TB, idiopathic pulmonary fibrosis, sarcoidosis, pneumoconiosis
Consolidation (XR) (see p. 497)	Silhouette sign If consolidation borders on a fissure, only 1 side of fissure will be visible Trachea and mediastinum may be pulled toward the side of shadow Air bronchogram may be present (see **Air Space Disease**)
Congestive heart failure (XR)	Cardiac shadow usually (not always) increased in size and shapelessness Pulmonary vascular engorgement into lung fields Bronchi become framed (peribronchial cuffing) in edema Lungs appear hazy due to interstitial edema; can get Kerley B lines
Emphysema (XR)	Hyperinflation of lungs Low, flattened diaphragm on lateral film In some patients, pulmonary fibrosis causes filamentous strands of increased opacity that radiate from hila Bullae – large air cysts enclosed by thin, dense walls
Lung Cancer (XR, CT, MRI)	May reveal an obvious mass, widening of the mediastinum (likely due to spread of lymph nodes), atelectasis, consolidation (pneumonia), or pleural effusion

APPROACH TO ABDOMINAL RADIOGRAPHY

Indications
- Plain film (PF) allows viewing of the entire abdomen and is used before proceeding to a more specific investigation
- PF lacks sensitivity and specificity and is being replaced by cross-sectional imaging modalities (CT, U/S) as they become more available
- Abdominal CT differentiates organ densities better than plain films and can detect abnormalities not found on abdominal radiographs
- Abdominal pain, distension, trauma, vomiting and diarrhea are common reasons for obtaining plain films
- Abdominal series usually includes supine (Kidney, Ureter, Bladder – KUB), upright or Left Lateral Decubitus (LLDB) ± erect CXR

> **Clinical Pearl**
> An abdominal series is often performed to aid the diagnosis of an acute abdomen. The series includes upright, supine and decubitus views of the abdomen.

General Approach to Abdominal Radiographs (ITS Free ABDO)

- **I**dentifying data
- **T**echnical factors
- **S**oft tissue (other)
- **Free** fluid
- **A**ir
- **B**owels
- **D**ensities (bones, calcifications)
- **O**rgans (solid and hollow)

Pathologies Assessed

- Intestinal obstruction/ileus*
- Foreign bodies*
- Perforation*
- Bowel ischemia
- Volvulus
- Calcifications (e.g. gallstones, renal stones, fecalith)
- Abnormal gas collection (free air, intramural air, biliary air)
- Ascites (plain films used less often)
- Bony abnormalities (e.g. fractures, metastases)

*Abdominal plain films are most clinically useful for the indicated pathologies

Interpretation

Identifying Data
- Date of exam, name, sex, age, history number, position (supine, decubitus, upright), view (e.g. AP, PA), markers (R and L)

Technical Factors
- Good coverage, appropriate penetration, identify view

Soft Tissues (other than bowels and organs)
- Flank stripe: extra-peritoneal fat; symmetry; neighbouring structures: colon, abdominal muscles (lateral)
- Psoas muscles: fat surrounds the muscles; right psoas often not seen

Free Fluid
- Assess: distance between lateral fat stripes and adjacent colon for evidence of free peritoneal fluid in paracolic gutters
- Check for: large amounts of fluid – diffuse increased opacification and bowel floats to centre of anterior abdominal wall (on supine film)

Air (Outside and Inside bowel)
- Outside bowel
  - Look for evidence of free intraperitoneal air, retroperitoneal air, branching air in the liver, abcesses, and air in bowel wall
- Inside bowel
  - Volvulus: twisting of bowel upon itself
    - Sigmoid: "coffee bean" sign; Cecal; Gastric; Small Bowel: "corkscrew" sign
  - Toxic Megacolon
    - Extreme dilatation of colon (>6.5 cm) with mucosal changes including foci of edema, ulceration and pseudopolyps, loss of normal haustral pattern

Bowels
- Wall thickening: increased soft tissue densities in bowel, "thumb printing" in bowel wall, picket-fence (or "stacked coin") appearance of valvulae conniventes
  - May indicate IBD, infection, ischemia, hypoproteinemic states, submucosal hemorrhage

Densities
- Bones
  - Assess: vertebrae (lower thoracic, lumbar, sacral), lower ribs, pelvis, upper femur
  - Check for: vertebrae and disc spaces, lytic or sclerotic lesions, rib (discontinuity in bony cortex or sharp line), features of osteoporosis (osteopenia, compression fracture, wedged)
  - To avoid confusing calcifications of costal cartilages with calcifications of the gallbladder, kidney or adrenal gland, trace the expected course of the rib
- Abnormal calcifications – see **Table 3**

Organs - solid
Check for: borders, masses, fat, shift in position, calcifications
- Liver
  - Upper border: adjacent to R hemidiaphragm
  - Lateral margin: visualized because of adjacent "flank stripe"
  - Postero-inferior border: defined by extraperitoneal fat
  - Antero-inferior border: defined by gas in adjacent transverse colon and hepatic flexure (may see depression of hepatic flexure (colon) with hepatomegaly)
  - Note: clinical estimation of liver size is more reliable than PF estimation of liver size due to its complex shape. The posterior liver border is consistently seen on PF but the anterior border is found by physical exam
- Spleen
  - Outlined by fat
  - Diagnosis of splenomegaly from PF is fairly accurate (medial displacement of gastric air bubble)
- Kidneys
  - Outlined by perirenal fat
  - Left higher than right (renal hila are located at L1 and L2 respectively)
  - Length: 8-15 cm in adult; 3.7 times the height of the second lumbar vertebrae in a growing child
- Gallbladder
  - Not usually seen on PF
  - May be seen as a shadow superimposed on the liver margin and right kidney
- Pancreas
  - Normal pancreas not visible on PF
- Aorta
  - Calcification is frequently seen in older patients
- Bladder
  - Visible because surrounded by fat
  - Filled: globular shadow
  - Empty: flattened oval shadow
- Ureters
  - Not visible on PF
  - Course to bladder along psoas (shadow)

- Uterus
    - Visible because surrounded by fat
    - Indents dome of the bladder
- Ovaries, Fallopian tubes, seminal vesicles and prostate
    - Not usually seen on PF

Organs - hollow

Check for: obstruction, intraperitoneal air (free air), intramural air
- Stomach
    - Immediately under the left hemidiaphragm
    - Normally contains "gastric air bubble" on upright PF
- Small Intestine
    - Adult: normally contains fluid and little gas
    - Infant: normally contains gas
- Colon
    - A distinctive speckled shadow outlined by gas and feces
- Splenic Flexure
    - Variable position: may be indented by spleen tip, partially overlap the spleen or extend over the spleen as high as the diaphragm
- Free intraperitoneal air (pneumoperitoneum)
    - Erect PA CXR: air under diaphragm

Table 3. Differential Diagnosis for Calcification

Location	Differential Diagnosis
RUQ	Renal stone, gallstone, calcified hepatic granuloma, adrenal calcification
RLQ	Stone in ureter, appendicolith
LUQ	Splenic vessel, renal stone, adrenal calcification, tail of pancreas
Central	Aorta, pancreas, lymph nodes
Pelvis	Phleboliths, fibroids, bladder, prostate

R/LUQ = right/left upper quadrant, RLQ = right lower quadrant

---

Clinical Pearl
Calcium, cystine and struvite stones are radioopaque and seen on abdominal x-rays. Uric acid stones are radiolucent and not seen on abdominal x-rays.

Detailed Abdominal Imaging Findings

Table 4. Abdominal Pathology and Radiographic Findings

Pathology	Typical Findings
Obstruction of small bowel (XR, CT) (see p. 498)	Dilated (>3 cm) small bowel loops with valvulae conniventes (plicae circulares) extending across full diameter of loop May see multiple air/fluid levels on upright and decubitus films If dilated, loops are fluid/gas filled ("string of pearls" sign) Check for gas in colon: if absent, suggests a high grade obstruction
Obstruction of colon (XR, CT)	Haustral indentations which extend only part-way across the diameter of the loop, are shallower but still visible More of the colon is continuously outlined with air Bowel dilated proximal to the obstructed segment No air distal to obstructed segment
Free air (XR, CT) (see p. 498)	Usually indicates GI tract perforation (e.g. peptic ulcer or colonic diverticulum) Upright radiograph is most sensitive Look for free air outlining under surface of hemidiaphragms, particularly on R Do not mistake a small amount of air in stomach on an upright PF as free air
Primary liver tumours (U/S, CT, MRI)	U/S shows hypo/iso/hyperechoic mass(es) CT/MRI shows solid/complex cystic mass(es). Some primary liver masses (e.g. hepatoma, focal nodular hyperplasia) are vascular in arterial phase of a dynamic study with less intensity during venous phase (washout) Look for evidence of cirrhosis (nodular contour, lobar redistribution, portal HTN)
Biliary tree obstruction (U/S, CT, MRI)	U/S shows dilated biliary system resulting in branching, tubular structures running along portal triads Establish level and cause of obstruction
Acute appendicitis (U/S, CT) (see p. 499)	U/S in young and asthenic patients, CT in obese patients and for complication Appendix >6 mm diameter Appendicolith, stranding of mesoappendix
Acute cholecystitis (US, Cholescintigraphy) (see p. 500)	U/S usually shows gallstones (rounded echogenic foci with posterior acoustic shadowing) Maximum tenderness over sonographically localized gallbladder Distended, thick-walled gallbladder Pericholecystic fluid outside the gallbladder wall
Acute diverticulitis (U/S, CT) (see p. 499)	Sigmoid colon most commonly affected U/S or CT shows multiple, air-filled out-pouchings Thickened colon wall with narrowed lumen Inflammation centred around involved diverticulum (site of maximal tenderness) May be evidence of local (or less commonly diffuse) perforation with perienteric abscess

Table 4. Abdominal Pathology and Radiographic Findings (continued)

Pathology	Typical Findings
Acute pancreatitis (U/S, CT) (see p. 500)	The pancreas may appear normal, or border may be irregular CT often shows edema and enlargement of the pancreas Inflammatory stranding in the surrounding soft tissue Pancreatic/peripancreatic fluid collections may be visible, along with pancreatic necrosis U/S: decrease in echogenicity but most helpful in diagnosing gallstones
Pancreatic tumour (U/S, CT, MRI)	Ductal adenocarcinoma is the most common with a very poor prognosis U/S or CT shows an ill-defined hypoechoic or hypoattenuating mass that usually obstructs pancreatic duct and causes atrophy of pancreas above level of mass If mass is situated in head of pancreas, there will often be associated biliary obstruction
Renal colic (CT)	Unenhanced spiral CT has replaced IVP as the imaging modality of choice Ureteric stones as small as 1-2 mm can be routinely detected Look for other evidence of ureteric obstruction: hydronephrosis, perirenal/periureteric streaking Can follow progress of larger ureteric stones with PF CT may show other causes for the pain if a ureteric stone is not present (e.g. appendicitis, diverticulitis)

PF = plain film, IVP = intravenous pyelogram

GI CONTRAST STUDIES

GI Contrast Studies (listed from Upper to Lower GI)
Cine Esophagogram
- Description: contrast agent swallowed
- Assessment: cervical esophagus

Barium Swallow
- Description: contrast swallowed under fluoroscopy, capture selective images
- Indications: dysphagia, r/o GERD, post esophageal surgery
- Assessment: thoracic esophagus

Upper GI Series
- Description: double contrast (1. Barium to coat mucosa; 2. Gas pill to distend)
- Indications: dyspepsia, r/o UGI bleed, weight loss, anemia, post gastric surgery
- Assessment: thoracic esophagus, stomach, duodenum

Small Bowel Follow Through (aka Small Bowel Series, Small Bowel Meal)
- Description: single contrast images - continuation of UGI series or separate study
- Indications: GI bleed (with UGI series/barium enema nondiagnostic), weight loss, anemia, diarrhea, IBD, malabsorption, abdominal pain, post small bowel surgery
- Assessment: small bowel

Enteroclysis (aka Small Bowel Enema)
- Description: Contrast infusion via tube inserted from nose to duodenum
  - (1) barium/methyl cellulose for fluoroscopic exam
  - (2) water infusion for CT enteroclysis
- Indications: IBD, malabsorption, weight loss, anemia, Meckel's diverticulum
- Assessment: small bowel

Hypaque Enema
- Description: retrograde filling with water soluble contrast
- Indications: post op to assess anastomoses for leak/obstruction/perforation
- Assessment: large bowel

Barium Enema (largely replaced by CT Colonography where available)
- Description: retrograde filling of colon with barium and gas (air or CO_2)
- Indications: altered bowel habits, r/o LGI bleed, weight loss, anemia, r/o large bowel obstruction, r/o perforation, check surgical anastamosis, history of polyps
- Assessment: large bowel

Virtual Colonoscopy/CT Colonography
- For evaluation of intraluminal colonic masses (i.e. polyps, tumours)
- CT scan of abdomen using air instillation after bowel prep and 3D lumen reconstruction
- Indications: after incomplete endoscopy, patients with elevated endoscopic risk or aversion, staging of identified colonic lesions
- Assessment: large bowel

Clinical Pearl
Do not use a barium contrast when suspecting a bowel perforation.
Consider using Hypaque contrast.

APPROACH TO MUSCULOSKELETAL RADIOGRAPHY

MSK X-Ray
- Always 2 x-rays at right angles to each other (AP + lateral)
- X-ray joint above and below the area of injury
- X-ray before and after reduction
- Shoulder injuries – always do trans-axillary lateral

Indications for X-Ray
- Ankle Rules: x-rays of ankle required if pain in the malleolar zone and any one of the following: bone tenderness along the posterior edge of the tibia OR tip of the medial malleolus OR bone tenderness along the posterior edge of the fibula OR tip of the lateral malleolus OR an inability to bear weight both immediately and in the emergency department (Stiell et al., JAMA 1993; 269:1127)
- Knee Rules: x-rays of the knee injury patients required if >55 yrs OR older OR isolated tenderness of the patella (no bone tenderness of knee other than patella) OR tenderness of head of fibula OR inability to flex 90° OR an inability to bear weight both immediately and in the emergency department (Stiell et al., JAMA 1996; 275:611)

- C-spine Rules (for alert and stable patients with concern of cervical spine injury): radiography of the C-spine when 1. high risk factors: ≥65 yrs OR dangerous mechanism OR paresthesia in extremities 2. Unable to perform safe assessment of range of motion 3. Unable to actively rotate neck (Stiell *et al., Canadian Journal of Emergency Medicine* 2002)

General Approach
- Alignment
- Bone
- Cartilage
- Fracture Pattern
- Soft Tissue Involvement

Pathologies Assessed
- Arthritis
- Cartilage defects
- Dislocations
- Fractures
- Ligamentous Injuries
- Tumour (benign, malignant)

Interpretation

Identifying Data
- Exam date, name, sex, age, history number, views (i.e. PA or lateral views)

Assess:
- Alignment – displacement (translation, angulation, rotation, impaction)
- Bone – site of bone fracture:
  - Epiphyseal: end of bone
  - Metaphyseal: flared portion of bone at the ends of the shaft
  - Diaphyseal: shaft of a long bone
  - Physis: growth plate
- Cartilage
  - Softening
  - Swelling
  - Fragmentation
  - Fissuring
  - Erosion
- Fracture Pattern (see **Musculoskeletal Exam** p. 145)
  - Butterfly: slight comminution at the fracture site resembling a butterfly
  - Comminuted: more than 2 fracture fragments
  - Compression/impacted: impaction of bone, e.g. vertebrae, proximal tibia
  - Green-stick: an incomplete fracture of one cortex, often in children
  - Intra-articular: fracture line crosses articular cartilage and enters joint
  - Oblique: angular fracture line
  - Pathologic: fracture through bone weakened by disease/tumour
  - Segmental: a separate segment of bone bordered by fracture lines – high energy
  - Spiral: complex, multi-planar fracture line, rotational force – low energy
  - Torus: a buckle fracture of one cortex, often in children
  - Transverse: perpendicular fracture line
- Soft Tissue Involvement
  - Closed: skin/soft tissue over fracture site is intact
  - Open: skin/soft tissue over fracture site is lacerated, fracture exposed to outside environment

Detailed Musculoskeletal Imaging Findings

Table 5. MSK Pathology and Radiographic Findings

Pathology	Typical Findings	
Anterior Shoulder Dislocation (XR)	Humeral head is anterior on axillary view	
Avascular Necrosis (XR, fMRI)	Reactive sclerosis of adjacent bone Subcondral fracture Flattening of weighbearing zones with eventual collapse	
Arthritis of Hip (XR)	Osteoarthritis Joint space narrowing Subchondral sclerosis Subchondral cysts Osteophytes	Rheumatoid Arthritis Bony erosions
Colles Fracture (XR)	Dorsal tilt Dorsal displacement of distal fragment Ulnar styloid facture	Radial displacement Radial tilt Shortening
Galeazzi Fracture (XR)	Fracture of distal radial shaft with disruption of the distal radioulnar joint (DRUJ) Shortening of distal radius >5 mm relative to the distal ulna Widening of the DRUJ space on AP view Dislocation of radius with respect to ulna on true lateral	
Multiple Myeloma (XR)	Punched-out lesions on x-ray at multiple bony sites	
Osteomyelitis (XR, fMRI)	Soft tissue swelling Lytic bone destruction Periosteal reaction	
Rotator Cuff Disease (XR, U/S, MRI)	AP view may show high riding humerus relative to glenoid (XR) Visible large cuff tears (U/S) Injected dye leaks out of joint through rotator cuff tear (MRI)	
Subcapital Hip Fractures (XR)	Disruption of Shenton's line (curved line formed by the top of the obturator foramen and the inner side of the neck of the femur, seen in a radiograph of the normal hip joint) Altered neck-shaft angle (normal is 120-130°)	

APPROACH TO NEUROIMAGING

Skull Films (X-Ray)
- No longer play a significant role in diagnosing neurological disease
- Indications: penetrating injury, destructive lesions, metabolic bone disease, congenital anomalies and postoperative changes
- Negative skull films do not exclude the possibility of significant intracranial injury

Table 6. Indications of CT and MRI of the Central Nervous System

Location	CT	MRI
Craniospinal trauma		
Acute head injury	*Assessment of hemorrhage, edema, herniation, depressed calvarial fractures	Delayed sequelae of trauma (encephalomalacia, hemosiderin deposition)
Spinal, vertebral or cord injury	Assessment of number and extent of fractures; narrowing of spinal canal	Associated disk herniations, epidural hematoma; Assesses spinal cord compression, edema, hematomyelia
Acute cerebrovascular disease		
Stroke; cerebral infarction; subarachnoid hemorrhage; intracerebral hematoma (see p. 503)	*Immediate assessment of hemorrhage in patients with acute stroke syndrome (infarct, hematoma, subarachnoid hemorrhage)	Assessment of posterior fossa infarct or hemorrhage after 24 hr; diffusion-weighted MRI
Arteriovenous malformation; aneurysm		Assessment of unruptured aneurysm using MR or CT angiography
Neoplasm		
Brain (intra-axial and extra-axial); spine; skull base; metastases	Detection of calcification, skull erosion, destruction, hyperostosis	*Best sensitivity; assessment of size, extent and effect on normal brain and spinal cord
Neurodegenerative disease	Exclusion of some treatable causes (e.g. hydrocephalus, chronic subdural hematoma)	*Best assessment of atrophy, white matter disease, old infarcts, iron deposits
Cysts and hydrocephalus	Follow up assessments of changes in ventricular size	*Assesses site of ventricular obstruction, extent of cyst
Myelopathy	CT plus myelography only if MRI contraindicated or unavailable	*All intrinsic spinal cord lesions; all causes of cord compression
Degenerative diseases of spine	Spinal stenosis, facet degeneration, osseous lesions	Disk herniation, spinal stenosis

CT

- Excellent for bony detail resolution and detection of calcification and hemorrhage
- Administration of contrast shows blood brain barrier disruption

MRI

- Excellent for visualization of vascular structures, imaging in any plane
- Clearly distinguishes white and grey matter
- T1 weighted scans: CSF/edema-dark (hypointense), fat-light (hyperintense), white matter-light, grey matter-dark
- T2 weighted scans: CSF/edema-light (hyperintense), fat-light (hyperintense), white matter-dark, grey matter-light

Clinical Pearl
TIAs are not associated with any radiological findings.

Detailed Neuroimaging Findings

Table 7. Neurological Pathology and Radiographic Findings

Pathology	Typical Findings
Cerebral edema (CT, MRI)	MRI is more sensitive for detecting edema Loss of white-grey matter differentiation Diffuse edema may show effacement of cerebral sulci and CSF-containing cisterns Can exhibit a mass effect
Hydrocephalus (CT, MRI)	Enlarged ventricles usually due to obstructed CSF flow Temporal horns are usually the first to enlarge May also have some periventricular edema Can be seen with both CT or MRI
Cerebral abscess (CT, MRI)	An area of low density on CT T1-weighted MRI shows low intensity signal; T2-weighted is hyperintense With contrast there is usually ring enhancement around its edges on CT and MRI May have surrounding edema and mass effect
Subarachnoid hemorrhage (SAH) (CT) (see p. 502)	Unenhanced CT shows high density blood in CSF spaces around the brainstem, Sylvian fissure and sometimes the ventricles Hydrocephalus is a common complication
Infarction (CT, MRI)	Changes usually do not appear for 6 to 24 hours Acute infarct: CT shows low density, wedge shaped area corresponding to vascular distribution, with little or no mass effect Hemorrhagic stroke or transformation will have areas of increased density (blood) on CT Subacute infarct: CT shows well defined area of lower density, prominent mass effect from edema (maximal at one week, then decreases) Chronic infarct: very low density on CT with parenchymal volume loss and dilatation of adjacent ventricles
Subdural hematoma (SDH) (CT) (see p. 502)	Acute: crescent-shaped area of increased density on CT between the dura and arachnoid The density on CT decreases with time and after about 3 weeks it is lower density than brain tissue Mass effect will be proportional to its size

Table 7. Neurological Pathology and Radiographic Findings (continued)

MEDICAL IMAGING

Pathology	Typical Findings
Epidural hematoma (CT) (see. p. 501)	CT: typically appears as biconvex high-density lesion between dura and skull Usually a larger mass effect than subdural hematoma
Intracerebral Hematoma (CT) (see p. 503)	Well defined area of high density on CT within cerebral or cerebellar cortex Mass effect proportional to its size
Multiple sclerosis (MRI)	T2-weighted MRI commonly shows round or ovoid white matter plaques Plaques often have periventricular or subcortical distribution Plaques tend to be hyperintense, confluent and >6 mm in diameter on T2-weighted MRI New lesions with active demyelination enhance with gadolinium contrast while old lesions do not
Tumours	**CT or MRI findings include:**
Gliomas	Low grade tumours are well defined, often calcified, have little associated edema, and show no contrast enhancement High grade tumours are often multifocal, ill-defined, show considerable edema and contrast enhancement
Meningiomas	Well-defined high density tumours that show marked contrast enhancement May be calcified
Metastases	Often multiple masses Usually at grey/white matter interface May have significant contrast enhancement, edema and virtually never calcified Most common primary site is the lungs

PF = plain film, IVP = intravenous pyelogram

BASICS OF NUCLEAR MEDICINE

Table 8. Nuclear Medicine and Radiographic Findings

Test	Typical Findings
Brain	
SPECT	Assesses cerebral blood flow DDx: CVA, dementia, vasculitis
PET	Assesses metabolic activity DDx: dementia, CVA, tumour
Thyroid	
Radioactive Iodine Uptake	Measures thyroid function Done in a fasting patient and measured as a percentage of administered thyroid taken up by the gland DDx for increased uptake: Graves, toxic adenoma, toxic multinodular goiter DDx for decreased uptake: hormone suppression, late Hashimoto's disease, subacute thyroiditis
Thyroid Imaging	Measures functional anatomic detail Three types of lesions: hot (hyperfunctioning), cold (hypofunctioning), cool DDx for Hot lesions: adenoma, toxic multinodular goiter, cancer very unlikely DDx for Cold lesions: cancer must be considered until biopsy is negative
Respiratory	
V/Q	Looks at lung areas where there is a ventilation/perfusion mismatch Ventilation scan: patient breathes radioactive gas through a closed system. Scan defects indicate: bronchospasm, airway obstruction, chronic lung disease, and obstruction due to mass Perfusion scan: radiotracer injected intravenously and gives an overview of pulmonary circulation. Scan defects indicate: reduced blood flow due to PE, COPD, asthma, bronchogenic carcinoma, inflammatory lung diseases, mediastinitis, mucus plug, vasculitis
Cardiac	
Myocardial Perfusion Scanning	Injected at peak exercise (physical stress) or after persantine challenge (vasodilator) and again later at rest DDx: angina, atypical chest pain, coronary artery disease, post bypass follow-up, to differentiate between reversible (ischemia) vs. irreversible (infarction) changes
Radionuclide Ventriculography	Radionuclide attached to RBCs Passes through right ventricle → pulmonary circulation → left ventricle Gives information about right ventricular function

Table 8. Nuclear Medicine and Radiographic Findings (continued)

Test	Typical Findings
Abdomen	
Liver/Spleen Scans	Intravenous injection DDx of "cold spots": tumour, cysts, abscess, hemangioma, infarct
Hepatobiliary IminoDiacetic Scan (HIDA)	Intravenous injection of HIDA binds to protein, is taken up and then excreted by hepatocyes into biliary system Normal: gallbladder visualized when cystic duct is patent Acute cholecystitis: no visualization of gallbladder at 4-hour or after administration of morphine at 1-hour Chronic cholecystitis: no visualization of gallbladder at 1-hour but seen at 4-hour or after morphine administration
RBC Scan	Used for GI bleed and liver lesion evaluation
Renal Scan	Renogram: to assess renal function and collecting system Morphological scan: to assess renal anatomy
Bone	
Bone Scan	Radioactive tracer binds to hydroxyapatite of bone matrix Increased binding when increased blood supply to the bone Positive bone scan: primary bone tumour, arthritis, fracture, infection, anemia, Paget's disease, bone metastases from breast, lung, thyroid, prostate
Inflammation and Infection	
Labelled WBC Scan	Tracer attached to WBCs Labeled WBCs accumulate in normal spleen, liver, bone marrow, sites of inflammation and infection

REFERENCES

Armstrong P, Wastie M. 2001. *A Concise Textbook of Radiology.* New York: Oxford University Press.

Brant W, Helms C (eds.) 2006. *Fundamentals of Diagnostic Radiology.* Lippincott Williams & Wilkins.

Dahnert W. 2003. *Radiology Review Manual.* Lippincott Williams & Wilkins.

Dugani S, Lam D (eds.) 2009. *The Toronto Notes 2009: Comprehensive Medical Reference.* Toronto: Toronto Notes for Medical Students, Inc.

Gelderen F. 2004. *Understanding X-Rays.* New York: Springer-Verlag.

Grainger DG, Allison D. 2001. *Diagnostic Radiology: A Textbook of Medical Imaging.* Churchill Livingstone.

Howlett D, Ayers B. 2004. *The hands-on guide to imaging.* Massachusetts: Blackwell Publishing.

Kember P. 2000. *Imaging for Junior Doctors – A survival guide.* Toronto: W.B. Saunders Company.

Laughlin S, Montanera W. 1998. Central nervous system imaging. *Postgraduate Medicine* 104(5):73-88.

Stiell IG, Greenberg GH, Wells GA, McDowell I, Cwinn AA, et al. 1996. Prospective validation of a decision rule for the use of radiography in acute knee injuries. *JAMA* 275(8):611-615.

Stiell IG, Greenberg GH, McKnight RD, Nair RC, McDowell I, et al. 1993. Decision rules for the use of radiography in acute ankle injuries. Refinement and prospective validation. *JAMA* 269(9):1127-1132.

Stiell IG, Wells GA, Vandemheen KL, Clement CM, Lesiuk H, et al. 2001. The Canadian C-spine rule for radiography in alert and stable trauma patients. *JAMA* 286(15):1841-1848.

DETAILED IMAGE FINDINGS

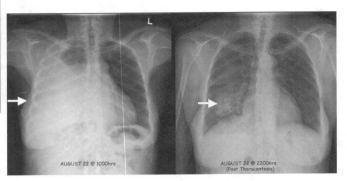

PLEURAL EFFUSION – CXR: (Left Image) Right hemithorax is opaque due to large right pleural effusion. (Right Image) The patient develops unilateral right alveolar pulmonary edema post rapid thoracentesis.
TEACHING POINT: DO NOT PERFORM A RAPID THORACENTESIS ON A PATIENT WITH LARGE PLEURAL EFFUSION.

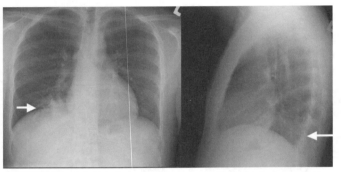

PNEUMONIA – CXR: Right lower lobe pneumonia. The right diaphragm edge is blurred (silhouette sign). The right heart margin remains distinct.

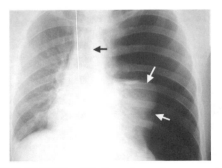

TENSION PNEUMOTHORAX – CXR: Signs of a tension pneumothorax seen here include a collapsed left lung (white arrows), a lucent/black left hemithorax, and a shift in the trachea (black arrow) towards the right and inferior displacement of left hemidiaphragm.

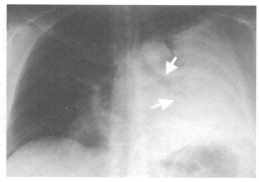

SIGN OF CONSOLIDATION – CXR: There is consolidation of left lower lobe with air bronchogram (arrows = tubular air structures within consolidated lung).

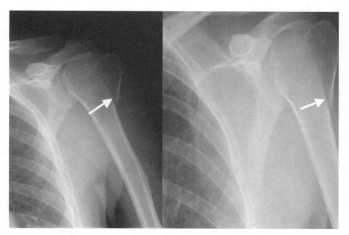

FRACTURE OF SHOULDER – Shoulder XR: AP view of Left shoulder shows avulsion fracture of the greater tuberosity.

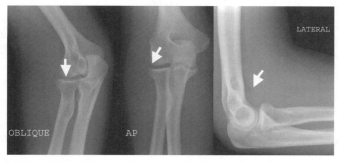

RADIAL HEAD FRACTURE – Elbow XR: Right elbow shows lucent fracture line on oblique view. Lateral view shows triangular fat pad sign anteriorly representing an effusion.

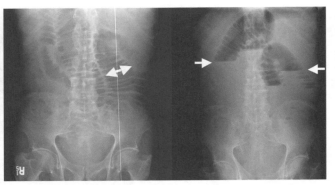

SMALL BOWEL OBSTRUCTION – Abdomen XR: The two views of the abdomen shows dilated small bowel (5 cm width – left image) with differential air fluid levels (right image) and no gas in colon.

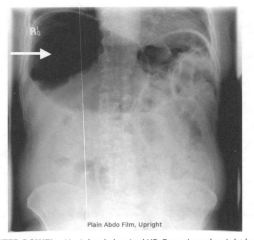

Plain Abdo Film, Upright

PERFORATED BOWEL – Upright abdominal XR: Free air under right hemidiaphragm from a perforated duodenal ulcer.

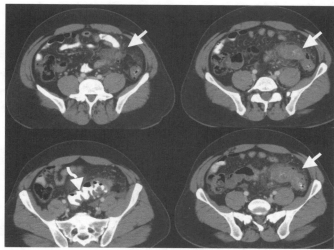

DIVERTICULITIS – CT Abdomen: Sigmoid colon shows marked thickening with few diverticula and mesenteric inflammation (straight arrows). Contrast can be seen in the sigmoid colon (curved arrow).

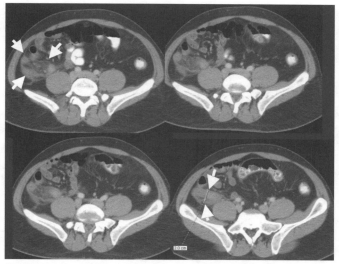

APPENDICITIS – CT Abdomen: Thickened and inflamed mesoappendix in top-left image. Thickened appendix in lower-right image measuring 2 cm.

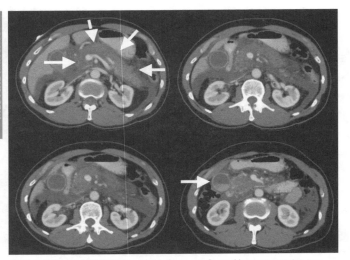

GALLSTONE PANCREATITIS – CT Abdomen: Inflamed low attenuation pancreas. Lower-right image shows gallbladder with stones inside it. Stones in bile duct are best seen on ultrasound.

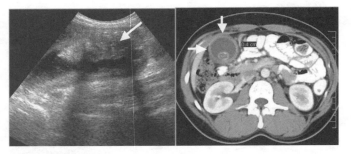

ACUTE CHOLECYSTITIS
(Left) US of Acute Suppurative Cholecystitis: Shows an inflamed and thick gallbladder wall (arrow).
(Right) Abdominal CT of Acute Cholecystitis: The gallbladder wall is thickened (0.4 cm thick) with calcified stone.

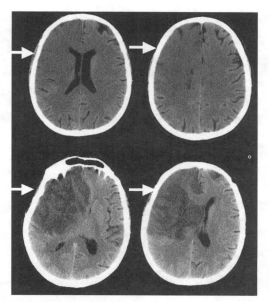

ISCHEMIC STROKE IN EVOLUTION:
CT Head (top images): Decreased attenuation of right cerebral hemisphere (right middle cerebral artery territory). Notice the decreased sulci on the right. CT Head with IV contrast (bottom images): Repeat CT scan with IV contrast 3 days later showing more pronounced low attenuation in the right cerebral hemisphere.

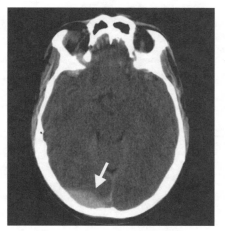

EPIDURAL HEMATOMA – CT Head: Biconvex lenticular shape high attenuation hemorrhage in the posterior epidural space.

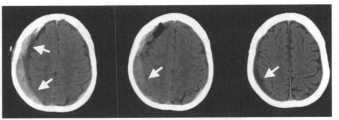

SUBDURAL HEMATOMA IN EVOLUTION – CT Head:
(Left Image) Classical crescentic shape, hyperdense blood in subdural space (<3 days).
(Middle Image) Subacute isodense blood (3-14 days).
(Right Image) Chronic hypodense blood (>14 days).

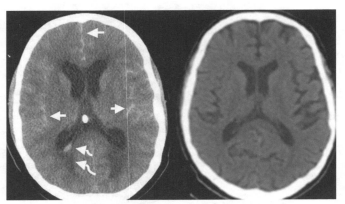

SUBARACHNOID HEMORRHAGE – CT Head (Image on left, Normal CT on right): There is diffuse high attenuation hemorrhage within the sulci of the cerebral hemispheres (straight arrows). There is also blood in the lateral ventricles (hyperdense newer blood floating on hypodense older blood (curved arrows).

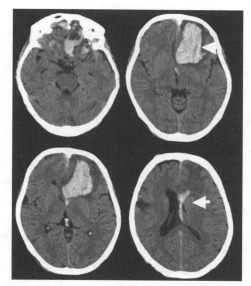

INTRACEREBRAL BLEED – CT Head: Large intracerebral bleed in the left frontal lobe (top right image) with extension into the lateral ventricle (lower right image)

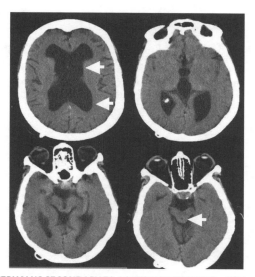

HYDROCEPHALUS SECONDARY TO AQUEDUCT STENOSIS – CT Head: Marked dilatation of the lateral, second and third cerebral ventricles with narrowing of the aqueduct (narrow aqueduct seen in lower right image)

CHEST IMAGING

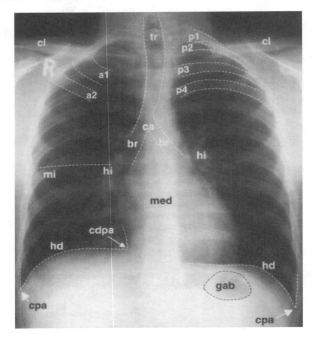

PA FILM

Normal PA film of a male. Note the right and left clavicles (cl), posterior (p1 4) and anterior (a1-2) ribs, right and left costophrenic angles (cpa), right cardio-phrenic angle (cdpa), right and left hemidiaphragms (hd), gastric air bubble (gab), trachea (tr), right and left mainstem bronchi (br), mediastinal shadow (med), carina (ca) and, right and left hila (hi). The normal position of the minor fissure (mi) is also indicated.

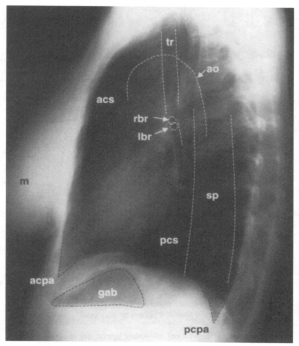

LATERAL FILM

This is a normal lateral film of a female patient. Note the spine (sp), anterior costophrenic angle (acpa), gastric air bubble (gab), trachea (tr), left mainstem bronchus (lbr), right mainstem bronchus (rbr), aortic arch (ao), anterior/retrosternal (acs) and posterior/retrocardiac (pcs) clear spaces and, breast shadow (m).

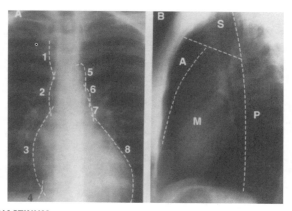

MEDIASTINUM

Components of the PA mediastinal shadow (A) include SVC (1), ascending aorta (2), RA (3), IVC (4), aortic arch (5), pulmonary trunk (6), LA appendage (7) and, LV (8). Mediastinal compartments on the lateral film (B) include: superior (S), anterior (A), middle (M) and posterior (P) compartments.

The Essentials of Oncology

Carlo Hojilla &
James Kennedy

Faculty Reviewers:
Natasha Leighl, MD, FRCP(C)
Richard Tsang, MD, FRCP(C)

ONCOLOGY

TABLE OF CONTENTS

Screening Guidelines 507
Colorectal Cancer 508
Prostate Cancer 509
Lung Cancer 509
Bladder Cancer 510
Breast Cancer (see *Breast Exam*) 510
Skin Cancer (see *Essentials of Dermatology*) 510
Lymphoma (see *Lymphatic System and Lymph Node Exam*) 510
Gynecological Cancer (see *Gynecological Exam*) 510
Fundamentals of Cancer Therapy 511
Oncologic Emergencies 512

SCREENING GUIDELINES

Primary prevention is essential in the management of cancer. **Table 1** lists the rank estimates of cancer cases by incidence and mortality. **Table 2** lists the current Canadian Screening Guidelines for some common cancer types.

Table 1. Canadian Cancer Statistics, 2008 Estimates

Incidence	Mortality
1. Prostate	1. Lung
2. Lung	2. Colorectal
3. Breast	3. Breast
4. Colorectal	4. Prostate
5. Non-Hodgkin's Lymphoma	5. Non-Hodgkin's Lymphoma
6. Bladder	6. Leukemia
7. Melanoma	7. Bladder

Table 2. Cancer Screening Guidelines

Cancer Type		Canadian Guidelines
Breast Cancer	Avg. risk	Mammography ± clinical breast exam every 1-2 years
	Family history	Screen every 1-2 years starting 10 years prior to index case (family history especially important if within 1st degree relative)
Colon Cancer	Avg. risk	Starting at age 50 • Fecal Occult Blood Test (FOBT) every 2 years • Air contrast barium enema every 5 years • Flexible sigmoidoscopy ± FOBT every 5 years • Colonoscopy every 10 years

Table 2. Cancer Screening Guidelines (continued)

Cancer Type	Canadian Guidelines	
Colon Cancer	Higher risk	FAP – annual sigmoidoscopy starting at 10-12 years of age HNPCC – colonoscopy at 20 years or 10 years before index case Previous colon cancer or polyps – colonoscopy every 3-5 years IBD – colonoscopy 8-10 years after diagnosis, then every 8-15 years depending on disease extent
Cervical Cancer	Pap smear • Start within 3 years of the onset of vaginal sexual activity • Perform yearly; every 3 years if 3 consecutive negative smears • Stop at age 70 if unremarkable Paps for 10 previous years	
Prostate Cancer	DRE + PSA starting at age 50 • Increases detection of early-stage cancers, but no evidence that screening decreases mortality • Consider screening after discussion of risks/benefits	

COLORECTAL CANCER

- History
  - Change in bowel habits: alternating constipation and diarrhea; decreased stool calibre (thinner)
  - Hematochezia/melena
  - Abdominal pain
  - Intestinal obstruction
  - Iron-deficiency anemia
  - Asymptomatic (detected by screening)
  - Constitutional: anorexia, fatigue, weight loss
- Risk Factors
  - Age >50
  - Smoking, diet (low fibre)
  - Family history
    - Familial adenomatous polyposis (FAP)
    - Hereditary non-polyposis colorectal cancer (HNPCC)
    - Non-syndromic familial colon cancer
  - Personal history
    - Colon cancer
    - Adenomatous polyps (especially if villous, >1 cm or multiple)
    - Inflammatory bowel disease
- Focused Physical Exam
  - Frequently the physical exam is completely normal
  - General appearance
    - Weight loss, cachexia
  - DRE (see *Urological Exam* p. 359)
    - Mass may be palpable if rectal involvement (poor overall sensitivity)
    - Bright red blood per rectum may be evident
  - Abdomen (see *Abdominal Exam*)
    - Palpable mass
    - With advanced disease may see:
      - Liver mass
      - Distension/ascites
- Investigations
  - Screening (see above)
  - May need to rule out upper GI bleed with upper endoscopy
  - Colonoscopy for lesion identification and biopsy
  - Metastatic workup: CXR, CT chest/abdomen/pelvis, possible head CT, bone scan, CEA

PROSTATE CANCER

- History
  - Frequently asymptomatic and detected by screening
  - If locally advanced:
    - Obstructive lower urinary tract symptoms: hesitancy, double voiding, intermittent/slow stream
    - Irritative lower urinary tract symptoms: frequency, urgency, nocturia, dysuria
  - If metastatic:
    - To bone: bone pain (frequently localized to back)
    - To pelvic nodes: lower extremity pain/edema (2° to lymphatic obstruction)
  - Constitutional: anorexia, fatigue, weight loss
- Risk Factors
  - Race: African-American
  - Family history
  - High dietary fat
  - Smoking
- Focused Physical Exam
  - General appearance: cachexia, weight loss, lower extremity edema
  - DRE (see *Urological Exam* p. 359)
    - Can present as hard, irregular nodule in peripheral zone of prostate
- Investigations
  - Screening (see above)
    - DRE, PSA, free/total PSA (<10% free PSA is suggestive of cancer)
    - Prediction algorithms can be of use in determining whether further testing is warranted
  - Transrectal ultrasound (TRUS) of the prostate
  - Metastatic Workup: CT, bone scan

LUNG CANCER

- History
  - Chronic cough, dyspnea
  - Hemoptysis
  - Chest pain
  - Persistent or recurrent pneumonia
  - Pleuritic chest pain (with peripheral tumours)
  - Constitutional: anorexia, fatigue, weight loss
- Associated Presentations
  - Due to locoregional spread:
    - Dysphagia (2° to esophageal compression)
    - Hoarseness (2° to recurrent laryngeal nerve paralysis)
    - Horner Syndrome (pancoast tumour)
    - Superior Vena Cava Syndrome (see **Oncologic Emergencies**)
  - Paraneoplastic syndromes:
    - Small Cell Carcinoma: SIADH, Cushing's (2° to ACTH), Lambert-Eaton
    - Squamous Cell Carcinoma: hypercalcemia (2° to PTH)
- Risk Factors
  - Cigarette smoking/second hand smoke exposure
  - Exposure to radon gas, asbestos
  - Uranium mining

- Focused Physical Exam
  - General appearance: cachexia, weight loss, clubbing
  - Respiratory exam
    - Variable findings: wheezing, atelectasis, pleural effusion
  - Head and neck exam
    - Supraclavicular lymphadenopathy
    - Horner's syndrome (ptosis, miosis, anhydrosis)
- Investigations
  - Imaging: CXR, CT
  - Sputum cytology
  - Biopsy (bronchoscopy or percutaneous) and histology
  - Metastatic Workup: LFTs (liver), calcium/ALP (bone), CT chest, abdo, bone scan, HPOA, and brain imaging

BLADDER CANCER

- History
  - Painless gross hematuria
  - Irritative LUTS
    - Dysuria, frequency, urgency
  - Obstructive LUTS 2° to clot retention
    - Hesitancy, double voiding, intermittent/weak stream
  - Ureter obstruction: uremia (nausea/vomiting, diarrhea), flank pain
  - Constitutional: anorexia, fatigue, weight loss
- Risk Factors
  - Environmental carcinogen exposure
    - Cigarette smoke
    - Chemicals (naphthylamine dyes)
    - Drugs (cyclophosphamide, phenacetin)
  - *Schistosoma hematobium*
  - Pelvic radiation
  - Chronic bladder inflammation (stones, cystitis)
- Focused Physical Exam
  - Abdominal Exam
    - Palpable midline pelvic mass (if invasion into bladder muscle) – rarely present
    - Inguinal lymphadenopathy
- Investigations
  - Urinalysis – chemical, culture/sensitivity and cytology
  - Cystoscopy, bladder washings and biopsy
  - Ultrasound to assess for hydronephrosis
  - Metastasis: LFTs, CT abdo (liver mets); bone scan; CXR

BREAST CANCER (see *Breast Exam*)

SKIN CANCER (see *Essentials of Dermatology* p. 396)

GYNECOLOGICAL CANCER (see *Gynecological Exam* p. 103)

FUNDAMENTALS OF CANCER THERAPY

Most cancers involve a multidisciplinary approach to treatment and management. A thorough discussion of each cancer-specific strategy is beyond the scope of this handbook. Below we outline the fields of medical, surgical, and radiation oncology.

A. Surgical Oncology

Surgery offers a multitude of procedures from the diagnosis to the management of cancer.

- Surgical oncology procedures for diagnosis and staging
  - Fine needle aspiration
  - Sentinel lymph node biopsy
- Surgical oncology procedures with curative extent
  - Surgery for preneoplastic conditions: e.g. FAP, cryptorchidism
  - Curative surgery for early-stage cancer
  - Standard oncological surgery
  - Surgery for locally advanced disease
  - Palliative surgery for metastatic disease

B. Medical Oncology

Medical oncology is a medical specialty involved in the systemic treatment of cancer, especially in the presence of metastatic dissemination. The types of systemic treatment regimens (see **Table 3**) are constantly changing and subject to ongoing research.

Table 3. Classes of Chemotherapeutic Agents

Class	Mechanism of Action
Alkylating agents	Inhibits DNA synthesis by cross-linking nucleotide bases (e.g. cyclophosphamide, cisplatin)
Anti-metabolites	Inhibits DNA synthesis as a nucleotide base analogues (e.g. fludarabine)
Microtubule inhibiting agents	Inhibits DNA synthesis by interfering with mitotic spindle (e.g. vinca alkaloids, taxanes)
Topoisomerase inhibitors	Inhibits DNA synthesis by interfering with DNA unwinding (e.g. camptothecin, etoposide, anthracycline)
Hormonal agents	Inhibits specific hormone synthesis for hormone-sensitive cancers (e.g. SERMs, aromatase inhibitors, GnRH agonists)
Tyrosine kinase inhibitors	Small molecule inhibitors that block ATP binding site of tyrosine kinase (e.g. imatinib, lapatinib, sutinitib)
Monoclonal antibodies	Antibodies directed at surface receptors blocking ligand blocking or receptor dimerization (e.g. trastuzumab, bevacizumab, panitumumab)

- Principles of Chemotherapy
  - *Adjuvant Chemotherapy:* for patients with successful initial treatment (no evidence of residual disease), but high risk for relapse (e.g. post-surgery)
  - *Neoadjuvant Chemotherapy:* for patients with bulky primary disease (not immediately amenable to initial therapy) with goal of reducing this bulk prior to initial treatment ("downstaging")

C. Radiation Oncology

Radiation oncology is a medical specialty in which ionizing radiation is used to treat patients with cancer. The goals of treatment are locoregional eradication of cancer while preserving the normal structure and function of surrounding tissues.

- Goals of radiation therapy
  - Treatment planning
  - Treatment with curative intent
  - Treatment with palliative intent
- Types of radiation therapy
  - External beam radiation therapy
  - Brachytherapy
  - Unsealed radionuclide therapy (e.g. ^{131}Iodine, free or tagged to MAb)
- Contraindications to radiation therapy
  - Previous radiation therapy to normal tissue tolerance
  - Pacemaker/defibrillator within the direct radiation field
- Side effects of radiation therapy
  - Early radiation-induced reactions: acute, local (e.g. local skin reactions, alopecia, nausea, mucositis, esophagitis) or constitutional (e.g. fatigue), and myelosuppression for large volume of bone marrow irradiation
  - Late radiation-induced reactions: dose-dependent (particularly sensitive to high dose per fraction), occurring months to years after treatment, progressive (e.g. lung fibrosis, bone necrosis, myelopathy)
  - Secondary malignancy: latency period generally >10 years, risk is higher in conjunction with chemotherapy

D. Palliative Care in Oncology

Palliative care integrates a proactive approach to honouring the patient's wishes, the care of symptoms, and improving patient quality of life

- Symptom Management
  - Pain control: use the WHO Pain Ladder as guide; manage analgesic-induced constipation
  - Respiratory symptoms: manage dyspnea and cough
  - Gastrointestinal symptoms: manage nausea and vomiting with antiemetics; provide nutritional support
  - Fatigue: consider EPO, planned activity programs
- End-of-Life Care Principles
  - Assess patient's wishes
  - Communicate with patient's family
  - Discuss legal documentation: living will, power of attorney, advanced directives

ONCOLOGIC EMERGENCIES

- Hypercalcemia (see *Essentials of Fluids, Electrolytes and Acid/Base Disturbances*)
  - Associated with the following cancers: breast, lung, thyroid, kidney, prostate, multiple myeloma
  - Can be from bony metastasis or ectopic production (PTH or PTHrP)
  - Symptoms:
    - Early: polyuria, polydipsia, nocturia, anorexia
    - Late: apathy, irritability, muscle weakness, nausea and vomiting
  - Investigations: serum calcium, phosphate, albumin, alkaline phosphatase levels; serum electrolytes; ECG
  - Management: hydration, bisphosphonate, calcitonin

- Tumour Lysis Syndrome
  - Massive release of potassium, phosphate, uric acid, and tumour breakdown products from successful chemotherapy
  - Occurs between hours and few days after treatment
  - Associated with acute leukemia, Burkitt's lymphoma, and other hematologic malignancies
  - Presents as electrolyte abnormalities (hypocalcemia, hyperphosphatemia, hyperkalemia, hyperuricemia)
  - Investigations and management options depend on the electrolyte abnormality but focus on hydration, and prophylaxis with allopurinol in high risk cases
- Febrile Neutropenia
  - Definition: Absolute neutrophil count <1.0, temperature >38.0°C × 1 hr or single temperature >38.5°C
  - Etiology: treat as infection until proven otherwise
  - Signs and symptoms: fever with associated granulocytopenia
  - Granulocytopenia carries risk of bacterial infection (usually patient's own endogenous flora) and fungal infection if prolonged
  - Management: septic workup; intravenous broad spectrum antibiotics, to include gram-negative coverage preferably with Pseudomonal coverage
    - If severe sepsis, can also add G-CSF (though onset of effect is delayed)
    - Also can consider oral antibiotics as outpatient if follow up is possible: observe for 18 hours with septic workup and antibiotics, then treat with ciprofloxacin + clavulanic acid
    - Can subsequently consider prophylactic antibiotics, dose reduction or G-CSF with next cycle
- Superior Vena Cava Obstruction Syndrome
  - Etiology: lung cancer (85%), advanced lymphoma (15%), metatstatic disease
  - Signs and symptoms: tachypnea, neck vein swelling, facial plethora, upper extremity edema, vocal cord paralysis, Horner's syndrome (rare)
  - Investigations: chest x-ray, spiral CT
  - Management: supportive, stenting, radiation therapy, chemotherapy for sensitive tumours (SCLC, lymphoma – but must obtain tissue diagnosis before treatment)
- Spinal Cord Compression
  - Etiology: metastasis to the spine (thoracic spine is the commonest site) involving the vertebral body, paravertebral tissue, or epidural space
  - Signs and symptoms: pain, neurological deficits (muscle weakness, bladder and bowel dysfunction, and sensory deficit)
  - Investigations: plain film, CT, MRI
  - Treatment: radiotherapy, neurosurgery opinion if single level; chemotherapy if sensitive tumour (SCLC, lymphoma)
  - Note that residual neurological deficit is related to time from symptom onset to treatment; therefore spinal cord compression must be diagnosed and treated quickly!
- Paraneoplastic Syndromes
  - Etiology: direct effect of the primary cancer or metastasis
  - Symptoms, investigations, and management depend on the following types:
    - Brain and neurological syndromes (e.g. encephalomyelitis, neuropathy)
    - Syndromes involving muscle (e.g. dermatomysoitis)
    - Syndromes involving skin (e.g. Paget's disease, acanthosis nigricans)

- Hematological syndromes (e.g. anemia of chronic disease, pancyto-penia)
- Paraneoplastic rheumatic syndromes
- Metabolic (e.g. electrolyte, uric acid, glucose, cortisol abnormalities)
  - Usual rule of thumb is that most get better with treatment of underlying disease, but supportive measures are also appropriate

REFERENCES

Cavalli F, European Society for Medical Oncology. 2009. *Textbook of Medical Oncology.* London: Informa Healthcare.

Chabner B, Lynch TJ, Longo DL. 2008. *Harrison's Manual of Oncology.* New York: McGraw-Hill Medical.

Feig BW, Berger DH, Fuhrman GM, University of Texas M.D. Anderson Cancer Center. Dept. of Surgical Oncology. 2006. *The M.D. Anderson Surgical Oncology Handbook.* Philadelphia: Lippincott Williams & Wilkins.

Govindan R. 2005. *Devita, Hellman, and Rosenberg's Cancer, Principles & Practice of Oncology Review.* Philadelphia: Lippincott Williams & Wilkins.

Gunderson LL, Tepper JE. 2007. *Clinical Radiation Oncology.* Philadelphia: Elsevier Churchill Livingstone.

Yeung S-CJ, Escalante CP, Holland JF, Frei E. 2002. *Holland Frei Oncologic Emergencies.* Hamilton: BC Decker.

The Essentials of Pain Management

Editors:
Monique Martin, Elena Qirjazi
& Bertha Wong

Faculty Reviewer:
Paul Tumbar, MD, FRCP(C)

TABLE OF CONTENTS

Pain Basics	515
Approach to the Pain History	517
Focused Physical Exam	517
Pharmacological Approaches to Pain	518
Medications	518
Routes of Delivery	521
Complementary and Alternative Therapies	525

PAIN BASICS

- Pain is an unpleasant sensory and emotional response to a noxious stimulus that is subjectively modified by past experiences and expectations

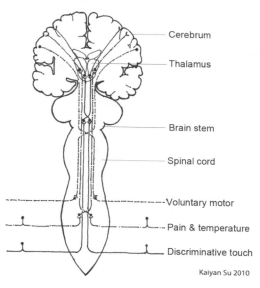

Kaiyan Su 2010

Figure 1. Sensory Pathways

Table 1. Pain Classification

Classification	Description	Example
Acute	Lasts minutes to weeks Usually concordant with degree of tissue damage (e.g. surgery, trauma, acute illness) and inflammation Expected to resolve spontaneously with tissue healing Often accompanied by anxiety	Dental infection Kidney stone Appendectomy Hip fracture Myocardial infarction
Chronic	Lasts >3-6 months Continuous or intermittent Low levels of identified underlying pathology that do not explain presence and/or extent of the pain Often accompanied by depression	**Recurrent:** Migraines **Persistent:** Osteoarthritis Painful diabetic neuropathy Chronic low back pain
Cancer	Strong relationship between tissue pathology and levels of pain Limited time frame that permits aggressive pain management Rarely involves medicolegal or disability issues	**Primary:** Inflammation from tumour **Metastatic:** Back pain from metastasis to vertebrae
Chronic non-cancer pain (CNCP)	Weak relationship between tissue pathology and pain levels Prolonged, potentially life-long pain May involve medical, legal, disability issues/conflicts, work or relationship problems, physical deconditioning, psychological symptoms	Complex regional pain syndromes (CRPS) Fibromyalgia Headaches (e.g. migraine, tension, cluster)
Nociceptive	Pain arising from normal activation of peripheral nociceptors by potentially noxious stimuli (e.g. heat, pressure, cold) Usually associated with actual or potential tissue damage Well-localized (more diffuse if deeper structures or involving viscera)	Soft tissue injuries (e.g. burn, laceration) Fracture Arthritis Abscess Ischemia
Neuropathic	Pain arising from direct injury to neural tissue and resulting in altered function of the central/peripheral nervous system Bypasses nociceptive pathways May or may not have visible tissue damage	**Peripheral syndromes:** Peripheral mononeuropathy Peripheral polyneuropathy Deafferentation (phantom limb) **Central syndromes:** Post-stroke pain Multiple sclerosis Spinal cord injury Trigeminal neuralgia

Common Pain Patterns

- **Localized pain**: pain confined to site of tissue injury (e.g. cutaneous pain, some visceral pain, arthritis, tendonitis)
- **Referred pain**: pain that is referred to a distant structure (e.g. pain produced by a heart attack may feel as if it is coming from the arm)
- **Projected (transmitted) pain**: pain transferred along the course of a nerve with a segmental distribution (e.g. herpes zoster) or a peripheral distribution (e.g. trigeminal neuralgia)
- **Dermatomal patterns**: peripheral neuropathic pain
- **Nondermatomal**: central neuropathic pain, fibromyalgia
- **No recognizable pattern**: complex regional pain syndrome

APPROACH TO THE PAIN HISTORY

In addition to general history taking, important aspects of the history include:

- Pain history: OPQRSTUVW
- Pain medication history (naturopathic, nonprescription, prescription):
    - Previous experience with opioid therapy
    - Effectiveness on pain and function
    - Compliance
    - Side effects of opioid therapy
    - Use of opioids for nonprescribed purposes (e.g. insomnia, stress, mood)
- Past medical history:
    - Illnesses that may require opioid therapy (e.g. respiratory, hepatic, renal disease)
    - Medical illnesses associated with substance abuse (e.g. hepatitis, HIV, TB, cellulitis)
    - Sexually transmitted diseases
    - Surgeries
    - Accidents, trauma, burns
- Psychiatric history:
    - Current or past mental illness
    - History of substance abuse, including alcohol and tobacco
- Family history:
    - Chronic pain
    - Substance abuse
- Psychosocial history:
    - Recent life stressors
- Patient's expectations and goals of treatment (pain intensity, daily activities, quality of life)

FOCUSED PHYSICAL EXAM

- Perform MSK and neurological exams of the painful body locations (look for tenderness, trigger points)
- Look specifically for signs of neuropathic pain (hyperalgesia, allodynia, parasthesia)
- Look for secondary consequences of chronic pain (e.g. stiffness, disuse muscle atrophy, weakness)
- Document any physical stigmata of a substance use disorder (e.g. skin tracks, spider nevi, hepatomegaly, etc.)
- Observe posture, gait, pain behaviours
- Assess the patient's pre-treatment mental status (e.g. MMSE)

- Screening tests for risk of substance abuse
- Urine medication monitoring
- Endocrine tests
- Other blood tests as appropriate
- Outside medical records

PHARMACOLOGICAL APPROACHES TO PAIN MANAGEMENT

- Treat the underlying cause where possible (e.g. steroids for polymyalgia rheumatica, appendectomy for appendicitis)
- Rate the pain as mild, moderate or severe
- World Health Organization (WHO) approach to pain management:
  - Begin with nonopioid drugs starting with acetaminophen and then nonsteroidal antiinflammatories (NSAIDs)
  - For continued uncontrolled pain of mild to moderate nature, add a weak opioid (e.g. tramadol, codeine, oxycodone)
  - For continued uncontrolled pain of a moderate to severe nature, use a stronger opioid (e.g. oxycodone, morphine, hydromorphone, fentanyl, methadone/buprenorphine)
- Choice of analgesic and delivery method depend on:
  - Type of pain
  - Underlying medical condition
  - Patient's desires
  - Requirement for future management or procedure
- Note: it is often necessary to switch therapies

MEDICATIONS

Acetaminophen
- First-line for mild acute pain (little placebo-controlled evidence in chronic pain)
- Analgesic and antipyretic but no antiinflammatory properties
- Unlike NSAIDs, no increased risk of gastrointestinal bleeding or ulceration
- Can be used in conjunction with opioid analgesia for moderate and severe pain
- Can be given at a dosage of 500-1000 mg orally every 6 hours (may be taken every 4 hours as long as the risk of hepatotoxicity is considered); doses should not exceed 4 g/d long-term or 2g/d in elderly patient or those with liver disease
- Potential side effect: liver failure (rare)

NSAIDs
- For mild to moderate acute pain
- Analgesic and antiinflammatory properties, thus efficacious for alleviating acute pain due to tissue damage and inflammation
- Significant variation in efficacy and side effects between individuals:
  - Aspirin: abdominal pain, bleeding, edema, mental status change, nausea/vomiting, pruritus/rash
  - Nonselective NSAIDs: abdominal pain, bleeding, congestive heart failure, constipation, edema, headache, hypertension, nausea/vomiting, pruritus/rash

- COX-2-selective NSAIDs: abdominal pain, congestive heart failure, edema, headache, hypertension, nausea/vomiting, pruritus/rash, cardiovascular thrombosis

> **Clinical Pearl**
> Use NSAIDs with caution in patients with asthma, coagulopathy, GI ulcers, renal insufficiency or in their third trimester.

Opioids
- In general, oral route is preferable, then transcutaneous, subcutaneous and, lastly, intravenous.
- **Mild to moderate acute pain**
  - Start with oral immediate release (IR)/short-acting (SA) opioids compounded with acetaminophen (e.g. Tylenol® #3 or Tramacet™) dosed q4-6h prn
  - Side effects of oral opioid analgesics: constipation and abdominal pain
  - If the acetaminophen dose exceeds 3-4 g/day, switch to a stronger compound (e.g. Percocet®) and titrate
- **Moderate to severe pain**
  - Start with either Percocet® or an oral opioid (e.g. oxycodone, morphine, hydromorphone) q4h prn
- **Severe pain**
  - Use IV opioid titrated q1-4h prn
  - Note: avoid IM opioid injections for acute, severe pain as absorption is too slow and erratic
  - Other methods of opioid administration which are more invasive, expensive and require very close monitoring:
    - Intrathecal administration (spinal block): use with caution as higher concentration of narcotics in the brainstem may lead to respiratory depression, sedation, nausea/vomiting, pruritus/rash
    - Continuous infusion into epidural space
- Switch to oral opioid when pain is under control and taper dose as the acute pain resolves
- Pay attention to and treat side effects: constipation, sedation, nausea
- Avoid sedating medication – especially benzodiazepines – in patients on opioids
- Use other medications for sleep if required: amitriptyline, doxepin, trazadone, cannabinoids, gabapentin, pregabalin, mirtazapine, quetiapine
- In palliative and end-of-life care: dose of morphine is titrated to patient's pain control requirements (no maximum dose); also, opioids may be used to manage dyspnea in patients

Indications for/Contraindications to Opioids
- Opioids should be considered for patients with chronic pain who are refractory to other treatments and who have shown responsiveness to opioids
- Relative contraindications to starting chronic opioid therapy: history of substance abuse, drug-seeking behaviours, personality disorders, hepatic insufficiency, renal insufficiency, severe respiratory disease with impaired respiratory drive, pre-existing constipation or urinary retention, suicidal tendency or cognitive impairment

- A useful tool to screen patients: **Screener and Opioid Assessment for Patients with Pain (SOAPP)**
  - Rate the following on scale of 0 to 4 (0 = never; 4 = usually or frequently):
    - How often do you have mood swings?
    - How often do you smoke a cigarette within an hour after you wake up?
    - How often have you taken medication other than in the way that it was prescribed?
    - How often have you used illegal drugs (e.g. marijuana, cocaine, etc.) in the past 5 years?
    - How often, in your lifetime, have you had legal problems or been arrested?
  - Total score >4 indicates patient is at risk

Adapted with permission from Butler SF, Budman SH, Fernandez K, Jamison RN. 2004. Pain 112:65-75.

> **Clinical Pearl**
> For opioid therapy in older patients or those with severe renal/liver disease:
> **Start LOW*, go SLOW**
> *Initial dose should be half the usual starting dose.

Opioid Analgesic Equivalencies
- When converting from one opioid to another, use 50-75% of the equivalent dose to allow for incomplete cross-tolerance. Rapid titration and prn use may be required to ensure effective analgesia for the first 24 hours
- Dose equivalencies provided in the **Table 2** are approximate; individual patients vary

Table 2. Opioid Equivalent Doses

Generic Name	Oral (mg)	IV (mg)	Comments
Morphine	30-60	10	Parenteral 10 mg morphine is standard for comparison Morphine PO:IV = 60:10 for opioid naïve patient, 30:10 for others Do not crush, break or chew oral controlled release morphine
Oxycodone	30	15	Often formulated in combination with acetaminophen/aspirin Use with caution if administering additional acetaminophen or aspirin
Hydromorphone	7.5	1.5	PO especially useful for initial dose titration with prn SC supplementation
Codeine	200	120	Limited by potential toxicities of acetaminophen with which it is often combined Use with caution if administering additional acetaminophen or aspirin
Hydrocodone	20	Not available	Often combined with other analgesics Use with caution if administering additional acetaminophen or aspirin

Table 2. Opioid Equivalent Doses (continued)

Generic Name	Oral (mg)	IV (mg)	Comments
Meperidine	300	75	Not a first-line opioid May cause seizures due to accumulation of normeperidine (metabolite) Should not be used longer than 48 h nor more than 600 mg/24 h Contraindicated with MAOI
Fentanyl	Not available	0.1	Common in ambulatory patients
Fentanyl (transdermal)	Transdermal 50 mcg/h patch = morphine 100 mg PO q24h = 16 mg PO q4h = 1.4 mg/h IV		Usually for stable pain, especially in patients with GI dysfunction
Methadone	20	10	Long, variable half-life, which may complicate titration
Levorphanol	4	2	Long half-life with relatively short dosing interval

Opioid Antagonists

- Opioid toxicity affects mainly CNS: manage ABCs!
- Mechanism of action of opioid antagonists: competitively inhibit opioid receptors, predominantly mu receptors
  - Naloxone is short acting ($t_{1/2} = 1$ h); effects of narcotic may return when naloxone wears off, therefore monitoring of patient is essential
  - Naltrexone is longer acting ($t_{1/2} = 10$ h); less likely to see return of narcotic effects
- Relative overdose of naloxone may cause symptoms of opioid withdrawal: nausea, agitation, sweating, tachycardia, hypertension, re-emergence of pain, pulmonary edema, seizures

Neuropathic Pain Management

- Neuropathic pain (e.g. postherpetic neuralgia, diabetic neuropathy) not usually relieved by typical analgesics (e.g. acetaminophen, NSAIDs, coxibs)
- Mexiletine, an orally administered form of lidocaine
- Topicals: capsaicin (substance P inhibitor), xylocaine
- Opioid analgesics can be effective, usually in conjunction with adjuvant medications
- Adjuvant medications:
  - Tricyclic antidepressant agents (TCAs):
    - Compared with the antidepressant effect, analgesic effect occurs at lower dosages and sooner
    - Dosing at night may help with insomnia
    - May treat co-existing depression, which can aggravate pain
  - Anticonvulsants (e.g. carbamazepine, phenytoin, valproic acid, gabapentin, clonazepam)
    - Compared with the anticonvulsant effect, analgesic effect occurs at equal (or lower) dosages
    - Gabapentin is relatively safe in accidental overdosage and may be preferred over TCAs for a patient with a history of congestive heart failure or arrhythmia or if there is a suicide risk

PAIN

- Serotonin and norepinephrine reuptake inhibitor (SNRI) (e.g. duloxetine) is approved for the treatment of diabetic neuropathy. To avoid nausea as a side effect, patients should be advised to take duloxetine on a full stomach

ROUTES OF DELIVERY

Local Analgesic Delivery
- Analgesic delivery techniques include:
  - Topical analgesia/anesthesia: minor pain relief
  - Injections: acute pain relief
  - Continuous infusions: continuous pain relief
  - Infusion pumps
  - Patient-controlled infusion pumps

> **Clinical Pearl**
> Analgesics can be administered similarly to and in combination with most regional anesthetic agents.

Patient-Controlled Analgesia (PCA)
- Use of computerized (usually parenteral) pumps that can deliver a constant infusion as well as bolus breakthrough doses of opioid analgesics
- Most commonly used agents for PCA are morphine and hydromorphone
- Shown to lessen post-operative pain, decrease complications, lead to earlier discharge and lessen the overall opiate level consumed
- PCA parameters: loading dose, bolus dose, lockout interval, continuous infusion (optional), maximum 4 h limit (optional)

Local/Regional Anesthesia
- Definition: blockade of nerve fibers that subserve pain and sensation to the region of interest by local anesthetics; prevents conduction of electrical impulses by the nerve
- Uses:
  - Diagnostic procedures
  - Minor surgical procedures
  - Peri-operative anesthesia
  - Post-operative analgesia
  - Chronic pain relief
- Benefits:
  - Avoids adverse effects of general anesthesia: myocardial and respiratory depression
  - Lower stress and mental confusion in the peri-operative period
  - Rapid functional recovery
- Side effects:
  - At low concentrations: drowsiness, light-headedness, visual/auditory disturbances, restlessness, circumoral and tongue numbness, metallic taste
  - At high concentrations:
    - CNS: nystagmus, muscular twitching, followed by overt tonic-clonic convulsions/seizures
    - Cardiovascular: arrhythmia, sudden death
    - Hematological: conversion of hemoglobin to methemoglobin with potential decomposition if pre-existing cardiac or pulmonary disease
  - Insufficient or excessive duration of anesthetic
  - Headaches with spinal anesthesia
  - Dizziness and hypotension

- Contraindications:
  - Infection at the block site
  - Allergy to anesthetics/analgesics
  - Patient reluctance to be awake during procedure
- Complications:
  - Injury of targeted nerve or nerve plexus
  - Inadvertent injection of agent intravascularly or around nontargeted neurological tissues
  - Damage to other tissues around injection site (e.g. pneumothorax for chest and abdomen blocks)
  - Infection
  - Perineural hematoma could result in patients under anticoagulation and/or antiplatelet therapy or who have an underlying bleeding disorder

Table 3. Regional Anesthesia Techniques

Regional Anaesthesia Technique	Main Uses
Local anesthesia	Small incisions, sutures and excisions of small lesions
Infiltration anesthesia	Small dermal surgeries/procedures
Bier block (IV regional anesthesia)	Short procedures in the distal limbs (<60 min)
Tumescent anesthesia	Liposuction procedures
Peripheral nerve blocks: Brachial plexus block	Shoulder and upper limb procedures
Paravertebral sympathetic ganglion block	Treatment of reflex sympathetic dystrophy
Chest and abdomen block	Abdominal and chest wall procedures
Lumbar plexus block	Pelvic girdle, knee and proximal tibia procedures
Femoral nerve block	Open knee procedures (total knee replacement)
Psoas compartment block	Hip procedures (total hip replacement)
Sciatic nerve block	Foot and distal lower limb procedures
Central neural blocks:* Spinal (subarachnoid) anesthesia	Procedures on anatomical structures below upper abdomen
Epidural anesthesia	Gynecological procedures, orthopedic surgery, general surgery, vascular surgery (for structures innervated by lumbar spine and below)

* There is a recent trend towards using combined spinal and epidural anesthesia

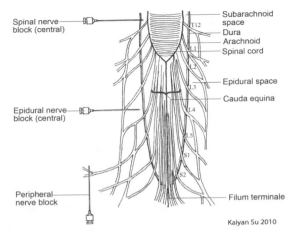

Spinal nerve block (central)

Subarachnoid space
Dura
Arachnoid
Spinal cord

Epidural space

Cauda equina

Epidural nerve block (central)

Peripheral nerve block

Filum terminale

Kaiyan Su 2010

Figure 2. Landmarks for Nerve Blocks

Systemic Analgesic Delivery
- Treatments include:
  - Oral analgesia/anesthesia (most commonly used)
  - IV injections
  - IV PCA
  - Inhalational analgesia
- Note: analgesic agents are administered similarly to anesthetic ones

General Anesthesia
- Definition: a reversible state of amnesia, analgesia, loss of consciousness, immobility and inhibition of sensory and autonomic reflexes
- Typical approach: induced with IV anesthetic agents and maintained with inhalational and/or IV anesthetics; used in combination with muscle relaxants
- Uses:
  - Surgical procedures
- Benefits:
  - Relatively low cost, reliable anesthesia for surgical procedures
- Side effects/toxicities:
  - Decrease in sympathetic tone and cardiac depression resulting in arrhythmias and hypotension
  - Respiratory depression
  - Nausea/vomiting and aspiration
  - Prolonged sedation/coma/death
  - Malignant hyperthermia
- Contraindications:
  - Allergies to anesthetic agent
  - Having ingested food or liquid in the last 8 hours
- Relative contraindications:
  - Cardiovascular disease
  - Lung disease
  - Renal disease
  - Obesity

- Stomach and esophageal problems
- Neurological conditions
- Pregnant patients: anesthetic causes fetal depression
- Alcohol and smoking

Neuroablative/Stimulatory Procedures
- These treatments are mostly used for chronic or neuropathic pain refractive to other pain management techniques
  - Central ablation:
    - Spinal tractotomy
    - Stereotactic thalamotomy
    - Dorsal root entry lesion
  - Peripheral ablation:
    - Paravertebral sympathetic ganglionectomy
    - Peripheral nerve lesion
  - Stimulatory:
    - Deep brain stimulation to the thalamus
    - Dorsal column neurostimulation
  - Stereotactic thalamic stimulation

COMPLEMENTARY AND ALTERNATIVE THERAPIES
- Medical conditions that have no conventional effective and well-tolerated treatments lead patients and physicians to look outside conventional medicine for effective and better tolerated treatments
- There is a lack of standardization complementary and alternative therapies making comparisons difficult. Nevertheless, they are being increasingly investigated for their potential to be nonpharmacological interventions for reducing pain. Uncontrolled pain has a high burden of disease and any treatment that offers the chance of improvement can be recommended without absolute proof of efficacy. Note, however, that there are certain circumstances where alternative therapy is contraindicated

Table 4. Examples of Complementary and Alternative Therapies

Mindful	Spiritual	Stimulation-based	Movement-based	Mechanical	Nutriceutical
Hypnosis	Prayer	TENS	Exercise	Chiropractic	Vitamins
Imagery	Spiritual	Acupuncture	Tai Chi	Osteopathy	Diet
Meditation	healing	Massage	Yoga	Massage	Herbal
Relaxation	Psychic	Aromatherapy			medicine
Biofeedback	healing	Therapeutic			Homeopathy
	Yoga	touch			Aromatherapy
	Music				

Belgrade MJ. Alternative and complementary therapies. In Jensen TS, Wilson PR, Rice ASC (eds.) 2003. *Clinical Pain Management: Chronic Pain.* London: Hodder Arnold

TENS (Transcutaneous Electrical Nerve Stimulation)
- Definition: application of electrical current through the skin for pain control
- Effect:
  - Activation of opioid reception in CNS (high frequency = delta opioid, low freqency = mu-opioid)
  - Reduces excitation of CNS nociceptive neurons
  - Reduces release of excitatory (glutamate) neurotransmitters
  - Increases release of inhibitory (GABA) neurotransmitters

- Activates muscarinic receptors (blocked pain gate)
- Release of serotonin, activation of serotonic receptors
- Meta-analyses have shown effectiveness in treating chronic and acute pain
- TENS should never be placed:
  - On or near the eyes or in the mouth
  - Transcerebrally (on each temple)
  - On the front of the neck (risk of acute hypotension due to vasovagal reflex)
  - On areas of numb skin/decreased sensation, broken skin areas or wounds
  - On or near the trigeminal nerve if there is a history of post-herpetic neuralgia
- TENS should be used with caution in:
  - People with epilepsy
  - Pregnant women
  - People with pacemakers

Psychotherapy
- Treatments include:
  - Counselling
  - Relaxation therapy
  - Biofeedback
  - Behavioural modification
  - Cognitive strategies
  - Hypnosis
  - CBT
  - Systematic reviews show the efficacy of CBT
  - There is strong evidence that psychological treatments can be effective without a therapist being physically present (e.g. over the internet)

Physiotherapy
- Effects:
  - Diminishes dysfunction of affected joints, muscles
  - Inhibits pain perception by stimulation of sensory afferents (gate-control theory)
  - Avoid painful movements by improvement in the quality of movement (muscle strength and coordination)
  - Normalizes autonomic nervous functions and lessens depression (functional adaptive process)
- Indicated in all pain syndromes where motor dysfunction is involved and in chronic pain (to reduce depression)
- Active therapy should start early
- Apply in combination with other treatments such as analgesic drugs

Acupuncture
- Definition: the technique of inserting and manipulating fine filiform needles into specific points on the body to relieve pain
- Effect: excites receptors and nerve fibres (mechanical activation of somatic afferents)
- "Ashi points" are used for the treatment of pain
  - Near the source of pain (local points)
  - On the forearms and lower legs (distal points)
- Meta-analyses have yet to show effectiveness

Table 5. Comparison of Acupuncture Use for Analgesia

Acupuncture Analgesia	Therapeutic Acupuncture
Immediate and strong hypoalgesia is the goal	Long-term hypoalgesia is the goal
Fast onset (minutes)	Slowly-induced symptom relief after a number of treatments
Stimulation felt very strongly; often painful and uncomfortable	Effects gradually increase after additional treatments over days to months
Used most often in different physiological experiments and for surgical hypoalgesia	Stimulation felt rather weakly; rarely painful and often relaxing
Often electro-acupuncture and pain threshold experiments on humans or animals	Used for clinical pain relief and other symptom relief
	Most often manual acupuncture but can also be electro-acupuncture

Massage
- Synonyms: effleurage, petrissage, friction, tapotement, vibration
- Mechanisms:
  - Stimulation of large diameter nerve fibers (gate-control theory)
  - Elevation of serum beta-endorphin levels for 1 h after cessation; motor neuron activity may be attenuated during application
  - Intramuscular temperature in superficial layers is increased after application
  - Blood flow is increased by dilatation of superficial blood vessels
  - Histamine release
  - Physical and mental relaxation
- Indications:
  - Back pain: massage therapy is among the most popular therapeutic strategies
  - Cancer-related pain: evidence exists that massage is beneficial for pain management
  - Chronic tension
  - Post-exercise muscle pain
- The most consistent proven effect is decreased anxiety and perception of tension
- Contraindications:
  - Any area of acute inflammation
  - Skin infection
  - Nonconsolidated fracture
  - DVT
  - Burns
  - Active cancer tumours
  - Advanced osteoporosis

REFERENCES

Belgrade MJ. Alternative and complementary therapies. In Jensen TS, Wilson PR, Rice ASC. 2003. *Clinical Pain Management: Chronic Pain.* London: Hodder Arnold.

Butler SF, Budman SH, Fernandez K, Jamison RN. 2004. Validation of a screener and opioid assessment measure for patients with chronic pain. *Pain* 112(1-2):65-75.

Rice ASC. 2008. *Clinical Pain Management.* London: Hodder Arnold.

Schmidt RF, Willis WD. 2007. *Encyclopedia of Pain.* Berlin; New York: Springer.

Swartz MH. 2006. *Textbook of Physical Diagnosis: History and Examination.* Philadelphia: Saunders Elsevier.

THE ESSENTIALS OF CLINICAL EXAMINATION HANDBOOK, 6TH ED.

Appendix 1: Concepts in Evidence-Based Medicine

Editors:
Zainab Abdurrahman &
Paul James

Faculty Reviewer:
Sharon Straus, MD, FRCP(C)

TABLE OF CONTENTS

What is Evidence-Based Medicine 529
Defining the Appropriate Question 529
Finding the Evidence 529
Evaluating the Evidence 530
Key Concepts 531
Summary of Key Formulae 532

WHAT IS EVIDENCE-BASED MEDICINE?

- Evidence-based medicine (EBM) is the conscientious, explicit and judicious use of the best current evidence in making patient-care decisions
- This section serves as a general guide to three steps involved in the EBM approach to searching for evidence regarding clinical questions: (1) defining the appropriate question, (2) finding the evidence, and (3) evaluating the evidence

DEFINING THE APPROPRIATE QUESTION

Defining the Question: the PICO Method

- A clinical question must be focused and well defined
- Use the PICO method to identify and classify key components of questions:
  - Patient/Population/Problem
  - Intervention
  - Comparison
  - Outcome

FINDING THE EVIDENCE

Systematic Reviews

- The Cochrane Library is an internationally respected resource for providing the gold standard in "what works and what doesn't," and is used by researchers and clinicians worldwide, and increasingly by patients and their families. It contains the most comprehensive collection of evidence on which interventions have been shown to work and which need more research.
- The Cochrane Library consists of various databases
  - Cochrane Database of Systematic Reviews
  - Database of Abstracts of Reviews of Effectiveness
  - Lighting Cochrane Central Register of Controlled Trials
  - National Health Services Economic Evaluation Database

Clinical Studies

- MEDLINE is the National Library of Medicine's premier bibliographic database covering the fields of medicine, nursing, dentistry, veterinary medicine, and the preclinical sciences. While this is the most up to date resource, its use requires that user to be able to critically appraise the original literature for its validity and importance. It is available through many portals including OVID and PubMed
- Ovid is an easy-to-use interface for searching databases such as MEDLINE that cover a wide range of disciplines. Most databases, index primarily journal articles, but some databases also cover conference proceedings, reports, meeting abstracts, and other publication formats.
- PubMed is a publicly accessible free service of the National Library of Medicine. PubMed includes links to many sites providing full text articles and other related resources. Search filters have been provided for questions of therapy, diagnosis, prognosis and harm

Database Searching Tips
- Establish the subject you want to find information about
- Determine the key elements of the topic
- Review synonyms for the key words describing the subject
- Consider alternative terminology and spelling that may be used to describe the subject (e.g. American versus British terminology and spelling)
- Determine which databases would best provide you with the information you need
- Develop a search strategy specific for the database you will be using; this includes how you intend to combine search terms and set limits to refine your search
- Be familiar with the functions of the databases you use regularly to optimize your search strategy

EVALUATING THE EVIDENCE

- Evaluating the evidence involves deciding whether the results being reviewed are valid, important and applicable to our individual patients. Evidence regarding both beneficial and harmful effects must be considered

1. Study Design: Are the results valid?
- Was the assignment of patients to treatment randomized?
- Was follow-up of patients sufficiently long and complete?
- Were all patients analyzed in the groups to which they were randomized?
- Were patients and clinicians kept blind to treatment?
- Were groups treated equally, apart from the experimental therapy?
- Were the groups similar at the start of the trial?
- Were potential confounding variables treated appropriately?

2. Effect Size and Precision: Are the results important?
- What is the magnitude of the treatment effect?
  - May be described by the odds ratio, relative risk, absolute risk, number needed to treat, etc.
- What is the precision of the treatment effect?
  - Mainly described by the confidence interval

3. Relevance: Do these results apply to your patient?
- Is your patient so different from those in the study that its results cannot apply?
- Is the treatment feasible in your setting?
- What are the potential benefits and harms of the therapy for your patient?
- Are your patient's values and preferences satisfied by the regimen and its consequences?

KEY CONCEPTS

- **Incidence:** the rate of occurrence of an event in a defined population. This is also the probability (or risk) of an event occurring in the defined population
- **Prevalence:** the proportion of individuals in a defined population with a particular disorder. This is also the pretest probability of anyone in the defined population having a particular disorder

Test Characteristics

- **Sensitivity:** a measure of how well a test detects a disorder when it is present (i.e. will test positively for a disorder when there is a disorder)
- **Specificity:** a measure of how well a test does not detect a disorder when it is not present (i.e. will test negatively for a disorder when there is not a disorder)
- **Positive Predictive Value (PPV):** the posttest probability of having a particular disorder when test results are positive i.e. the proportion of people with a positive test that have the disorder. PPV = TP / (TP + FP)
- **Negative Predictive Value (NPV):** the posttest probability of not having a particular disorder when test results are negative i.e. the proportion of people with a negative test who do not have the disorder. NPV = TN / (TN + FN)
- Predictive values vary with changes in the prevalence of a particular disorder, while sensitivity and specificity do not

SUMMARY: Sensitivity and Specificity

	Disease Present	Disease Absent
Test Positive	True Positive (TP)	False Positive (FP)
Test Negative	False Negative (FN)	True Negative (TN)

Sensitivity = TP / (TP + FN)
Specificity = TN / (TN + FP)

A very sensitive test with a negative result will help you rule out a condition (SnNout). A very specific test that produces a positive result will help you rule in a condition (SpPin).

Likelihood Ratio

- **Likelihood Ratio (LR):** the odds that a specific test result will be obtained in a patient with the condition compared to a person without the condition. If the LR is greater than 1, the finding is more likely among patients with the condition than patients without the condition. If the LR is less than 1, the finding is less likely among patients with the condition than patients without the condition
- The likelihood ratio for a negative test result (LR –):
  - LR – = (1 – sensitivity) / (specificity)
- The likelihood ratio for a positive test result (LR +):
  - LR + = (sensitivity) / (1 – specificity)
- The LR + multiplied by the Pretest Odds of having a particular condition yields the posttest odds of having a particular disorder. This value can then be converted to the posttest probability using the formula:
  - Posttest probability of having disorder = Posttest Odds / (Posttest Odds +1)

- Pretest Odds of having a particular disorder (i.e. before the patient has the diagnostic test):
  - Pretest Odds = Probability of having disorder / Probability of not having disorder
  - Alternatively, monograms have been created to skip the need to calculate posttest probabilities from prevalence and likelihood ratio calculations

Effect Descriptors

- **Odds**: ratio of probability of event occurring to probability of event not occurring
  - Odds of A being present when B is present = P (A and B) / P (not A and B) probability of A being present and B being present) / (probability of A not being present and B being present)
  - Where A and B can be any event or exposure
- **Odds Ratio**: ratio of the odds of event A among the exposed population compared to the odds of event A among the unexposed population
  - Where event A can be any defined outcome, including disease or illness
  - For rare diseases, the odds ratio is an estimate of the relative risk, but as the prevalence of the outcome increases, the odds ratio becomes a poor approximation of the relative risk
- **Relative Risk**: the risk of event A in a population exposed to X divided by the risk of event A in a population not exposed to X. One needs to have sampled the population prior to exposure. Thus the relative risk can be calculated from cohort studies, randomized trials, and controlled clinical trials, but cannot be calculated from case control studies or surveys
- **Absolute Risk**: the risk of event A in a population exposed to X minus the risk of event A in a population not exposed to X
- **Absolute Risk Reduction (ARR):** the risk of adverse event B in a population exposed to the protective effects of X compared to the risk of adverse event B in a population not exposed to X
- **Absolute Risk Increase (ARI):** the risk of adverse event C in a population exposed to the deleterious effects of X compared to the risk of adverse event C in a population not exposed to X
- **Number needed to treat (NNT):** the number of patients that would have to be treated with X in order for one patient to benefit by avoiding one harmful outcome
- **Number needed to harm (NNH):** the number of patients that would have to be treated with X in order for one patient to experience one harmful outcome
  - Where X is a defined exposure or intervention and A can be any defined outcome, including disease or illness
  - For a therapy that is associated with equally beneficial and harmful effects, NNT < NNH indicates that more patients will benefit than be harmed by the therapy.
- **Statistical significance**: the probability that a result occurred by chance. This concept is used to demonstrate whether a calculated or measured value represents a true effect and is not just the product of random variation. By convention this pre-determined cut-off probability is less than 5%. In other words, the result would be observed once every 20 measurements if it is determined by chance alone. This cut-off value of 0.05 is arbitrary and has no relationship to the magnitude of the effect
- **Clinical significance**: the importance allotted to the magnitude of the measured or calculated effect. This term implies that the practical meaning of the estimated values to health care professionals and their patients.

- **Confidence Interval**: the range of values in which one can be confident a measured or calculated value will reside if the measurement or calculation is repeated. A confidence interval provides a summary of the precision of an estimate, that is, how much variability exists around a given estimate (e.g. for a 95% confidence interval, 19 of every 20 repeated measurements or calculations would produce a value that lies within this interval)

SUMMARY OF KEY FORMULAE

Table 1. Summary of Key Formulae in Evidence-Based Medicine

Concept	Formula
Sensitivity	$\text{Sensitivity} = \dfrac{TP}{TP + FN}$
Specificity	$\text{Specificity} = \dfrac{TN}{TN + FP}$
Positive Predictive Value (PPV)	$PPV = \dfrac{TP}{TP + FP}$
Negative Predictive Value (NPV)	$NPV = \dfrac{TN}{TN + FN}$
Likelihood Ratio for a negative result (LR–)	$LR- = \dfrac{1 - \text{sensitivity}}{\text{specificity}}$
Likelihood Ratio for a positive result (LR+)	$LR+ = \dfrac{\text{sensitivity}}{1 - \text{specificity}}$
Pretest Odds (of having a particular disorder)	$\text{Pretest Odds} = \dfrac{P(\text{having disorder})}{P(\text{not having disorder})}$
Posttest Odds (of having a particular disorder)	$\text{Posttest Odds} = (\text{Pretest Odds}) \times (LR+)$
Posttest Probability (of having a particular disorder)	$\text{Posttest Probability} = \dfrac{\text{Posttest Odds}}{\text{Posttest Odds} + 1}$
Odds Ratio	$\text{Odds Ratio} = \dfrac{\text{Odds(Event A in Exposed Population)}}{\text{Odds(Event A in Unexposed Population)}}$
Relative Risk (RR)	$RR = \dfrac{\text{Risk of Event A in Exposed Population}}{\text{Risk of Event A in Unexposed Population}}$
Absolute Risk (AR)	$AR = (\text{Risk of Event A in Exposed Population}) - (\text{Risk of Event A in Unexposed Population})$
Number needed to treat (NNT)	$NNT = \dfrac{1}{ARR}$
Number needed to harm (NNH)	$NNH = \dfrac{1}{ARI}$

Appendix 2:
Commonly Used Drugs

Editors:
Alex Cheng & Janine Hutson

COMMONLY USED PHARMACOLOGICAL AGENTS BY SUBCATEGORY OR CLINICAL SCENARIO

Category	Subcategory/Clinical Scenario	Examples
Analgesia	Nonsteriodal Anti-Inflammatories (NSAIDs)	acetylsalicylic acid (Aspirin®), diclofenac, ibuprofen (Motrin®, Advil®), indomethacin, ketorolac, meloxicam, naproxen, piroxicam
	NSAIDs – COX 2 specific Inhibitors	celecoxib (Celebrex®), valdecoxib (Bextra®)
	Opioid Analgesics (Narcotics)	codeine, morphine, meperidine, oxycodone, hydrocodone, fentanyl, sufentanyl, alfentanyl, hydromorphone
	Opioid Antagonists	naloxone (Narcan®), naltrexone, nalmefene
	Other Analgesics	acetaminophen (Tylenol®), acetaminophen with codeine (Tylenol #2®, Tylenol #3®)
Anesthesia/ Sedation	General Anesthetics – IV	ketamine, propofol (Diprivan®), thiopental
	General Anesthetics – Inhalation	enflurane, halothane, isoflurane, nitrous oxide, sevoflurane
	Muscle Relaxants	succinylcholine, neostigmine, atracurium, pancuronium
	Sedatives – Benzodiazepines	diazepam (Valium®), lorazepam (Ativan®), midazolam (Versed®), oxazepam, temazepam, triazolam
	Sedatives – Other	zaleplon, zopiclone, chloral hydrate
Cardiology	ACE Inhibitors	captopril, enalapril (Vasotec®), fosinopril, lisinopril, ramipril (Altace®), perinopril
	Angiotensin II Blocker (ARB)	candesartan, irbesartan, losartan, telmisartan, valsartan
	Anti-adrenergics	clonidine, methyldopa, prazosin, reserpine
	Anticoagulant	heparin, warfarin, LMWH – dalteparin (Fragmin®), enoxaparin (Lovenox®), tinzaparin (Innohep®)
	Agents for dyslipidemia – Bile Acid Sequestrants	cholestyramine, colestipol
	Agents for dyslipidemia – HMG CoA Reductase Inhibitors (Statins)	atorvastatin (Lipitor®), lovastatin, pravastatin, rosuvastatin (Crestor®), simvastatin (Zocor®), fluvastatin
	Agents for dyslipidemia – Cholesterol Absorption Inhibitor	Ezetimibe (Ezetrol®)

APPENDIX: DRUGS

Category	Subcategory/Clinical Scenario	Examples
Cardiology	Agents for dyslipidemia – Fibrates	fenofibrate, gemfibrozil
	Agents for dyslipidemia – Nicotinic Acid	niacin
	Antiplatelet Agents	ASA, clopidogrel (Plavix®), dipyridamole/ASA (Aggrenox®)
	Beta-Blockers	metoprolol, atenolol, acebutolol, propranolol, nadolol, timolol
	Calcium Channel Blockers	amlodipine (Norvasc®), nifedipine, diltiazem, verapamil
	Diuretics – Carbonic Anhydrase Inhibitors	acetazolamide
	Diuretics – Loop	furosemide (Lasix®), bumetanide, ethacrynic acid, torsemide
	Diuretics – Osmotic	mannitol, glycerol, urea
	Diuretics – K^+ Sparing	amiloride, spironolactone (Aldactone®)
	Diuretics – Thiazide and related	hydrochlorothiazide (HCTZ), chlorthalidone
	Inotropes (increase contractility)	Cardiac glycosides: digoxin Sympathomimetic amines: norepinephrine, epinephrine, dopamine, dobutamine Phosphodiesterase inhibitors: amrinone, milrinone
	Nitrates	nitroglycerin, isosorbide dinitrate, isosorbide mononitrate
	Thrombolytics (lytics)	alteplase (tPA), reteplase, streptokinase, tenecteplase, urokinase
	Acute Myocardial Infarction (Clinical scenario)	ASA, nitroglycerin, morphine, β-blocker, ACE inhibitor, thrombolytics, heparin
	Angina Pectoris (Clinical scenario)	ASA, β-blocker, nitrates, calcium channel blockers
	Congestive Heart Failure (Clinical scenario)	diuretic, ACE inhibitor, angiotensin receptor antagonist, digoxin, β-blocker
	Hypertension (Clinical scenario)	diuretic, ACE inhibitor, angiotensin receptor antagonist, calcium channel blockers, β-blocker
Endocrinology	Addison's Disease (Clinical scenario)	hydrocortisone, fludrocortisone
	Diabetes Mellitus Type I (Clinical scenario)	insulin – rapid (aspart, lispro), short (insulin), intermediate (NPH, lente), long (ultralente, glargine)
	Diabetes Mellitus Type 2 (Clinical scenario)	Sulfonylureas: glyburide (DiaBeta®), glyclazide, glimepiride, chlorpropamide Biguanides: metformin α-Glucosidase inhibitor: acarbose Thiazolidinediones: pioglitazone, rosiglitazone Meglitinides: nateglinide, repaglinide Insulin
	Hypercalcemia (Clinical scenario)	Bisphosphonates, Osteoclast RNA synthesis inhibitors (mithramycin), calcitonin, Bone reabsorption inhibitor (gallium nitrate), Precipitating Agents (potassium phosphate), Calcimimetic agent (cinacalcet)

Category	Subcategory/Clinical Scenario	Examples
Endocrinology	Hyperkalemia (Clinical scenario)	Electrolyte supplements (calcium chloride, calcium gluconate), insulin with dextrose, sodium bicarbonate, β agonists, furosemide, potassium binding resins (sodium polystyrene sulfonate)
	Hyperthyroidism (Clinical scenario)	methimazole, propylthiouracil, sodium iodide I-131, β-blocker to alleviate symptoms
	Hypothyroidism (Clinical scenario)	levothyroxine (T4, Synthroid®, Eltroxin®), liothyronine (T3, Cytomel®) can be used in conjunction with levothyroxine
Gastroenterology	Antacids	aluminum hydroxide, calcium carbonate, OTC preparations (Alka-Seltzer®, Gaviscon®, Maalox®, Mylanta®, Rolaids®)
	Anti-emetics	dolasetron, ondansetron, granisetron, dimenhydrinate (Gravol®), metoclopramide, prochlorperazine, scopolamine
	H2 – Antagonists	cimetadine, famotidine (Pepcid®), ranitidine (Zantac®), nizatidine
	Proton-Pump Inhibitors (PPIs)	esomeprazole, lansoprazole (Prevacid®), omeprazole (Losec®), rabeprazole, pantoprazole
	Constipation (Clinical scenario)	psyllium, senna, bisacodyl, magnesium hydroxide, magnesium citrate, lactulose, mineral oil, docusate
	Diarrhea (Clinical scenario)	Oral rehydration therapy, loperamide, psyllium, cholestyramine, diphenoxylate, bismuth subsalicylate, attapulgite, octreotide
	GI Bleed (Clinical scenario)	pantoprazole
	Irritable Bowel Syndrome (Clinical scenario)	tegaserod, cholestyramine, psyllium, loperamide, TCA for pain
	Inflammatory Bowel Disease (Clinical scenario)	Steroids: prednisone, budesonide, hydrocortisone Other: sulfasalazine, 5-aminosalicylic acid, azathioprine, 6-mercaptopurine, methotrexate, cyclosporine, infliximab
Geriatrics	Palliative – Analgesic	Indomethacin, Ketorolac, Meperidine, Methylnaltrexone
	Psychiatry – antidepressants	Fluoxetine, cyclic antidepressants
	Psychiatry – antipsychotics	Thioridazine, mesoridazine
	Psychiatry – sedative hypnotics	Alprazolam, lorazepam, oxazepam, temazepam, triazolam
	Cardiology – antiarrythmics	Amiodarone, digoxin
	Cardiology – antihypertensive	Clonidine, methyldopa
	Endocrinology – hypoglycemic	Chlorpropramide, sitagliptin
	Gastroenterology – laxatives	Bisacodyl, cascara, neoloid

Category	Subcategory/Clinical Scenario	Examples
Geriatrics	Gastroenterology – antispasmodics	Belladonna alkaloids, Clidinium/ chlordiazepoxide, Dicyclomine, Hyocyamine, Propantheline
	Gastroenterology – anti-emetics	Prochlorperazine, Ondansetron, Granisetron, Scopolamine
	MSK – muscle relaxants	Carisoprodol, Chlorzoxazone, Cyclobenzaprine
	Urinary Incontinency-stress incontinence i.e. weak urinary sphincter (Clinical scenario)	α-adrenergic drugs (pseudoephedrine hydrochloride), estrogen, and tricyclic antidepressant agents (imipramine, amitriptyline, desipramine)
	Urinary Incontinency-urge incontinence i.e. hyperactive bladder (Clinical scenario)	Anticholinergic drugs (propantheline bromide, dicyclomine hydrochloride) antispasmodics (oxybutynin chloride, tolterodine, trospium) and tricyclic antidepressant agents (imipramine, amitriptyline)
Head and Neck	Bell's Palsy (Clinical scenario)	Oral antivirals (acyclovir), corticosteroids, artificial tears, ocular ointment, eye patch for eye protection
	Acute Otitis Externa (Clinical scenario)	Otic drops: ciprofloxacin, ofloxacin, garasone; Analgesics
	Sudden Sensorineural Hearing Loss (Clinical scenario)	Corticosteroids: oral/IV/intra-tympanic
	Otitis Media (Clinical scenario)	Antibiotics First Line: Amoxicillin, macrolides (clarithromycin, azithromycin), trimethoprim-sulphamethoxazole Second Line (for amoxicillin failures): amoxicillin-clavulinic acid (Clavulin), cephalosporins Symptomatic Rx: analgesics, antipyretics
	Vertigo (Clinical scenario)	meclizine hydrochloride, diphenhydramine, phenothiazine, transdermal scopolamine, diazepam (Valium) ± diuretics (if Meniere's), betahistine hydrochloride, ± corticosteroids
	Rhinorrhea (Clinical scenario)	Anti-histamines (loratadine, desloratadine, fexofenadine, diphenhydramine) Topical/systemic decongestants (phenylephrine, pseudoephedrine) Topical glucocorticoids (fluticasone, mometasone, budesonide, cicesonide), ± antibiotics ± ipatropium bromide
	Anterior Epistaxis (Clinical scenario)	Topical vasoconstrictor (oxymetazoline, cocaine hydrochloride)
Infectious Diseases – Anti-bacterial	Cell Wall Synthesis Inhibitors	penicillins cephalosporins carbapenems glycopeptides – vancomycin
	DNA Complex Agents	metronidazole
	DNA-directed RNA Polymerase Inhibitors	rifampin
	DNA Gyrase Inhibitors	fluroquinolones
	Folic Acid Metabolism Inhibitors	trimethoprin, sulfamethoxazole

Category	Subcategory/Clinical Scenario	Examples
Infectious Diseases – Anti-bacterial	Protein Synthesis Inhibitors (50S Ribosomes)	Chloramphenicol Clindamycin Macrolides
	Protein Synthesis Inhibitors (30S Ribosomes)	Aminoglycosides Tetracyclines
	Community-Acquired Pneumonia (Clinical scenario)	macrolide, quinolones (gatifloxaxin, levofloxacin, moxifloxacin), amoxicillin/clavulinic acid, cephalosporin, doxycycline
	Otitis Media (Clinical scenario)	amoxicillin, amoxicllin/clavulinic acid, cefuroxime, cefprozil, cefixime, trimethoprim/sulfamethoxazole (Septra®)
	TB (Clinical scenario)	isoniazid (INH), rifampin, ethambutol, pyrazinamide, streptomycin
	UTI (Clinical scenario)	Quinolones (norfloxacin, ciprofloxacin), trimethoprim/sulfamethoxazole (Septra®), cephalosporin (cephalexin – Keflex®), nitrofurantoin, amoxicillin, amoxicillin/clavulinic acid
Infectious Diseases – Anti-fungal	Polyene	amphotericin B, nystatin
	Imidazoles	Clotrimazole Ketoconazole Miconazole
	Triazole	Fluconazole
Infectious Diseases – Anti-viral	Nucleoside/nucleotide reverse transcriptase inhibitors	zidovudine (AZT), lamivudine (3TC), stavudine (d4T), abacavir (ABC)
	Nucleoside polymerase inhibitors	acyclovir, ganciclovir
	Non-nucleoside reverse transcriptase inhibitors (NNRTIs)	efavirenz, nevirapine, delavirdine
	Protease inhibitors	ritonavir, saquinavir, nelfinavir, indinavir, lopinavir, amprenavir, atazanavir
	Integrase inhibitors	raltegravir
	Combination anti-retrovirals	Combivir (Zidovudine + Lamivudine) Trizivir (Abacavir + Zidovudine + Lamivudine)
	Fusion inhibitors	Enfuvirtide, maraviroc
	Other anti-virals	ribavirin, amantadine, oseltamivir (Tamiflu)
	HIV (Clinical scenario)	NNRTIs (non-nucleoside reverse transcriptase inhibitors), NRTIs (nucleoside reverse transcriptase inhibitors), protease inhibitors, fusion inhibitors
MSK	Osteoarthritis (Clinical scenario)	acetaminophen, NSAIDs, selective cox-2 inhibitors, intra-articular glucocorticoid injection, intraarticular hyaluronan injection, opioids, capsaicin topical
	Osteoporosis (Clinical scenario)	calcium and vitamin D supplementation, bisphosphonates (alendronate, risedronate, etidronate), raloxifene, tamoxifen, calcitonin, parathyroid hormone, estrogen

Category	Subcategory/Clinical Scenario	Examples
MSK	Rheumatoid Arthritis (Clinical scenario)	NSAIDs, disease modifying therapy (methotrexate, gold compounds, D-penicillamine, antimalarials or sulfasalazine), systemic glucocorticoid therapy, anti-cytokine agents, immunosuppressive therapy (azathioprine, leflunomide, cyclosporine, and cyclophosphamide)
Neurology	Alzheimer's Disease (Clinical scenario)	Cholinesterase inhibitors: donezepil, rivastigmine, galantamine
	CVA/TIA (Clinical scenario)	tPA, clopidogrel, ASA, dipyridamole/aspirin (Aggrenox®), warfarin
	Epilepsy (Clinical scenario)	carbamazepine, phenytoin, phenobarbital, valproic acid, ethosuximide, gabapentin, lamotrigene, topiramate, vigabatrin, lorazepam, diazepam
	Multiple Sclerosis (Clinical scenario)	glucocorticoids, interferon-beta-1a or 1b, glatiramer acetate, cladribine
	Parkinson's Disease (Clinical scenario)	levodopa/carbidopa (Sinemet®) Dopamine agonists: bromocriptine, pergolide, pramipexole, ropinirole, cabergoline Other: MAO-B inhibitors (selegiline), anticholinergics (benztropine), NMDA antagonists (amantadine), COMT inhibitors (entacapone)
Obstetrics and Gynecology	Nutritional Supplementation (Clinical scenario)	Folic acid, multivitamins (e.g. Materna)
	Anti-nausea (Clinical scenario)	Diclectin, diclectin + gravol, phenothiazines, benzamides
	Hypertension (Clinical scenario)	For severe HTN (>160 systolic or >90 diastolic) – labetolol, nifedipine, hydralazine For non-severe HTN – methyldopa, labetolol, other β-blockers
	Inducing Agents (Clinical scenario)	Prostaglandin E2, oxytocin
	Medical Abortion (Clinical scenario)	methotrexate and misoprostol
	Rh- mother and Rh+ or unknown fetus (Clinical scenario)	RHO Immune Globulin (RhoGAM®)
Psychiatry	Antidepressants	Tricyclic Antidepressants (TCAs): amitriptyline, imipramine, clomipramine, doxepin, nortriptyline, trimipramine, desipramine Selective Serotonin Reuptake Inhibitors (SSRIs): fluoxetine, paroxetine, citalopram, escitalopram, sertraline, fluvoxamine Serotonin-Norepinephrine Reuptake Inhibitors (SNRIs): venlafaxine, duloxetine Monoamine Oxidase Inhibitors (MAOIs): phenelzine, tranylcypromine Other: bupropion, mirtazapine, tryptophan
	Antipsychotics	Typical: haloperidol, chlorpromazine, perphenazine, flupenthixol Atypical: olanzapine, risperidone, quetiapine, clozapine, ziprasidone

Category	Subcategory/Clinical Scenario	Examples
Psychiatry	Anti-Anxiety Agents	SSRIs, TCAs, MAOIs Benzodiazepines: alprazolam, lorazepam, clonazepam β-blockers: propranolol, atenolol, oxprenolol, pindolol Other: venlafaxine, buspirone, hydroxyzine, pregabalin
	Mood Stabilizers (for bipolar disorder)	Lithium Anti-convulsants: valproic acid, carbamazepine, lamotrigene
	Opiate Agonist	Methadone Buprenorphine

Notes for psychiatry:
1. Cognitive behavioural therapy is an effective first line treatment for mild to moderate depression and anxiety disorders.
2. Electroconvulsive therapy is indicated and effective for severe and medically refractory depression.

Category	Subcategory/Clinical Scenario	Examples
Respirology	Asthma (Clinical scenario)	Relief Medications – β-agonists (salbutamol (Ventolin®), epinephrine, isoproterenol, and terbutaline), Methylxanthines (theophylline), Anticholinergics (ipratropium bromide) Long-term Control Medications – inhaled glucocorticoids (beclomethasone, fluticasone (Flovent®), budesonide), leukotriene inhibitors (montelukast, zileuton), mast cell-stabilizing agents (cromolyn sodium and nedocromil sodium)
	COPD (Clinical scenario)	Anticholinergics (ipratropium bromide, tiotropium bromide), β-agonists (salmeterol, salbutamol) Methylxanthines (theophylline), inhaled glucocorticoids (beclomethasone, fluticasone (Flovent®), budesonide)
Urology	Benign Prostatic Hyperplasia (Clinical scenario)	doxazosin, finasteride, tamsulosin (Flomax®)
	Chronic Renal Failure (Clinical scenario)	Protein restriction, ACE inhibitors, angiotensin receptor blockers
	Erectile Dysfunction (Clinical scenario)	sildenafil (Viagra®), tadalafil (Cialis®), vardenafil (Levitra®)
Vascular	DVT/PE (Clinical scenario)	heparin, warfarin, LMWH (dalteparin, enoxaparin, tinzaparin)
	Temporal Arteritis (GCA) (Clinical scenario)	Prednisone (high dose, start at 60 mg po minimum)

THE ESSENTIALS OF CLINICAL EXAMINATION HANDBOOK, 6TH ED.

Appendix 3: Common Laboratory Values

HEMATOLOGY

Test	Conventional Units	SI Units
Complete Blood Count (CBC)		
Hemoglobin (Hb)	M: 13.5-17.5 g/dL F: 12.0-16.0 g/dL	M: 135 – 175 g/L F: 120 – 160 g/L
Hematocrit (Hct)	M: 39-49% F: 35-45%	M: 0.39-0.49 F: 0.35-0.45
Mean corpuscular Hb concentration (MCHC)	31-37% Hb/cell	4.81-5.74 mmol Hb/L
Mean corpuscular volume (MCV)	78-100 fL	78-100 μm^3
Erythrocyte count (RBC)	M: $4.50\text{-}5.90 \times 10^6/mm^3$ F: $4.00\text{-}5.20 \times 10^6/mm^3$	M: $4.50\text{-}5.90 \times 10^{12}/L$ F: $4.00\text{-}5.20 \times 10^{12}/L$
Leukocyte count (WBC)	$4.5\text{-}11.0 \times 10^3/\mu L$	$4.5\text{-}11.0 \times 10^9/L$
Differential count 　Neutrophils 　Bands 　Segmented 　Lymphocytes 　Monocytes 　Eosinophils 　Basophils	Percent (%) 57-67 3-5 54-62 23-33 3-7 1-3 0-0.75	Cells $\times 10^9/L$ 3.15-6.20 0.15-0.40 3.0-5.8 1.5-3.0 0.29-0.50 0.05-0.25 0.015-0.05
Platelet count	$150\text{-}450 \times 10^3/\mu L$	$150\text{-}450 \times 10^9/L$
Miscellaneous Hematology Values		
Erythrocyte sedimentation rate (ESR)	M: 0-17 mm/h F: 1-25 mm/h	M: 0-17 mm/h F: 1-25 mm/h
Reticulocyte count	0.5-1.5% of erythrocytes	0.005-0.015 of erythrocytes

COAGULATION

Test	Conventional Units	SI Units
International normalized ratio (INR)	0.9-1.1	0.9-1.1
Prothrombin time (PT)	9-13 sec	9-13 sec
Partial thromboplastin time (PTT)	60-85 sec	60-85 sec
Activated partial thromboplastin time (aPTT)	25-35 sec	25-35 sec
Bleeding time	2-9.5 min	2-9.5 min

ARTERIAL BLOOD GASES

Test	Conventional Units	SI Units
pH	7.35-7.45	7.35-7.45
pCO_2	35-45 mmHg	35-45 mmHg
pO_2	83-100 mmHg	83-100 mmHg
SaO_2	95-98%	0.95-0.98

SERUM CHEMISTRY

Test	Conventional Units	SI Units
Electrolytes		
Sodium	136-146 mEq/L	136-146 mmol/L
Potassium	3.5-5.1 mEq/L	3.5-5.1 mmol/L
Chloride	98-106 mEq/L	98-106 mmol/L
Bicarbonate (HCO_3)	18-23 mEq/L	18-23 mmol/L
Anion gap [$Na-(Cl+HCO_3)$]	7-14 mEq/L	7-14 mmol/L
Calcium		
Total	8.4-10.2 mg/dL	2.1-2.55 mmol/L
Ionized	4.65-5.28 mg/dL	1.16-1.32 mmol/L
Magnesium	1.3-2.1 mEq/L	0.65-1.05 mmol/L
Phosphorus	2.7-4.5 mg/dL	0.87-1.45 mmol/L
Non-Electrolytes		
Blood urea nitrogen (BUN)	7-18 mg/dL	2.5-6.4 mmol/L
Creatinine	M: 0.7-1.3 mg/dL	M: 62-115 µmol/ L
	F: 0.6-1.1 mg/dL	F: 53-97 µmol/ L
Uric acid	M: 3.5-7.2 mg/dL	M: 210 – 420 µmol/L
	F: 2.6-6.0 mg/dL	F: 150 – 350 µmol/L
Glucose (fasting)	70-105 mg/dL	3.9-5.8 mmol/L
Osmolality	275-295 mOsm/kg	275-295 mOsm/kg
Osmolal gap	<10 mOsm/kg	<10 mOsm/kg
Liver/Pancreas Tests		
Alanine aminotransferase (ALT)	8-20 U/L	8-20 U/L
Aspartate aminotransferase (AST)	10-30 U/L	10-30 U/L
γ-Glutamyltransferase (GGT)	M: 9-50 U/L	M: 9-50 U/L
	F: 8-40 U/L	F: 8-40 U/L
Alkaline phosphatase (ALP)	M: 53-128 U/L	M: 53-128 U/L
	F: 42-98 U/L	F: 42-98 U/L
Bilirubin		
Total	0.3-1.0 mg/dL	5.1-17 µmol/L
Conjugated (Direct)	0.1-0.3 mg/dL	1.7-5.1 µmol/L
Unconjugated (Indirect)	0.2-0.7 mg/dL	3.4-12 µmol/L
Amylase	25-125 U/L	25-125 U/L
Lipase	10-140 U/L	10-140 U/L
Albumin	3.5-5.0 g/dL	35-50 g/L
Lipids		
Total cholesterol		
Recommended	<200 mg/dL	<5.2 mmol/L
Moderate risk	200-239 mg/dL	5.2-6.2 mmol/L
High risk	≥240 mg/dL	≥6.2 mmol/L
HDL-cholesterol	M: >29 mg/dL	M: >0.75 mmol/L
	F: >35 mg/dL	F: >0.91 mmol/L

SERUM CHEMISTRY

Test	Conventional Units	SI Units
Lipids		
LDL-cholesterol		
Recommended	<130 mg/dL	<3.37 mmol/L
Moderate risk	130-159 mg/dL	3.37-4.12 mmol/L
High risk	≥160 mg/dL	≥4.14 mmol/L
Free fatty acids (FFAs)	8-25 mg/dL	0.28-0.89 mmol/L
Triglycerides (TG)	M: 40-160 mg/dL	M: 0.45-1.81 mmol/L
	F: 35-135 mg/dL	F: 0.40-1.52 mmol/L
Apolipoprotein A-1	119-240 mg/dL	1.2-2.4 g/L
Apolipoprotein B	52-163 mg/dL	0.52-1.63 g/L
Serum Proteins		
Albumin	3.5-5.0 g/dL	35-50 g/L
Immunoglobulins	IgA: 40-350 mg/dL	IgA: 0.4-3.5 g/L
	IgD: 0-8 mg/dL	IgD: 0-0.08 g/L
	IgE: 0-380 mg/dL	IgE: 0-3.8 g/L
	IgG: 650-1600 mg/dL	IgG: 6.5-16 g/L
	IgM: 55-300 mg/dL	IgM: 0.55-3.0 g/L
Protein		
Total	6.4-8.3 g/dL	64-83 g/L
Electrophoresis	α_1-globulin: 0.1-0.3 g/dL	α1-globulin: 1-3 g/L
	α_2-globulin: 0.6-1.0 g/dL	α2-globulin: 6-10 g/L
	β-globulin: 0.7-1.1 g/dL	β-globulin: 7-11 g/L
	γ-globulin: 0.8-1.6 g/dL	γ-globulin: 8-16 g/L
C-reactive protein (CRP)	<0.8 mg/dL	<8.0 mg/L
Markers for Neoplasia		
α-Fetoprotein (αFP)	<10 ng/mL	<10 µg/L
Carcinoembryonic antigen (CEA)	Non-smokers: <2.5 ng/mL	Non-smokers: <2.5 µg/L
Prostate specific antigen (PSA)	0-4.0 ng/mL	0-4.0 µg/L
CA-125	0-35 U/mL	0-35 kU/L
Markers for Cardiac/Skeletal Muscle Injury		
Lactate dehydrogenase (LDH)	208-378 U/L	208-378 U/L
Isoenzymes	Fraction 1: 18-33%	Fraction 1: 0.18-0.33
	Fraction 2: 28-40%	Fraction 2: 0.28-0.40
	Fraction 3: 18-30%	Fraction 3: 0.18-0.30
	Fraction 4: 6-16%	Fraction 4: 0.06-0.16
	Fraction 5: 2-13%	Fraction 5: 0.02-0.13
Creatine kinase (CK)	M: 1.00-6.67 µkat/L	M: 60-400 U/L
	F: 0.67-2.50 µkat/L	F: 40-150 U/L
CK-MB Isoenzyme	0-7 ng/mL	0-7 µg/L
Myoglobin	M: 19-92 µg/L	M: 19-92 µg/L
	F: 12-76 µg/L	F: 12-76 µg/L
Troponin I (depends on the vendor)	0-0.4 ng/mL	0-0.4 µg/L
Troponin T	0-0.1 ng/mL	0-0.1 µg/L
Nutrition		
Folate		
Serum	3-16 ng/mL	7-36 nmol/L
Erythrocytes	130-628 ng/mL packed cells	294-1422 nmol/L
Iron	50-150 µg/dL	9-27 µmol/L

SERUM ENDOCRINE TESTS

Test	Conventional Units	SI Units
Adrenocorticotropin hormone (ACTH)		
0800 hours	8-79 pg/mL	1.8-17.4 pmol/L
1600 hours	7-30 pg/mL	1.5-6.6 pmol/L
Aldosterone		
Supine	3-10 ng/dL	80-280 pmol/L
Upright	5-30 ng/dL	410-830 pmol/L
β-human chorionic gonadotrophin (β-hCG)	<5.0 mIU/mL	<5.0 IU/L
Cortisol		
0800 hours	5-23 µg/dL	138-635 nmol/L
1600 hours	3-15 µg/dL	82-413 nmol/L
C-peptide	0.78-1.89 ng/mL	260-620 pmol/L
Dehydroepiandrosterone sulfate (DHEAS)		
M:	10-619 µg/dL	0.9 – 17 µmol/L
F: Premenopausal	12-535 µg/dL	0.9 – 9.9 µmol/L
F: Postmenopausal	30-260 µg/dL	<4.8 µmol/L
Estradiol		
M	<20 pg/mL	<184 pmol/L
F: Follicular phase	20-145 pg/mL	184-532 pmol/L
F: Ovulatory peak	112-443 pg/mL	411-1626 pmol/L
F: Luteal phase	20-241 pg/mL	184-885 pmol/L
F: Postmenopausal	<59 pg/mL	<217 pmol/L
Follicle stimulating hormone (FSH)		
M	1.0-12.0 IU/L	1.0-12.0 IU/L
F: Follicular phase	3.0-20.0 IU/L	3.0-20.0 IU/L
F: Ovulatory peak	9.0-26.0 IU/L	9.0-26.0 IU/L
F: Luteal phase	1.0-12.0 IU/L	1.0-12.0 IU/L
F: Postmenopausal	18.0-153.0 IU/L	18.0-153.0 IU/L
Growth hormone (GH)	M: <2 ng/mL	M: <2 µg/L
	F: <10 ng/mL	F: <10 µg/L
Hemoglobin A_{1c} (HbA$_{1c}$)	<5.6% of total Hb	< 0.056 of total Hb
Luteinizing hormone (LH)		
M	2.0-12.0 IU/L	2.0-12.0 IU/L
F: Follicular phase	2.0-15.0 IU/L	2.0-15.0 IU/L
F: Ovulatory peak	22.0-105.0 IU/L	22.0-105.0 IU/L
F: Luteal phase	0.6-19.0 IU/L	0.6-19.0 IU/L
F: Postmenopausal	16.0-64.0 IU/L	16.0-64.0 IU/L
Progesterone		
M	<1.0 ng/mL	<3.18 nmol/L
F: Follicular phase	<1.0 ng/mL	<3.18 nmol/L
F: Luteal phase	3-20 ng/mL	9.54-63.6 nmol/L

SERUM ENDOCRINE TESTS

Test	Conventional Units	SI Units
Prolactin		
M	2-18 ng/mL	2-18 µg/L
F: Non-pregnant	3-30 ng/mL	3-30 µg/L
F: Pregnant	10-209 ng/mL	10-209 µg/L
F: Postmenopausal	2-20 ng/mL	2-20 µg/L
Parathyroid hormone (PTH)	10-60 pg/mL	1.4-7.6 pmol/L
Serotonin (5-HT)	50-200 ng/mL	<1140 nmol/L
Testosterone		
Free	M: 52-280 pg/mL	M: 180.4-971.6 pmol/L
	F: 1.6-6.3 pg/mL	F: 5.6-21.9 pmol/L
Total	M: 300-1000 ng/dL	M: 10.4-34.7 nmol/L
	F: 20-75 ng/dL	F: 0.69-2.6 nmol/L
Thyroid stimulating hormone (TSH)	2-10 µU/mL	2-10 mU/L
Thyroxine (T_4)		
Free	0.8-2.4 ng/dL	10-31 pmol/L
Total	5-12 µg/dL	65-155 nmol/L
Triiodothyronine (T_3)		
Free	1.4-4.4 pg/mL	2.2-6.78 pmol/L
Total	60-181 ng/dL	0.92-2.78 nmol/L
Vasoactive intestinal polypeptide (VIP)	<75 pg/mL	<75 ng/L

URINE

Test	Conventional Units	SI Units
Urinalysis		
pH	5.0-9.0	5.0-9.0
Specific gravity	1.001-1.035	1.001-1.035
Osmolality	50-1200 mOsm/kg	50-1200 mOsm/kg
Creatinine	1.0-1.6 g/day	8.8-14 mmol/day
Creatinine clearance	M: 82-125 mL/min	M: 1.37-2.08 mL/sec
	F: 75-115 mL/min	F: 1.25-1.92 mL/sec
Urea nitrogen	6-17 g/day	214-607 mmol/day
Sodium	100-260 mEq/day	100-260 mmol/day
Potassium	25-100 mEq/day	25-100 mmol/day
Calcium	<300 mg/day	<7.5 mmol/day
Phosphate	400-1300 mg/day	12.9-42.0 mmol/day
Uric acid	250-800 mg/day	1.49-4.76 mmol/day
Glucose	50-300 mg/day	0.3-1.7 mmol/day
Albumin	10-100 mg/day	0.01-0.1 g/day
Protein	<150 mg/day	<0.15 g/day
Urine sediment		
Leukocytes	0-2/high power field	0-2/high power field
Erythrocytes	0-2/high power field	0-2/high power field
Urinary Catecholamines	<100 µg/day	<5.91 nmol/day
Dopamine	65-400 µg/day	424-2612 nmol/day
Epinephrine	0-20 µg/day	0-109 nmol/day
Norepinephrine	15-80 µg/day	89-473 nmol/day

CEREBROSPINAL FLUID (CSF)

Test	Conventional Units	SI Units
Cell count	0-5 cells/mm^3	0-5 cells/mm^3
Chloride	120-130 mEq/L	120-130 mmol/L
Glucose	40-70 mg/dL	2.2-3.9 mmol/L
Opening pressure	50-180 mmH$_2$O	50-180 mmH$_2$O
Protein		
Albumin	6.6-44.2 mg/dL	0.066-0.442 g/L
IgG	0.9-5.7 mg/dL	0.009-0.057 g/L
Lumbar	15-50 mg/dL	0.15-0.5 g/L
Cisternal	15-25 mg/dL	0.15-0.25 g/L
Ventricular	6-15 mg/dL	0.06-0.15 g/L

ASCITIC FLUID

Condition	Gross Appearance	Protein, g/L	Cell Count Red Blood Cells, 10,000/μL	Cell Count White Blood Cells, per μL	Other Tests
Transudates Serum	Serum albumin − ascites albumin difference >11 g/L				
Cirrhosis	Straw-coloured or bile-stained	<25 (95%)	1%	<250 (90%); predominantly mesothelial	
Congestive heart failure	Straw-coloured	Variable, 15–53	10%	<1000 (90%); usually mesothelial, mononuclear	
Exudates	Serum albumin − ascites albumin difference <11 g/L				
Neoplasm	Straw-coloured, hemorrhagic, mucinous, or chylous	>25 (75%)	20%	>1000 (50%); variable cell types	Cytology, cell block, peritoneal biopsy
Tuberculous peritonitis	Clear, turbid, hemorrhagic, chylous	>25 (50%)	7%	>1000 (70%); usually >70% lymphocytes	Peritoneal biopsy, stain and culture for acid-fast bacilli
Pyogenic peritonitis	Turbid or purulent	If purulent, >25	Unusual	Predominantly neutrophils	Positive Gram's stain, culture
Nephrosis	Straw-coloured or chylous	<25 (100%)	Unusual	<250; mesothelial, mononuclear	If chylous, ether extraction, Sudan staining
Pancreatic ascites (pancreatitis, pseudocyst)	Turbid, hemorrhagic, or chylous	Variable, often >25	Variable, may be blood-stained	Variable	Increased amylase in ascitic fluid and serum

Condition	Gross Appearance	pH	Glucose mmol/L	Amylase PF:Serum	Red Blood Cells (1000/mm³)	White Blood Cells (1000/mm³)
Transudates	pleural fluid/serum protein <0.5 OR pleural fluid/serum LDH < 0.6 OR pleural fluid LDH < 2/3 upper normal serum limit					
Congestive heart failure	Clear, straw	>7.4	>3.3	≤1	0-1	<1 predominantly mononuclear
Cirrhosis	Clear, straw	>7.4	>3.3	≤1	<1	<0.5 predominantly mononuclear
Pulmonary embolus: atelectasis	Clear, straw	>7.3	>3.3	≤1	<5	5-15 predominantly mononuclear
Exudates	pleural fluid/serum protein >0.5 OR pleural fluid/serum LDH >0.6 OR pleural fluid LDH >2/3 upper normal serum limit					
Pulmonary embolus: infarction	Turbid to hemorrhagic, small volume	>7.3	>3.3	≤1	bloody in 1/3 to 2/3 of patients	5-15 predominantly neutrophils; may show many mesothelial cells
Pneumonia	Turbid	≥7.3	>3.3	≤1	<5	5-40 predominantly neutrophils
Empyema	Turbid or purulent	5.50-7.29	<3.3	≤1	<5	25-100 predominantly neutrophils
TB	Straw; sero-sanguineous in 15%	<7.3 (20%)	1.7-3.3 (20%)	≤1	>10	5-10 predominantly mononuclear
Malignancy	Straw to turbid to bloody	<7.3 (30%)	<3.3 (30%)	≤1	1 to >100	<10 predominantly neutrophils
RA effusion	Turbid or green or yellow	<7.3; usually ~7.0	<1.7 (95%)	≤1	<1	1-20 neutrophils in acute; mononuclear in chronic
SLE	Straw to turbid	<7.3 (30%)	<3.3 (30%)	>2		Neutrophils in acute; mononuclear in chronic
Rupture off esophagus	Purulent	6.0	N or D	Salivary type		Predominantly neutrophils
Pancreatitis	Serous to turbid to serosanguineous	>7.3	>3.3	>2	1-10	5-20 predominantly neutrophils

Note: Normal values may vary. Check the normal values established by your laboratory.

Index

A

Abdominal aortic
   aneurysm 309-310, 408
Abdominal pain 30, 407
Abdominal series 482, 498-500
Abruptio placenta 207
Acetaminophen 518
Acne vulgaris 391
Acoustic neuroma 111
Acromegaly 418
Acupuncture 526
Acute pain 516
Addison's disease 420
ADLs 82
Adnexa, examination of 97
Adolescent physical examination .277-283
Adrenal hyperfunction 419-420
Adrenal hypofunction 420-421
Age-related macular degeneration 244
Agoraphobia 327
Air bronchogram 480
Air space disease 481
Allen test 305
Alzheimer's disease 199
Amblyopia 228
Amniocentesis 216
Anaphylaxis/Anaphyloid 402
Angina 60
Angiography 67, 306
Ankle brachial index 306
Anorexia nervosa 293, 330
Anosmia 115
Anti-phospholipid
   antibody syndrome 316
Anxiety disorders 292, 326
Aortic dissection 410
Aortic stenosis 68, 410
APGAR 222
Appendicitis 43
   Acute 486,499
Arrhythmias 74
Arterial blood gases 343
Ascites 36, 44
Asthma 284, 346, 347
Atherosclerosis risk factors 300
Atrial fibrillation 69
Attention deficit/hyperactivity
   disorder 293
Autism spectrum disorders 293
Avascular necrosis 166

B

Bacterial vaginosis 106
Barium enema 488
Barium swallow 487
Barlow's test 270
Basal cell carcinoma 396
Batwing sign 480
Benign prostatic hyperplasia 362
Bimanual examination 97
Biophysical profile 217
Bipolar disorder 326
Bladder cancer 510
Blood pressure
   Measurement 20
   Classification 21
   Errors 22
Body mass index 22
Bouchard's nodes 156
Boutonniere deformity 156
Brain tumours 198
Braxton-Hicks contractions 217
Breast cancer
   Risk factors 50, 51
Breastfeeding 225
Breast mass 52, 53, 55
Brodie-Trendelenburg maneuver 306
Bulimia nervosa 293, 331
Burns 405

C

Cancer pain 516
Cancer therapy 511-512
Candidiasis, vaginal 106
Cardiac tamponade 410-411
Cardiovascular examination
   Pediatric 263-266
Carotid artery disease 311-312
Carpal tunnel syndrome 155
Cataracts 243
Cauda equina syndrome 166
Celiac disease 43
Cervical cancer 103-104
Cervical dilatation 218
Cervix, examination of 94
Chemotherapy 511
Chest pain 410
Cheyne-Stokes breathing 340
Child abuse 294-296
Chlamydia 454
Cholecystitis 408
   Acute 486, 500

INDEX

Chorionic villus sampling 216
Chronic pain 516
Claudication
    Intermittent 309
Clubbing 339
Colles fracture 490
Colorectal cancer 508
Colour vision 234
Common cold 447
Compartment syndrome 145
Conductive hearing loss 111
Congestive heart failure 68, 482
Consolidation 482
Contraception 100-101
Coordination 194
COPD 347, 348
Cough 116, 284-285
Cranial nerves 181
    CN IX, CN X, CN XII 119
Cushing's disease 418
Cushing's syndrome 419
Cysts 394-395

D

Delirium 331
Dementia 331
Dependency, see pallor on elevation
    Chronic arterial 301, 303, 308
    Chronic deep vein 314
    Venous 302, 305
Depression 293
Depressive disorder 325
Dermatitis 391-392
    Atopic 392
    Contact 392
Dermatological examination 273
Dermatology
    Arrangement 388-389
    Colour 387
Diabetes mellitus 415-416
Diabetic neuropathy 199
Diarrhea 41, 457
Digital rectal examination 359
Diverticulitis 486, 499
Dizziness 125
Drawer tests 171-172
Driving competency; Elderly Fitness to
    Drive assessment 88
Drug interactions 377
Dupuytren's contracture 156
Dysphagia 117
Dyspnea 338

E

Ear
    Discharge 110
    Pain 109
Eating disorders 293
Echocardiography 67
ECG 67
ECG interpretation 71-78
Ectopic pregnancy 408
Eczema 391-392
Edema 305
Elder abuse 86
Elephantiasis (lymphatic filariasis) 138
Emphysema 347-348, 482
Encephalopathy 44
Endometrial carcinoma 104
Endometriosis 105
Endometritis 224
Eneuresis 287
Enteroclysis 488
Epistaxis 126-127
Epstein-Barr virus mononucleosis 137
Erectile dysfunction (impotence) .356-357
Esophageal rupture 411
External ocular examination 236
Extraocular muscle examination 236
Eye complications in
    diabetes mellitus 244-245

F

Facial pain 115
Falls – elderly 85
Family tree 10
Febrile neutropenia 513
Febrile seizures 289
Fetal heart rate (FHR) monitoring 220
Fetus
    Delivery 222
    Position 219
    Station 219
Fibroadenoma 55
Fibroids (leiomyomata) 103
Fluid loss 427
Fluid wave 36
Fracture 145
Functional inquiry 11
Fundoscopy 239-240
Fungal infections 393-394

G

Galactorrhea 418
Galeazzi fracture 490
Gastrointestinal examination
    Pediatric 266-268
General survey and vitals 254-256
Generalized anxiety disorder 328

Genetic disorders.....................................292
Genital warts..456
Genitourinary and reproductive
    examination.................................268-269
Geriatrics
    Drug Safety..376
    Geriatric Giants..................................80
Gestational trophoblastic
    neoplasms.........................100-101, 102
GI obstruction....................409, 486, 498
Glasgow coma scale..............195-196, 400
Glaucoma...242-243
Gliomas...493
Goldman cardiac risk factors................442
Golfer's elbow (medial epicondylitis) ..153
Gonorrhea..454
Gynecological Cancer 103

H

Hair..390
Head & Neck examination
    Pediatric......................................257-262
Headache 198, 412
Hearing loss..111
Heat
    Cramps...404
    Edema 404
    Exhaustion...404
    Stroke 404
    Syncope..404
Heart
    Axis...71-72
    Failure 285
    Rate...72
    Rhythm...72
    Sounds..65
    Valves 64-65
Heave...64
Hematuria 361, 365
Hemoptysis...338
Hepatitis..460
Hepatobiliary iminodiacetic scan.........495
Hepatojugular reflux 63
Heberden's nodes...................................156
Hernias
    (direct, indirect, femoral) 358,359
Herpes simplex 456
Herpes simplex encephalitis 201
HIV...451
HIV sero-positivity 137
Hoarseness...128
HPV vaccination 102
Hypaque Enema 488
Hypercalcemia 433, 512
Hypercoaguability
    History 300, 312
    Testing..308

Hyperkalemia...431
Hypermagnesemia 436
Hypernatremia 429
Hyperphosphatemia................................435
Hyperthermia...404
Hyperthyroidism 418, 422
Hypocalcemia 432
Hypokalemia 430
Hypomagnesemia.....................................435
Hyponatremia...428
Hypophosphatemia 434
Hypopituitarism 418
Hypothermia...403
Hypothyroidism..............................423-424

I

IADLs..82
Incontinence............................... 287, 366
Increased ICP..412
Infective endocarditis..............................69
Infertility..105
Inflammatory bowel
    Disease/syndrome 46
Insufficiency
    Acute arterial.....................................307
    Allen test, see Allen test
    Arterial...................................... 302, 305
Integrated prenatal screen 216
Interstitial disease...................................482
Intravenous fluids 440
Ischemia
    Symptoms of
        Arterial....................................... 301, 307
        ECG findings...76
Ischemic bowel..409

J

Jaundice 32
    Newborn...286
JVP...62-63

K

Kerley B lines..480
Kussmaul's sign 63

L

Labour...217-223
    False...217
    First stage...219
    Second stage.......................................221
    Third stage...223
    Fourth stage.......................................223
Lichen sclerosus......................................103
Lymphadenitis, suppurative...................137
Lymphangitis..137

INDEX

Localized pain	517
Lochia	224
Lumbar disc prolapse	201
Lung cancer	509
Lymphadenopathy	131, 136
Lymphangiography	135
Lymphedema	131, 132, 134, 135

M

Malaria	472, 473
Malignancies	
Dermatology	396
Mallet	
Finger	156
Thumb	156
Massage therapy	527
Mastitis	56
Mediastinal mass	479
Medical oncology	511
Melanoma	396-397
Menarche	99
Meningiomas	493
Meningitis	412, 463
Menopause	93, 101
Menstrual bleeding, abnormal	93
Menstruation	99
Metabolic acidosis	438
Metabolic alkalosis	438
MI/ACS	67, 410
Mini-mental status exam	322
Mitral prolapse	411
Mitral regurgitation	69
Mitral stenosis	68
Mood disorder	324
Motor examination	187
Multiple sclerosis	200, 493
Murmur	65-66
Muscle tone	188
Musculoskeletal examination	
Pediatric	269
Mycoplasma infection	136
Myocardial perfusion scanning	494

N

Nails	16, 18, 391
Nasal obstruction	114
Nasopharynx	118
Neck mass	121
Neurological examination	
Pediatric	271
Neuropathic Pain	516
Nevi	395
Nipple changes	50, 52
Peau d'orange	52
Retraction	52
Nociceptive pain	516
Non-cancer pain	516

Non-stress test	217
NSAIDs	518
NYHA classification	61

O

Obesity, pediatric	297
Obsessive-compulsive disorder	327
Obstructive lung disease	345, 346
Oncologic emergencies	512-514
Operative delivery	223
Operative note	442
Opioids	519
Prescribing	89
Oppositional defiant disorder	294
Oral cavity	118
Ortolani's test	270
Osteoarthritis	146
Osteomyelitis	467
Osteoporosis	146
Otalgia	109
Otitis media	124, 283
Otorrhea	110
Otoscopic exam	113
Ovarian cancer	104

P

Palliative care	512
Pallor on elevation/	
rubor on dependency	305
Pancreatitis	42, 487
Panic	
Attack	326
Disorder	327
Pap smear	95-96
Paraneoplastic syndromes	513
Parkinson's disease	200
Patello femoral syndrome	169
Patient controlled analgesia	522
Pediatrics	
Drug dosing	376
Pelvic examination	94-98
Pelvic inflammatory disease	102
Pelvic organ prolapse	370-371
Peripheral nerve blocks	524
Personality disorder	332
Peyer's patch	131
Pharmacokinetic formulae	376
Pharyngitis	116, 283
Pituitary	
Hyperfunction	417-418
Hypofunction	418-419
Placental separation	223
Plasma anion gap	438
Pleural effusion	496
Poisoning	380
Pneumonia	348, 349
Pneumothorax	411, 481, 496

Polycystic ovarian syndrome 424-425
Postnatal examination 253-254
Postoperative orders..............................444
Postpartum
    "Baby" Blues.................................224
    Depression (PPD).........................224
    Hemorrhage (PPH) 224
    Psychosis.......................................225
Post-term labour..................................217
Power...189
Precordial exam 64
Pregnancy
    Drug Safety...................................379
Prescription writing 374
Preterm labour......................................217
Primitive reflexes 289
Prostate cancer......................361, 362, 509
Psoriasis...392-393
    Guttate...393
    Flexural..393
    Pustular..393
Psychosis...328
Puerperium 224
Pulmonary embolism 350, 411
Pulmonary function tests 344
Pulmonary nodules...............................481
Pulse
    Palpation..303
    Description.....................................303
Pulse oximetry......................................343
Pupil examination 234
Pupillary dilation..................................237

R

Radiation oncology 512
Radionuclide ventriculography 494
Rapid primary survey 399-401
Rash, pediatric 290-291
Recreational drugs................................381
Rectal bleeding.....................................286
Rectovaginal examination 98
Referred pain...517
Reflexes 190
Reflux (see peptic ulcer disease) 47
Regional anesthetic 523
Renal colic 487
Respiratory acidosis 437
Respiratory alkalosis 437
Restrictive lung disease................. 345,346
Retinal detachment 241-242
Review of systems...................................11
Rheumatoid arthritis.............................146
Rhinorrhea 114-447
Ringworm..393-394
Ringing in ears 107
Rinne test..113
Rosacea 391
Rupture of membranes 219

S

Salivary apparatus.................................118
Scars 395
Schizophrenia 329
Sciatica..166
Screening guidelines, cancer................507
Seizures 199
Sensorineural hearing loss 111
Sensory examination.............................192
Sepsis...465
Shock...400
Silhouette sign......................................480
Sinus pain 115
Skin cancer 396
Sleep disorders 293
Slit lamp examination 237-239
Social phobia...327
Speculum examination 95-96
Speculum, nasal 115
SPIKES approach......................................7
Squamous cell carcinoma.....................396
Strep throat.................................... 119, 448
Spinal cord compression.......................513
Spinal cord disorders 202
Spleen..132
Splenic injury 408
Spousal abuse 23
ST segment changes 77
Stroke 197
Subarachnoid hemorrhage ... 413, 492, 502
Subdural hematoma 492, 502
Substance abuse, dependence 330
Superior vena cava obstruction 513
Surgical oncology 511
Sutures...443
Swan neck deformity.............................156
Syphilis.................................... 134, 136, 457
Systemic diseases, dermatological
    manifestation 398
Systemic lupus erythematosus 134, 138

T

Tactile fremitus 340
Temporal arteritis 413
Tennis elbow (lateral epicondylitis) 153
Term labour...217
Testicular torsion 363
Thoracic outlet syndrome.....................166
Thrill...64
Thrombophlebitis, superficial...............313
Thrombosis
    Arterial..307
    Deep Vein 312-313
    Risk Factors 300
Thrush..283
Thyroid..123
Thyroiditis 422
Thyrotoxicosis................................422-423

Tine 394
Tinnitus..110
Tonsillitis 283
Tonsils (palatine) 118
Toxic megacolon..............................483
Toxic syndromes..............................380
Transcutaneous electrical nerve
   stimulation 525
Transient ischemic attack 311
Trichomonas 456
Tuberculosis 448
Tumour lysis syndrome 513
Tympanic membrane 108, 110, 111

U

Ulcer
   Arterial.......................................302
   Venous..302
   History 301
Incontinence – elderly 85
Urinary tract infection 287, 368
Uterus
   Examination of 97

V

Varicose veins...................................314
Vasculitis................................. 302, 315-316
   Anti-phospholipid antibody 316
   Behçet's disease....................................315
   Buerger's disease 308, 315
   History 300
   Polyarteritis nodosa.............................316
   Raynaud's phenomenon/
   disease 302, 308 316
   Temporal (giant cell) arteritis 315
   Takayasu's arteritis.............................316

Venous insufficiency
   See insufficiency.....................................302
   Incompetent saphenous vein
   testing.......................................306
Venous obstruction 302
Ventilation perfusion scanning 343
Virchow's triad 312
Virtual colonoscopy/
   CT colongraphy 488
Visual acuity...................................233
Visual field testing 234
Vital signs 19
Volume depletion 427
Volume overload.....................................427
Vulvar malignancies................................103

W

Waldeyer's ring.......................................132
Webber test..112
Whisper test 112
Wound care 406

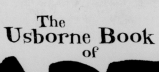

The Usborne Book of ART skills

Fiona Watt

Designed and illustrated by
Antonia Miller, Katrina Fearn,
Natacha Goransky and Vici Leyhane

Additional illustrations by
Felicity House and Jan McCafferty
Photographs by Howard Allman

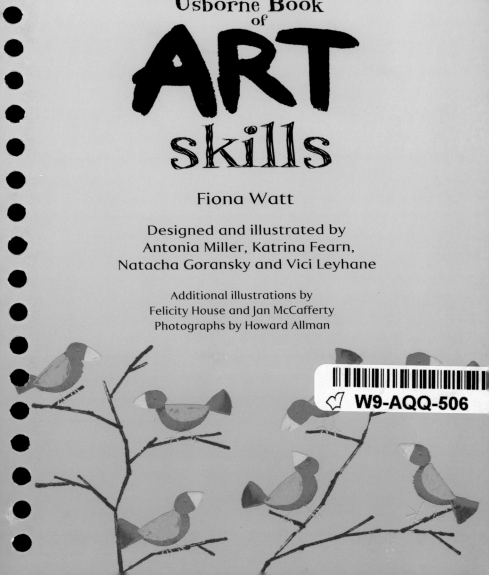

W9-AQQ-506

Contents

4 Materials
6 Tissue paper collage
8 Oil pastel resist
10 Collage with ink drawing
12 Dragged paint
14 Tissue paper rubbings
16 Cardboard and potato printing
18 Cut paper
20 Techniques for trees
24 Printing with a sponge

26 Fingerpainting
28 Pastel and ink resist
30 Creating textured papers
32 Brushstrokes
34 Techniques for skies
38 Mixed media collage
40 Painted patterns
42 Patterns with plastic foodwrap
44 Watercolour washes
46 Tissue paper and glue collage
48 Printing with an eraser

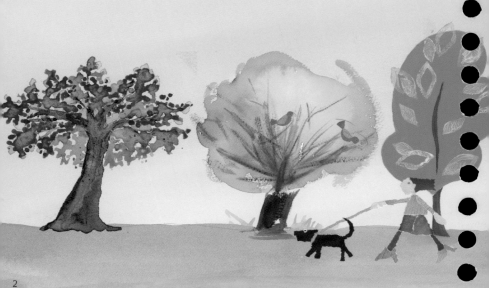

50	Techniques for water	74	Paper collage
54	Wet inks and chalk pastels	76	Oil pastel resist and spattering
56	Blow-painting	78	Techniques for feathers
58	Adding gold highlights	80	Watercolour effects
60	Tessellating and transforming shapes	82	Chalk pastels
62	Continuous line drawing	84	Lifting off watercolour paint
64	Techniques for fur	86	Scratched paint and pastels
68	Wet-on-wet painting	88	Collage with found objects
70	Magazine paper collage	90	Pencil and eraser drawings
72	Wax resist and spattering	92	More ideas
		96	Index

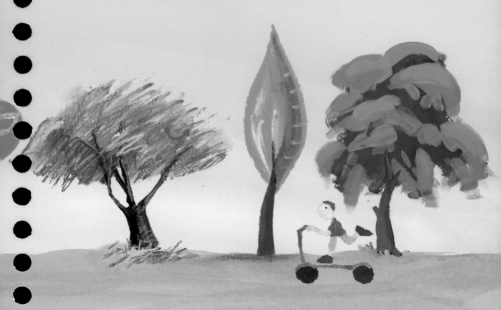

Materials

The techniques in this book use materials which can be found in art shops and most stationers. These two pages give information on some of the materials and how to use them.

Paint

The types of paint used in this book are watercolour paint, acrylic paint, poster paint and gouache.

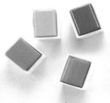

You can buy watercolour paints in tubes or in solid blocks called pans. Mix the paints with water before you use them.

Gouache and poster paints are quite thick and opaque. They can be used without mixing with water.

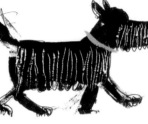

Acrylic paints come in tubes or bottles. Squeeze them onto an old plate or palette. You can add water to make them thinner and more transparent.

This dog was painted with acrylic paint. See page 67 for this technique.

Pastels

In the book, there are several techniques which use oil pastels or chalk pastels. These are usually sold in sets.

Oil pastels

Oil pastels give a brighter effect than chalk pastels. Chalk pastels are good for techniques where colours are blended.

Chalk pastels

Wax crayons can be substituted for oil pastels. They are good for rubbing and resist techniques.

You'll find this scratched pastel technique on page 86.

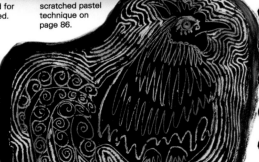

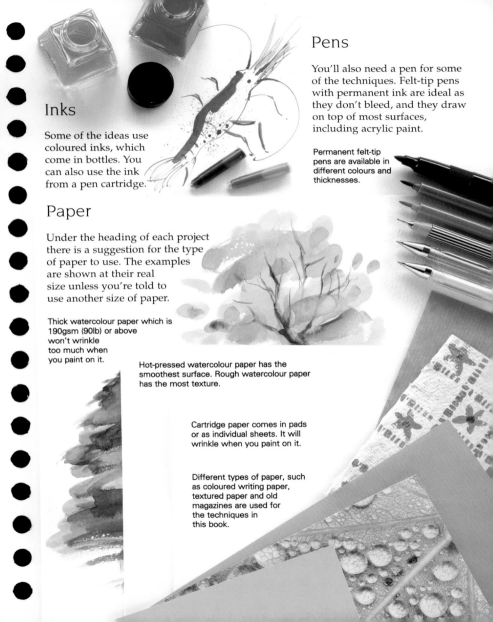

Inks

Some of the ideas use coloured inks, which come in bottles. You can also use the ink from a pen cartridge.

Pens

You'll also need a pen for some of the techniques. Felt-tip pens with permanent ink are ideal as they don't bleed, and they draw on top of most surfaces, including acrylic paint.

Permanent felt-tip pens are available in different colours and thicknesses.

Paper

Under the heading of each project there is a suggestion for the type of paper to use. The examples are shown at their real size unless you're told to use another size of paper.

Thick watercolour paper which is 190gsm (90lb) or above won't wrinkle too much when you paint on it.

Hot-pressed watercolour paper has the smoothest surface. Rough watercolour paper has the most texture.

Cartridge paper comes in pads or as individual sheets. It will wrinkle when you paint on it.

Different types of paper, such as coloured writing paper, textured paper and old magazines are used for the techniques in this book.

Tissue paper flowers

CARTRIDGE PAPER OR WHITE CARDBOARD

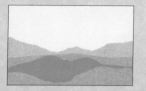

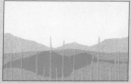

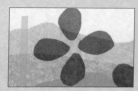

1. Rip some strips of blue tissue paper. Glue them across a piece of paper, making them overlap.

2. Cut some thin strips of green tissue paper for the stems and glue them at the bottom of the paper.

3. Cut out some red petals. Glue four petals around the top of some of the stems.

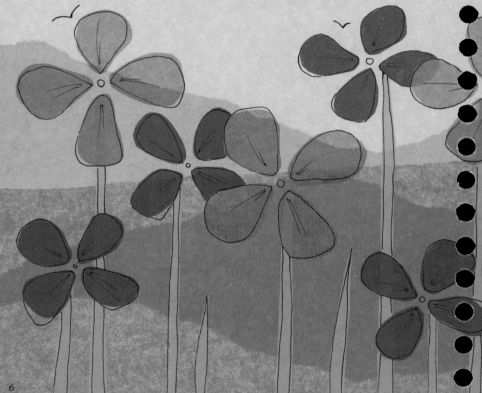

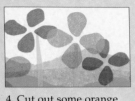

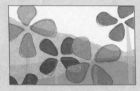

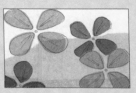

4. Cut out some orange petals. Glue them around other stems, overlapping some of the red petals.

5. Use a thin felt-tip pen to draw a line around each petal. It doesn't need to be too accurate.

6. Draw a small circle in the middle of each flower, then add two or three lines to each petal.

These flowers also have outlines drawn along their stems.

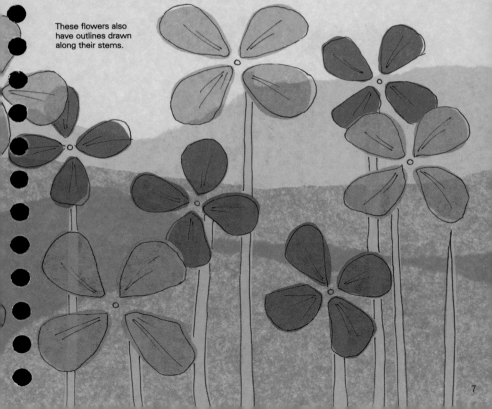

Reflections in water

GREY OR ANOTHER PALE COLOUR OF PAPER

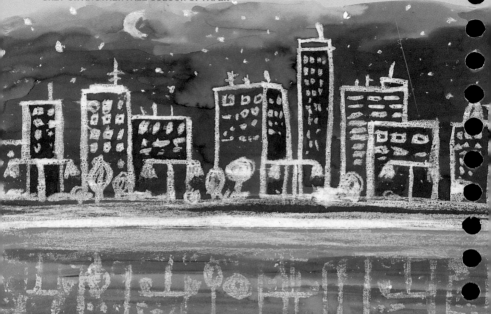

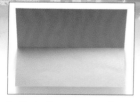

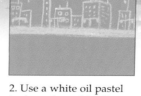

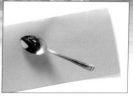

1. Cut a large rectangle of grey paper, then fold it in half with its long sides together. Crease the fold then open the paper.

2. Use a white oil pastel to draw three thick lines above the fold. Draw lots of buildings, trees, street lights, a moon and stars.

3. Fold the paper again, then rub all over it with the back of a spoon. This transfers your drawing to the other half.

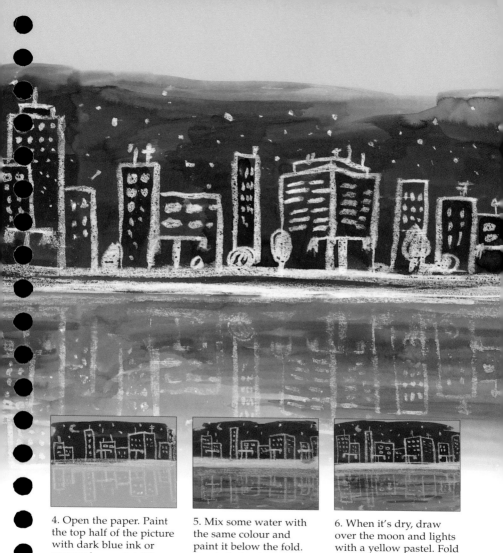

4. Open the paper. Paint
the top half of the picture
with dark blue ink or
watercolour paint. The
pastel will resist the paint.

5. Mix some water with
the same colour and
paint it below the fold.
Brush darker lines on top
to make it look like water.

6. When it's dry, draw
over the moon and lights
with a yellow pastel. Fold
the paper and rub over it
to make yellow reflections.

Simple figures
THICK BRIGHT PAPER OR CARDBOARD

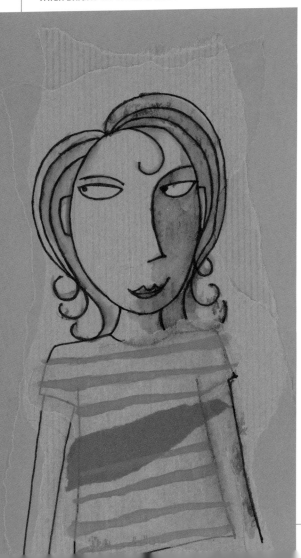

1. Cut a piece of thick paper or cardboard. Rip a rectangle from some brown wrapping paper and glue it in the middle.

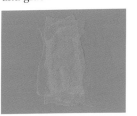

2. Rip a slightly wider rectangle from a bright piece of tissue paper and glue it over the brown wrapping paper.

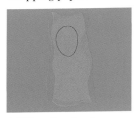

3. When the glue has dried, use a water-based felt-tip pen or a fountain pen to draw an oval for the face.

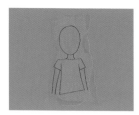

4. Draw two lines for the neck and a round-necked T-shirt. Add lines for the arms, but don't worry about drawing hands.

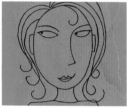

5. Draw a curved line for the eyebrow and nose, then add the other eyebrow and eyes. Draw the ears, hair and lips.

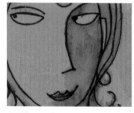

6. Then, dip a paintbrush into some clean water. Paint the water along some of the lines to make the ink run a little.

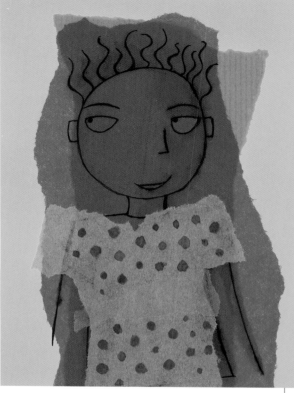

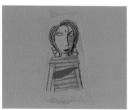

7. Rip a rough T-shirt shape from tissue paper and glue it over your drawing. Add a torn paper stripe, too.

8. Finally, when the glue has dried, paint thin stripes across the T-shirt using a bright colour of watercolour paint.

Fantasy castle

CARTRIDGE PAPER OR THIN CARDBOARD

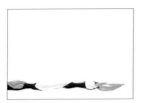

1. Squeeze a line of acrylic paint along the bottom of the paper, straight from the tube. Use blue, turquoise and white.

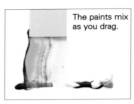

The paints mix as you drag.

2. Cut pieces of thick cardboard, making them different widths. Place a piece below the paint, then drag it upwards.

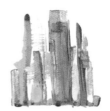

3. Then, use the other pieces of cardboard to drag more towers, making them different heights. Leave it to dry.

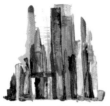

4. Put some black paint onto a plate and dip the edge of another piece of cardboard into it. Drag it over the dried paint.

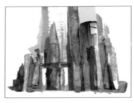

5. Dip the edge of the cardboard into the black paint again and use it to print lines for bridges between the towers.

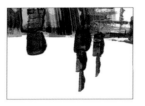

6. Dip a narrow piece of cardboard into the paint. Drag small rectangles under the towers, to give them shadows.

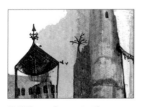

7. When the paint has dried, use a black felt-tip pen to draw bridges, trees, turrets, windows and weather vanes.

This sunset scene was created using the same technique.

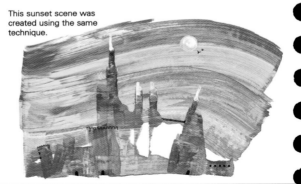

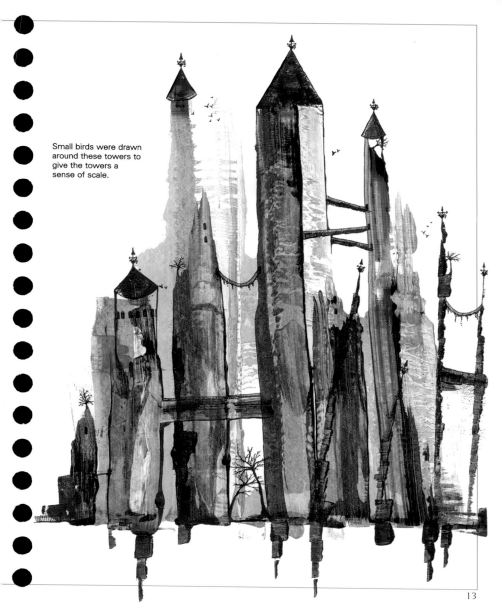

Small birds were drawn
around these towers to
give the towers a
sense of scale.

13

Tissue paper fruit

TISSUE PAPER

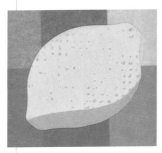

Orange

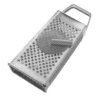

1. Cut a circle from orange tissue paper. Then, cut a curved strip of tissue paper and glue it along one side.

2. Lay the tissue paper orange on a grater. Then, rub the side of an orange oil pastel or wax crayon gently over the paper.

Apple

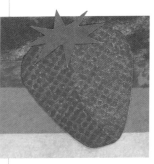

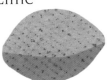

3. Carry on rubbing until the orange is covered with texture. Then, use a fine black felt-tip pen to add a stalk to the top.

Cut an apple shape from green tissue paper. Rub it with a green pastel around one side and at the top. Glue on a stalk.

Lemon

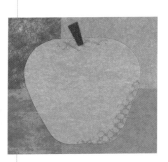

Lime

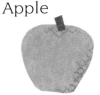

Cut a lemon from yellow tissue paper. Glue a green strip along one edge. Rub it with a yellow oil pastel, then a light green one.

Cut the shape of a lime from green tissue paper. Add a green strip along one edge, then rub it all over with a green pastel.

Try using different sides of the grater to get different textures.

Strawberry

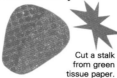

Cut a stalk from green tissue paper.

Cut a strawberry from red tissue paper. Add a red strip covering about half of the shape. Rub it with a yellow oil pastel.

Grapefruit

Cut a circle from yellow tissue paper and add a pale green strip. Rub it with a yellow, then a light green pastel. Add a stalk.

Pear

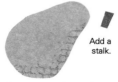

Add a stalk.

Cut a pear shape from green tissue paper. Rub down one side with a green pastel. Then, glue on a stalk.

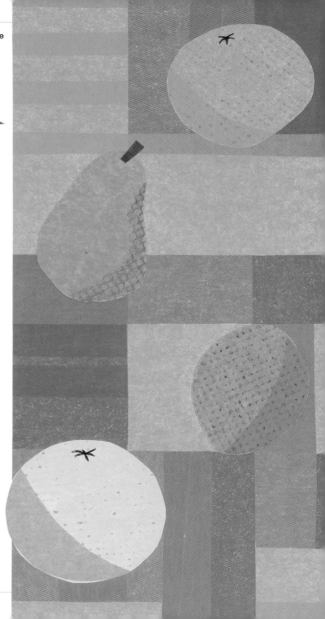

Printed birds in a tree

ANY TYPE OF THICK PAPER

1. For the branches, pour some brown poster paint onto an old plate, then dip the edge of a strip of thick cardboard into it.

2. Press the painted edge onto your paper. Dip the cardboard into the paint, then print another branch, joining the first one.

The bodies and heads of these birds were printed at different angles to make them look animated.

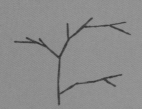

3. Dip different widths of cardboard into the paint and print more branches. Leave spaces between them for the birds.

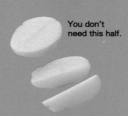

4. While the branches are drying, cut a small potato in half, lengthways. Then, cut one piece in half again.

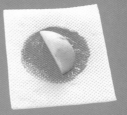

You don't need this half.

5. For the birds' bodies, spread red paint on some paper towels. Press the cut side of one of the pieces of potato onto it.

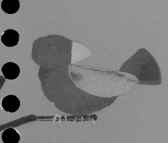

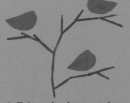

6. Print a body onto the paper, with the straight edge at the top. Print more bodies in the spaces between the branches.

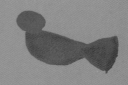

7. For the tails, dip the edge of some cardboard into the paint. Put it at the end of the body and twist it. Fingerprint the heads.

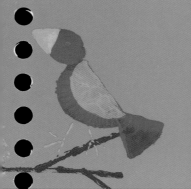

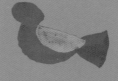

8. For the wings, cut a slice off the other small piece of potato. Press it in orange paint and print it on the body.

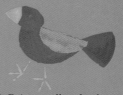

9. Paint a yellow beak and a blue eye on each bird. Then, paint short yellow lines for the legs, using a thin brush.

Paper shapes

ANY KIND OF COLOURED PAPER

Spiral

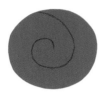

1. Cut a circle from coloured paper, then draw a spiral from the edge of the circle to the middle of it.

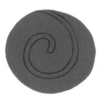

2. At the middle of the circle, curve the line around a little, then draw another line out to the edge of the circle.

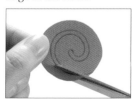

3. Cut along one of the lines of the spiral, turning the paper as you cut. Carry on cutting until you reach the edge again.

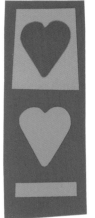

4. Cut the pointed end off the spiral and trim any wobbly bits from around the edges. Glue it onto another colour of paper.

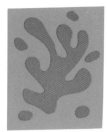

Build up layers of different shapes on top of each other.

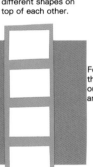

For a sun, cut a circle, then cut small triangles out of its edge. Glue another circle on top.

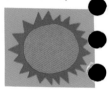

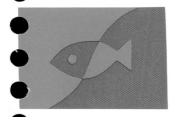

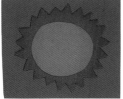

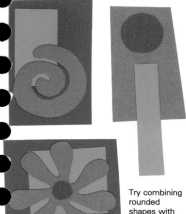

The shapes below could be used on a Valentine's card.

Try combining rounded shapes with squares and rectangles.

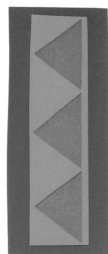

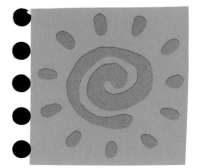

Fish

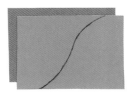

1. Cut two rectangles, the same size, from blue and orange paper. Then, draw a wavy line across the blue one.

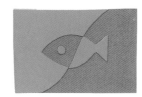

2. Draw a simple outline of a fish across the line. Cut along the line, then cut out the front part of the fish, like this.

3. Glue the front part onto the orange rectangle. Then, cut out the back of the blue fish and glue it on. Glue on a blue eye.

Techniques for trees

The next four pages show you lots of different ways of drawing, painting and printing trees. When you try any of these techniques, you will get a better result if you make your tree bigger than the ones shown.

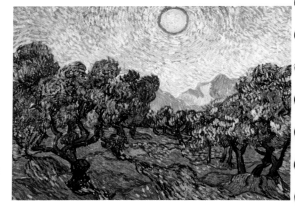

This oil painting of olive trees, by Vincent van Gogh, was painted in 1889. Van Gogh used lots of short lines to build up the shape and colour of the trees and the sky.

Oil pastel trees

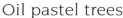

1. Draw a twisted tree trunk using dark brown oil pastels. Add several short branches.

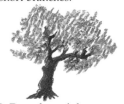

2. Draw lots of short diagonal lines with a green oil pastel, overlapping the branches.

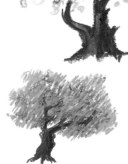

This tree was filled in with dots, instead of short lines.

3. Add more diagonal lines for the leaves, using a lighter green and a lime green pastel.

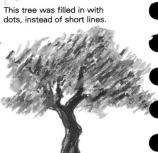

Use orange, brown and rusty pastels for autumn leaves on a tree.

Pen and ink

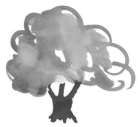

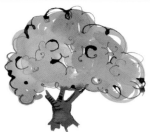

1. Use brown ink to paint a very simple trunk with three thick branches coming from it.

2. Use green ink to paint a wavy line for the top of the tree. Then fill it in, leaving some small gaps.

3. Use a felt-tip or an ink pen to draw loopy lines around the edge of the tree and around the gaps.

Brushed branches

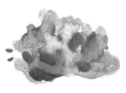

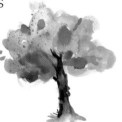

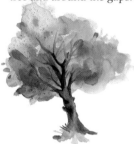

1. Paint a patch of green and brown watercolour paint. Spatter it by flicking the bristles of your brush.

2. Leave it to dry, then use different shades of brown watercolour paint to paint the trunk.

3. While the trunk is still wet, paint the branches by brushing the paint up onto the leaves.

Chalk pastel leaves

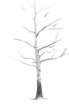

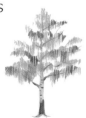

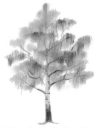

1. Paint a trunk with yellowy-brown watercolour paint. Add some branches, too.

2. Draw lines using a light green chalk pastel. Add some darker green lines on top.

3. Gently rub the tip of your little finger down the lines to smudge the chalks together.

More techniques for trees

Sponged leaves

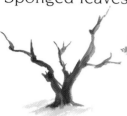 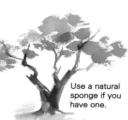 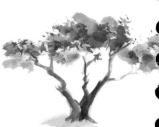

Use a natural sponge if you have one.

1. Use the tip of a brush to paint the trunk and twisted branches of a tree, using watercolour paint or ink.

2. Dampen a piece of sponge, then dip it into some red paint. Dab it gently around the tops of the branches.

3. Wash the sponge, then squeeze as much water out as you can. Dip it into purple paint, then dab it around the branches.

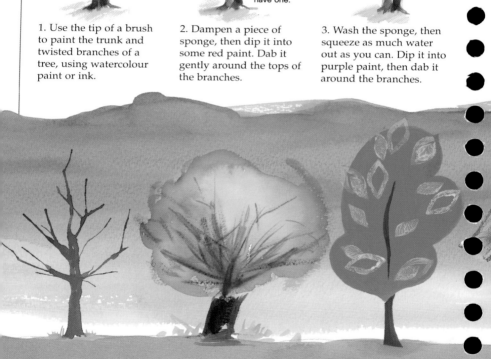

This tree was blow-painted through a straw (see pages 56-57). Use this technique for a tree in winter.

Dip the hard end of a paintbrush in paint, then drag it across a patch of wet watercolour paint to make branches.

The leaves on this tree were printed with an eraser which had been cut into leaf shapes (see page 48 for this technique).

Zigzag trees

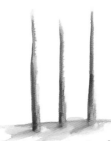

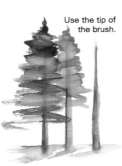

Use the tip of the brush.

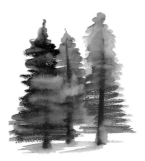

1. Paint three tree trunks using green watercolour paint. Make them get thinner towards the top. Add some ground.

2. Put the tip of your brush at the top of a tree and paint a zigzag down the trunk. Make it get wider as you paint.

3. Carry on painting, but leave part of the trunk showing at the bottom. Then, zigzag some clean water over the top.

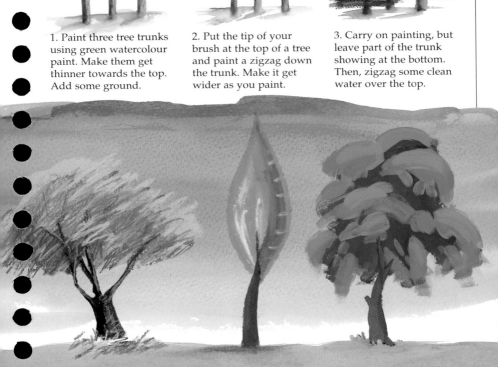

Draw a trunk with brown chalk pastels. Scribble pastels for the leaves. Smudge them in a few places.

This stylized tree was drawn with chalk pastels. The leaves were drawn first then the trunk was added.

These leaves were painted first in dark green acrylic, then lighter green was added on top.

Sponge-printed snails

ANY TYPE OF PAPER

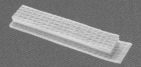 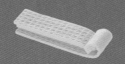

This is the end you print with.

1. Cut a piece of kitchen sponge 17 x 4 cm and two pieces 15 x 3 cm. Lay them together, matching the top edges, like this.

2. Cut a long piece of tape, so that it is ready to use. Fold the end of the long piece of sponge over the end of the shorter pieces.

3. Roll up the pieces of sponge carefully but not too tightly, keeping the edges even. Secure the sponge with the tape.

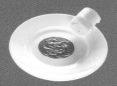 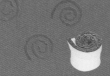

4. Pour blue acrylic paint onto an old plate and spread it a little. Then, dip the end of the sponge into the paint.

5. Print spirals all over a piece of paper. Press the sponge into the paint again each time you print a spiral.

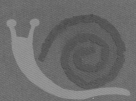 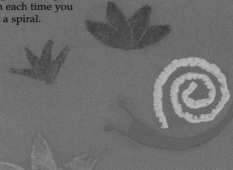

6. When the paint is dry, paint a snail's body below each spiral. Then, use a thin paintbrush to paint the antennae.

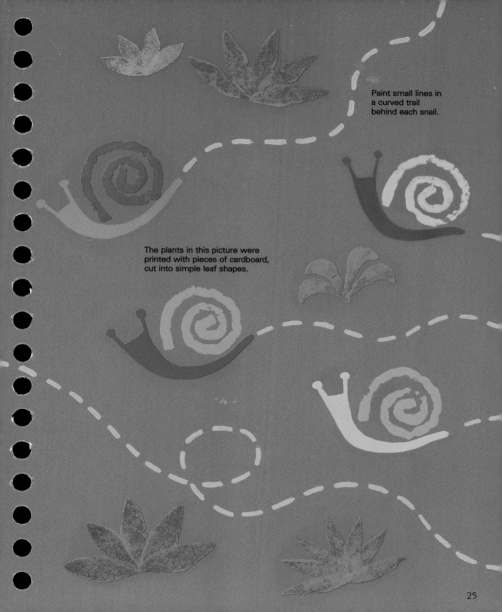

Paint small lines in a curved trail behind each snail.

The plants in this picture were printed with pieces of cardboard, cut into simple leaf shapes.

25

Fingerpainted flowers

CARTRIDGE PAPER

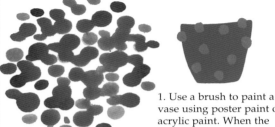

The stem, leaves and pot of this flower were painted with a brush, then the flower head was fingerpainted on top.

1. Use a brush to paint a vase using poster paint or acrylic paint. When the paint is dry, fingerpaint some dots on the vase.

Drag your finger towards the middle each time.

2. For a daffodil, dip a fingertip in yellow paint. Then, drag six lines for the petals, making them join in the middle.

3. Do several more daffodils above the vase. When the paint is dry, fingerpaint a star shape in the middle of the petals.

4. For a tulip, fingerpaint a curved line with bright red paint. Do another line that meets the first one at the bottom.

5. For the blue flowers, dip a fingertip in paint and print a small dot. Add lots more dots in a rough triangular shape.

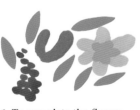

6. To complete the flower arrangement, use a paintbrush to paint green leaves in the spaces between the flowers.

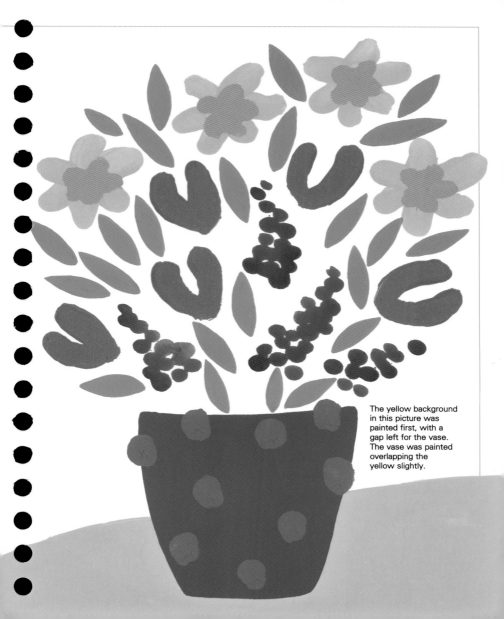

The yellow background in this picture was painted first, with a gap left for the vase. The vase was painted overlapping the yellow slightly.

Oil pastel lizards

ANY THICK WHITE PAPER

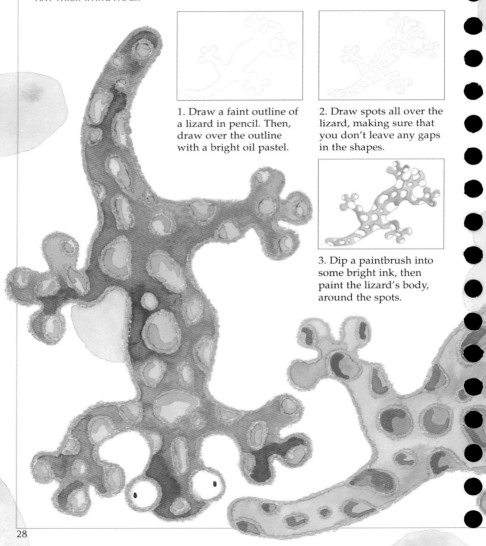

1. Draw a faint outline of a lizard in pencil. Then, draw over the outline with a bright oil pastel.

2. Draw spots all over the lizard, making sure that you don't leave any gaps in the shapes.

3. Dip a paintbrush into some bright ink, then paint the lizard's body, around the spots.

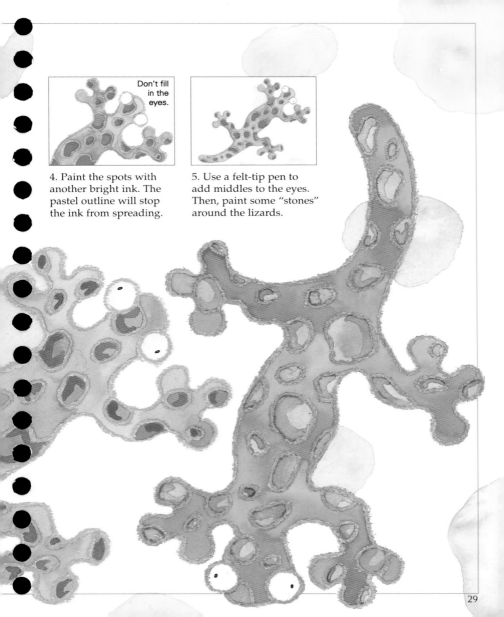

4. Paint the spots with another bright ink. The pastel outline will stop the ink from spreading.

Don't fill in the eyes.

5. Use a felt-tip pen to add middles to the eyes. Then, paint some "stones" around the lizards.

29

Textured houses

THIN WHITE CARDBOARD

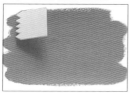

1. Cut a zigzag at one end of a strip of cardboard. Then, paint a rectangle of acrylic paint on another piece of cardboard.

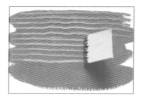

2. Drag the zigzag end of the cardboard across the paint again and again to make textured lines. Leave the paint to dry.

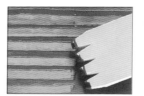

3. Cut several small triangles into the end of another cardboard strip. Drag it across another rectangle of paint.

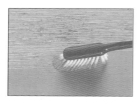

4. For a very fine texture, drag the end of an old toothbrush across a rectangle of paint, again and again.

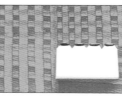

5. Do some more textured patches of paint by experimenting with different shapes cut into strips of cardboard.

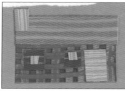

6. Cut rectangles from the textures for the buildings, windows, doors and roofs. Glue them on another piece of cardboard.

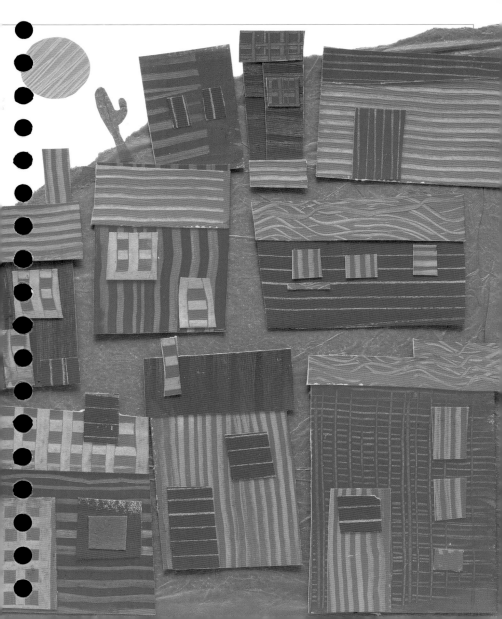

Patterned reptiles

CARTRIDGE PAPER OR WATERCOLOUR PAPER

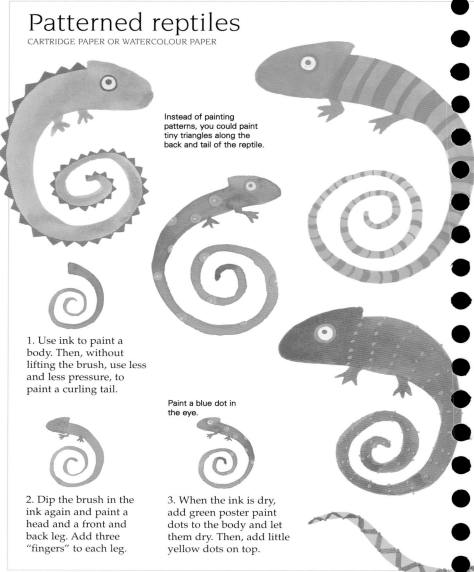

Instead of painting patterns, you could paint tiny triangles along the back and tail of the reptile.

1. Use ink to paint a body. Then, without lifting the brush, use less and less pressure, to paint a curling tail.

Paint a blue dot in the eye.

2. Dip the brush in the ink again and paint a head and a front and back leg. Add three "fingers" to each leg.

3. When the ink is dry, add green poster paint dots to the body and let them dry. Then, add little yellow dots on top.

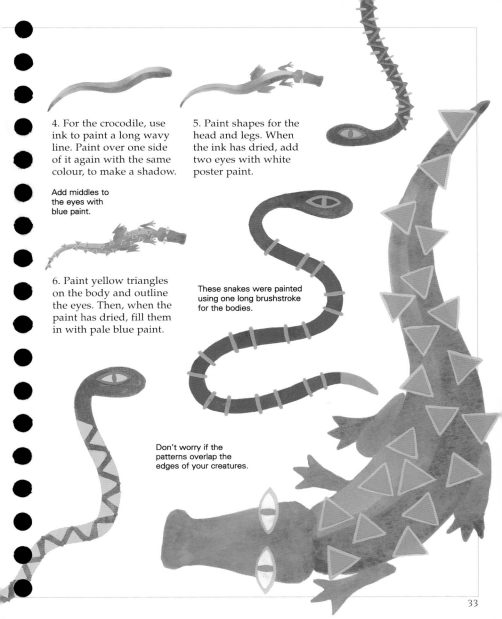

4. For the crocodile, use ink to paint a long wavy line. Paint over one side of it again with the same colour, to make a shadow.

Add middles to the eyes with blue paint.

5. Paint shapes for the head and legs. When the ink has dried, add two eyes with white poster paint.

6. Paint yellow triangles on the body and outline the eyes. Then, when the paint has dried, fill them in with pale blue paint.

These snakes were painted using one long brushstroke for the bodies.

Don't worry if the patterns overlap the edges of your creatures.

33

Techniques for skies

On the next four pages you will find different techniques and tips for drawing and painting skies and clouds. Watercolour paints are very good for creating atmospheric skies.

This picture, called Rain, Steam and Speed, was painted in oil paints by J.M.W. Turner in 1844. The sky is stormy, but Turner painted bright areas on some of the clouds, which makes it look as if the sun is about to break through.

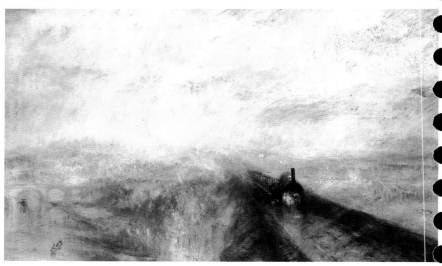

Watery clouds

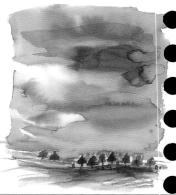

1. Brush clean water onto a piece of watercolour paper. Then, use the tip of a brush to blob on patches of blue watercolour paint.

2. The paint will run. Then, press the brush a little bit more firmly in some places to make darker patches of sky.

Summer sky

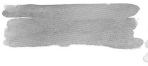

1. Mix enough cobalt blue watercolour paint to cover a piece of watercolour paper. Paint a stripe across the top.

2. Paint another stripe below the first one before it has had a chance to dry. Paint quickly and make the stripes overlap.

3. Carry on painting overlapping stripes all the way down the paper. This technique is known as 'painting a wash'.

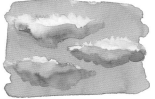

4. Before the paint has dried, scrunch up a paper tissue and dab it in several areas on the paper to lift some paint off.

5. When the paint has dried, mix some darker blue. Paint it along the bottom of each cloud to make shadows.

More techniques for skies

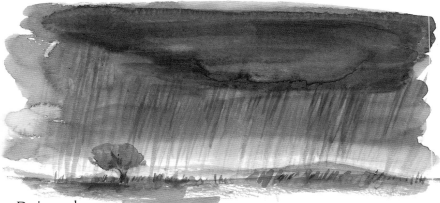

Rainy sky

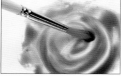

1. Wet some watercolour paper with clean water. Then, mix Prussian blue watercolour paint with brown to make dark grey.

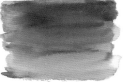

2. Paint overlapping stripes across the top of the paper. They don't need to be even or to start in the same place.

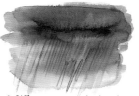

3. While the paint is still quite wet, add blue stripes across the middle, then grey ones at the bottom of the paper.

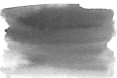

This creates a misty effect.

4. Before the paint has dried, swipe a cotton bud across the paint so that the bottom is almost white. Leave it to dry.

5. While it is drying, practise painting some fine lines for the rain, using grey paint on a piece of scrap paper.

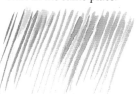

6. When your painting is completely dry, paint fine lines for the rain, coming from the grey area near the top of the paper.

Starry night

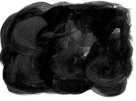 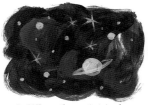 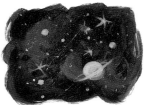

1. Paint a piece of cardboard with dark blue acrylic paint. Move the brush around in a circle to get an uneven finish.

2. When the paint is dry, paint some planets with pale yellow acrylic paint. Then, add several stars around them.

3. For the tiny stars, dip a paintbrush into the yellow paint, then spatter it all over, following the steps on page 73.

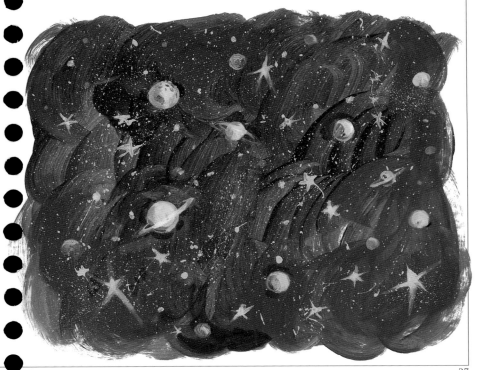

Leaf collage
THICK PAPER OR CARDBOARD

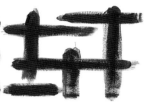

1. Use dark paint and a thick paintbrush to paint vertical and horizontal lines on your paper.

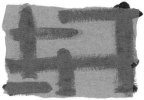

2. When the paint has dried, cut a piece of tissue paper to cover the lines, and glue it on.

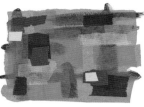

3. Rip some squares and rectangles from different colours of tissue paper and glue them on.

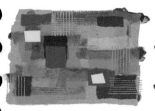

4. Cut a square of corrugated cardboard. Press it into some paint and print it several times.

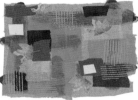

5. Either cut out leaves from a picture in a magazine, or cut some leaf shapes from paper.

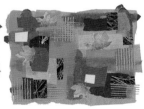

6. Cut small rectangles from a magazine picture of leaves or grass. Glue them on.

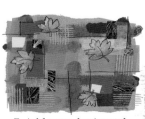

7. Add some horizontal and vertical lines with a felt-tip pen. Then, outline the leaves, loosely.

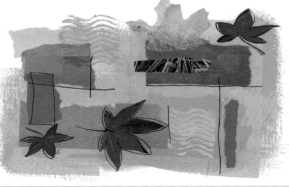

Doodle painting
BROWN WRAPPING PAPER

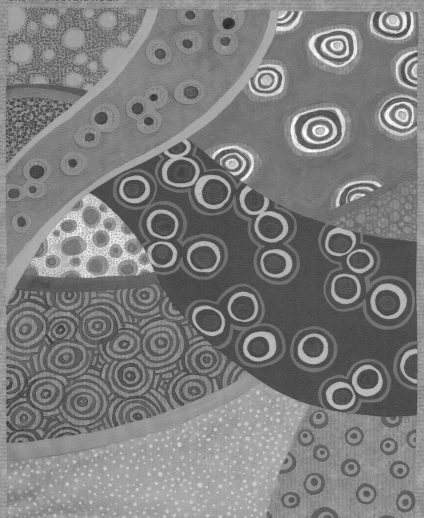

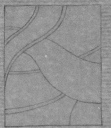

Leave a space around each circle.

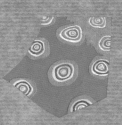

1. Use a pencil to draw a rectangle on some brown wrapping paper. Draw curving lines to separate the rectangle into sections.

2. In one section, paint pale blue spots a little way apart. Fill in the spaces around them with lots of darker blue dots.

3. Paint white circles, one inside another. Add purple, blue and yellow inside them. Fill around the circles in light blue.

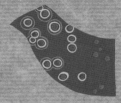

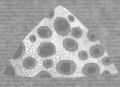

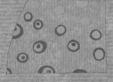

4. Fill one section with blue. When it's dry, add purple spots, then paint yellow and light blue circles around them.

5. In another section, paint blue spots. Fill in around them with white paint, leaving a space. Add tiny blue dots.

6. Paint light blue spots. Outline them in darker blue, then add a purple dot. Add a circle of pale blue dots around each one.

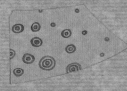

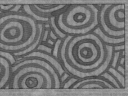

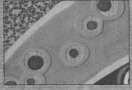

7. Use the tip of a thin brush to paint small purple circles. Paint more circles around them, leaving gaps in between.

8. Then, fill in the spaces between the circles with curved lines, following the shapes of the circles, like this.

9. Fill in the rest of the sections with different patterns of circles, spots and dots. Fill in thick lines between some sections.

Random patterns

THICK CARTRIDGE OR WATERCOLOUR PAPER

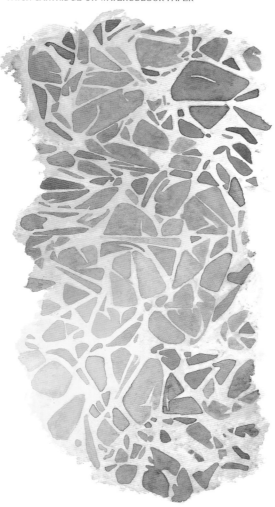

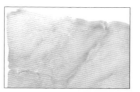

1. Mix different colours of watercolour paint. Make them quite watery. Paint them in patches close to each other.

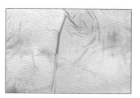

2. Before the paint has dried, cut a piece of plastic foodwrap larger than your painting. Then, lay it over the paint.

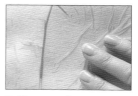

3. Use your fingers to move the paint under the foodwrap, to make patterns and blend the colours together.

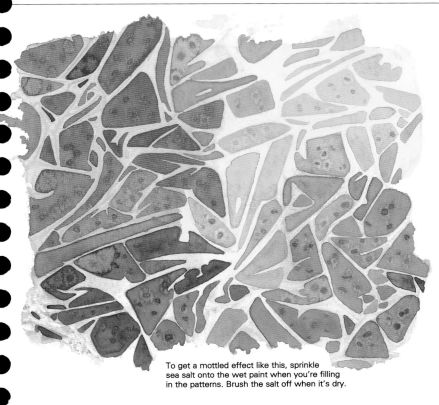

To get a mottled effect like this, sprinkle sea salt onto the wet paint when you're filling in the patterns. Brush the salt off when it's dry.

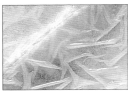

4. Leave the foodwrap on top of the paint and let the paint dry completely. Then, carefully peel off the foodwrap.

5. Use watercolour paints to fill in lots of the patterns left by the foodwrap. Leave a space around each shape.

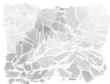

6. Carry on filling in the patterns using some strong colours and some paler ones. Leave some of the patterns unfilled.

Autumn leaves

WATERCOLOUR PAPER

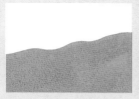

1. Mix a little red and yellow watercolour paint to make orange. Paint it evenly across the bottom of the paper, like this.

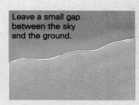

Leave a small gap between the sky and the ground.

2. Mix lots of Prussian blue watercolour paint with water. Paint across the top of the paper for the sky.

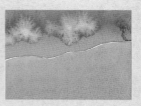

3. Before the sky has dried, dip a paintbrush into water, then let it drip onto the sky. The paint will spread a little.

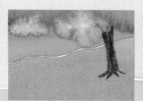

4. Mix red and green acrylic paint to make brown. Drag your brush down several times to paint the tree trunk.

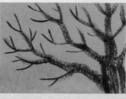

5. Add some branches in the same way, then use a thinner paintbrush to paint finer twigs at the ends of the branches.

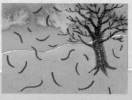

6. When the paint is dry, use a brown oil pastel or wax crayon to draw wavy lines for the middle veins of the leaves.

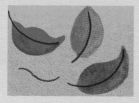

7. Mix red and yellow watercolour paint to make shades of orange. Paint a leaf shape around each line.

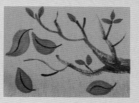

8. Paint a few little leaves on the tree and some in the sky. This will make it look as if the leaves are blowing in the wind.

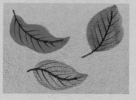

9. When all the leaves are dry, use a fine brush to paint lots of thin, dark brown lines on each of the large leaves.

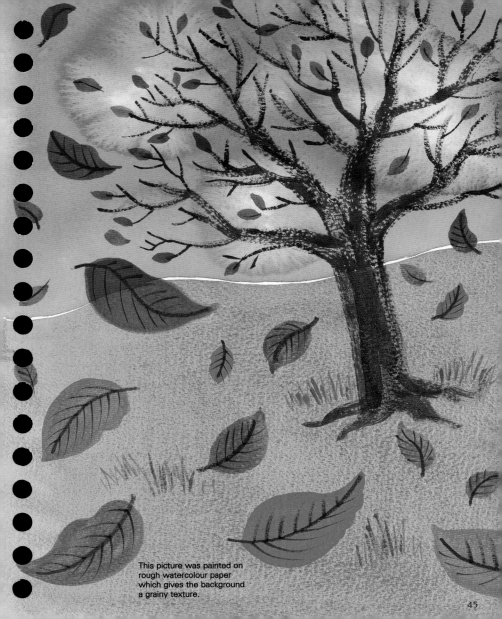

This picture was painted on
rough watercolour paper
which gives the background
a grainy texture.

Tissue paper pond

TISSUE PAPER

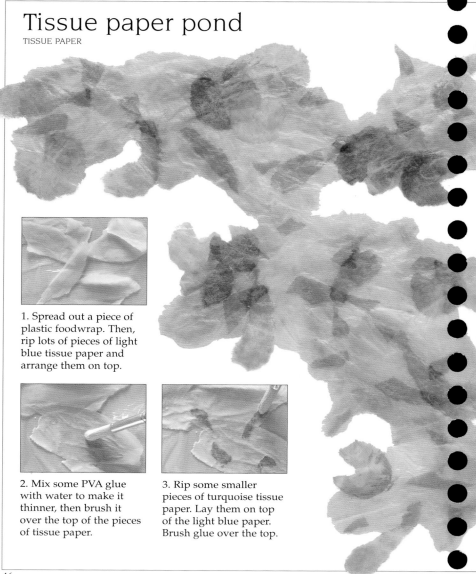

1. Spread out a piece of plastic foodwrap. Then, rip lots of pieces of light blue tissue paper and arrange them on top.

2. Mix some PVA glue with water to make it thinner, then brush it over the top of the pieces of tissue paper.

3. Rip some smaller pieces of turquoise tissue paper. Lay them on top of the light blue paper. Brush glue over the top.

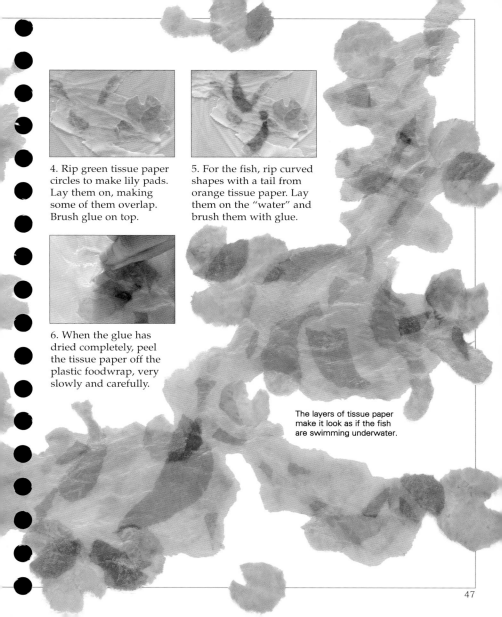

4. Rip green tissue paper circles to make lily pads. Lay them on, making some of them overlap. Brush glue on top.

5. For the fish, rip curved shapes with a tail from orange tissue paper. Lay them on the "water" and brush them with glue.

6. When the glue has dried completely, peel the tissue paper off the plastic foodwrap, very slowly and carefully.

The layers of tissue paper make it look as if the fish are swimming underwater.

Geometric prints

ANY PAPER

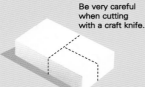

Be very careful when cutting with a craft knife.

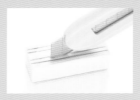

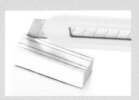

1. Use a craft knife to cut a long eraser in half. Then, cut one of the pieces of eraser in half lengthways.

2. Draw sets of parallel lines along the eraser. Then, holding the knife at an angle, make a clean cut along one line.

3. Turn the eraser around and cut along the other side of the line to make a groove. Cut the other line in the same way.

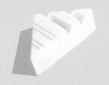

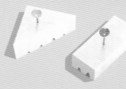

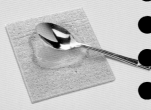

4. Cut the corners off the other half of the eraser to make a triangle. Draw four lines on it, then cut along them as before.

5. Push a map pin or an ordinary pin into the back of both pieces of eraser. This makes them easier to hold when you print.

6. Wet a piece of sponge cloth, then squeeze out as much water as you can. Spread acrylic paint on it with the back of a spoon.

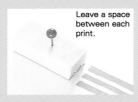

Leave a space between each print.

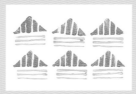

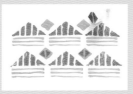

7. Press the first eraser into the paint, then onto some paper. Press it in the paint again before you do another print.

8. Then, do a triangle print above each set of line prints. Repeat these rows of prints several times on your paper.

9. Cut a small square of eraser and print it between each triangle. Then, cut a line across another square of eraser and print it on top.

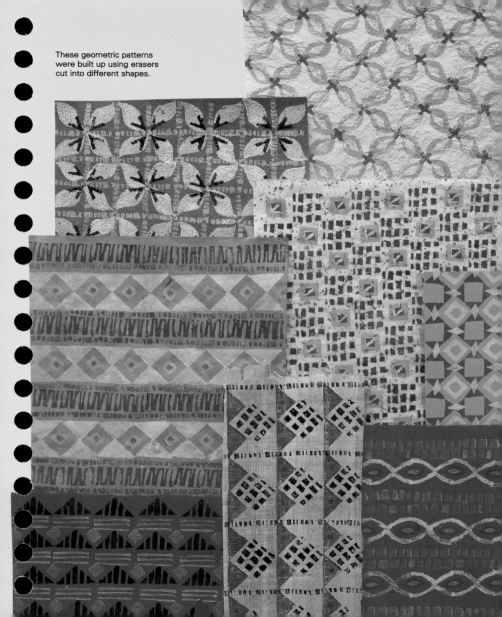

These geometric patterns were built up using erasers cut into different shapes.

Techniques for water

On the next four pages you will find different techniques for drawing and painting water. There are ideas for waves, rippling water and reflections of moonlight on water.

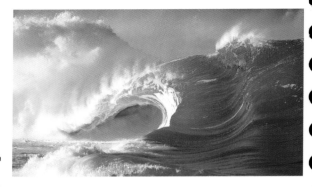

This photograph of a crashing wave shows different shapes, patterns and colours which can be found in water.

Soapy painting

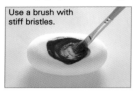

Use a brush with stiff bristles.

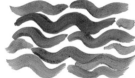

1. Dip a brush into some blue watercolour paint. Then, move the bristles around on an old block of soap.

2. Paint the soapy paint straight onto a piece of watercolour paper, moving the brush in a wavy pattern.

3. Dip the brush into a different shade of blue paint and then on the soap again. Paint more waves, overlapping them.

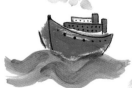

The soap helps to show the marks made by the paintbrush.

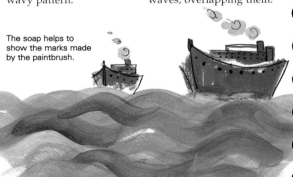

4. Paint a boat with thick red and blue watercolour paint. Add an outline with a fine felt-tip pen.

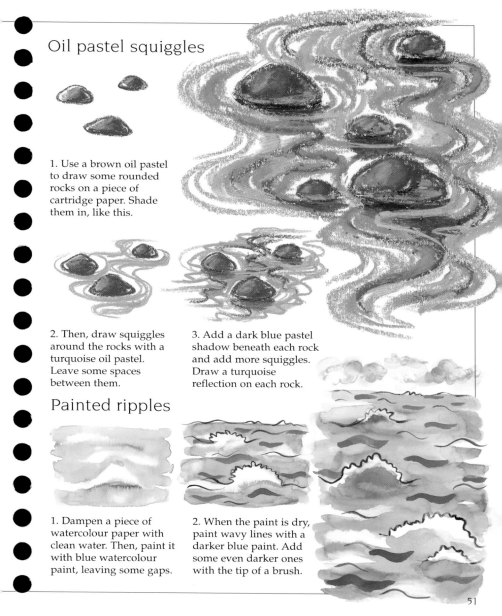

Oil pastel squiggles

1. Use a brown oil pastel to draw some rounded rocks on a piece of cartridge paper. Shade them in, like this.

2. Then, draw squiggles around the rocks with a turquoise oil pastel. Leave some spaces between them.

3. Add a dark blue pastel shadow beneath each rock and add more squiggles. Draw a turquoise reflection on each rock.

Painted ripples

1. Dampen a piece of watercolour paper with clean water. Then, paint it with blue watercolour paint, leaving some gaps.

2. When the paint is dry, paint wavy lines with a darker blue paint. Add some even darker ones with the tip of a brush.

51

More techniques for water
Sea collage

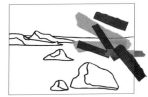

1. Draw some rocks on some thick cardboard and add a line for the horizon. Then, rip strips of blue tissue paper.

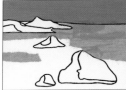

2. Paint the sky with blue acrylic paint. When the sky is dry, glue pieces of pale blue paper around the rocks for the sea.

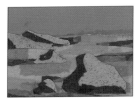

3. Glue on some darker shades of blue paper. Rip paper shapes for rocks and glue them on. Add tissue paper shadows.

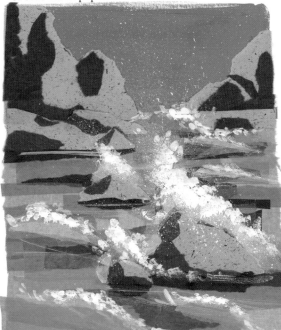

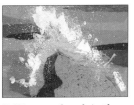

4. For the waves, glue on pieces of white tissue paper. Dab white acrylic or poster paint along the top of each wave.

5. Dip your brush in the paint again, then spatter it over the top of a wave by following steps 5 and 6 on page 73.

52

Wax resist reflections

1. Draw a moon with a white oil pastel on watercolour paper. It's shown here in yellow so that you can see it.

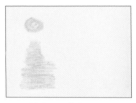

2. Add lots of short lines, starting about a third of the way down the paper. Make each line a little longer than the one before.

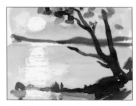

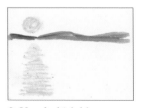

3. Use darkish blue watercolour paint to paint a line of distant hills between the moon and the lines on the water.

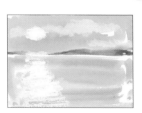

4. Then paint the sky and the water with yellow watercolour. Use a tissue to lift patches of paint off the sky, for clouds.

5. When the paint is dry, paint a strip of land. Paint a tree trunk, then dab on leaves with the tip of a brush and a sponge.

Ink and pastel pets

WATERCOLOUR PAPER

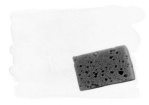

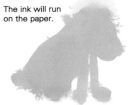

The ink will run on the paper.

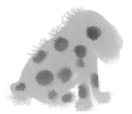

1. Use a clean sponge or a wide paintbrush to wet a piece of watercolour paper.

2. Dip a thick paintbrush into some bright ink and paint lines for the head, ear, body, legs and tail.

3. While the ink is still wet, use the tip of a brush to add spots. Do one on the head for the eye.

Fill in around the dog with another colour of ink.

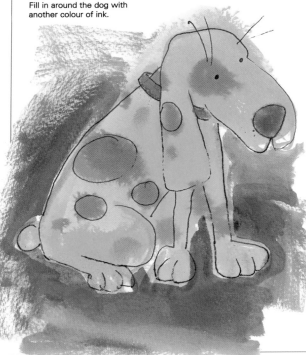

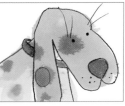

4. When it's dry, outline the body with a black felt-tip pen. Add a nose, eyes and lines on the paws.

5. Draw on a few dots and hairs, too. Fill in the nose and draw a collar with chalk pastels.

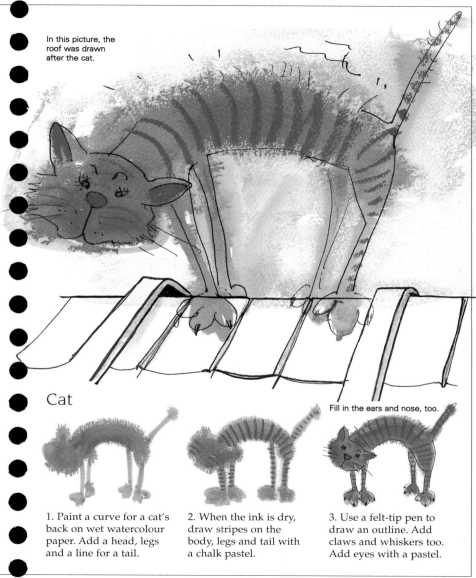

In this picture, the roof was drawn after the cat.

Cat

1. Paint a curve for a cat's back on wet watercolour paper. Add a head, legs and a line for a tail.

2. When the ink is dry, draw stripes on the body, legs and tail with a chalk pastel.

3. Use a felt-tip pen to draw an outline. Add claws and whiskers too. Add eyes with a pastel.

Fill in the ears and nose, too.

Blow-painted trees

THICK CARTRIDGE PAPER OR WATERCOLOUR PAPER

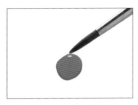

1. Dip a paintbrush into some bright ink and paint a thick blob for the tree trunk.

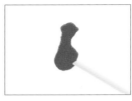

2. Blow through a drinking straw so that you extend the ink up the paper for the trunk.

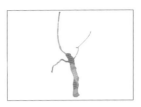

3. Then, use the end of the straw to pull little lines of ink away from the trunk.

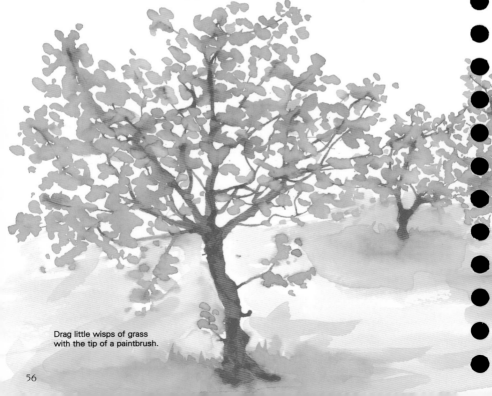

Drag little wisps of grass with the tip of a paintbrush.

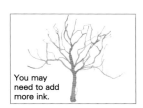

You may need to add more ink.

4. Blow the lines of ink to make the branches. Then, paint and blow more trees in the same way.

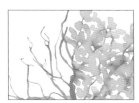

5. For the leaves, mix orange ink with water. Dab it over the branches again and again.

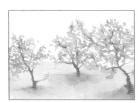

6. For the ground, mix more watery ink and paint it around the bottom of the trees.

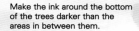

Make the ink around the bottom of the trees darker than the areas in between them.

57

Domed buildings
WATERCOLOUR PAPER OR THICK CARTRIDGE PAPER

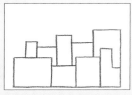

1. Use a pencil to draw several large rectangles on your paper. Make them different sizes.

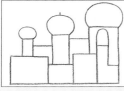

2. Add some domes and turrets. Make them different sizes and shapes, too.

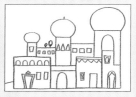

3. Add lots of different shapes of windows, doorways, columns and arches to the buildings.

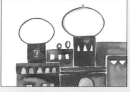

4. Use watercolour paints or inks to fill in the buildings. Leave a small gap between each part.

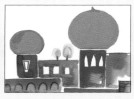

5. When the paint or ink is dry, fill in the domes with a gold felt-tip pen or gold paint.

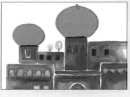

6. Draw around some of the windows and add patterns to the buildings, with a gold pen.

The sky and landscape in this picture were added after the buildings were painted.

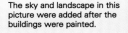

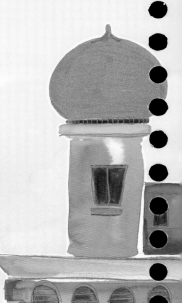

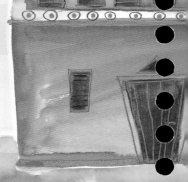

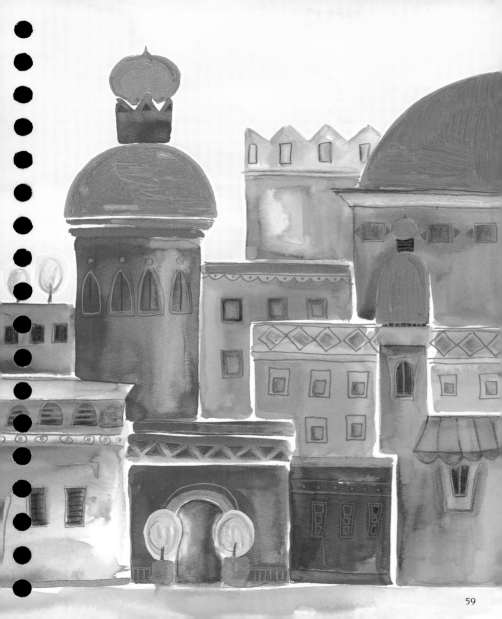

59

Animal shapes

THIN CARDBOARD

Tessellating bird

1. Cut a corner off a square of thin cardboard. Then, tape the triangle along the top edge of the square, like this.

> Shapes like these, which fit together exactly to form repeating patterns, are called tessellations.

2. Cut the other bottom corner off the square and tape it along the top, so that the two triangles meet in the middle.

3. To make the beak, cut a long v-shape into the left-hand side. Tape the shape onto the triangle at the top.

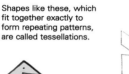 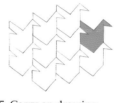

4. Draw around the bird shape. Then, move the shape so that the beak fits under the wing. Draw around it again.

5. Carry on drawing around the shape so that you build up a pattern of birds which fit into each other on all sides.

> These birds were painted with gouache, then outlined with a black felt-tip pen.

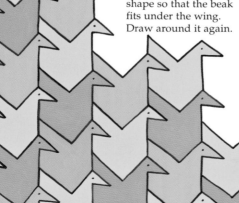

Transformations

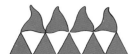

1. Draw a row of five tall triangles and fill them in. Add four triangles above them, making their sides curve slightly.

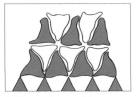

2. Draw three white curvy triangles in the spaces. Add more blue ones and white ones on top. Make the shapes curve, like this.

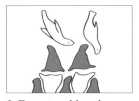

3. Draw two blue shapes which look like sitting seals. Then, draw several swimming seals. Add flippers and eyes.

The shapes gradually transform, or change, from one thing into another.

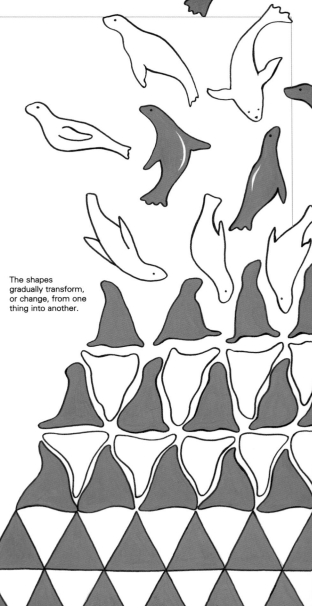

Street scene

A PIECE OF THICK CARDBOARD

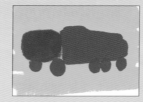

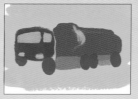

1. Make a pale apricot colour by mixing white and orange acrylic paint. Brush it all over a large piece of cardboard.

2. When the paint has dried, paint a blue shape for the cab of a truck. Paint a brown tank and add dark blue wheels.

3. Use the apricot paint to add windows and headlights. Paint a curve on the tank, and two small tanks below. Let it dry.

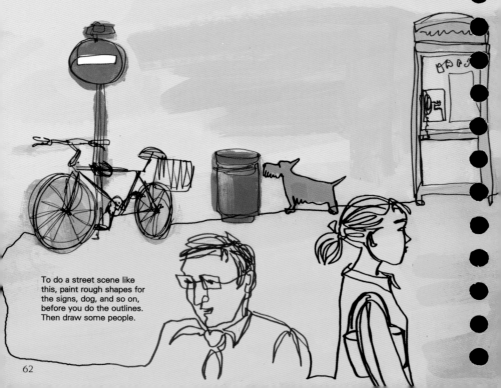

To do a street scene like this, paint rough shapes for the signs, dog, and so on, before you do the outlines. Then draw some people.

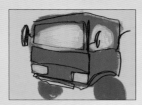

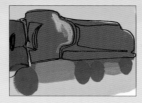

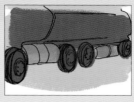

4. Without lifting your pen, outline the whole cab with a black felt-tip pen. You may need to go over some lines twice.

5. Continue the line onto the brown tank. Draw a shape for the flat part at the front of the tank, then outline the back part.

6. Continue the line around and around for the wheels and along the two small tanks under the truck, too.

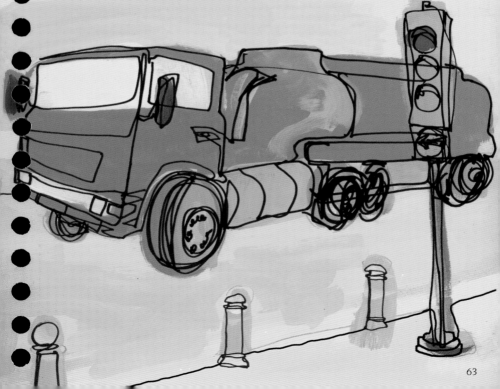

Techniques for fur

Some animals have long hairy fur, curly fur, or smooth skin. They can also be one colour or have amazing patterned fur. Here are a few suggestions of different ways to draw animal fur:

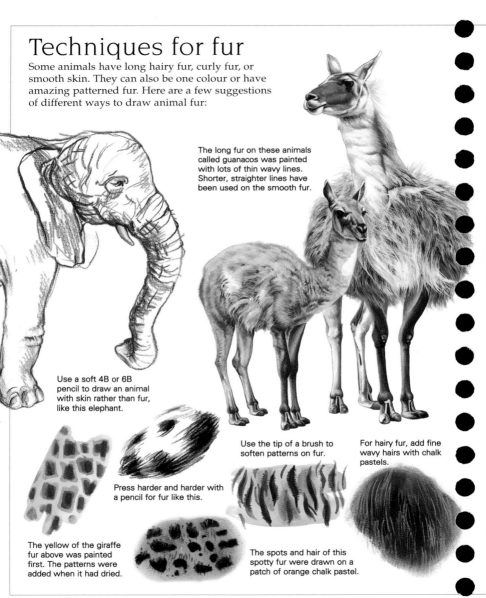

The long fur on these animals called guanacos was painted with lots of thin wavy lines. Shorter, straighter lines have been used on the smooth fur.

Use a soft 4B or 6B pencil to draw an animal with skin rather than fur, like this elephant.

Press harder and harder with a pencil for fur like this.

The yellow of the giraffe fur above was painted first. The patterns were added when it had dried.

Use the tip of a brush to soften patterns on fur.

For hairy fur, add fine wavy hairs with chalk pastels.

The spots and hair of this spotty fur were drawn on a patch of orange chalk pastel.

Pencil and paint

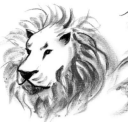

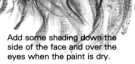

1. Use a soft 6B pencil to draw a lion's eyes, ears and nose. Add some curved lines for the mane.

2. Paint lines in shades of orange between the pencil lines, but don't put too much paint on your brush.

Add some shading down the side of the face and over the eyes when the paint is dry.

Chalk pastel leopard

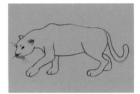

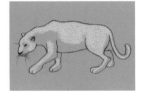

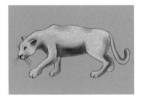

1. Use a pencil to draw a faint outline of a leopard on coloured paper. Fill in its nose and eyes and add some long whiskers.

2. Using a chalk pastel, fill in areas on the leopard's head, along the neck and back, and down the legs and tail.

3. Use a darker pastel to fill in shadows under the chin and on the tail, legs and tummy. Smudge the pastel with a finger.

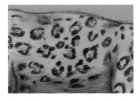

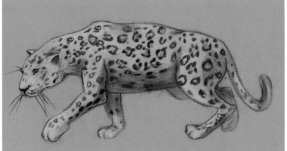

4. Add spots on the head, back, tail and legs. Then, outline the leopard and its eyes and nose with a black pastel.

65

More techniques for fur

Watercolour seal

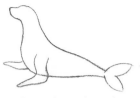

1. Draw the outline of a seal's body with a pencil on watercolour paper. Add the flippers.

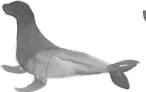

2. Fill in your outline with blue watercolour paint. Use Prussian blue if you have it.

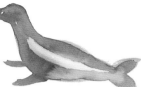

3. Before the paint has dried, lift off a line of paint along the body with a tissue or a dry brush.

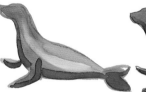

4. Paint darker blue lines for shadows along the neck, flippers, tummy, and on the tail.

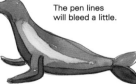

The pen lines will bleed a little.

5. Before the lines have dried, outline the seal with a water-based felt-tip pen.

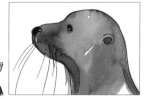

6. Use the pen to add an eye, ear and nose. Draw some dots on the chin and add long whiskers.

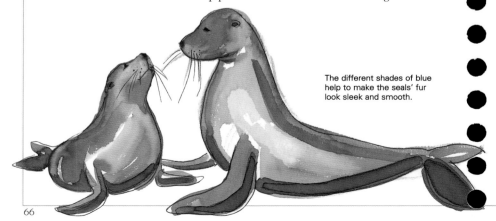

The different shades of blue help to make the seals' fur look sleek and smooth.

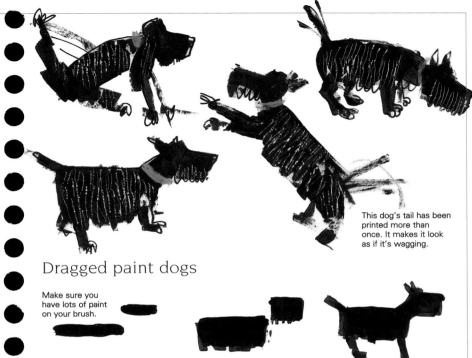

This dog's tail has been printed more than once. It makes it look as if it's wagging.

Dragged paint dogs

Make sure you have lots of paint on your brush.

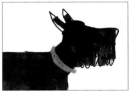

1. Paint two lines of really thick black acrylic paint for the dog's back and head.

2. Use the edge of a piece of cardboard to drag the paint downwards to make the head and body.

3. Use the corner of the cardboard to drag the paint to make the ears, legs and tail.

Use a ballpoint or felt-tip pen.

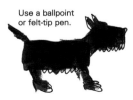

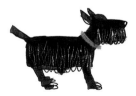

4. When the paint is dry, draw wavy lines under the head and body. Add lines to the ears and feet.

5. Draw a curved line for a collar around the dog's neck with a bright chalk pastel or oil pastel.

6. Then, use a craft knife to scratch vertical lines into the paint on the dog's head and body.

Wet paper watercolour

WATERCOLOUR PAPER

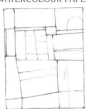

1. Do a plan on some scrap paper before you start. Draw a rectangle and fill it with shapes, like this.

2. Paint a rectangle of watercolour paper with clean water. Following your plan, fill in the main shapes with pale colours.

3. When the paint has dried, fill some of the shapes with a stronger colour. Paint patterns in some of the shapes.

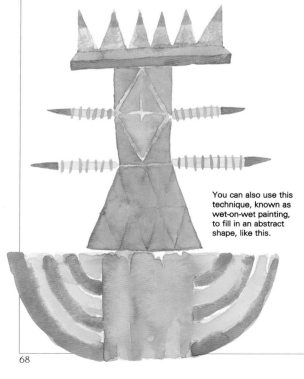

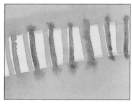

4. While the paint is still wet, add small lines in different colours, letting the paints bleed into each other.

You can also use this technique, known as wet-on-wet painting, to fill in an abstract shape, like this.

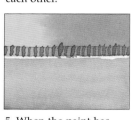

5. When the paint has dried, paint some more little lines. The colours won't bleed as they did when the paint was wet.

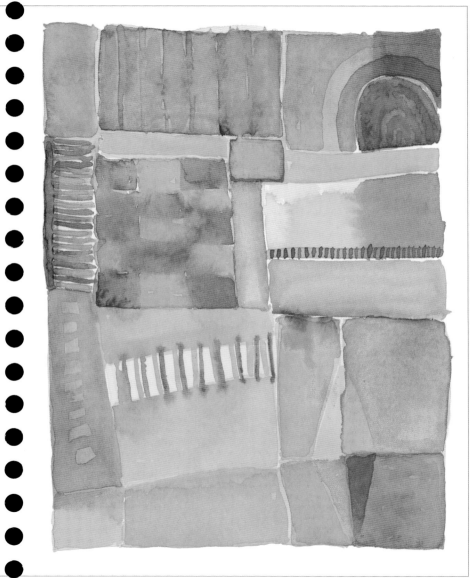

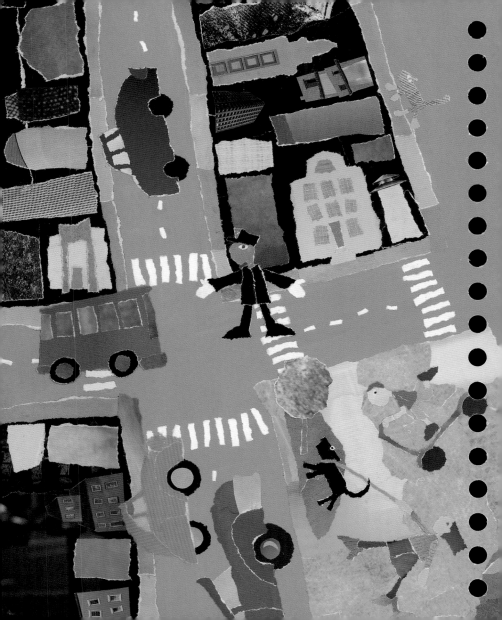

Town collage
CARTRIDGE PAPER OR CARDBOARD

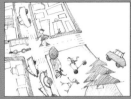

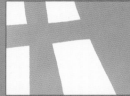

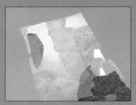

1. Make a rough plan for your collage on a piece of scrap paper. Mark on the position of roads, a park, buildings, cars, and so on.

2. On a large piece of paper or cardboard, paint the shapes which are the roads on your plan, with acrylic or poster paint.

3. For the park, rip pieces of light-coloured paper from old magazines and glue them. Add green paper for grass.

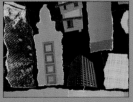

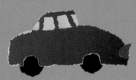

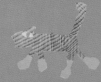

4. Fill in the areas for the buildings with dark pieces of paper. Rip shapes for the buildings and add some windows.

5. For the cars, rip a shape for the body, with wheel arches ripped out. Glue two wheels behind and windows on top.

6. For a cat, rip the body from magazine paper which has a texture on it. Glue on paws. Cut out an eye and glue it on, too.

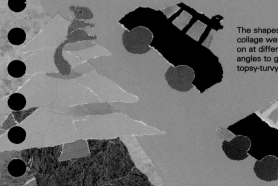

The shapes in this collage were glued on at different angles to give it a topsy-turvy effect.

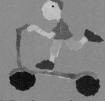

7. For the people, rip all the parts of the body and the clothes. Glue the pieces together, then glue them onto the collage.

71

Wax resist fish and butterflies

CARTRIDGE PAPER

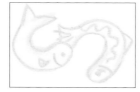

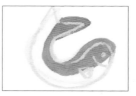

1. Draw the outline of some fish with a pale yellow wax crayon. Add eyes, fins and some patterns on the bodies.

2. Mix some orange watercolour paint and paint part of each fish. Don't worry if you overlap the outline a little.

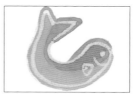

3. Mix a paler yellowy-orange paint and fill in the rest of the fish. The wax crayon lines will resist the paint.

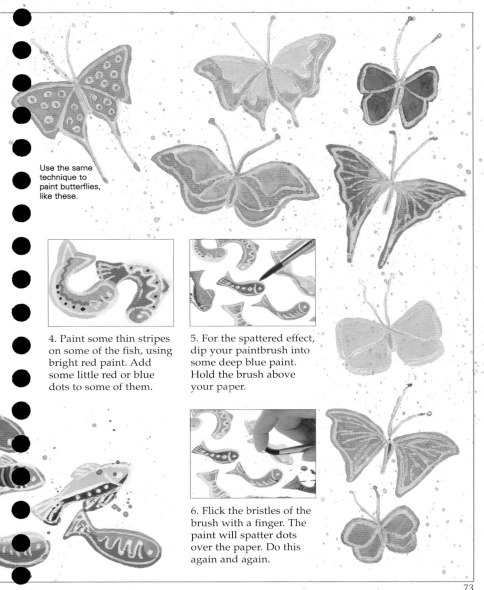

Use the same technique to paint butterflies, like these.

4. Paint some thin stripes on some of the fish, using bright red paint. Add some little red or blue dots to some of them.

5. For the spattered effect, dip your paintbrush into some deep blue paint. Hold the brush above your paper.

6. Flick the bristles of the brush with a finger. The paint will spatter dots over the paper. Do this again and again.

Cityscape

WHITE OR COLOURED PAPER OR CARDBOARD

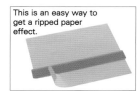

1. For the road, lay a ruler on a piece of paper. Press firmly on the ruler and rip the paper along its edge.

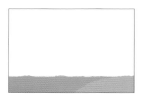

2. Glue the road along the bottom of a large piece of paper. Rip another piece, with an angle at one end, and glue it on.

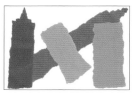

3. For the buildings, rip rectangles from lots of different kinds of paper. Rip tower shapes on one end of some of them.

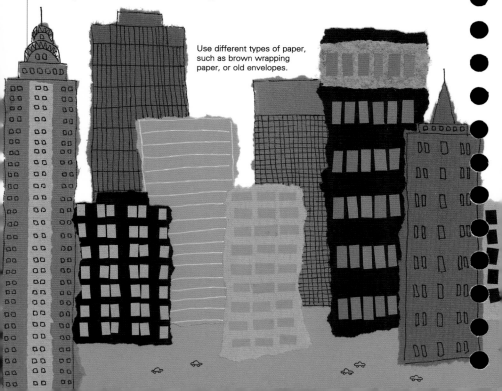

Use different types of paper, such as brown wrapping paper, or old envelopes.

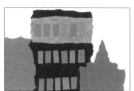

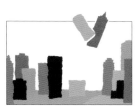

4. Arrange the rectangles of paper along the road, then glue them on. Overlap some of them to get a 3-D effect.

5. Cut out and glue lots of windows on some of the buildings. Glue some strips of white tissue paper on some, too.

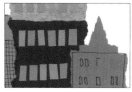

6. Draw an outline around a few of the buildings with a black felt-tip pen. Draw windows on some of them, too.

Draw some tiny cars. This helps to make the buildings look massive.

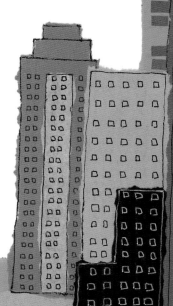

75

Sheep on a hill

THICK CARTRIDGE OR WATERCOLOUR PAPER

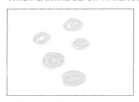

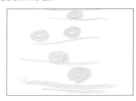

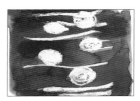

1. Use a white oil pastel to draw ovals for the sheep's bodies. They are shown here in yellow so that you can see them.

2. Use the pastel to draw some horizontal lines in front of the ovals. Add some thinner lines between the sheep, too.

3. Then, brush a rectangle of watery purple and pink watercolour paint on top. The pastel resists the paint.

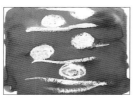

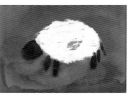

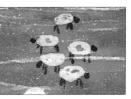

4. Hold the paper and gently tilt it from side to side so that the colours blend together. Then, leave it to dry.

5. Mix some dark blue paint or ink and paint a little oval on each sheep's body for a head. Add four stick legs, too.

6. Dip your paintbrush into thick white paint and spatter the snow by following steps 5 and 6 on page 73.

Other ideas

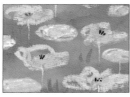

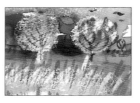

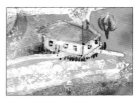

Draw flowers with white and yellow oil pastels. Paint green watercolour on top, then scratch the stalks with a craft knife.

Draw trees, grass and clouds in white. Paint over the sky, trees and grass. When the paint's dry, scratch across the pastel.

Draw buildings with oil pastels. Add white roads and hills. Paint over them with blue, then sponge thick white paint on top.

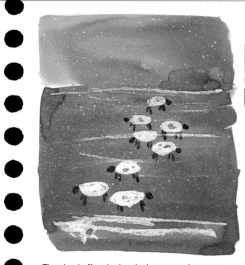

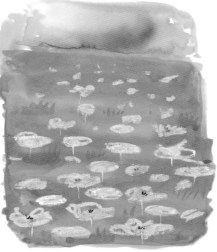

The cloud effect in the sky happens when you tilt the paper and the colours blend together.

The tufts of grass were painted in a slightly darker green once the background had dried.

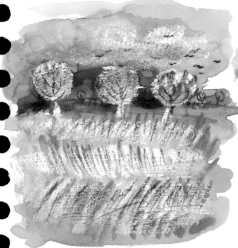

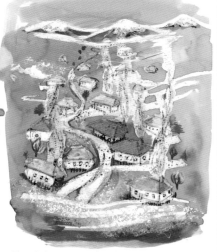

If you scratch the paint away with a craft knife, the pastel and paper are revealed underneath.

The windows were painted over the pastel, which resisted the paint, making uneven lines.

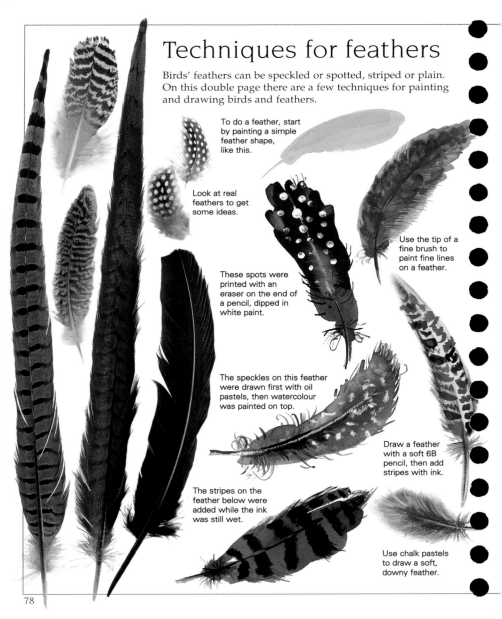

Techniques for feathers

Birds' feathers can be speckled or spotted, striped or plain. On this double page there are a few techniques for painting and drawing birds and feathers.

To do a feather, start by painting a simple feather shape, like this.

Look at real feathers to get some ideas.

Use the tip of a fine brush to paint fine lines on a feather.

These spots were printed with an eraser on the end of a pencil, dipped in white paint.

The speckles on this feather were drawn first with oil pastels, then watercolour was painted on top.

Draw a feather with a soft 6B pencil, then add stripes with ink.

The stripes on the feather below were added while the ink was still wet.

Use chalk pastels to draw a soft, downy feather.

Pheasant

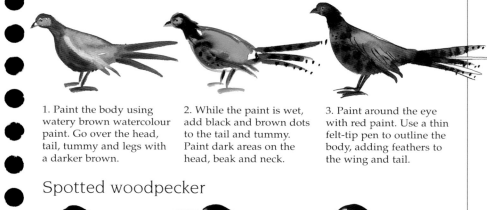

1. Paint the body using watery brown watercolour paint. Go over the head, tail, tummy and legs with a darker brown.

2. While the paint is wet, add black and brown dots to the tail and tummy. Paint dark areas on the head, beak and neck.

3. Paint around the eye with red paint. Use a thin felt-tip pen to outline the body, adding feathers to the wing and tail.

Spotted woodpecker

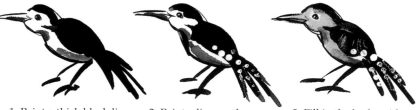

1. Paint a thick black line for the head, back and tail. Then use finer lines for the rest of the body.

2. Paint a line on the tummy with watery ink. Fingerpaint spots on the tail with acrylic paint.

3. Fill in the body with a peach-coloured chalk pastel. Add markings on the back and wing.

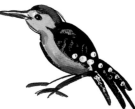

4. Draw a red chalk patch on the head and tummy. Smudge the pastel a little with your finger.

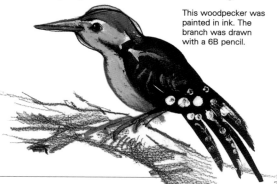

This woodpecker was painted in ink. The branch was drawn with a 6B pencil.

Swimming turtles

WATERCOLOUR PAPER

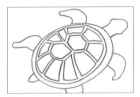

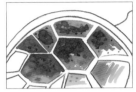

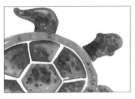

1. Use a blue pencil to draw a faint outline of a turtle's shell. Add a head, flippers, a tail and markings on the shell.

2. Paint markings on the shell with turquoise watercolour paint. Before the shapes dry, add a few dots. The paint will run.

3. Fill in the head, tail and flippers with turquoise paint. Then, add dots of paint to them before they have dried.

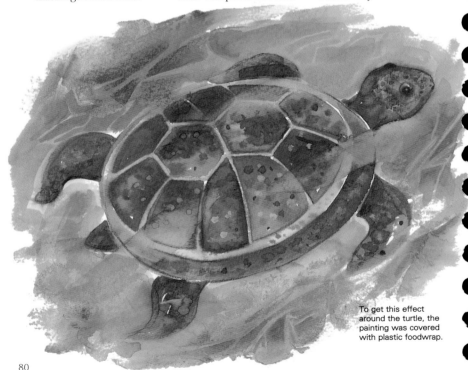

To get this effect around the turtle, the painting was covered with plastic foodwrap.

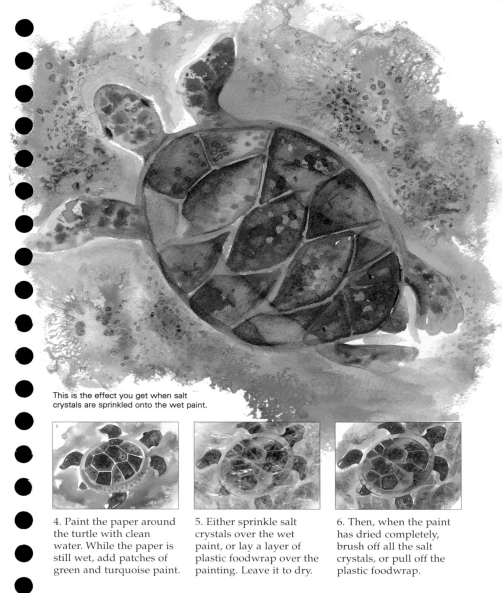

This is the effect you get when salt crystals are sprinkled onto the wet paint.

4. Paint the paper around the turtle with clean water. While the paper is still wet, add patches of green and turquoise paint.

5. Either sprinkle salt crystals over the wet paint, or lay a layer of plastic foodwrap over the painting. Leave it to dry.

6. Then, when the paint has dried completely, brush off all the salt crystals, or pull off the plastic foodwrap.

Pastel landscape

ANY TYPE OF YELLOW OR BEIGE PAPER

1. Using a pencil, draw a plan for your pastel landscape on a large piece of yellow or beige coloured paper.

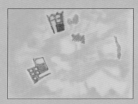

2. Make the pencil lighter with an eraser. Then, fill in the background with a mustard-coloured chalk pastel. Fill in some shapes.

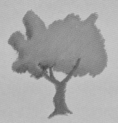

3. Draw a tree trunk with a brown pastel. Add green leaves, then add shadows and highlights with dark and light green pastels.

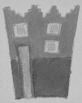

4. For the buildings, fill in the main part with chalk pastels, leaving gaps for the window frames and door, then fill them in.

5. Draw green stems and leaves for the sunflowers. Add darker lines. Use yellow for the flowers and add orange on top.

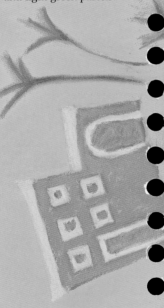

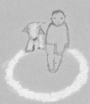

6. Draw a white oval for the fountain. Outline the boy and the dog in blue, then fill them in. Fill in the water last of all.

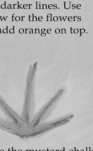

7. Use the mustard chalk pastel to go over parts of the background again, around each of the things you have drawn.

To stop pastels smudging, you can fix them with fixative spray or hair spray.

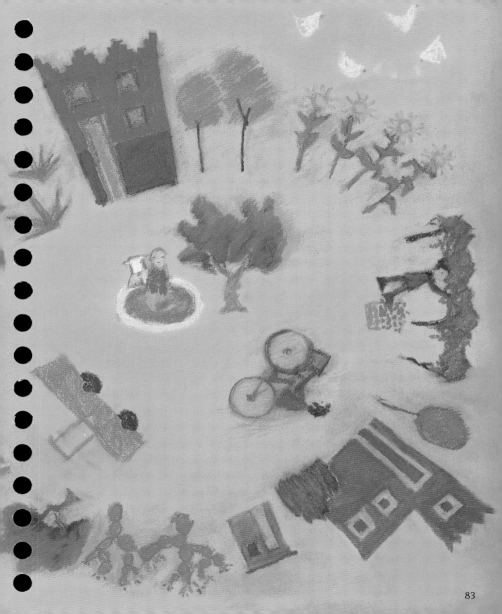

83

Cloud people

WATERCOLOUR PAPER

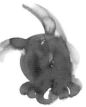

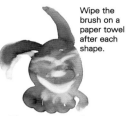

Wipe the brush on a paper towel after each shape.

1. Mix some watery dark blue watercolour paint, then use a thick brush to paint a large patch of colour, like this.

2. Brush some of the paint away from the patch to make the shapes for the clown's hat and collar. Let the patch dry a little.

3. Then, using a clean, dry brush, lift off a curve of paint for the clown's chin and shapes for the nose and eyebrows.

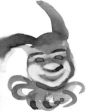

4. Leave the paint to dry completely, then use dark blue paint to add shadows under the nose and chin.

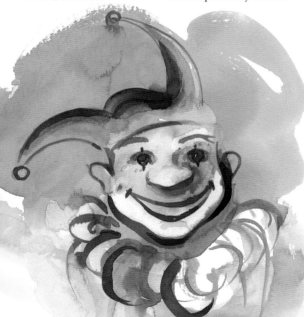

5. Add lines for the eyebrows and the eyes. Then, paint a line for the side of the face and some curved lines on the collar.

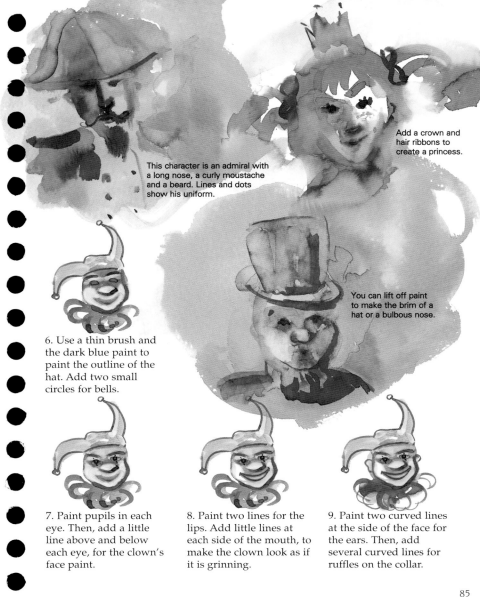

This character is an admiral with a long nose, a curly moustache and a beard. Lines and dots show his uniform.

Add a crown and hair ribbons to create a princess.

You can lift off paint to make the brim of a hat or a bulbous nose.

6. Use a thin brush and the dark blue paint to paint the outline of the hat. Add two small circles for bells.

7. Paint pupils in each eye. Then, add a little line above and below each eye, for the clown's face paint.

8. Paint two lines for the lips. Add little lines at each side of the mouth, to make the clown look as if it is grinning.

9. Paint two curved lines at the side of the face for the ears. Then, add several curved lines for ruffles on the collar.

85

Scratched patterns

CARTRIDGE PAPER

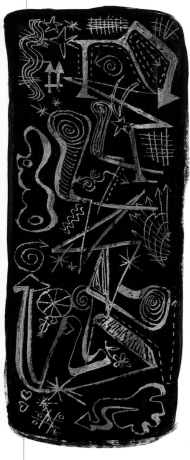

This patch was scratched with random shapes and patterns.

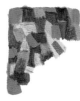

1. Use different oil pastels to draw patches of colour on a piece of cartridge paper. Make sure that the patches join together.

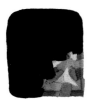

2. Mix a little water with black acrylic paint, but don't make it too thin. Cover the oil pastel completely with the paint.

3. Leave the paint until it is almost dry. Then, use a screwdriver to scratch lines, revealing the pastel underneath.

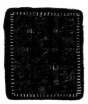

4. Scratch several more lines down the paint, then scratch lines across to make a large grid. Scratch a border, too.

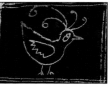

5. Draw a simple outline of a bird in part of the grid. Add curved lines for feathers, a wing, an eye and a beak.

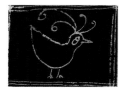

6. If you make a mistake, paint some of the black acrylic paint on top and let it dry a little before scratching it again.

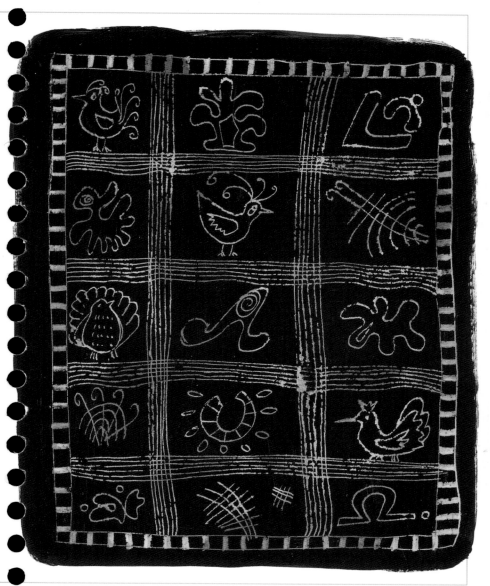

Giraffe collage

A LARGE PIECE OF CARDBOARD

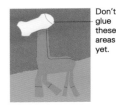

Don't glue these areas yet.

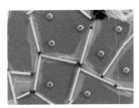

1. Glue a piece of brown wrapping paper onto some cardboard. Then, rip another piece of paper. Glue it across the bottom.

2. Cut out a giraffe's body and legs. Cut a head from corrugated cardboard. Glue the pieces to the background, like this.

3. Rip lots of patches from brown paper and glue them onto the body. Glue matchsticks around them. Add beads or dried beans.

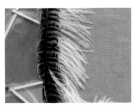

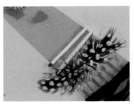

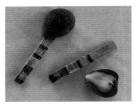

4. Glue fluffy feathers or lots of pieces of wool down the neck for the mane. Glue long feathers over the top.

5. Wrap black wool around each hoof and glue on things like matchsticks, feathers and pieces of shiny paper.

6. For the giraffe's antlers, twist the wire off an old peg. Glue a large, dried seed or bean onto the end of each peg.

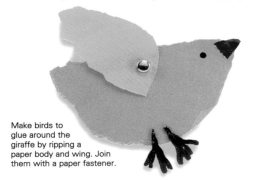

Make birds to glue around the giraffe by ripping a paper body and wing. Join them with a paper fastener.

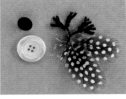

7. For eyes, glue together things such as feathers, dried plants and buttons. Stick them on, then stick the rest of the body down.

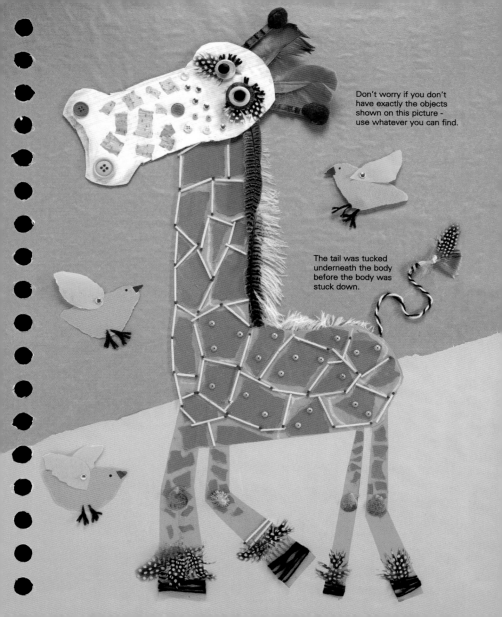

Don't worry if you don't have exactly the objects shown on this picture - use whatever you can find.

The tail was tucked underneath the body before the body was stuck down.

Pencil bugs

ANY PAPER WITH A SMOOTH SURFACE

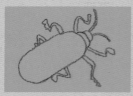

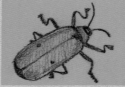

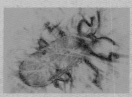

1. Use a pencil with a soft lead (a 6B pencil is ideal) to draw a simple outline of an insect on your paper.

2. Shade the insect's body, making it darker close to the edges. Fill in the head and legs. Add any spots or patterns, too.

3. Rub lines across your drawing with an eraser to smudge the pencil a little. Rub the lines in different directions.

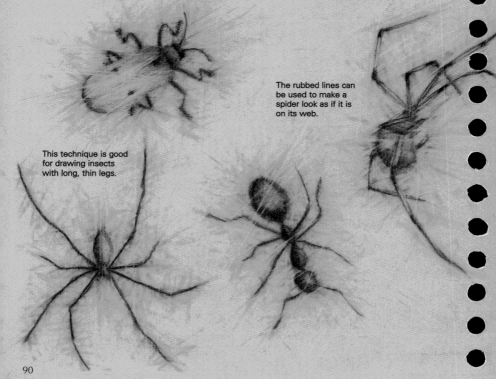

The rubbed lines can be used to make a spider look as if it is on its web.

This technique is good for drawing insects with long, thin legs.

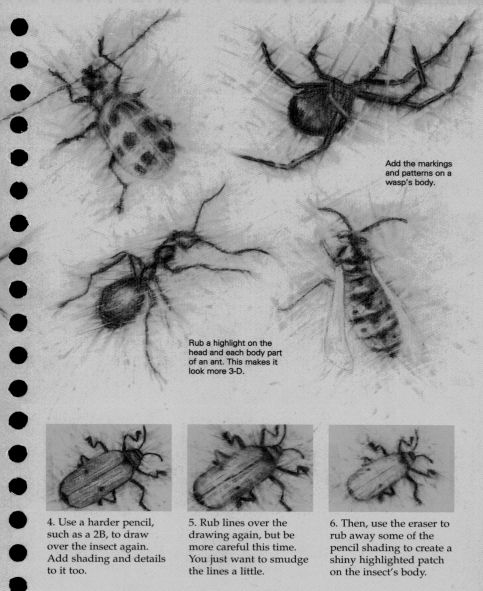

Add the markings and patterns on a wasp's body.

Rub a highlight on the head and each body part of an ant. This makes it look more 3-D.

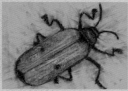

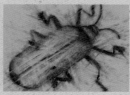

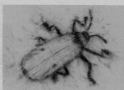

4. Use a harder pencil, such as a 2B, to draw over the insect again. Add shading and details to it too.

5. Rub lines over the drawing again, but be more careful this time. You just want to smudge the lines a little.

6. Then, use the eraser to rub away some of the pencil shading to create a shiny highlighted patch on the insect's body.

More ideas

Over the next four pages there are lots more ideas for using the techniques in this book. Turn back to the pages which are mentioned to find out how they were done.

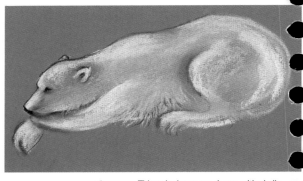

This polar bear was drawn with chalk pastels, like the leopard on page 65.

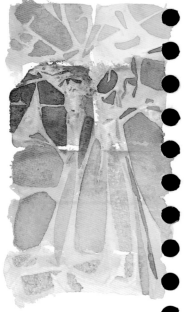

These birds were made with ripped paper from old magazines (see pages 70-71).

This pattern was created with plastic foodwrap (see pages 42-43).

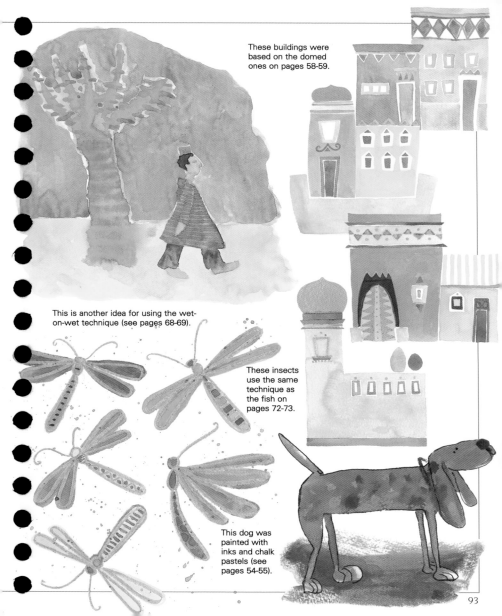

These buildings were based on the domed ones on pages 58-59.

This is another idea for using the wet-on-wet technique (see pages 68-69).

These insects use the same technique as the fish on pages 72-73.

This dog was painted with inks and chalk pastels (see pages 54-55).

93

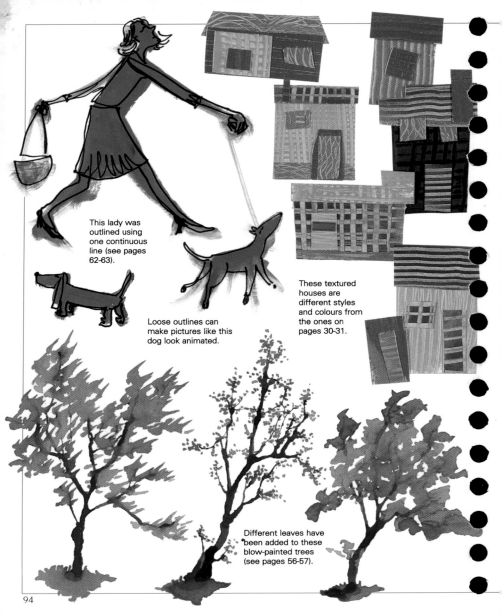

This lady was outlined using one continuous line (see pages 62-63).

Loose outlines can make pictures like this dog look animated.

These textured houses are different styles and colours from the ones on pages 30-31.

Different leaves have been added to these blow-painted trees (see pages 56-57).

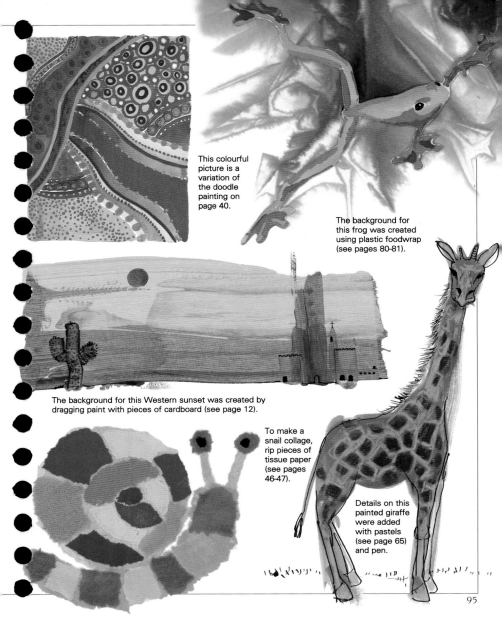

This colourful picture is a variation of the doodle painting on page 40.

The background for this frog was created using plastic foodwrap (see pages 80-81).

The background for this Western sunset was created by dragging paint with pieces of cardboard (see page 12).

To make a snail collage, rip pieces of tissue paper (see pages 46-47).

Details on this painted giraffe were added with pastels (see page 65) and pen.

95

Index

blow-painting, 56-57, 94
brushstrokes, 32-33

cardboard and potato printing, 16-17
chalk pastels, 4, 82-83, 92, 95
  and wet inks, 54-55, 93
collage,
  glue and tissue paper, 46-47
  magazine paper, 70-71, 92
  mixed media, 38-39
  paper, 74-75
  tissue paper, 6-7
  with found objects, 88-89
  with ink drawing, 10-11
continuous line drawing, 62-63, 94
cut paper, 18-19

dragged paint, 12-13
drawing,
  collage with ink, 10-11
  continuous line, 62-63
  eraser and pencil, 90-91

eraser,
  and pencil drawings, 90-91
  printing, 48-49

feathers, techniques, 78-79
fingerpainting, 26-27
foodwrap patterns, 40-41, 92
found object collage, 88-89
fur, techniques, 64-65, 66-67

glue and tissue paper collage, 46-47
gold highlights, adding, 58-59

ink drawing with collage, 10-11
inks, 4
  with chalk pastels, 54

lifting off watercolour paints, 84-85

line drawing, continuous, 62-63

magazine paper collage, 70-71
materials, 4-5
mixed media collage, 38-39
mixing paints, 4

oil pastel,
  and spattering, 76-77
  resist, 8-9
  squiggles, 51
oil pastels, 4

paint, 4
  acrylic, 4
  dragged, 12-13
  gouache, 4
  poster, 4
  scratched, with pastel, 86-87
  watercolour, 4
painted patterns, 40-41
painting,
  blow-, 56-57
  doodle, 40-41, 95
  plastic foodwrap, 42-43, 80-81
  soapy, 50
  wet-on-wet, 68-69
paper, 5
  cartridge, 5
  collage, 74-75
  cut, 18-19
  textured, 30-31
  watercolour, 5
pastel and ink resist, 28-29
pastels, 4
  scratched paint and, 86-87
patterns,
  painted, 40-41
  with plastic foodwrap, 42-43
pencil and eraser drawings, 90-91
pens, 5
plastic foodwrap painting, 80-81, 95
potato and cardboard printing, 16-17

printing,
  cardboard and potato, 16-17
  with an eraser, 48-49
  with a sponge, 24-25
resist,
  oil pastel, 8-9
  oil pastel and spattering, 76-77
  pastel and ink, 28-29
  wax, 53
  wax and spattering, 72-73
rubbings, tissue paper, 14-15

scratched paint and pastels, 86-87
shapes,
  cut paper, 18-19
  tessellating, 60
  transforming, 61
skies, techniques, 34-35, 36-37
spattering, 73, 76-77
sponge printing, 24-25

tessellating shapes, 60
textured papers, 30-31, 94
tissue paper,
  and glue collage, 46-47, 95
  collage, 6-7
  rubbings, 14-15
transforming shapes, 61
trees, techniques, 20-21, 22-23, 56-57, 94

washes, watercolour, 44-45
water, techniques, 50-51, 52-53
watercolour,
  effects, 80-81
  lifting off, 84-85
  paper, 5
  washes, 44-45
wax,
  crayons, 4
  resist and spattering, 72-73
wet inks and chalk pastels, 54-55, 93
wet-on-wet painting, 68-69, 93

Acknowledgements

Every effort has been made to trace the copyright holders of the material in this book. If any rights have been omitted, the publishers offer their sincere apologies and will rectify this in any subsequent edition following notification. The publishers are grateful to the following organisations and individuals for their contributions and permission to reproduce material.
Page 20 Vincent van Gogh 'Olive Orchard with Mountains' © Francis G. Mayer/CORBIS. Page 34 J.M.W. Turner 'Rain, Steam, and Speed - The Great Western Railway' © The National Gallery, London.
Page 50 Waves © Digital Vision. Page 64 Guanacos - Ian Jackson.